GERIATRIC & NURSING Healthy Aging

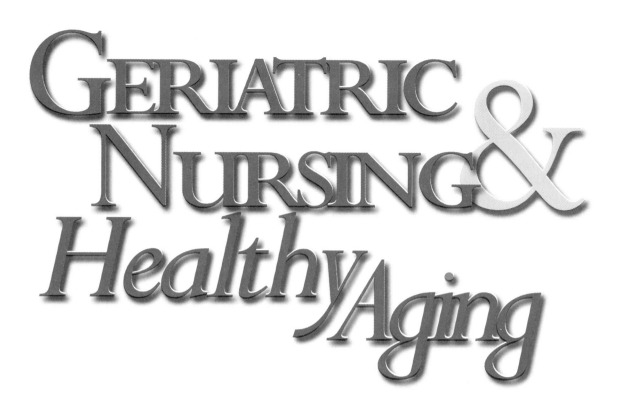

GERIATRIC NURSING & Healthy Aging

PRISCILLA EBERSOLE, PhD, RN, FAAN
Professor Emerita
San Francisco State University
San Francisco, California

PATRICIA HESS, PhD, RN, GNP-CS, NAP
Professor of Nursing
San Francisco State University
San Francisco, California

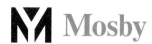 Mosby

A Harcourt Health Sciences Company

St. Louis   London   Philadelphia   Sydney   Toronto

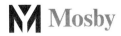

A Harcourt Health Sciences Company

Vice President, Nursing Editorial Director: Sally Schrefer
Senior Editor: Michael S. Ledbetter
Senior Developmental Editor: Laurie K. Muench
Project Manager: John Rogers
Project Specialist: Betty Hazelwood
Designer: Liz Rudder
Cover Designer: Kathi Gosche

Mosby, Inc.
A Harcourt Health Sciences Company
11830 Westline Industrial Drive
St. Louis, Missouri 63146

Printed in the United States of America

International Standard Book Number 0-323-01062-8

00 01 02 03 04 GW/FF 9 8 7 6 5 4 3 2 1

REVIEWERS

Nancy Batchelor, MSN
Assistant Professor
Northern Kentucky University
Highland Heights, Kentucky

Barbara P. Daniel, MEd, MS, RNCS, RCNP
Professor of Nursing
Cecil Community College
North East, Maryland

Joanne M. Flanders, MS, RN
Assistant Professor
Midwestern State University
Wichita Falls, Texas

Kim A. Heim, MSN, RN, GNP
Nursing Instructor
Milwaukee Area Technical College
Milwaukee, Wisconsin

Sharon Lambert, DNS, RN
Assistant Professor
McKendree College
Lebanon, Illinois

Betty A. Maxwell, MSN, RN
Nursing Instructor
St. Clair County Community College
Port Huron, Michigan

Margaret A. McGinty, MS, RN
Associate Professor
Anne Arundel Community College
Arnold, Maryland

Ouida Anne Miller, BSN, MA, RN.C
Director, Nursing Program
Valencia Community College
Orlando, Florida

Anna Marcia Smitherman, MSN, RN
Instructor, School of Nursing
Wallace Community College
Selma, Alabama

Pat Woodbery, ARNP-C, MSN
Professor of Nursing
Valencia Community College
Orlando, Florida

PREFACE

This text is designed for nurses, faculty, and students working with older adults. Experiences that allow sufficient time to identify client problems, design nursing interventions, and evaluate outcomes are expected. Content will be most applicable to clinical practice in long-term care settings: nursing homes, rehabilitation centers, life care and retirement communities, assisted living, specialty units such as Alzheimer's, subacute units, hospice, and home care. Most information is equally useful for the care of older adults in acute care, but the rapid discharge rate and intense demands of daily care seldom allow full attention to more extended applications.

Examples illuminate the concepts; glossaries in each chapter provide for ease of student understanding. Key concepts and learning activities and discussion questions at the end of each chapter summarize the most important points presented and relate directly to the objectives of the chapter. Examples are presented with consideration of gender and ethnicity whenever significant. Resources are provided for the reader who may wish to seek additional help with specific problems of an elder.

An added feature, entirely unique to this text, is phenomenologic consideration of the lived experience of an elder in a given situation. These provide the feeling tone of the individual encountering the elder in those situations.

We are very aware of the fads and fashions in being politically correct, but we believe the sensitivity to the older person is shown in genuine interaction rather than simply in words. In many cases one term has been singled out as being appropriate and, by implication, all others are disrespectful in some way. This is absurd and only confirms that we cannot look the person fully in the face but must carefully tiptoe around him or her.

What could possibly be more discriminating? This is the most insidious form of ageism. Throughout this text we have used several terms to refer to individuals who are chronologically advanced in years: aged, client, elder, elderly, old, patient, resident, and aging or aged adult. The usage somewhat depends on the context.

The intent of the text throughout is to facilitate the healthiest adaptation possible for any elder, regardless of situation and disease process. The majority of the text is devoted to discussing the significant problems that may occur as one grows old and methods that nurses may use to make these problems more bearable, to solve some, and to help the elder find the best possible resolution to attain maximal life satisfaction. That is healthy aging, and that is our quest (mission). Search with us for the most livable and exciting journey of and for the old. They are us, and we are them. It is only the particular linear thinking of our scientific minds that insists we categorize people, events, things, eras, and epochs.

Acknowledgments

Throughout the production of this text, the able assistance of our long-term editors, Michael Ledbetter and Laurie Muench, is reflected in the quality, coherence, and accuracy of the text. They are consistent in their guidance and sensitivity to the topic. We wish also to thank our reviewers, who have helped us streamline the text and make it practical and useful for clinical application. These are the folks who let us know how concepts jibe with realities. We are again very grateful to be able to present our ideas and those of others, upon whose shoulders we stand, for the aged who are entrusted to us for the best possible nursing care.

Priscilla Ebersole
Patricia Hess

CONTENTS

chapter

1

Introduction to Aging

►LEARNING OBJECTIVES

Upon completion of this chapter, the reader will be able to:

- Relate at least three factors that contribute to ageism and stigmatization of the elderly.
- Describe the needs and developmental tasks in late life.
- Define health and wellness.
- Delineate dimensions of wellness.
- Explain wellness in the context of chronic illness.
- Explain how some of the goals of wellness for elders are being accomplished.
- Discuss nursing as it relates to the care of the aged.

►GLOSSARY

Accoutrements Necessary equipment or implements as used in this chapter.

Assimilate To absorb into a cultural tradition not of one's origin.

Authenticate To prove genuine.

Contemplate To consider with continued attention.

Cumbersome An awkward burden that weighs one down.

Hindrance Something that holds back or slows progress.

Ineptitude Lacking fitness, inappropriate, out of place, bungling.

Innovation The introduction of a new idea, method, or device.

Metaphor A figure of speech in which one subject or idea is meant to suggest a likeness to another; for example, "the wind sighs through the trees."

Migratory Moving from one country, place, or locality to another.

Patriarchal A system in which males are revered as leaders and heads of families.

Proliferate To grow or increase rapidly.

Residual Pertaining to the portion that remains after an activity that removes the bulk of the substance, problem, or issue; for example, the urine that remains in the bladder after urination, or the limp that remains after the healing of a fractured foot.

Stereotype Considered to lack individuality, trite, repeated without variation.

►THE LIVED EXPERIENCE

I believe a human life is like a river, meandering through its course, rushing through rapids, flowing placidly over the plains, twisting and turning through countless bends until it spends itself. It is the same river; yet it looks very different from one place to another. So it is with our lives; circumstances vary from one time to another in the course of a life, but I think each stage has its own value.

Georgia, a 35-year-old woman

It is so strange! I only realize I'm considered old when I'm automatically given a senior discount without even asking. Sometimes I will catch a glance from someone who seems as if they are afraid I may need help, and of course my children notice if I forget something and are kind enough to not mention it. As if they never forget anything!! But the worst is when I catch a glimpse of a wrinkled old lady and realize it is my own reflection. How can that be?

Reba, a 75-year-old

1

AGING

In this introductory chapter we set out to launch students of aging, particularly nurses, into a mind-set that recognizes the individuality, uniqueness, and potential for wellness of every person of whatever age. Brief background information is provided here that will orient the reader to critical issues affecting the present and future of the aged and the nurse's role in their care. All of these issues are addressed in more depth throughout the text.

Attitudes

Ageism and stereotypes are at the root of many myths and misunderstandings about our elders. *Ageism* is a term coined by Robert Butler, the first Director of the Institute on Aging, to describe the discrimination that often accompanies old age and is based solely on age. Cole (1992) examined the historic roots of ageism in America and concluded that the erosion of the patriarchal and hierarchical systems of inheritance, in which male elders held power of ownership based on age, was a significant factor. In crowded and land-poor countries committed to the notion that the young were to serve and the old were to rule, old men were venerated. Early in U.S. history the general availability of land and the need for youthful power and vigor reduced the elder's power base. With the shift to urban industrialism, emphasis on productivity, and shifting philosophies in government, old men lost some of their influence. In a consumer-oriented society it is inevitable that those who purchase less will receive less attention (Box 1-1). In our society a specific type of ageist marketing exists. The old are aggressively marketed for health aids, funeral plans, and fraudulent schemes.

Ageism exists among some health care professionals, undoubtedly somewhat influenced by the fact that providers often see older persons who need help or are ill. The influence these negative perceptions have on potential therapeutic outcomes has been largely ignored. The realization that aging is the greatest challenge one will ever face is a reality for the very old. For some, the challenge is exciting; for others, a test of the human spirit. As long as old age represents proximity to death, it will be embraced with reluctance by those who love life.

Stereotypes

Stereotypes are at the base of ageism and are ideas that set individuals apart based on supposed characteristic qualities. Positive stereotypes may be just as damaging as negative ones if the positive stereotypes impose unre-

---

Box 1-1	SEVEN CONTRIBUTORS TO AGEISM

Seven factors account for the majority of ageism in advertising, according to "Ageism in Advertising: A Study of Advertising Agency Attitudes Towards Maturing and Mature Consumers." According to the report's author, Richard A. Lee of High-Yield Marketing, based in Roseville, Minn., "Take them away, and ageism in advertising largely goes away with them."

1. The majority of advertising-agency professionals are in early adulthood, when empathetic understanding for people of different generations is relatively uncommon.
2. Most agency professionals are most comfortable advertising to younger consumers like themselves.
3. Advertising-agency culture and output reflect the tastes and values of a relatively narrow slice of society—young adults in their 20s and 30s.
4. Advertising professionals don't believe that Baby Boomers are maturing (and will mature) as people always have.
5. Not wanting to be educated about older consumers, rather than lack of informational and educational resources, perpetuates common misperceptions among agency professionals about older consumers.
6. Although ageism in advertising is most visible in relation to "seniors"—what we see is actually the culmination of a long process that starts with consumers in their 40s.
7. There is scant internal pressure within agencies to "break the lock" of ageism—and external pressure, although rising, is still at minimal levels.

Modified from Lee RA: Seven contributors to ageism, *Aging Today* 16(5):11, 1995.

---

alistic expectations. Stereotypes of the elderly held by young, middle-age, and elderly adults vary significantly and become more complex as the individuals age (Hummert et al, 1994). In other words, the older one becomes, the more likely one is to see old age as complex and with many more facets than younger persons view it. Distinct differences in stereotypical thinking among young adults and older adults are seen in Table 1-1.

Gender stereotypes exist as well (DeAngelis, 1994). Women are thought to be more concerned about maintaining appearance, and men more concerned about maintaining status and power. Also, stereotypes exist about older women who marry younger men and about very young women who marry older men. These stereotypes are changing as the opportunities and expectations of both men and women of all ages are be-

Table 1-1

Frequently Named* Traits in Additional Category

Trait	Age-group			
	Young (n = 40)	Middle-aged (n = 40)	Elderly (n = 40)	Trait valence
Conservative	7.5	20.0	2.5	Positive
Depressed	12.5	20.0	7.5	Negative
Determined	2.5	20.0	17.5	Positive
Eager to learn and experience	0.0	17.5	25.0	Positive
Has sense of humor	12.5	15.0	12.5	Positive
Health-conscious	15.0	45.0	30.0	Positive
Independent	5.0	25.0	22.5	Positive
Likes social activities	25.0	20.0	17.5	Positive
Move after retirement	22.5	10.0	2.5	Positive
Politically aware and active	22.5	17.5	17.5	Positive
Pursues a hobby	30.0	30.0	27.5	Positive
Religious	12.5	32.5	20.0	Positive
Scared of becoming sick and incompetent	0.0	35.0	52.5	Negative
Successful	12.5	25.0	5.0	Positive
Timid	5.0	27.5	7.5	Negative
Tired	25.0	17.5	2.5	Negative
Travels often	10.0	20.0	32.5	Positive
Trustworthy	2.5	20.0	5.0	Positive
Well-groomed	5.0	17.5	20.0	Positive
Worried about finances	7.5	5.0	35.0	Negative

From Hummert ML et al: Stereotypes of the elderly held by young, middle-aged, and elderly adults, *J Gerontol* 49(5):P240, 1994.
*Named by 20% or more informants in at least one age-group or by 10% or more of informants in all three age-groups.

coming less rigid. Personal contact with elders provides continual illumination of their variability.

In the United States today there are rural aged in small communities and on farms; urban aged in ghettos and exclusive penthouses; suburban aged living with family, spouse, or alone; and elders living in congregate communities, retirement settlements, nursing care centers, and assisted living complexes. No profile of older persons fits; there are no norms.

Influences of History

To demonstrate the amazing variations in personality, needs, and concerns of the aged, one must think in terms of generational, geographic, cultural, and gender differences, as well as the impact of educational and economic opportunities. My (P.E.) grandmother lived in a small farm community from 1902 until her death in 1934 at age 67. During the depths of the Great Depression, neighbors relied on each other for survival and many lost their farms; some went to the "poor farm." Social Security, Medicare, or services for the aged did not

exist. Medical care was so primitive in some rural areas as to often do more harm than good. Most labor was physical, and heavy, hearty meals were expected. The majority of the diet consisted of home-grown fruits and vegetables, and meat was a rare luxury although chickens and eggs usually were plentiful. We could easily contend that the five dimensions of wellness—self-responsibility, exercise, nutritional awareness, stress management, and environmental sensitivity (discussed later in this chapter)—were evident in this cohort but the overriding factors of medical ineptitude and economic deprivations brought on the ravages of "old age" early.

Influences of Cohort

A cohort is a group born at approximately the same time, usually within a particular decade. Thus the men born between 1920 and 1930 were very likely to have been active participants in World War II and the Korean War. These experiences made an impact on their lives in a manner different from that of men born earlier or later. Likewise, women born between 1930 and 1940

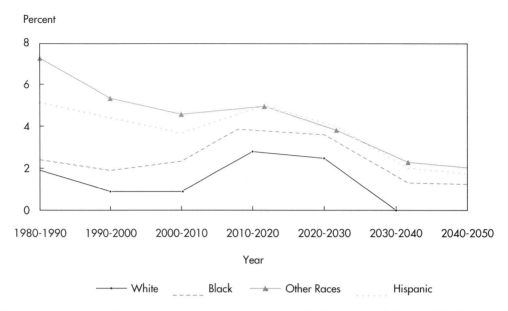

Percent

Fig. 1-1   Annual rate of increase in elderly population by race and ethnicity: 1980-2050. (Modified from Angel JL, Hogan DP: The demography of minority aging populations. In *Minority aging,* The Gerontological Society of America, Washington, DC, 1994, The Society.)

were coming of age as the feminist revolution took wing. They were somewhat less likely than their sisters, born a decade earlier, to believe that being a model homemaker was their major life function. However, there are no set responses to major cohort events. Each elder should be asked what major events in his or her early life affected him or her and how.

Influences of Culture
The United States is experiencing a "gerontologic explosion" of ethnically diverse adults. The cultural impact on recent émigrés who have left their homelands late in life to come to the United States is evident in their special needs and attributes. It is estimated that within 30 years minority elders will comprise 25% of the aged population. Fig. 1-1 depicts the projected ethnic changes in the elderly population by the year 2050. The present and expected growth and diversity of the elderly population mean that nurses will be caring for a significant number of minority elders who have varied cultural backgrounds and geographically distinct influences. Standard care approaches will not necessarily be appropriate for those so diverse in needs, abilities, and resources. This is discussed more fully in Chapter 4.

Influences of Gender
Women and men have very particular needs that emerge during later life. Women survive longer and thus de-

velop more economic and physical dependencies and much more frequently live alone; men become more suicidal as they age, particularly white men. They are more likely to marry after widowhood. In general, women have developed larger social networks apart from the work environment and may find more readily available social supports than do men. And, gender-related health problems emerge: women increasingly confront osteoporosis and breast and uterine cancer, whereas men are vulnerable to prostate enlargement and cancer. Cardiac problems afflict both genders about equally, but women are treated less aggressively than are men. Gender significant variations are presented in Table 1-2.

Human Needs

Maslow's theories of the hierarchy of human needs provide an excellent organizing framework for understanding individuals and their concerns at any particular time. The most basic needs must be adequately met: pain alleviated and biologic processes reasonably efficient. If not, the individual remains insecure and anxious. When basic needs are met and the individual feels secure, a sense of belonging and being cared for develops. Building on the awareness that he or she is cared for, the person's self-esteem rises. Feeling listened to and respected allows the person to free energies previ-

Table 1-2

Gender Differences

	Male	Female
Mental disorders	Addiction Personality disorders	Neuroses Depression
Cognitive function (specific capacities)	Spatial ability Accuracy Mathematics	Processing information Verbal skills
Personality	Both sexes are thought to become more androgenous—"gender free"	
Role behaviors (most likely troublesome)	Work transition	Poverty
Living situation		
With spouse	74.3%	40.1%
Alone	15.9%	40.9%
With relative(s)	8.4%	17.8%
With nonrelative	1.4%	1.2%

ously bound in other concerns and to transcend the immediate difficulties. The energies to achieve the highest possible level of adaptation and wellness are then available to the person. We health care providers must address the need of most concern to the elder if we expect a positive and growing response to the problems that we may have identified.

Health and Wellness in Aging

Medically, health is thought to be only the absence of disease. The strong emergence of the holistic health movement has resulted in broader definitions of health, to include wellness. Wellness involves one's whole being—physical, emotional, mental, and spiritual—all of which are vital components. A shift in any of these influences the wholeness of the person. In addition, wellness includes the cultural expectations and these must be given adequate consideration in the definitions and attainment of wellness. A positive approach to health emphasizes strengths, resilience, resources, and capabilities rather than focuses on existing pathology. Box 1-2 enumerates the traits of a healthy person. Wellness is based on the belief that every person has an optimal level of function regardless of his or her situation. Even in chronic illness and dying, some levels of well-being are attainable when supports and encouragement allow the individual to make meaning out of the present situation.

Wellness involves achieving a balance between one's internal and external environment and one's emo-

Box 1-2   TRAITS OF A HEALTHY PERSON

Attuned to mind-body signals of pain and pleasure as well as fatigue, anger, sadness.
Can confide one's secrets, traumas, and feelings to others instead of keeping them locked inside.
Exhibits control over own health and quality of life.
Exhibits a strong commitment to work, creative activities, or relationships.
Can see stress as a challenge rather than a threat.
Demonstrates appropriate assertiveness concerning needs and feelings.
Forms relationships based on unconditional love rather than power.
Is altruistically committed to helping others.
Is willing to explore many different facets of own personality, which will provide strength to fall back on if one fails.

Modified from Dreher H: *The immune power personality: seven traits you can develop to stay healthy,* New York, 1995, Dutton.

tional, spiritual, social, cultural, and physical processes. The interrelationship of these facets is shown in Fig. 1-2. It is the mission of nursing to assist the individual to achieve the highest level of adaptation to whatever situation exists. Throughout this text it is apparent that wellness must be assessed and is always a goal for which to strive.

The long-existing concepts of illness prevention and health promotion are coming to the fore as consumers take charge of their care through alternative health methods and internet information sources. Elderly individuals are now encouraged to take personal responsibility for their own health by seeking knowledge and making behavioral changes. Terms frequently heard in the health arena now are *empowerment of the individual, prevention of illness,* and *health promotion.*

Wellness in Chronic Illness

Chronic disorders and acute illness cannot really be separated because so many conditions are intricately intertwined; acute disorders leave chronic problems, and many of the commonly identified disorders tend to flare up intermittently and then go into remission. Many elders have several chronic disorders simultaneously and have great difficulty managing the complexity of the overlapping and often contradictory demands and restrictions. The management of chronic illness relies primarily on the client and family caregiver because health care coverage usually is limited and available only when a particular measurably improved outcome is expected.

Physical disabilities are often multiple and serious but need not kill the spirit or define the person. The challenge to the aged individual with multiple disabilities and chronic problems may simply become overwhelming. However, with disability, the aged can still achieve a high level of wellness if the emphasis of care is placed on the promotion of function in the least restrictive environment.

"Well" elders mourn their losses and talk about them but not to the exclusion of other interests and events in their lives. They know they are more than just the body that sustains their functions. They believe in being responsible and responsive to their community. They be-

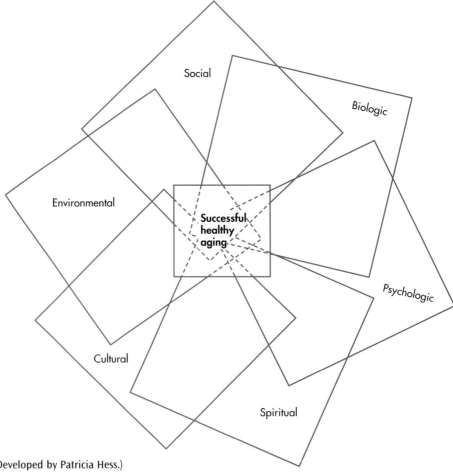

Fig. 1-2   Healthy aging. (Developed by Patricia Hess.)

lieve competition and conviction undergird their remarkable survival capacity. They have earned many past and present laurels but will not rest on them. Although they argue about the possibility of wellness during illness, they demonstrate wellness in their approach to life. They know that chronic disorders do not define them.

The ultimate goals of wellness for the elderly are to delay illness, prevent the ill from developing residual disabilities, and assist those who are disabled to function at maximally comfortable levels and prevent further disability. This often involves improving muscle strength and endurance, increasing range of motion, maintaining mobility, and redesigning activities of daily living.

One of the earliest geriatric nurse pioneers, Eldonna Shields, said, "Old age is a losing game when focused on function" (Ebersole, 1990). We, as nurses, are challenged to authenticate necessary dependency and to respect those who have the courage to let go of certain functions when necessary. The things nurses "do" and the order in which they are done are probably far less important in chronic disease management than attitudes framed in illness or wellness.

Achieving Wellness

The emergence of the holistic health movement has reintroduced a definition of and an approach to health that expands the definition of "health." Dunn (1961) defined the holistic approach to health as "an integrated method of functioning which is oriented toward maximizing the potential of which the individual is capable within the environment where he is functioning." The holistic definition does not limit health to just its physical or mental or even social aspects but, rather, incorporates all these facets into the total picture. Well-being for those older than 60 years is strongly related to health but is affected also by socioeconomic factors, degree of social interaction, marital status, and aspects of one's living situation and environment. Needs of the old and the very old differ in kind and degree, reflecting different cultural styles and physical and social environment.

To achieve wellness or assist an individual to attain wellness potential, one needs to consider the dimensions of wellness: self-responsibility, nutritional awareness, physical fitness, stress management, and environmental sensitivity (Pender, 1996). In Box 1-3 these are explained more fully, and each of these elements is discussed later in this text.

Box 1-3	DIMENSIONS OF WELLNESS
Self-responsibility (self-efficacy)	"How you maintain your body is your choice." Involvement in self-help groups for self-help strategies. Learn own body signals, and take action accordingly. Read about health promotion and maintenance. Talk with knowledgeable persons. Seek periodic health checkups for health promotion, disease prevention, and health maintenance. Follow universal self-care requirements (Box 1-4).
Nutrition awareness	Learn about foods that make the body respond in a physically and emotionally healthy way. Decrease fat, sugar, and salt intake. Read; seek counsel and classes on healthy nutrition for the older adult.
Physical fitness	Learn the benefits of physical fitness. Engage in aerobic exercise, balance, and flexibility exercise. These can be accomplished actively (e.g., walking, biking, golfing, swimming), in chair, or, for bedbound, in bed.
Stress management	Balance adequate rest and activity. Learn and implement relaxation techniques, meditation, biofeedback, and/or autogenic training. Learn to be selfish. Create a support network.
Environmental sensitivity (encompasses the world, neighborhood, home, and room)	Arrange the environment (personal space): sights, sounds, colors, furnishings. Establish friend and support networks.

Modified from Pender N: *Health promotion in nursing practice,* ed 3, Stamford, Conn, 1996, Appleton & Lange.

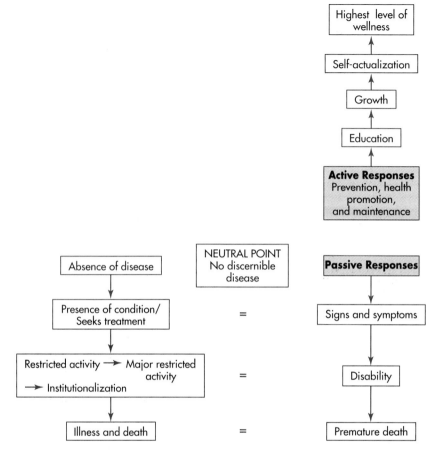

Fig. 1-3 Illness-wellness continuum.

Wellness begins with the individual and stimulates the desire for growth and change. This means nurturing the physical self, expressing emotions more freely, improving personal decision making, becoming more creative with others, staying in touch with the environment despite physical incapacities, and improving health practices (Hey, 1996). The wellness continuum picks up where the traditional medical model leaves off. Instead of a downward negative trajectory for the health of the aged, focused on deterioration, the wellness model rises and moves in a positive direction (Fig. 1-3). Hey (1996) contends that the aged can achieve high-level wellness through the promotion of productivity, self-actualization, self-respect, self-determination, and continued personal growth.

When one considers the wellness or holistic approach as an appropriate model for the aged, one re-

gards the illness and wellness continuum from a positive direction and the role of the individual as active. Wellness is within the grasp of all persons, no matter what age. The significance for the aged is a new and positive approach to what the nurse and other caregivers call "healthy." Wellness is a state of being and feeling that one strives to achieve through motivation and positive health practices. An individual must work hard to achieve wellness just as he or she must work hard to perform competently at a job. In working toward wellness, an individual may reach plateaus in his or her ascension to higher-level wellness. The person may also regress because of an illness event or simply the various cycles of life, but these events can be a stimulus for growth potential and a return to moving up the wellness continuum. Table 1-3 depicts self-management in acute and chronic care models.

Table 1-3

Comparison of Acute Care (Medical Model) and Chronic Care (Self-Management Model)

Characteristics	Acute	Chronic
Onset	Rapid	Gradual
Cause	Generally one thing	Multiple causes
Duration	Short	Indefinite
Diagnosis	Usually accurate	Often uncertain
Treatment	Cure	Cure is rare
Role of professional	Selects and conducts therapy	Teaches and is in partnership with patient
Role of patient	Follows orders	Explains symptoms accurately
Partnership with professionals for daily management

The nurse can, through knowledge and affirmation, empower, enhance, and support the aged person's movement toward self-responsibility by exploring with the aged the underlying situations that may be creating a wellness imbalance and discussing with the aged the alternatives available to them. Given sufficient unbiased information, the aged can, in most instances, make meaningful decisions. Self-responsibility incorporates universal self-care requirements as shown in Box 1-4.

Healthy People 2000, an effort by the U.S. Department of Health and Human Services (USDHHS) to establish and publish goals for health, was meant to prevent health risks, unnecessary disease, disability, and death. The goals set forth by that report included (1) increasing the span of healthy life for Americans, (2) reducing health disparity among Americans, and (3) achieving access to preventive services for all Americans through health promotion, protection, and preventive services. These recommendations are now updated in a recent report, *Healthy People 2010.* A summary of the *Healthy People 2010* (2000) objectives for adults 65 years of age and older appears in Box 1-5. The intent of these goals is not only lengthening of life but, more important, improving the functional independence of the aged and the quality of life. We did not reach the desired outcomes in the past decade, century, or millenium, but the shift in direction is significant. There is a small but important movement toward health. The present concern we have is that those who are now coping with chronic illness be provided sufficient support, assistance, accoutrements, and comforts to enjoy the extended life span that is more and more possible for the aging population (see Bibliography).

This text and particularly this chapter are devoted to those ends.

Alternative Health Care

Individuals are increasingly taking charge of their own health through the use of complementary/alternative health strategies. Because of public interest and citizen involvement, the National Institutes of Health (NIH) established in 1992 the National Center for Complementary and Alternative Medicine. Recent estimates are that almost one half of U.S. residents use some form of complementary medicine—often because they are dissatisfied with conventional medical approaches (Lorenzi, 1999). These strategies include focusing or transferring of positive energies through meditation, visualization, touch, massage, acupressure, acupuncture, magnets, crystals, aromas, and colors. Also, numerous nutritional supplements and dietary aberrations are popular. Some of these are legitimate, and some are fads. The aged are very vulnerable to fads because they are especially likely to have chronic disorders and energy depletion. Nutritionists, nurses, doctors, acupuncturists, and chiropractors are only a few of the providers that offer services to the public. It is a nursing function to discuss the use of alternative/complementary therapies with each individual because these are such an important aspect of an individual's treatment. The nurse should discuss the problem the individual experiences and the alternative therapy being used or considered. What is the expectation? Most important, the nurse should not recommend any specific therapy but, instead, alert the individual to the fact that the responses to alternative therapeutic in-

Box 1-4	UNIVERSAL SELF-CARE REQUIREMENTS

1. Maintaining sufficient intakes of air, water, food
   a. Taking in that quantity required for normal functioning with adjustments for internal and external factors that can affect the requirement, or, under conditions of scarcity, adjusting consumption to bring the most advantageous return to integrated functioning
   b. Preserving the integrity of associated anatomic structures and physiologic processes
   c. Enjoying the pleasurable experiences of breathing, drinking, and eating without abuses
2. Provision of care associated with eliminative processes and excrements
   a. Bringing about and maintaining internal and external conditions necessary for the regulation of eliminative processes
   b. Managing the processes of elimination (including protection of the structures and processes involved) and disposal of excrements
   c. Providing subsequent hygienic care of body surfaces and parts
   d. Caring for the environment as needed to maintain sanitary conditions
3. Maintenance of body temperature and personal hygiene
   a. Bringing about and/or maintaining internal and external conditions necessary for regulating body temperature processes

   b. Using personal capabilities and values as well as culturally prescribed norms as bases for maintaining personal hygiene
   c. Caring for the environment to maintain a healthy living condition
4. Maintenance of a balance between activity and rest
   a. Selecting activities that stimulate, engage, and keep in balance physical movement, affective responses, intellectual effort, and social interaction
   b. Recognizing and attending to manifestations of needs for rest and activity
   c. Using personal capabilities, interests, and values as well as culturally prescribed norms as bases for development of a rest-activity pattern
5. Maintenance of a balance between solitude and social interaction
   a. Maintaining that quality and balance necessary for the development of personal autonomy and enduring social relations that foster effective functioning of individuals
   b. Fostering bonds of affection, love, and friendship; effectively managing impulses to use others for selfish purposes, disregarding their individuality, integrity, and rights
   c. Providing conditions of social warmth and closeness essential for continuing development and adjustment
   d. Promoting individual autonomy as well as group membership

From Department of Health and Human Services: *Toward a plan for the chronically mentally ill.* Report to the Secretary of Health and Human Services, Washington, DC, 1980, The Department.

terventions vary. A method effective for one person may not be for another. Individuals are psychologically and biologically unique, and responses to any therapy vary greatly. This is not sufficiently considered among medical or alternative providers. We caution individuals to thoroughly investigate the qualifications of the provider, research the method being considered, use only one new therapy at a time, and allow sufficient time to identify reactions.

ROLE DEVELOPMENT IN GERIATRIC NURSING

Nursing is most important in the care of the aged. The survival and quality of life more often than not depend on nursing care and expertise. Sporadically since 1904, when the American Journal of Nursing published an article on old age and disease, a few visionary nurses

have been drawn to gerontologic nursing as they recognized that a body of nursing knowledge and skills related to nursing care for older persons was distinguishable within the full scope of nursing practice. These nurses also recognized that institutional settings such as old-age homes or boardinghouses—all predecessors of today's nursing homes—were settings in which nurses could best provide homelike nursing services for older persons who did not need the acute care services of a hospital. The best of these were truly homes. However, it was not until 1966 that the ANA formed a Division of Geriatric Nursing and in 1970 developed the Standards of Geriatric Nursing Practice. In 1976 the Division of Geriatric Nursing changed its name to the Gerontological Nursing Division to reflect the broad role nurses play in the management of the elderly. In 1984 the Council of Gerontological Nursing was formed and certification in the specialty became available. Since the mid-1970s geriatric nursing service has flourished

Box 1-5	HEALTHY PEOPLE 2010

Goals

Goal #1: Increase Quality and Years of Healthy Life: To help individuals of all ages increase life expectancy *and* improve their quality of life.

Goal #2: Eliminate Health Disparities: To eliminate health disparities among different segments of the population.

Focus Areas and Objectives

The nation's progress in achieving the two overarching goals of *Healthy People 2010* will be monitored through 467 objectives in 28 focus areas. Many objectives focus on interventions designed to reduce or eliminate illness, disability, and premature death among individuals and communities. Others focus on broader issues, such as improving access to quality health care, strengthening public health services, and improving the availability and dissemination of health-related information. Each objective has a target for specific improvements to be achieved by the year 2010.

Healthy People 2010 Focus Areas

- Access to quality health services
- Arthritis, osteoporosis, and chronic back conditions
- Cancer
- Chronic kidney disease
- Diabetes
- Disability and secondary conditions
- Educational and community-based programs
- Environmental health
- Family planning
- Food safety
- Health communication
- Heart disease and stroke
- Human immunodeficiency virus (HIV)
- Immunization and infectious diseases
- Injury and violence prevention
- Maternal, infant, and child health
- Medical product safety
- Mental health and mental disorders
- Nutrition and overweight
- Occupational safety and health
- Oral health
- Physical activity and fitness
- Public health infrastructure
- Respiratory diseases
- Sexually transmitted diseases
- Substance abuse
- Tobacco use
- Vision and hearing

Source: http://www.health.gov/healthypeople

and now includes nursing opportunities anywhere within the continuum of aging services. In the care of the aged, which relies on carefully orchestrated care (the foundation of nursing knowledge), the nurse functions as a key member of the health care team and, in many cases, functions autonomously. Terry Fulmer, codirector of the John A Hartford Foundation Institute for Geriatric Nursing, says, "Long ago I realized that, in the arena of caring for the aged, I could have an autonomous nursing practice that would make a real difference in medical outcomes. I could practice the full scope of nursing. It gave me a great sense of freedom and accomplishment" (Ebersole, 1999).

THE FUTURE OF AGING IN THE UNITED STATES

"Baby boomers" are expected to carry their particular energies and expectations into old age and will change the face of aging in America. Articles about menopause proliferate, midlife crises abound, and anxiety about the future is rampant. Will there be income support, adequate retirement, available health care, disability benefits, and all the things the present generation of the old have relied on? At present the major concerns of baby boomers are health, finances, job security, children, and parents. They are the "sandwich generation," trying to meet the needs of college-age children, elderly parents, and, in many cases, grandparents. Gerontologists, marketing strategists, and the age industry are preparing for the anticipated challenges (Wylde, 1995).

The last members of the celebrated baby boom cohort will die around the year 2080 (National Academy On Aging, 1995), and more than 1.5 million of them will live to 100 years of age. Although it has been fashionable to consider the baby boomers en masse, they are extremely diverse, differing by as much as 19 birth years and separated by race, culture, and socioeconomic status. To plan well for their retirement years, we must consider the following:

- Their diversity
- The uncertain political and economic future
- Potential major shifts in life-style expectations

- Radical differences in health care delivery systems
- Progress in technology and medical management of some disorders
- Shifts in values and ethics that will profoundly affect daily life

This segment of the population is characterized by its affluence, relative good health, and vitality. The most potent influences on their development are the almost universal opportunities for higher education, inflationary economics, political participation, urban and suburban life-styles, assimilation of myriad cultures into the mainstream of American life, technologic innovations, youth-centered family life, and now the increasing responsibility for elderly parents. One of the major concerns is based in the shift of life-styles away from the traditional family. Single parents, blended families, limited parenthood, unmarried parents, and gay parents all represent life-styles that may or may not produce children willing or available to assist parents as they age (Cornman, Kingson, 1996). Yet, in the middle of the twentieth century, there was much concern about the break-up of the extended family (Hashimoto, 1993); however, this has not deterred adult children in nuclear families from caring for their elderly parents.

Migratory tendencies and travel opportunities throughout baby boomers' working lives have led to sophistication and a world focus. The increasing migration of "snowbirds" for half of each year and the enormous population shifts in the United States (U.S. retirees emigrating to other countries; retirement-age adults from other countries emigrating to the United States) are presenting additional challenges to policy planners.

Thus these space-age children can only wonder what the future holds for their own later years. They seem more concerned about healthful life-styles than previous generations were, are better educated, have higher expectations of themselves (and others), and are forming the core of the "moral majority." Although formal religion seems to have been supplanted by a sense of personal responsibility, many have sought leadership or inspiration among gurus, charismatic personalities, cults, and mystics. Many uncertainties remain about the conditions, status, and benefits baby boomers will experience.

Metaphors of Aging

The "sandwich" metaphor provides a clear picture of the dilemma of the middle-age population, caught between adult children and aging parents. The "machine" conveys the image of wear and tear, even to the analogy of oil in the joints drying up, and the need for mainte-nance. The "over the hill" image has been a popular one for decades and is still held by some. If the hill we visualize is somewhat like a bell curve, attaining the peak of everything good occurs at age 38. "Stages of life" provide a picture of sequential steps toward goodness, wisdom, heaven, or whatever one believes must be achieved in a progressive manner. Often the life course is seen as a race that the individual is trying to win or as a river that ultimately brings the elder back to the source of all life. In all of these images, a model or some type of trajectory shapes our thoughts (Cirillo, 1993). Literature, theater, and the media contribute to these images (Holstein, 1994).

Variations on the metaphors of aging throughout the world seem infinite. What we make of aging, it seems, depends on how we see it. Bernice Neugarten (Neugarten et al, 1968), the foremost gerontologic theorist, recently predicted that we are rapidly moving into an age-irrelevant society. Our goal throughout this text is to present age in its many faces; to focus on the diversity and potential for wellness of each elder encountered within our nursing practices, regardless of the situation or obstacles.

▶ KEY CONCEPTS

- Aging is a gradual process of change over the course of time. Each species has an expected life span, and that of the human species as presently understood is limited to approximately 120 years.
- Although the population as a whole is aging, the greatest categoric increase by group percentage is occurring among those 85 years old and older.
- Studies of exceptional longevity in various geographic pockets show the importance of diet, exercise, environment, and, most important, adequate documentation of age. Those studies of individuals thought to be older than 150 years have proved to be questionable because of unverified birth records.
- The number of centenarians is increasing rapidly, and many scientists and lay persons are fascinated by the study of their lives.
- The study of gerontology in the United States is comparatively new, with serious study and research going back only about 35 years.
- Old age must be studied as a complex phenomenon with biopsychosocial and spiritual aspects affecting the manner in which an individual ages.
- It is unknown at this time what changes over time are specifically the result of aging, disease, life-style, or

environmental impact. In other words, the changes caused purely by the aging process are unknown.

- Theories of aging are particularly culture and cohort bound and must be studied with that in mind.
- Each aged cohort is in some ways distinctly different from others, and individual aged persons become more unique the longer they live. Thus one must be cautious in attributing any specific characteristics to "old age."
- Political actions and appropriations have had far-reaching influence on the individual experience of aging, chiefly through Medicare, Medicaid, and Social Security.
- With the advance of medical science, there has been a tendency to prolong the lives of the old and to consider their medical needs predominant.
- Nursing leads the field in gerontology; nurses were the first professionals in the nation to be certified as geriatric specialists.

▶ Activities and Discussion Questions

1. Discuss the reasons underlying ageist attitudes.
2. Interview an older person, and ask how he or she has changed since being 25 years old.
3. Discuss health and wellness with your peers. Develop a definition applicable to an aged person.
4. Discuss the dimensions of wellness and which you think may be most important.
5. Explain wellness in the context of chronic illness.
6. Discuss how you seek wellness in your own life.
7. Discuss nursing as it relates to the care of the aged.

REFERENCES

Cirillo L: Verbal imagery of aging in the news magazines, *Generations* 17(2):91-93, 1993.

Cole TR: *The journey of life: a cultural history of aging in America,* Cambridge, 1992, Cambridge University Press.

Cornman JM, Kingson ER: Trends, issues, perspectives, and values for the aging of the baby boom cohorts, *Gerontologist* 36(1):15-26, 1996.

DeAngelis T: Researchers explore roots of ageism, *Aging Today* 15(1):12, 1994.

Dunn HL: *High-level wellness,* Arlington, Va, 1961, Beatty.

Ebersole P: Leaders in geriatric nursing: the dynamic duo: Mathy Mezey and Terry Fulmer, *Geriatr Nurs* 20(2):106-107, 1999.

Ebersole P: *Geriatric nurse pioneers,* Personal interviews, Cleveland, Ohio, 1990, Unpublished data.

Hashimoto A: Family relations in later life: a cross-cultural perspective, *Generations* 17(4):24-26, 1993.

Healthy People 2000: US Department of Health and Human Services, Public Health Services, US Government Printing Office, Washington, DC, Pub No (PHS) 91-50212, 1-8; 22-27; 587-591, 1991.

Healthy People 2000 Midcourse Review and 1995 Revisions: US Department of Health and Human Services, Public Health Service, US Government Printing Office, Washington, DC, 1995.

Healthy People 2010: US Department of Health and Human Services, Public Health Service, US Government Printing Office, Washington, DC, 2000.

Hey RP: Healthy, wealthy, and wise, *AARP Bull* 37(7):6, 1996.

Holstein M: Taking next steps: gerontological education, research and the literary imagination, *Gerontologist* 34(6):822-827, 1994.

Hummert ML et al: Stereotypes of the elderly held by young, middle-aged, and elderly adults, *J Gerontol* 49(5):P240, 1994.

Lorenzi EA: Complementary/alternative therapies: so many choices, *Geriatr Nurs* 20(3):125-133, 1999.

National Academy on Aging: What do people want to know about population aging? *Public Policy Aging Report* 7(1):11, 1995.

Neugarten B, Havighurst R, Tobin S: Personality and patterns of aging. In Neugarten B, editor: *Middle age and aging,* Chicago, 1968, University of Chicago Press.

Pender N: *Health promotion in nursing practice,* ed 3, Stamford, Conn, 1996, Appleton & Lange.

Wylde MA: How to size up the current and future markets: technology and the older adult, *Generations* 19(1):15-19, 1995

BIBLIOGRAPHY

Burggraf V, Barry R: *Gerontological nursing,* Thorofare, NJ, 1996, Slack.

Carlson E, Crowley S: The Friedan mystique: feminist leader sees radical change in attitudes on aging, *AARP Bull* 33(8):20, 1992.

Cole TR: What have we "made" of aging? *J Gerontol* 50B(6):S341-S343, 1995.

Heidrich SM: Mechanisms related to psychological well-being in older women with chronic illnesses: age and disease comparisons, *Res Nurs Health* 19(3):225, 1996.

Heinemann GD: In geriatrics, the team approach, *Generations* 19(2):20-22, 1995.

Hendricks J: The social power of professional knowledge in aging, *Generations* 19(2):51-53, 1995.

Maslow A: *Motivation and personality,* ed 2, New York, 1970, Harper & Row.

Modern Maturity: *Boomers: the babies face fifty, entire issue focus,* Washington, DC, 1996, American Association of Retired Persons.

National Academy on Aging: Facts on The Older Americans Act, Gerontology News, Washington, DC, *National Academy on Aging* 7(5):14, 1996.

Communication, Education, and Geriatric Nursing Roles

chapter 2

▶ LEARNING OBJECTIVES

Upon completion of this chapter, the reader will be able to:

- Describe several gerontic nursing roles and the educational preparation.
- Identify elements of the most recent American Nurses Association Standards of Practice for Gerontological Nursing.
- Discuss formal geriatric organizations and their significance to the geriatric nurse.
- Recognize and discuss the importance of certification.
- Identify factors that have influenced the progress of gerontologic nursing as a specialty practice.
- Understand the importance of nurse-to-nurse communication.

▶ THE LIVED EXPERIENCE

I really dread being evaluated today. It seems like, no matter how hard I try, more is expected. I don't think these RNs have any idea how hard it is to keep going day after day and take care of wealthy residents every day when my own mother is so poor and ill and my kids are home alone each day after school. They don't know how lucky they are to be in such a nice place. Does anyone ask what my life is like? Does anyone care?

Amy, a 30-year-old nursing assistant

I really dread doing Amy's evaluation today. She is late so often, and it seems like she is getting short with the residents. I know hers is a difficult job and residents can be demanding, but she just goes around scowling much of the time. After all, we have a reputation to keep up here. These residents pay a lot to get top-notch service, and we must be sure that happens.

Amy's supervisor

NURSE-TO-NURSE COMMUNICATION

True communication rests in one's ability to declare and respond with sensitivity to the position of oneself and the other at a given moment in time. This applies to every situation in which real communication exists. Communication in its most distilled sense involves communion, dedication to a common purpose, and sharing thoughts, feelings, and information with others. Reciprocity is essential to the completion of the process. Mechanically, communication is often reduced to sender, medium of message, and receiver. However, true communication is never a unidirectional process but is, by virtue of the root word (common), necessarily cyclic. Meaning is structured by the co-creating of reality through the use of language and images (Parse, 1998). This reality involves both *revealing* and *concealing*. Concealing may be done in respect for self or another, and revealing is that which enhances understanding. Meaning and reality are changing constantly throughout the process of communication. In a sense, we re-create ourselves and others through communication. Communication is at the heart of nursing.

This chapter addresses organizations, education, roles, and communication attributes that increase satisfaction and effective geriatric practice. These include the following:

- Focus on useful, satisfying, and enriching communication
- An increased understanding of education and the various practice roles
- Group strategies for management of staff morale
- Special attention to the needs of the paraprofessionals, aides, and LPNs/LVNs

In all areas of practice, nurses complain about the lack of professional supports, inadequate time, and fragmentation of care. Nurses must consciously seek appropriate education and practice settings that allow them to find satisfaction in nursing. Many have found their place in long-term care and community settings where contact with clients and residents is ongoing. Increasing numbers of students are choosing to specialize in the care of the aged because of the possibility of sustained and meaningful relationships.

This chapter examines the foundations of gerontic nursing, the educational needs of gerontic nurses, the developing roles, and supportive interactions. Historically, nurses have always been in the frontlines caring for the aged. They have provided hands-on care, supervision, administration, program development, teaching, and research and are, to a great extent, responsible for the rapid advance of gerontology as a profession.

GERONTOLOGIC NURSING AND ORGANIZATIONS

To develop accurate and informed attitudes, gerontologic nursing organizations have established standards, legitimized the specialty, upgraded the knowledge base, enhanced the image of gerontologic nurses, and identified the benefits of working with the aged. Nursing is the first of the professions to develop standards of gerontologic care and the first to provide a certification mechanism to ensure specific professional expertise through credentialing. We are proud to be the standard-bearers of excellence in the care of the aged (Box 2-1).

Box 2-1	PROFESSIONALIZATION OF GERONTIC NURSING

1904	First article published in *American Journal of Nursing* (AJN) on care of the aged	1979	*Education for Gerontic Nursing* written by Gunter and Estes; suggested curricula for all levels of nursing education
1925	AJN considers geriatric nursing as a possible specialty in nursing		ANA Council of Long Term Care Nurses established; group first chaired by Ella Kick
1950	Newton and Anderson publish first geriatric nursing textbook	1980	*Geriatric Nursing* first published by *AJN;* Cynthia Kelly, editor
	Geriatrics becomes a specialization in nursing	1981	ANA Division of Gerontological Nursing issues statement regarding scope of practice
1962	ANA forms a national geriatric nursing group	1983	Florence Cellar Endowed Gerontological Nursing Chair established at Case Western Reserve University, first in the nation; Doreen Norton first scholar to occupy chair
1966	ANA creates the Division of Geriatric Nursing		
1970	ANA establishes Standards of Practice for Geriatric Nursing committee, chaired by Dorothy Moses; included Lois Knowles and Mary Shaunnessey		
1973	ANA defined Standards of Practice for Geriatric Nursing	1984	National Gerontological Nurses Association established
1974	Certification in geriatric nursing practice offered through ANA; process implemented by Laurie Gunter and Virginia Stone		Division of Gerontological Nursing Practice becomes Council on Gerontological Nursing (councils established for all practice specialties)
1975	*Journal of Gerontological Nursing* published by Slack; first editor, Edna Stilwell	1986	ANA publishes survey of gerontologic nurses in clinical practice
1976	ANA renames Geriatric Division: "Gerontological"	1987	ANA revises and issues Standards and Scope of Gerontological Nursing Practice
	ANA publishes Standards for Gerontological Nursing Practice; committee chaired by Barbara Allen Davis	1989	ANA certifies gerontologic clinical nurse specialists
	ANA begins certifying geriatric nurse practitioners	1990	ANA establishes a Division of Long Term Care within the Council of Gerontological Nursing
	Nursing and the Aged edited by Burnside and published by McGraw-Hill	1992	ANA redefines long term care to include life-span approach
1977	First gerontologic nursing track funded by Division of Nursing and established by Sr. Rose Therese Bahr at University of Kansas School of Nursing	1993	National Institute of Nursing Research established as separate entity
		1994	ANA redefines Standards and Scope of Gerontological Nursing Practice

ANA and the Geriatric Standards of Practice

In 1973 the American Nurses Association (ANA) first defined standards of geriatric care. In 1976 and 1987 these were redefined as standards of gerontologic nursing practice.

In 1994 the ANA updated the scope of gerontologic nursing practice, which now focuses on "assessing the health and functional status of aging adults, planning and providing appropriate nursing and other health care services, and evaluating the effectiveness of such care" (American Nurses Association, 1995). The ANA standards further emphasize health, dignity, and comfort as the undergirding goals of all care of the elderly. The current standards of practice address the following:

- The ramifications of the aging process
- The different rates at which people age
- The multiplicity and collectiveness of an older person's losses
- The grief work necessary in accepting losses
- The interrelationship among the social, economic, psychologic, and biologic factors
- The frequently atypical response of the aged to disease and to the treatment of disease
- The accumulated disabling effects of multiple chronic illnesses and/or degenerative processes

Although most working nurses (more than 2 million employed nurses) (US Bureau of the Census, 1998) are involved in the care of the aged in some manner, only slightly more than 15,000 gerontologic nurses are certified by the ANA. In addition, several thousand advance practice nurses specializing in the care of the aged are certified as Geriatric Nurse Practitioners, Adult Nurse Practitioners, Family Nurse Practitioners, and Geriatric Clinical Nurse Specialists. Certification is the beginning step toward expertise, recognition, and satisfaction in the field.

Certification

Certification is a means of ensuring the public that the certified individual has pursued some specialized study in a given area, has successfully demonstrated requisite knowledge, and has been awarded recognition of this achievement. However, certificates of achievement are variable and there is little consistency in quality or meaning.

ANA certification in gerontologic nursing is one evidence of professional competency and a sign to health care administrators of a commitment by nurses to the care of older adults (Gaines, 1994). The certification program for gerontic nurses began in 1975. The original protocol has since been expanded to include nurse practitioners, clinical specialists, geriatric consultants, researchers, administrators, and educators. In October 1989 the first ANA examination for certification of gerontologic nurse clinical specialists was given. This was a major step toward recognition of this specialized practice arena. Approximately 15,000 geriatric generalists, 3500 gerontologic nurse practitioners, and 900 geriatric clinical nurse specialists are certified. For additional information on certification and specialty practice contact, see Resources at the end of this chapter.

Graduate nursing programs in gerontology prepare nurses to be credentialed as the following:
1. Geriatric nurse practitioners
2. Gerontologic nurse clinical specialists
3. Geriatric case managers for acute and long-term care
4. Nurse administrators in acute and long-term care
5. Gerontologic faculty and staff development roles
6. Geropsychiatric specialists

Canadian Gerontologic Nurses Association

Our neighbors, the Canadian Gerontologic Nurses Association (CGNA), have grown enormously in strength and purpose in recent years. Although the percentage of their elder population in most provinces is somewhat less than ours, the social services and functional aids provide (at no cost to those over 65 years of age) a model toward which we may strive. In addition, more than one half of their members are certified by the Canadian Nurses Association (CNA).

The seven standards and criteria of CGNA are as follows (Canadian Gerontological Nursing Association, 1987):
1. Respect for the uniqueness of each older person
2. Promotion of function and maximum independence
3. Assistance toward environmental mastery
4. Practice based on the specific and evolving knowledge of aging
5. Emphasis on sustaining interpersonal relationships
6. Advocacy on behalf of the rights and responsibilities of elders
7. The application of nursing process

National Gerontological Nursing Association

The National Gerontological Nursing Association (NGNA), organized in 1984, is the first and only national association created specifically for all levels of nurses specializing in the delivery of health care to the elderly. This nonprofit association comprises registered nurses (RNs), licensed practical nurses/licensed vocational nurses (LPNs/ LVNs), and certified nurse assistants (CNAs); however, the great majority of the nearly 2000 members are RNs. The functions of the NGNA are listed in Box 2-2.

NGNA has recently demonstrated its commitment to gerontologic nursing growth and elder care by completing a Delphi study that encompassed critical issues, problems, future directions, and priorities of gerontologic nursing. The results indicated major concerns regarding insufficient emphasis on gerontology in nursing curricula, too few well-prepared and enthusiastic faculty, uncertainty of federal legislative supports for elder care, and too little emphasis on health and wellness (Luggen, 1997).

National Conference of Gerontological Nurse Practitioners

The National Conference of Gerontological Nurse Practitioners (NCGNP) is an organization devoted solely to the promotion of high standards of health care for older persons through advanced gerontologic nursing practice (AGNP), education, and research. Its goals are to further opportunities for advanced nursing practice through continuing education of professionals and consumers.

National Association of Directors of Nursing Administration in Long-Term Care

The National Association of Directors of Nursing Administration in Long-Term Care (NADONA/LTC) specifically addresses the concerns of directors of nursing (DONs). Their mission is to build a strong network of DONs and assistant DONs through education, communication, and service to the members.

Gerontological Society of America and American Society on Aging

The Gerontological Society of America (GSA) and the American Society on Aging (ASA) are interdisciplinary organizations devoted to the development and promotion of progress in research and service to the aged. Both of these organizations have large contingents of nurse members. Nurses form the largest group of professionals belonging to GSA.

Long-term care nurses are particularly active in two other national organizations, the American Association of Homes and Services for the Aging (AAHSA) and the American Health Care Association (AHCA) (see Organizations at the end of this chapter for addresses). These organizations are highly visible in promoting legislation to strengthen the stature and practice opportunities in long-term care in numerous venues.

STAFF DEVELOPMENT

Staff development is an increasingly important part of the responsibility of every professional nurse. Equipment requirements, regulations, acuity level of clients, and expectations from the public change daily. Each health care organization should form a "vision statement" (philosophy) that becomes the framework to guide leadership and management in that particularly unique setting (Rodriguez, 1996). Within the parameters of the vision statement, specific objectives and programs should be written, prioritized, and periodically evaluated. An example of a philosophy statement is shown in Box 2-3. From that are derived the responsibilities of the Director of Staff Development. A model of these is shown in Table 2-1. For a detailed explanation, worksheets, and requirements of the staff development role, we recommend the *Manual of Staff Development,* listed in the Resources at the end of this chapter.

| Box 2-2 | NGNA FUNCTIONS |

- Provide a forum for identifying and exploring gerontologic nursing issues
- Sponsor and conduct lectures, seminars, debates, and similar educational programs for gerontology nurses, health care providers, and the general public
- Disseminate information and research results related to gerontologic nursing
- Promote activities designed to educate and inform the general public about health care issues with emphasis on those issues affecting the elderly
- Formulate programs designed to demonstrate innovative techniques and approaches in gerontologic health care to enable nurses and others to better meet the needs of America's aging population
- Advocate for elders for gerontologic health care through public policy and governmental involvement

Box 2-3   PHILOSOPHY STATEMENT EXAMPLE

Philosophy Statement

Camino Healthcare System Education Department

We, the Education Department of the Camino Healthcare System, believe in providing education and training for staff and patients. In order to do this:

- We acknowledge the rapidly changing health care environment that demands a balance between financial responsibility and caring and compassion for human beings.
- We recognize that cost-effective education, training, and development goals must be achieved and results measured.
- We believe that lifelong learning is a dynamic process, the responsibility of every individual, and is increasingly important in this rapidly changing environment.
- We possess the combined ability, talent, expertise, and creativity to meet the many challenges of this environment.

We will utilize these to serve employees and health care consumers while being guided by the strategic goals of the organization. We believe that adults learn through participation and in many different ways. The learner is accountable for seeking, acquiring, retaining, and reinforcing the knowledge and skills needed to function as a competent individual.

We are accountable to ourselves, our professions, our customers, the organization, and to the community. We intend to provide opportunities and resources for learning and development and intend to do this by collaborating with individuals to meet their learning needs. We are committed to the mission and the success of the organization.

From Rodriguez L et al: *Manual of staff development,* St Louis, 1996, Mosby.

Certified Nursing Assistants and Nurse Aides

Although it is necessary to promote professional nursing regarding institutionalized elders, most of their care and quality of life directly depend on CNAs or nurse aides. Geriatric nursing, to be satisfying for the professional and adequate for the patient, must begin at the bottom of the status ladder and work upward. When the aides are satisfied and feel truly appreciated, it is reflected in the professionalism of the entire service milieu. But, who is their advocate? Who is concerned about the quality of their lives? Who listens to the aide's story? Who provides a time and place for mourning the loss of loved residents? Who provides health care for those aides as they give health care services to elders? Until we health care professionals and our society make a real commitment to providing adequate wages and individual supports, both psychologic and material, these neglected workers cannot be expected to have the energy or incentive to extend to elders in their care. Regardless of our credentials, our success as professionals in geriatric nursing will depend largely on how effectively we interact with these frontline workers.

Ragland (1997) has produced a book, *Instant Teaching Treasures for Patient Education,* which is stimulating and enjoyable. These "instant patient teaching treasures" are adaptable and can be used to teach aides as well as patients. Examples of these are shown in "Caregiver Storm Warning" and "'Hats Off' to the Caregiver" (Figs. 2-1 and 2-2). We highly recommend these for fun and creative learning (see Resources at the end of this chapter). In tandem with these is *The Long-Term Care Nursing Assistant Training Manual* (Anderson et al, 1996), which provides detailed instructions with graphic illustrations of all the nursing activities an LPN/LVN or aide may be called on to perform. These would be useful also for all beginning nursing students.

Performance Evaluations

One of the most neglected areas of staff communication is that of performance evaluations. These may be a time of growth and inspiration or, too frequently, create an atmosphere of antagonism. The Joint Commission on Accreditation of Healthcare Organizations (JCAHO) has prepared a summary of Definitions of Dimensions of Performance (Box 2-4, p. 22). This is a particularly useful list of client-focused activities by which an employee could evaluate self and discuss areas where improvement may be desirable. The important elements are self-evaluation and the opportunity for discussing this in an open and responsive interaction.

Staff Support Groups

Group support activities can and should be built into the structure of the workday. These provide an opportunity for developing support without the necessity of intimate sharing or confrontation. They may begin by focusing on one specific goal for each meeting. Goals for employee groups include any of the following:

1. Increased functional levels
2. Environmental enrichment

Table 2-1

The Responsibilities of the Director of Staff Development*

Areas of responsibility	Focus for staff development
Strategic management	Design, implement, and influence the staff development direction. Develop goals congruent with the organization and nursing's strategic direction and needs.
Professional practice	Create an environment to promote excellence in education and clinical practice. Define and evaluate competencies of staff developers. Contribute to professional and scholarly nursing and educational activities including speaking and publishing.
Patient care management	Assist with development, implementation, and evaluation/revision of patient care standards. Provide educational programs in response to practice needs, organizational changes, and new program/products.
Quality management	Assist with continuous quality improvement projects including training of teams. Design educational programs in response to quality improvement needs.
Research	Create an environment supportive to critiquing, using, and participating in research. Use current professional educational research in practice and in teaching.
Human resources management	Create an environment for innovation, creativity, and empowerment. Support the self/peer assessment of staff development needs and growth opportunities. Collaborate in providing education to achieve competence.
Financial management	Plan and forecast financial needs (both operation and capital) and effectively manage the staff development budget. Implement cost containment and revenue generating programs. Facilitate budget/financial workshops for managers and staff.
Professional development	Provide courses in professional development, critical thinking, publishing, speaking, and lobbying for professional development. Contribute to the profession, community activities, and schools of health care professionals through outreach programs.

From Rodriguez L et al: *Manual of staff development,* St Louis, 1996, Mosby.
*Based on model by Organization of Nurse Executives of California, 1991.

3. Motivational strategies
4. Behavioral management
5. Staff morale
6. Autonomy

Needs Assessment

We advise organizing staff groups to meet needs at any level of Maslow's hierarchy. Even though most groups meet multiple needs, a primary focus should be established. Using the assessment of human needs as basic guides, one can begin to determine the type of group most suitable in a given situation. What is the primary need in the particular facility at that particular time? First, on the most basic level, the survival needs of staff, such as health care and child care, must be adequately met. Problem solving around these issues may be the major goal, in which each member shares methods he or she uses to meet survival needs. Some facilities, because of purchasing in large quantities, pass savings on to personnel, allowing them to purchase food and other items at cost. Many facilities now offer some assistance with child care.

CAREGIVER STORM WARNING

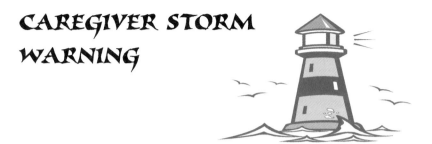

Directions: Answer the following questions by marking the best answer in the columns to the right.

	Always	Sometimes	Never	Rarely
1. I am the only person in the world in this situation.				
2. Nothing I do is ever enough.				
3. I feel all alone.				
4. I always seem to be exhausted.				
5. I resent my present situation.				
6. Caregiving responsibilities are now interfering with my work/social life.				
7. I never have a chance to be alone.				
8. I never get time just for me.				
9. I'm overeating.				
10. I never think of myself; that would be selfish.				
11. I no longer feel good about myself.				
12. There are no more happy times.				

Fig. 2-1 "Caregiver Storm Warning." (From Ragland G: *Instant teaching treasures for patient education,* St Louis, 1997, Mosby.)

At the second level, job security is fundamental. Informal or legal contracts should be supplied for every worker, regardless of status in the hierarchy of help. The contract should go beyond the standard job description to include the goals and expectations of the employee as well as those of the organization. The activity of negotiating these contracts not only provides a sense of security but simultaneously raises the employees' self-esteem and sense of autonomy.

On the third level of the hierarchy, the sense of belonging can be cultivated in any group in which the leader focuses on commonalities rather than differences. What are the common gripes of the group? What are the satisfactions experienced in the work environment?

Self-esteem, the fourth level of Maslow's hierarchy, is built when specific contributions of an employee are recognized by the group and when each feels his or her participation is recognized and deemed important. The pinnacle of Maslow's hierarchy of needs is in reaching for self-actualization and transcendence. This is a lifelong pursuit and one each individual identifies in his or

"HATS OFF" TO THE CAREGIVER

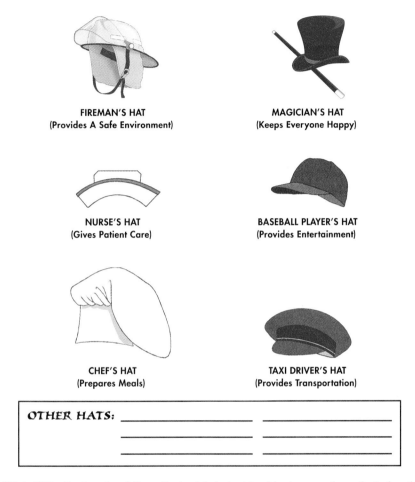

FIREMAN'S HAT
(Provides A Safe Environment)

MAGICIAN'S HAT
(Keeps Everyone Happy)

NURSE'S HAT
(Gives Patient Care)

BASEBALL PLAYER'S HAT
(Provides Entertainment)

CHEF'S HAT
(Prepares Meals)

TAXI DRIVER'S HAT
(Provides Transportation)

OTHER HATS: _____ _____
_____ _____
_____ _____

Fig. 2-2   "'Hats Off' to the Caregiver." (From Ragland G: *Instant teaching treasures for patient education,* St Louis, 1997, Mosby.)

her own creative manner. It is often enlightening to ask members to share experiences of deep personal significance that have occurred in the care of a resident.

Informal Groups

Informal groups are those that naturally arise and have restrictions, expectations, or goals. Small groups of staff who cluster together in long-term care or residential settings may be encouraged and supported by augmenting these spontaneous groups to form the core of working groups.

Formal Groups

Formal groups are defined by their expectations, dependability, and goals. The intensity of interpersonal exchange varies in accordance with the members' and group's goals. The group should maintain its goals and function despite variation in membership.

Focus Groups

Focus groups have been used successfully in many organizations to thoroughly explore various perceptions and solutions around specific issues. These are not casual exchanges but, rather, require prior preparation of all participants, ideally selected to represent an array of concerned or interested parties. Kerschner (1998) suggests certain steps to conducting a productive focus group. The first essential step is selecting a facilitator who is an effective communicator, has a sense of humor, and is interested in others' opinions. The facilitator should get to know each participant and reinforce the importance of each one's opinion. It is useful to give each participant a printed copy of established rules. These rules include the order of responses, how each will be addressed, and how they will be recorded. Each participant is expected to be prepared to focus on the material that was given before the meeting and to express clearly and concisely an opinion concerning it. Much information is available regarding the use of focus groups. The significant elements are the orderliness of the process and respect for each participant, regardless of position.

The following are some guidelines for evaluating the success of a group:

1. *Evaluation of goal accomplishment.* How were goals established and by whom? Did positive results occur that were not expected? What were they? Identify portions of goal accomplished, serendipity, group progress toward goals, and modification of goals as necessary when planning for next meeting.
2. *Process.* What was the mood of the group at the beginning? Were effects present of unusual events in the setting, in the community, or in the nation? Were there a significant number of deaths, accidents, staffing changes, upset in ward or agency routines, or new people in setting?
3. *Themes.* What were the major themes expressed in group: ineffectiveness, lethargy, anger, overload, satisfaction, accomplishment?
4. *Problems expressed.* How were they handled? Was the approach effective? Who contributed to problem solving?

Box 2-4   DEFINITIONS OF DIMENSIONS OF PERFORMANCE

Doing the Right Thing

- The efficacy of the procedure or treatment in relation to the patient's condition
- The degree to which the care or service for the patient has been shown to accomplish the desired or projected outcome(s)
- The appropriateness of a specific test, procedure, or service to meet the patient's needs
- The degree to which the care provided is relevant to the patient's clinical needs, given the current state of knowledge

Doing the Right Thing Well

- The availability of a needed test, procedure, treatment, or service to the patient who needs it
- The degree to which appropriate care is available to meet the patient's needs
- The timeliness with which a needed test, procedure, treatment, or service is provided to the patient
- The degree to which the care is provided to the patient at the most beneficial or necessary time
- The effectiveness with which tests, procedures, treatments, and services are provided

- The degree to which the care is provided in the correct manner, given the current state of knowledge, to achieve the desired or projected outcome for the patient
- The continuity of the services provided over time to the patient with respect to other services, clinicians, and providers
- The degree to which the care of the patient is coordinated among services, among organizations, and across time
- The safety of the patient (and others) to whom the services are provided
- The degree to which the risk of an intervention and risk in the care environment are reduced for the patient and others, including the staff members
- The efficacy with which services are provided
- The relationship between the outcomes (results of care) and the resources used to deliver patient care
- The respect and caring with which services are provided
- The degree to which the patient or a designee is involved in his or her own care decisions and to which those providing services do so with sensitivity and respect for the patient's needs, expectations, and individual differences

From Joint Commission on Accreditation of Healthcare Organizations: *1995 Accreditation manual for home care,* vol 1, *Standards,* Oakbrook Terrace, Ill, 1994, The Commission.

This brief discussion of possible groups and effects shows the versatility and potential of group work with employees and the potential it holds for strengthening bonds in the work environment.

Mentoring for Professional Growth and Development

In gerontologic nursing, mentoring has played a predominant role. The field is comparatively new, and many nursing programs do not have strong courses in gerontology or certified faculty geriatric specialists. Many individuals entered the field of aging without any particular professional preparation but have been individually guided toward professional competence by the efforts and inspiration of a dedicated mentor. The numerous needs of the aged and the special nature of their care require the most devoted and sophisticated nurses.

ROLES IN GERIATRIC NURSING

A geriatric nurse may be a generalist or a specialist. The generalist functions in a variety of settings—hospital, home, community—providing nursing care to individuals and their families. The generalist works in various models of care provision and draws on the expertise of the specialist in planning and evaluating care (Box 2-5).

The geriatric specialist has advanced preparation and performs all of the functions of the generalist but has additional education and developed clinical expertise, as well as an understanding of health and social policy and

---

Box 2-5	**ACUTE CARE MODEL 2—HOPE (HOSPITAL OUTCOMES PROJECT FOR THE ELDERLY)**

A cluster of five models that focus primarily on nursing care.

Geriatric Resource Nurse (GRN)—Integrating Expertise

A team composed of primary nurses, trained geriatric resource nurse, gerontologic nurse specialist, and geriatric physicians helps staff with specific problems of the elderly, such as delirium, physical functioning, incontinence, etc.

Implemented nationally. Originated in New England area, 1980s.

Acute Care of the Elderly (ACE)—Designed Environments

A 29-bed specialty unit designed for acutely ill older patients with attention to physical needs of older patients; appropriate colors, carpeting, art, music, activity room, and recliners in patient rooms.

Team of nurses, gerontologic nurse specialist, social workers, nutritionists, and physical therapist to prevent functional decline and multiple clinical problems.

Developed by University Hospitals of Cleveland conjointly with Frances Payne Bolton School of Nursing at Case Western Reserve University. An innovative though expensive model that has demonstrated rapid implementation, which is accomplished easily because of the interdisciplinary team.

Geriatric Nurse Specialist (GNS)—Targeting Common Problems

Clinical specialist who consults and educates staff about specific problems of the aged. NICHE project used this inexpensive way to focus on nursing care and issues of delirium.

Developed by University of Chicago hospitals. Disadvantage: immediate access to GNS not available.

Comprehensive Discharge Planning (CDP)—Planning Ahead

Focus of GNS is on high-risk older patients and caregivers. Assessment occurs at admission and every 48 hours thereafter. Available to family members and patients 7 days a week. Continuity of care continues after discharge.

Developed by University of Pennsylvania Hospital for continuity of care while minimizing readmissions. Findings concur success; extended time between discharge and readmission.

Case Management—Multidisciplinary Approach

A multidisciplinary case management model for patients with complex conditions, high acuity, and increased potential for complications, noncompliance, and absence of a support system.

Developed at Beth Israel Medical Center, New York.

Compiled from Strumpf NE: Innovative gerontological practices as models for health care delivery, *Nurs Health Care* 15(10):522, 1994; NICHE Project Faculty: Geriatric models of care: which one's right for your institution? *Am J Nurs* 94(7):21, 1994.

proficiency in planning, implementing, and evaluating health programs. To understand the variations of these categories and the progression of specialization see Fig. 2-3. Table 2-2 shows the organization of nursing relating to care of the elderly (Mezey, Fulmer, 1995).

Geriatric Nurse Practitioner

One of the most important roles emerging in the past few decades is that of the geriatric nurse practitioner. Originally the development of the gerontologic or geriatric nurse practitioner (GNP) emerged to meet the

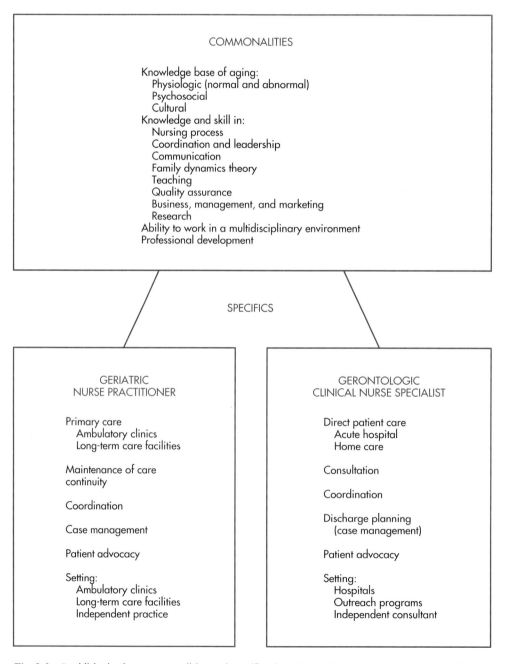

Fig. 2-3   Established roles: commonalities and specifics. (Developed by Patricia Hess and Helen Monea.)

need for consistent, accessible, quality primary care for persons in underserved areas such as nursing homes or remote rural areas. Today, with increasingly strong federal legislation to support advanced nursing practice, GNPs and geriatric clinical specialists are involved in nursing homes, acute care and subacute care facilities, retirement complexes, health maintenance organizations (HMOs), day care settings, community clinics, physicians' offices, independent practices, and in any situation requiring expert nursing in combination with midlevel medical practitioner skills. There are presently a full range of opportunities and roles to be filled.

GERIATRIC NURSING EDUCATION

It was recommended that by the year 2000 all undergraduate nursing programs should have a separate geriatric nursing course, all basic nursing programs should contain core content in gerontologic nursing, and accreditation should be contingent on meeting this re-

quirement. Content issues that are sorely neglected and need to be included are mental health, elder abuse, acute care of the aged, long-term care, and minority and rural aging (Klein, 1995). NGNA members, guided by Ann Luggen, have produced an extensive and detailed core curriculum for gerontologic nursing (Luggen, 1996). This provides sufficient information for the development of nursing courses at any level and in any program. A specialty in geriatrics in master's programs and a geriatric minor in other advanced programs should be available also.

We believe those in the field of nursing education must seriously consider specific minimum requirements at each level of education to fulfill the responsibility of nurses to the public and the profession. One is not limited in geriatric education to the acute care setting or the nursing home for clinical practice sites. Creative faculty consider sites such as retirement homes, private practice with families, nutrition centers, home care agencies, day care centers, and housing complexes. Learning in these sites to understand the living situations and truly communicate with elders is the first

Table 2-2

Organization of Nursing Relating to Care of the Elderly

Title	No. years education	Degree	Responsibilities related to care of the elderly
Professors of geriatric nursing	8 plus	PhD, Ed D, or DNS	Research Teaching
Geriatric nurse practitioners	6	MS	Both medical and nursing functions in ambulatory and institutional settings Case managers
Gerontologic nurse specialists	6	MS	Specialized nursing care of elderly clients Teachers and role models Case managers
Registered nurse—baccalaureate level	4-5	BS	Community health, hospital, home health agencies, nursing homes Case managers
Registered nurse—associate level	2-3	ADN	Hospital and nursing home staff nurses
Licensed practical nurses	1-1½		Nursing home staff Home nursing staff
Nursing aides and orderlies	0-6 mo		Nursing home staff Hospital staff

From Mezey MD, Fulmer TT: Nursing. In Maddox GL, editor: *The encyclopedia of aging,* ed 2, New York, 1995, Springer. Sources: U.S. Bureau of the Census: *Statistical abstract of the United States,* 1998, ed 118, Washington, DC, US Government Printing Office; American Nurses Association: *Facts about nursing,* Kansas City, Mo, 1992-1993, ANA, pp 1-4.

step to providing appropriate care. Acute care hospitals and nursing homes are integral to the total picture but might be included later in the students' learning experience after they have worked with elders who have less acute or complex conditions. Nursing homes provide special opportunities for leadership training and research application for more advanced students (Matzo, 1994; Sears, Wilson, 1996).

GERIATRIC NURSES CARING FOR EACH OTHER

Nurses derive their interpersonal satisfactions from co-workers, residents, and professional organizations. Ongoing knowledge should be readily available and is integral to an encouraging work milieu. Throughout this chapter our intent is to convey the importance of nurses working together and caring for each other as we care for the aged. We share in some of the most moving and profound life events. These cannot be taken lightly or held quietly and comfortably inside. In these situations, the close ties with co-workers and elders become especially significant. Opportunities to recognize and share the significance of these connections should be conscientiously developed. Only as nurses value and care for each other and feel valued can we reach out whole-heartedly and fully appreciate the elders in our care.

▶ KEY CONCEPTS

- Certification assures the public of nurses' commitment to specialized education and qualification for the care of the aged.
- Nursing programs should show solid evidence of geriatric content as a requirement for accreditation.
- The major changes in health care delivery have resulted in numerous revised, refined, and emergent roles for nurses in the field of gerontology.
- Advanced practice nurses have either nurse practitioner qualifications or clinical nurse specialist education.
- Advanced practice role opportunities for nurses are numerous and offer more independence, are cost effective, and facilitate more holistic health care.
- Gerontic nursing at its best requires specialized education, maturity, commitment, and sensitivity.

▶ Activities and Discussion Questions

1. Consider and discuss with classmates the various gerontic nursing roles that you find most interesting and stimulating.
2. Discuss what you consider the most important elements of the most recent American Nurses Association Standards of Practice for Gerontological Nursing.
3. Discuss the formal geriatric organizations and their significance to the practicing nurse.
4. Identify and discuss the working relationships that have had the most significance for you.
5. Identify factors that have influenced the progress of gerontologic nursing as a specialty practice.
6. What do you think are the most important issues in geriatric nursing education at this time?

RESOURCES
Publications
Manual of Staff Development
   Rodriguez L et al
   St Louis, 1996, Mosby, ISBN 0-8016-6609-0
Instant Teaching Treasures for Patient Education
   Ragland G
   St Louis, 1997, Mosby, ISBN 0-8151-4699-X
The Long-Term Care Nursing Assistant Training Manual, ed 2
   Anderson MA, Beaver KW, Culliton KR
   Baltimore, 1996, Health Professions Press, ISBN 1-878812-28-9

Organizations
American Association of Homes and Services for the Aging
   901 E Street NW, Suite 500
   Washington, DC 20004-2037
   (301) 490-0677
National League for Nursing (NLN)
   Accreditation Board
   10 Columbus Circle
   New York, NY 10019
American Health Care Association
   1201 L Street NW
   Washington, DC 20005
   (202) 842-8444
American Nurses Association (ANA)
   Accreditation Board
   600 Maryland Avenue SW, Suite 100 W
   Washington DC 20024-2571
   (202) 554-4444
American Nurses' Credentialing Center
   600 Maryland Avenue SW, Suite 100 W
   Washington, DC 20024-2571
   (800) 284-CERT

American Society on Aging
   833 Market Street, Suite 511
   San Francisco, CA 94103-1824
   (415) 974-9600
Canadian Gerontological Nursing Association
   PO Box 368, Postal Station K
   Toronto, Ontario M4P 2GT
Gerontological Society of America
   1275 K Street NW, Suite 350
   Washington, DC 20005-4006
   (202) 842-1275
National Gerontological Nursing Association (NGNA) Puetz Enterprises
   7794 Grow Drive
   Pensacola, FL 32514-7072
   (800) 723-0560; (850) 484-8762 (fax)
Because of the rapid development of numerous graduate, undergraduate, and certificate programs in gerontic nursing throughout the United States, it is advisable to contact the accrediting bodies directly for current information. Information regarding certificate and degree programs (undergraduate and graduate) in gerontology, standards, guidelines, and program directories are available.

REFERENCES

American Nurses Association: *Scope and standards of gerontological nursing practice,* Washington, DC, 1995, The Association.

Anderson MA, Beaver KW, Culliton KR: *The long-term care nursing assistant training manual,* ed 2, Baltimore, 1996, Health Professions Press.

Canadian Gerontological Nursing Association, Toronto, Ontario, 1987.

Gaines JE: Here comes everybody in APN, *Advanced Practice Nurse,* Spring/Summer, p 42, 1994.

Kerschner H: Ten easy steps to conducting focus group research, *Aging Today* 19(6):7, 1998.

Klein S: *A national agenda for geriatric education: white papers,* Washington, DC, 1995, US Department of Health and Human Services, Public Health Service, Health Resources and Services Administration, Bureau of Health Professions.

Luggen AS, editor: *Core curriculum for gerontologic nursing,* St Louis, 1996, Mosby.

Luggen AS: NGNA's strategic plan, *Geriatr Nurs* 18(1):33, 1997.

Matzo M: Baccalaureate nursing students as research clinicians in long-term care, *Geriatr Nurs* 15:250, 1994.

Mezey MD, Fulmer TT: Nursing. In Maddox Gl, editor: *The encyclopedia of aging,* New York, 1995, Springer.

Parse RR: *The human becoming school of thought: a perspective for nurses and other health professionals,* Thousand Oaks, Calif, 1998, Sage.

Ragland G: *Instant teaching treasures for patient education,* St Louis, 1997, Mosby.

Rodriguez L et al: *Manual of staff development,* St Louis, 1996, Mosby.

Sears LE, Wilson CS: Leadership experience in gerontological nursing for associate degree students in long-term care, *Geriatr Nurs* 17:128, 1996.

US Bureau of the Census: *Statistical abstract of the United States, 1998,* ed 118, Washington, DC, 1998, The Bureau.

3

Communicating With Elders

Upon completion of this chapter, the reader will be able to:

• Relate interventions that facilitate communication individually and in groups.
• Discuss various methods of communicating with distressed elders.
• Specify several teaching/learning strategies to facilitate elders' understanding and goal accomplishment.
• Identify several communication needs and goals for elders who have special communication problems.
• Describe ways to communicate with the hearing impaired.

▶GLOSSARY

Anomia An inability to name objects; a form of aphasia caused by a lesion in the temporal lobe of the brain.

Aphasia A neurologic condition in which language function is defective or absent because of injury to certain areas of the brain.

Apraxia An impairment in the ability to manipulate objects or perform purposeful acts.

Ataxia An inability to coordinate movement, which results in abnormal gait and staggering.

Catastrophic reaction Uncoordinated response to stressful situation beyond one's coping capacity.

Constrained Stiff, unnatural, or uneasy actions.

Dysarthria Poorly articulated speech resulting from interference with the speech mechanism.

Flaccidity Weak, soft, flabby; lacking normal muscle tone.

Hyperkinesia Abnormally reactive motor responses.

Hypokinesia Abnormally diminished motor activity.

Idiom Language peculiar to a particular person, group, or class of people.

Infarction A localized area of tissue death resulting from an interruption of the blood supply.

Phonation The production of speech through the vibration of the vocal cords.

Presbycusis Loss of hearing sensitivity related to the aging neurosensory system.

Prophylactic An agent or action that prevents the occurrence of disease and disorders.

Resonance A sound emitted by an item or organ vibrating to a particular compatible energy frequency.

▶THE LIVED EXPERIENCE

It is so terrible. For a whole year I haven't been able to tell anyone how I feel, how afraid I am of another stroke. My family talks around me and about me as if I'm not alive. I am alive, and I must be understood! They just don't have any idea that I can understand but simply can't get the words out.

Andy, after stroke

He always seems so angry, sputtering and spitting, and I just don't know what he wants. Sometimes I feel it is just hopeless. If I don't know what he wants and he can't tell me, I guess it is best just to let him alone and maybe he won't be so angry.

Andy's caregiver

COMMUNICATION WITH ELDERS

Genuine communication with elders has profound effects on caregivers as we develop a close-up view of aging with all its changes. It can be both threatening and a time of discovery if there is an open exchange of thoughts and feeling. Stephanie Nagley says, "Nursing care of the aged brings one in touch with the most basic and profound questions of human existence: the meanings of life and death; sources of strength and survival skills; and beginnings, endings, and reasons for being. It is a commitment to discovery of the self—and of the self I am becoming as I age" (Nagley, 1988). The very old are acutely aware of their limited time and, given the opportunity, generally are willing to talk about it and the problems they experience, as well as their satisfactions.

Basic communication strategies that apply to all situations in nursing, such as attending, listening, clarifying, giving information, seeking validation of understanding, keeping focus, and using open-ended questions, are all applicable in communicating with the aged. Some situational modifications must be considered, as well as some special circumstances. A discussion of the common problems, disorders, and impediments to communication that older adults often experience is the focus of this chapter. Communication with those experiencing mental health disorders is addressed in Chapter 25.

Basically, elders may need more time to give information or answer questions, simply because they have a larger life experience to draw from. Sorting through thoughts requires intervals of silence, and therefore listening carefully without rushing the elder is very important. Word retrieval may be slower, particularly for nouns and names. This is thought to relate to age-associated memory impairment (AAMI), which is discussed in Chapter 8. If you are sure of the word the individual is searching for, it may be helpful to supply it after waiting a few moments.

Thoughts unstated are often as important as those that are verbalized. You may ask, "What are you thinking about right now?" Clarification is essential to ensure that you and the elder have the same framework of understanding. Many generational and regional differences in speech patterns and idioms exist. Frequently seek validation of whatever you think you heard.

Open-ended questions are useful but difficult for some elders. Those who wish to please, especially when feeling vulnerable or somewhat dependent, may wonder what it is you want to hear rather than what it is they would like to say. When using closed questioning to obtain specific information, be aware that the elder may feel on the spot and the appropriate information may not be immediately forthcoming. This is especially true when asking questions to determine mental status. The elder may develop a mental block because of anxiety or become angry if questions are asked in a quizzing or demeaning manner. And, finally, communicate with the elder as with a potential friend; share a bit of your own perceptions, thoughts, and experience when it will facilitate mutual understanding and increase rapport. Benefits from verbalization of problems may be minimal if the caregiver maintains distance based on age or a patronizing attitude.

Communication that is most productive will initially focus on the issue of major concern to the elder, regardless of nursing priority assessments. Nursing interventions should include verbal anticipatory rehearsal of any event expected to be stressful. The identification of a reliable and ongoing support system that will be available to the individual before and after any especially demanding event is essential. In addition, options and alternatives related to the particular adjustment should be thoroughly discussed and considered. This will reduce the sense of helplessness and irreversibility.

Communication is the single most important capacity of human beings—the ability that gives us a special place in the animal kingdom. Little is more dehumanizing than the inability to reach out to others verbally. The following section of the chapter addresses neurologic disorders that impair the ability to verbalize in meaningful ways.

LANGUAGE DISORDERS ASSOCIATED WITH NEUROLOGIC DISRUPTIONS

Three major categories of impaired verbal communication arise from neurologic disturbances: (1) reception, (2) perception, and (3) articulation. Reception is impaired by anxiety related to a specific disorder, hearing deficits, and altered levels of consciousness. Perception is distorted by stroke, dementia, and delirium. Articulation is hampered by mechanical difficulties such as dysarthria, respiratory disease, destruction of the larynx, and cerebral infarction with neuromuscular effects. Specific difficulties include the following:

1. *Anomia.* Word retrieval difficulties during spontaneous speech and naming tasks.
2. *Aphasia.* An acquired impairment of language processes underlying receptive and expressive

modalities caused by damage to areas of the brain that are primarily responsible for language processes.

3. *Dysarthria.* Impairment in the ability to articulate words as the result of damage to the central or peripheral nervous system that affects the speech mechanism.

Difficulty in articulating words or selecting and comprehending appropriate words is caused by neuromotor disturbances that may be transient, longstanding, reversible, or irreversible. Prophylactic, or primary, prevention of these disorders is complex because so many problems can occur; however, much can be done in aggressive speech retraining programs to regain intelligible conversational ability.

Aphasia

The most common language disorder after a stroke is aphasia; it is a significant problem for the elderly. When a cerebrovascular accident damages the dominant half of the brain (left side in right-handed people), some disruption will occur in the "word factory." The two major categories of aphasia are *receptive* and *expressive* (Fig. 3-1). Aphasic persons with receptive problems cannot understand language; it is as if they are in a foreign land. They may recognize objects and their uses. Expressive aphasic patients can understand verbal and written communication but cannot organize concepts into words or meaningful expressions. Broca and

Wernicke areas of the left cerebral cortex are integral to the expression and understanding of language. These lie within the distribution of the left cerebral artery surrounding the sylvian fissure (Fig. 3-2) of the brain. Following are several types of aphasia that the nurse may encounter with elderly persons:

- *Wernicke* aphasia is the result of a lesion in the superior temporal gyrus. Wernicke area lies adjacent to the primary auditory cortex. Persons with Wernicke aphasia speak easily but in a repetitive jargon that is poorly understood. Unrelated words may be strung together or syllables repeated. These persons also have difficulty understanding spoken language.
- *Broca* aphasia typically involves damage to the posteroinferior portions of the dominant frontal lobe. Persons with Broca aphasia understand others but speak very slowly and use minimal words. They often struggle to articulate a word and seem to have lost the ability to voluntarily control the movements of speech. This is often called "apraxia of speech."
- *Conductive* aphasics understand speech and may speak fluently but may substitute sounds and words for the ones they wish to use.
- *Anomic* aphasia is associated with lesions of the dominant temporoparietal regions of the brain, although no single locus has been identified. Persons with anomic aphasia understand and speak readily but may have severe word-finding difficulty. They may be unable to remember crucial content words. This is

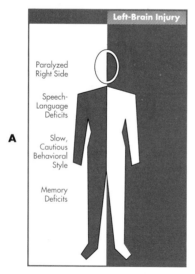
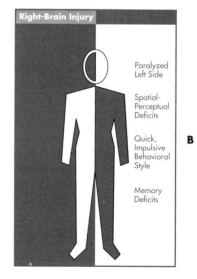

Fig. 3-1   Receptive and expressive aphasia arising from left (**A**) and right (**B**) brain injury. (From American Heart Association: *How stroke affects behavior*, Dallas, 1994, The Association.)

a frequent form of aphasia characterized by the inability to name objects. The individual struggles to come forth with the correct noun and often becomes angry at his or her inability to do so.

• *Global* aphasia is the result of large left hemisphere lesions and affects most of the language areas of the brain. Persons with global aphasia cannot understand words or speak intelligibly. They may use meaningless syllables repetitiously.

The capacities of the right hemisphere include selective attention, visual perceptions, orientation to time and place, and understanding of the subtleties of communication. Behaviors of patients with right hemisphere stroke are often very similar to those diagnosed with dementia and include five major deficits: attention, orientation, perception, retention, and integration. See suggestions in Box 3-1 for communicating with aphasic patients.

Box 3-1   COMMUNICATING WITH APHASIC PATIENTS

• Explain situations, treatments, and anything else that is pertinent to the patient because he or she may understand; the sounds of normal speech tend to be rehabilitative even if the words are not understood. Talk as if the person understands.
• Avoid patronizing and childish phrases.
• The aphasic patient may be especially sensitive to feelings of annoyance; remain calm and patient.
• Speak slowly, ask one question at a time, and wait for a response.

• Ask questions in a way that can be answered with a nod or the blink of an eye; if the patient cannot verbally respond, instruct him or her in nonverbal responses.
• Speak of things familiar and of interest to the patient.
• Use visual cues, objects, pictures, and gestures as well as words.
• Organize the environment to be as predictable as possible.
• Encourage articulation even if words convey no meaning.
• Show interest in the patient as an individual.

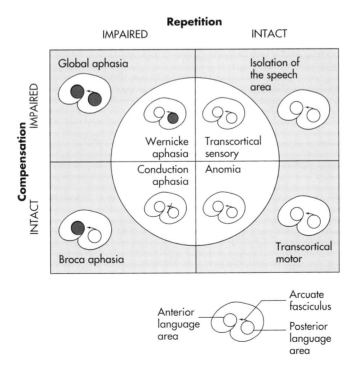

Fig. 3-2 Aphasia diagram: the three components of language function to be tested are comprehension, fluency, and repetition. Aphasias depicted within the circle are the fluent aphasias. (From Gallo JJ, Reichel W, Anderson L: *Handbook of geriatric assessment,* ed 2, Gaithersburg, Md, 1995, Aspen.)

A qualified speech pathologist should be consulted for each type of aphasia to develop appropriate rehabilitative plans as soon as the individual is physiologically stabilized. The speech pathologist can identify the areas of language that remain relatively unimpaired and can capitalize on the remaining strengths. The prognosis for recovery of speech is summarized in Table 3-1.

Nurses are responsible for accurately observing and recording the speech and word recognition patterns of the client and for consistently implementing the recommendations of the speech pathologist. Staff interest is increased when techniques that are being used have audible results.

Communication tools exist for every imaginable type of language disability, and a number of electronic tools are available: electromechanical boards, electronic boards, sentence structure boards, and computer programs. For individuals with hemiplegic or paraplegic conditions, these can be activated by specially designed switches. The following are some types of these switches:
1. *Thumb-depressed switch.* Requires some ability to move thumb.
2. *Minimal pressure switch.* Any finger is sufficient to activate switch.
3. *Photoelectric switch.* A beam of light interrupted by any object will activate switch (tongue, card, finger).
4. *Superminimal pressure switch.* May be touched from any angle at any place along bar; activated by slight contact with ear, nose, chin.
5. *Probe switch.* Designed for a patient who cannot open his or her hand.

To be generally useful, devices must be simply constructed, inexpensive, portable, and connected to a signaling device to attract attention when the individual wishes to communicate.

Dysarthria

Dysarthria is a condition arising from central or peripheral neuromuscular disorders that interfere with the clarity of speech and pronunciation. Dysarthria is second only to aphasia as a communication disorder of the aged and may be the result of neuromuscular flaccidity, spasticity, ataxia, hypokinesia, or hyperkinesia. It may be a mixture of any of these and often will involve several mechanisms of speech, such as respiration, phonation, resonance, articulation, and prosody (the meter, rhythm of speech). Dysarthria is characterized by one or more of the following:
1. Organic voice tremor produces a quavering articulation arising from tremors of the larynx muscles, lips, tongue, and diaphragm.

Table 3-1

Prognostic Variables in Aphasia

Variable	Summary
Age at onset	Younger patients have a better prognosis
Premorbid education, intelligence, and language abilities	Undetermined influence on prognosis
Associated defects and health during recovery	Patients with no associated deficits or illness have a better prognosis
Social milieu	Undetermined influence on prognosis
Cause	Nonpenetrating trauma has a better prognosis than penetrating trauma, vascular accident, tumor, and infection
Size and site of lesion	Small lesions not in temporoparietal area have a better prognosis
Time after onset	Patients with brief duration of aphasia have a better prognosis
Severity and type of aphasia	Mild aphasia and the absence of significant auditory comprehension deficits and severe apraxia of speech are favorable prognostic signs
Nonlanguage behavior	Awareness, high motivation, and high aspiration are favorable prognostic signs
Length and intensity of treatment	Participation in a longer, more intense treatment program is more likely to achieve prognosis

From Ginsberg S: *Prognostic variables in aphasia.* Unpublished paper, Cleveland, 1988, Case Western Reserve University.

2. Transient tremulous articulation; may be the result of tranquilizers, particularly phenothiazines.
3. A slow, unsteady speech pattern may be the result of cerebellar degeneration. In this case the gait also will be halting and wide based.
4. Uncontrolled movement of lips, face, and tongue may be an indication of Parkinson disease. Speech may be slurred and jumpy, the expression flat, and the voice tone monotonous, sometimes hardly audible.
5. Spastic dysarthria is found in 12% of stroke patients. Words are correct, but flow of speech is tight, constrained, and laborious.

To attain or maintain the highest practicable level of speech articulation after an acute episode, such as stroke or surgery, a comprehensive treatment program must be developed by a speech pathologist, neurologist, and physical medicine/rehabilitation therapist. In progressive neurologic disease the treatment begins early and is ongoing as the person is encouraged to maintain speech as long as possible (Lee, Itoh, 1990).

Most important are immediate rehabilitation efforts, as noted in the following episodes:

• A 59-year-old radio broadcaster had a left cerebrovascular accident. As his confusion lifted in the first few days of hospitalization, his nonverbal agony was heartrending. He sputtered meaningless sounds, pounded with his clenched left fist, and cried. His devastation was apparent to everyone who was with him. Fortunately, an active rehabilitation team began working with him immediately, and his progress was rapid.

• However, another situation involved an aged man in a senior center who could speak intelligently 3 years after a cerebrovascular accident. He shared the feelings of agony he experienced for 2 years, before active rehabilitation efforts, when he understood everything going on around him but did not have the capacity to make himself understood. He said for those 2 years he was treated as an imbecile. Finally he was properly evaluated, and his potential for recovering speech was facilitated. The task was arduous, but he was determined. This demonstrates that we must never assume that improvement cannot be made, because we know so little about human potential and motivation.

Laryngectomy

After laryngectomy surgery, the patient has no voice. The three options for the laryngectomy patient are reconstructive surgery, esophageal speech, or an electrolarynx. A pharyngolaryngologist is the appropriate professional to evaluate whether reconstructive surgery is advisable. Some individuals may learn to master esophageal speech, and others may prefer the electrolarynx even though the sound emitted is robotic. All clients should be given the opportunity to communicate with a member of the Lost Chord Club, a self-help group that offers advice and emotional support.

During the initial surgical recovery period the nurse will need to anticipate and articulate the intense feelings the elder can no longer express. The patient cannot even cry audibly. The nurse will need to seek corroboration by nonverbal gestures. The laryngectomee will be best motivated toward speech training by the ongoing verbal involvement of others.

HEARING AND HEARING IMPAIRMENT IN THE OLDER PERSON

Older persons are often unaware of hearing loss because of the gradual manner in which it usually develops. They usually believe others are mumbling and may become irritated at individuals around them who they perceive as not speaking up. Some are aware of a hearing loss and are disturbed by misperceptions and distortions, often imagining derogatory remarks are being said about them. However, knowing that one has a hearing loss is not sufficient. Testing must be done to determine the nature of the loss, how much it interferes with communication, whether it is treatable (as may be the case with metabolic alterations or middle ear structural changes), and whether a hearing aid will be useful. The recent advances in hearing aid technology make it possible to find appropriate hearing aids for some who have not found them satisfactory in the past.

The influences of genetics, noise exposure, cardiovascular status, central processing capacity, systemic disease, certain medications, smoking, diet, personality, and stress have all been implicated to varying degrees in the etiology of hearing impairment.

Older persons with presbycusis have difficulty filtering out background noise. This problem needs attention. Institutions are teeming with distracting sounds: intercoms, clattering equipment, meal and medication carts, vacuum cleaners, elders calling out or moaning, and "canned" music. The general high level of extraneous noise causes further difficulty for those with moderate hearing impairment and those wearing a hearing aid, particularly in congregate dining rooms. Seating at small tables arranged in quiet alcoves would be helpful for the hearing impaired.

In all communication with elders, fully facing the individual, articulating carefully, and speaking at a normal pace and in normal volume will greatly facilitate hearing and understanding. Elders have said they often cannot hear when a speaker has his or her head lowered to read material or has hands fluttering about in front of the face. Simple and thoughtful considerations allow the elder to hear and respond more effectively. An in-depth discussion of hearing impairment is in Chapter 9.

COMMUNICATING WITH THE COGNITIVELY IMPAIRED

Communicating with a patient in the moderate or advanced stage of cognitive impairment is extremely difficult. Memory loss, aphasia, apraxia, agnosia, and overwhelming disorientation make much verbal communication unintelligible. Bartol's classic studies (1979) identified misunderstood communication as the root problem in many adverse reactions of confused elders. Threatening gestures, increased voice volume, restlessness, agitation, hostility, behavioral problems, and strik-

ing out are definitely messages, whether or not they are fully understood. The nurse must recognize that feelings of distress may linger in a patient long after he or she has forgotten the precipitant. The object of nursing care is to prevent these reactions, but when they occur the nurse should avoid responding with anger or impatience. Communicating with the cognitively disturbed elder requires special skills and patience. Nurses need an appropriate outlet to express annoyance and frustration in these difficult situations. As noted in Chapter 2, staff groups can provide opportunities for such ventilation.

The nurse's calm concern will help alleviate anxiety and cultivate client and family responsiveness (Box 3-2). The sound of communication is a humanizing factor, even though words may not be understood. Actions will have more influence than words, although soft, soothing speech and music can settle many anxious or agitated elders. Some guidelines for communicating with individuals who have memory problems but can still respond verbally are shown in Box 3-3.

Even extremely disoriented persons may respond briefly with warmth and pleasure when they sense a caring person. For those persons the goal is not orienta-

Box 3-2 COMMUNICATING WITH THE COGNITIVELY DISTURBED

Be patient; the individual may lack comprehension but may respond to repeated and varied attempts to communicate.

Keep routines the same, and provide written reminders. Repetition is often necessary.

Introduce one idea, and allow time for response. A demented person may require inordinate amounts of time to respond.

Use the active tense when speaking; e.g., "Eat this apple."

Demonstrate and give pictures of eating the apple or whatever you wish the person to do.

Additional and specific information may tap some element of comprehension. Use redundant cueing; e.g., "Bite the apple with your teeth."

Ask closed, specific questions; e.g., "Do you want to eat the apple?" If the individual does not answer, offer another alternative after waiting for a response; e.g., "Are you hungry?"

Remember: the patient is likely to become even more frustrated than you when messages are not understood. Intersperse verbal activities with periods of quiet touch or stroking.

Box 3-3 GUIDELINES FOR COMMUNICATING WITH THE MEMORY IMPAIRED

1. Introduce yourself, and explain why you are there. Ask if the person can hear you clearly. Reach out to shake hands, and note the response to touch.
2. Sit closely, facing the person at eye level. If the response to the initial touch was positive, take the person's hand again and hold it.
3. Explain that you want to make the person comfortable before proceeding with conversation. Ask if anything is distracting: e.g., environmental noise, vacuuming, roommates.
4. Assume a pleasant, relaxed attitude, and convey your interest in the person through body language such as nodding, gentle yet clearly articulated speech, touching, and eye contact.
5. Ask, "Is there an early memory that you can tell me about?" Wait for the answer.
6. Use simple, clear statements to obtain information, and wait for an answer.
7. When leaving, thank the person for his or her time and attention as well as information. Touch as appropriate, depending on initial response.
8. Remember that the quality of the interaction is basic to all communication success.

tion but, rather, human contact. Listening with respectful attention to any attempts to communicate is most important. This can lead to reminiscing. Even though patients may not remember the names of their spouse or children, certain life events usually will remain in memory. See Chapter 5 for further discussion.

Bartol's thorough nursing care perspective is a beacon to those working with the extremely cerebrally impaired. Her work was conducted in a research unit well staffed with physicians, clinical specialists, and primary care nurses. The quality of life when caring for impaired elders depends directly on the skill and interest of care providers. A major nursing function for those in less ideal settings is to recruit and train qualified personnel. Because there are no known cures for progressive dementias, nursing function is to provide care and comfort in the present moment in the lives of cognitively impaired elders.

COMMUNICATION IN GROUPS

Group work with the aged has been used extensively in institutional settings to meet myriad needs in an economic manner. Many groups can be managed effectively by staff with clear goals and minimal guidance and training. Some of the possibilities for designing groups to meet special needs are shown in Box 3-4. Groups may be recreation or service oriented, inspirational, informative, or constrained by specific needs or goals. Groups providing interactional support may be formal or informal. Either may function well or poorly,

Box 3-4	CHOOSING A GROUP ACCORDING TO NEED	

Needs and Problems	**Suggested Group**
Biologic integrity	
Confusion—disorientation	Reality orientation
Loss of sexual satisfaction or opportunity	Male/female groups
Poor nutrition	Mealtime groups
Drugs—inadequate rest	Relaxation groups
Body preoccupation	Health monitoring groups (e.g., blood pressure or feet and mouth examinations)
Safety and security	
Impaired sensory perception	Sensory awareness training
Immobility	Movement groups
Translocation	Patient councils, environmental planning groups
Belonging	
Isolation	Socialization
Rejection of cohorts	Activities
Alienation from family	Family groups, cohort groups
Loss of significant others	Grief group
Self-esteem	
Uselessness	Reminiscing groups
Lack of work	Productive groups
Lack of love objects	Remotivation groups
Lack of recognition	Discussion groups
Depression	Therapy groups, expressive groups
Self-actualization	
Stimulation deprivation	Most groups, particularly those using touch
Apathy	Interest groups
Acceptance of cultural myths ("Old dogs can't learn new tricks.")	Discussions, debates, educational groups, creative/expressive groups

depending on the needs of the aged participants and the skill of the group leader.

Informal Groups

Informal groups are those that naturally occur and have few restrictions, expectations, or goals. The following are examples of such groups:
- Groups of the aged that spontaneously arise at nutrition sites
- Gatherings of old people in city parks
- Participants in senior citizen activities (these often have formal and informal components)
- Groups that cluster together in long-term care or residential settings
- Any group that occurs sporadically for the purpose of socialization, discussion, or participation in a particular activity

These groupings should be supported in whatever way possible.

Formal Groups

Formal groups are defined by their expectations, dependability, and goals. The intensity of interpersonal exchange varies in accordance with the members' and group's goals. The development and maintenance of aged peer groups are particularly important when friends are no longer available. The advantage of group affiliations for the aged is in the diffusion of relationship intensity and the constancy over time. A reliable group maintains its function despite the loss or addition of members. This is an important consideration when working with the very old.

Needs Assessment

Groups can be organized to meet any level of human need; some meet multiple needs (Fig. 3-3). Using the assessment of social climate and human needs as basic guides, one can begin to determine the type of group most suitable in a given situation.

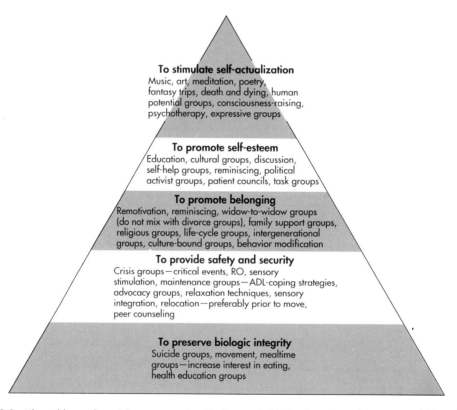

Fig. 3-3 Hierarchic needs met in group work with the aged. *RO,* Reality orientation; *ADL,* activities of daily living.

At least three types of groups exist: (1) those that accomplish some identifiable goal; (2) those designed to be psychotherapeutic; and (3) those that facilitate positive communication patterns. The distinction between the second and third types is in the readiness of members. Therapy groups imply some psychologic disturbance or conflict and should be led by qualified personnel. Nurses with training in psychotherapy often do an excellent job in such groups. The third type of group does not explore deep psychologic needs but, rather, assists individuals in overcoming some communication barriers. Some basic assessment parameters may help define particular levels of need of the aged (see Box 3-4).

Group Goals

Functional goals for groups of aged include combinations of the following:
- Socialization—interpersonal exchange
- Therapeutic—healing through group
- Entertainment
- Cohort affiliation
- Increased functional levels
- Stimulation/environmental enrichment
- Activation/movement
- Behavioral management
- Staff morale support
- Family morale support
- Increased autonomy

These might all be included in six major purposes: (1) reality orientation, (2) remotivation, (3) reminiscence, (4) recognition, (5) recreation, and (6) released potential.

Group Structure

Implementing a group follows a thorough assessment of environment, needs, and potential for various group strategies. Major decisions regarding goals will influence the strategy selected. For instance, several aged diabetics in an acute care setting may need health care teaching regarding diabetes. The nurse sees the major goal as restoring order (or control) in each individual's life-style. The strategy best suited for that would be motivational, or remotivation.

Guide for Evaluation of Group Meetings

The following are some factors used to evaluate effectiveness of group meetings:
1. *Setting.* Seating arrangement, room comfort, activities carried on in area, facilities; note movement of chairs, reseating, and objects that facilitate or distract.
2. *Goal.* How was it established? Who was included in the decision about goals? Is the goal flexible in response to changing needs?
3. *Participants.* Evaluate attendees, age, physical problems of importance to group, sex, mobility, and consistency of attendance.
4. *Types of interactions.* Dyads? Triads? Miniconversations, monologues, effects of place in the group, response to leader, roles of members?
5. *Process.* Mood of group at beginning, unusual events in setting, in community, nation, deaths, accidents, upset in ward or agency routines, new people in setting.
6. *Themes.* Outstanding themes expressed in group; usually not more than three or four: loneliness, power or lack of autonomy, rejection, universality, independence.
7. *Problems.* How were they handled? Was the approach effective? If problems occur again, what could be done?
8. *Significant content.* Identify goal-directed and effective interventions. Identify unsatisfactory interventions, and discuss what would have been more helpful.
9. *Evaluation of goal accomplishment.* What portions of the goal were accomplished? Evaluate group progress; make plans for the next meeting relative to evaluation of previous group meeting.

Groups of the aged have some unique aspects that require an extraordinary commitment on the part of the leader:
1. They often need assistance or transportation in getting to the group.
2. They may need more stimulation and be less self-motivating. (This is, of course, not true of self-help and senior activist groups such as the Gray Panthers.)
3. Many aged people likely to be in need of groups are depressed. The depression can be contagious, and leaders should be selected with that in mind. A leader prone to depression would not be appropriate.
4. Leaders must be prepared for some members to become ill, deteriorate, and die. Plans regarding recognition of missing members will need to be clear.
5. Leaders are continually confronted with their own aging and attitudes toward it. Group leaders need to plan in advance to incorporate a consistent support person in the group if possible. Co-leaders are ideal. If this is not feasible, someone must be available for planning and recapitulation of group sessions. Stu-

Table 3-2

Differences in Reality Orientation, Resocialization, and Remotivation

Reality orientation	Resocialization	Remotivation
1. Correct position or relation with the existing situation in a community; maximum use of assets	1. Continuation of reality living situation in a community	1. Orientation to reality for community living; present oriented
2. Called reality orientation, RO, and classroom reality orientation program	2. Called discussion group or resocialization to differentiate a social function from a therapeutic need	2. Called *remotivation*
3. Structured	3. Unstructured	3. Definite structure
4. Refreshments and/or food may be served for identification	4. Refreshments served	4. Refreshments not served
5. Appreciation of the work of the world; constantly reminded of who he is, where he is, why he is here, and what is expected of him	5. Appreciation of the work of the world; reliving happy experiences; encourages participation in home activities relating to subject	5. Appreciation of the work of the group stimulates the desire to return to function in society
6. Class range from 3-5, depending on degree/level of confusion or disorientation from any cause	6. Group range from 5-17, depending on mental and physical capabilities	6. Group size: 5-12 patients
7. Meeting $\frac{1}{2}$ hour daily at same time in same place	7. Meetings three times weekly for $\frac{1}{2}$-1 hour	7. Meeting once to twice weekly for 1 hour
8. Planned procedures: reality-centered objects	8. No planned topic; group centered feelings	8. Preselected and reality-centered objects
9. Consistency of approach/ response of resident responsibility of teacher	9. Clarification and interpretation in responsibility of leader	9. No exploration of feelings
10. Periodic reality orientation test pertaining to residents' level of confusion or disorientation	10. Periodic progress notes pertaining to residents' enjoyment and improvements	10. Progress ratings
11. Emphasis on time, place, person orientation	11. Any topic freely discussed	11. Topic: no discussion of religion, politics, or death
12. Use of portion of mind function still intact	12. Vast stockpile of memories and experiences	12. Untouched area of the mind
13. Resident greeted by name, thanked for coming, and extended handshake and/or physical contact according to attitude approach in group	13. Resident greeted on arrival, thanked, and extended handshake upon leaving	13. No physical contact permitted; acceptance and acknowledgment of everyone's contribution
14. Conducted by trained aides and activity assistants	14. Conducted by RN, LPN/LVN, aides, and program assistants	14. Conducted by trained psychiatric aides

From Barns E, Sack A, Shore H: Guidelines to treatment approaches, *Gerontologist* 13:513, 1973.

dents generally should work in pairs and will need supervision. Skills in developing and implementing groups for the aged improve with experience. Even though the effort is sometimes draining, there are many rewards.

Reality orientation (RO), remotivation, and resocialization are the main types of groups that have been used in institutional long-term care settings serving the aged. Reality orientation has been used with varying degrees of success, depending on the degree of cognitive impairment of the participants and the frequency and consistency of its use. Remotivation and resocialization have been adapted for many uses. All rely on including elders in communication with others and can be an effective and economic means of reaching withdrawn or confused elders.

The five guidelines emphasized in remotivation groups (Butler et al, 1991) are useful in any of the groups formed with the intent of increasing an elder's communication and participation with others in the setting. These guidelines, with numerous modifications, are as follows:

1. Establish a warm and friendly climate of acceptance of each member.
2. Keep in touch with current events; use as vehicle for information sharing.
3. Provide opportunities for in-depth or creative exploration of topics of interest.
4. Stimulate elders to think about their contribution to the world in general and to the present.
5. Show appreciation and enjoyment of the group and each member's contribution.

Remotivation for the aged in long-term care situations may be successfully used by individuals with little training. Student experiences in using remotivation group techniques can be very gratifying. The students learn to appreciate the aged, and the elders in turn become more interested in life, less irritable, better groomed, and motivated toward interpersonal contacts. Table 3-2 provides some guidelines and comparisons of reality orientation, resocialization, and remotivation groups.

LEARNING AND GROWING IN LATER LIFE

In this era of health care restrictions it is imperative that providers and elders understand each other and that necessary information is shared accurately and in a timely fashion. Reaching some elders with information that is understood and beneficial presents special challenges. Low literacy skills of some elders may create problems. More than 90 million adults have limited ability to read and understand directions on prescriptions, appointment slips, consent documents, insurance forms, and educational materials (Gerontological Society of America, 1999). Cultural and cohort variations have produced great differences in receptivity to health information. Many elders still have special learning needs based on education deprivation in their early years and consequent anxiety about formalized learning. Box 3-5 summarizes some ways to overcome these problems.

Box 3-5   ELDERLY CLIENT'S SPECIAL LEARNING NEEDS

- Make sure the client is ready to learn before trying to teach. Watch for clues that would indicate that the client is preoccupied or too anxious to comprehend the material.
- Sit facing the client so that he or she can watch your lip movements and facial expressions.
- Speak slowly.
- Keep your tone of voice low; elderly persons can hear low sounds better than high-frequency sounds.
- Present one idea at a time.
- Emphasize concrete rather than abstract material.
- Give the client enough time in which to respond because elderly persons' reaction times are longer than those of younger persons.
- Focus on a single topic to help the client concentrate.
- Keep environmental distractions to a minimum.
- Defer teaching if the client becomes distracted or tired or cannot concentrate for other reasons.
- Invite another member of the household to join the discussion.
- Use audio, visual, and tactile cues to enhance learning and help the client remember information.
- Ask for feedback to ensure that the information has been understood.
- Use past experience; connect new learning to that already learned.
- Compensate for physical discomfort and sensory decrements.
- Support a positive self-image in the learner.
- Use creative teaching strategies.
- Respond to identified interests of learners.
- Emphasize and integrate emotional and personal values in the acquisition of skills and ideas.

Modified from Fielo S, Rizzolo M: Handle with caring: meeting elderly clients' special learning needs, *Nurs Health Care* 9(4):193, 1988.

The nurse's role extends beyond simply giving information. To be useful the nurse must discover the preferred learning mode and setting appropriate to the needs and desires of the elder (Fig. 3-4). Also, the nurse should provide the elder with information about media resources that may make knowledge readily available and palatable. Because many older adults spend much time watching television, this is a particularly effective avenue of learning. Increasingly, elders are taking charge of their own learning and scanning the internet for information about health and life-styles. Nurses are beginning to recognize the necessity of revising the traditional teaching/learning strategies, which often are limited to giving information in the form of brochures and mini-lectures with return demonstrations. Follow-up to determine how much information was actually comprehended and used has been insufficient.

Numerous opportunities exist for older learners within the established educational institutions or in special programs. Many universities have "senior scholar" programs designed especially for elders. At the McGill Institute for Learning in Retirement, students design their own course of study (Clark, 1995-1996). Discussing latent interests with elders can be very useful. The nurse's role should include providing suggestions of resources available to the elder.

Throughout this chapter we have tried to convey the potential for honest and hopeful communication regardless of the condition of the elder. We must break through the barriers and continue to reach toward the humanity of the individual with the belief that communication is the most vital service we can offer. This is the heart of nursing.

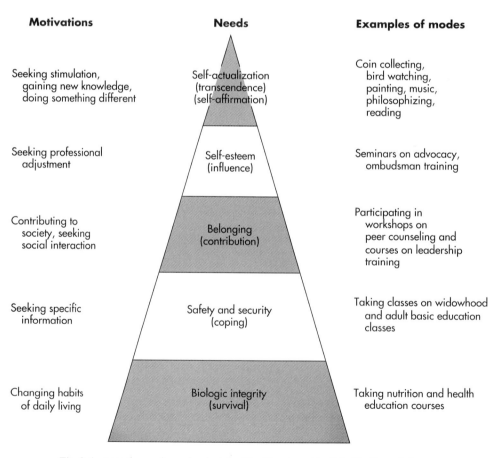

Fig. 3-4 Learning and growing in later life. (Developed by Priscilla Ebersole.)

▶ KEY CONCEPTS

- Communication is sometimes slowed by age-associated memory impairment (AAMI). This refers to the common forgetfulness that many elders experience. This is usually attributed to distraction, preoccupation, or performance anxiety. It is poorly understood but must be met with reassurance that this is not an evidence of impending dementia.
- Individuals who are mentally impaired respond best to calmness, few demands, clear communication, and predictable routines. They are hypersensitive to chaotic situations and may develop catastrophic reactions when demands exceed their ability.
- Individuals need opportunities for exposure to and discussion of various experiences and diverse ideas.
- Intergenerational contact between elders and youth often tends to increase communication and appreciation in both groups.
- Nursing functions related to communication and learning are focused mainly on providing necessary information, encouraging individuals to express personal interests and preferences, and, when function is impeded, assuring that basic needs are mutually recognized, discussed, and met to the greatest extent possible.

NANDA and Wellness Diagnoses

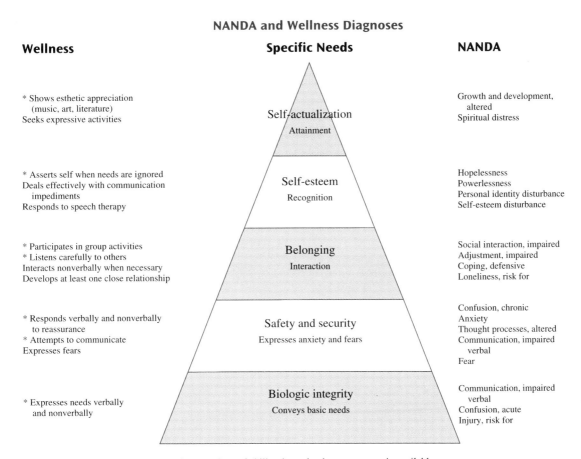

Wellness	Specific Needs	NANDA
* Shows esthetic appreciation (music, art, literature) Seeks expressive activities	**Self-actualization** Attainment	Growth and development, altered Spiritual distress
* Asserts self when needs are ignored Deals effectively with communication impediments Responds to speech therapy	Self-esteem Recognition	Hopelessness Powerlessness Personal identity disturbance Self-esteem disturbance
* Participates in group activities * Listens carefully to others Interacts nonverbally when necessary Develops at least one close relationship	**Belonging** Interaction	Social interaction, impaired Adjustment, impaired Coping, defensive Loneliness, risk for
* Responds verbally and nonverbally to reassurance * Attempts to communicate Expresses fears	Safety and security Expresses anxiety and fears	Confusion, chronic Anxiety Thought processes, altered Communication, impaired verbal Fear
* Expresses needs verbally and nonverbally	**Biologic integrity** Conveys basic needs	Communication, impaired verbal Confusion, acute Injury, risk for

* Wellness when individual communicates to best of ability through whatever means is available.

These are not all of the possible wellness or NANDA diagnoses that may be identified. The above are frequent examples of nursing diagnoses that should be considered when planning care for the older adult in whatever setting.

▶ **Activities and Discussion Questions**

1. Discuss interventions that facilitate communication with aphasic individuals.
2. Discuss your experiences with hearing-impaired persons and the actions you found most effective.
3. Discuss various methods of communicating with distressed elders that might have a calming effect.
4. With a partner, plan and discuss a communication activity that would be appropriate for an individual with moderate levels of dementia.
5. Role-play a simulated group discussion for individuals who are withdrawn and need remotivation.

RESOURCES

Films and Videos

Seasons of the Mind. A concise and excellent report on two septuagenarians who, on entering the university, relish the intensity, face the difficult challenges, and perhaps most surprisingly, find that they are welcomed and accepted by their younger fellows. To watch the expression of an 82-year-old lady accepting her Bachelor of Arts degree after 7 years of study is to know the truth (21 minutes). J. Rowe, Filmmakers Library, New York.

Communication Strategies for Alzheimer's Patients. Presents methods of maintaining patient dignity and self-respect while communicating effectively. Utilizes actual scenes with patients, family, and staff. Available from Geriatric Video Productions, PO Box 1757, Shavertown, PA 18708-0757, (800) 621-9181.

Problem Behaviors in Geriatrics: Agitation and Restlessness. Discusses triggers and preventive strategies to eliminate the behaviors without the use of physical and chemical restraints. Available from Geriatric Video Productions, PO Box 1757, Shavertown, PA 18708-0757, (800) 621-9181.

Working with the Confused Elderly. Presents verbal and nonverbal techniques that increase skills in coping with problem behaviors associated with chronic confusion in the elderly. The work presents some revolutionary methods to deal with problems such as wandering, paranoia, and disorientation (21-minute video). Dr. Joyce Colling, Oregon Health Sciences University, Nursing School, 3181 SW Sam Jackson Park Road, Portland, OR 97201.

Adult Education

Elderhostel, 50 Federal Street, Boston, MA 02110, (617) 426-8056. To receive catalogs, write ELDERHOSTEL, PO Box 1959, Wakefield, MA O1880-5959.

AARP's free Directory of Centers for Older Learners. The state-by-state listing includes the names, addresses, phone numbers, and sponsors of educational programs around the country, designed for older students. To receive copies, send a postcard requesting stock number 13973 to AARP Fulfillment, EE0233, PO Box 2400, Long Beach, CA 90801-2400.

Lifelong Learning: The Adult Years. Journal contains articles on adult education and is published monthly (except July and August) by the Adult Education Association of the IJSA, 810 18th Street NW, Washington, DC 20000.

Senior Learning Times. Journal is published by the College Board and AARP and is available to individuals and groups. Single copies are $1.50; multiple orders are available. To receive copies, send check, payable to the College Board, to the College Board, PO Box C749, Pratt Street Station, Brooklyn, NY 11205.

Institutes for Lifetime Learning. A service of the American Association of Retired Persons (AARP) National Retired Teachers Association (NRTA), it provides classes at institute centers throughout the country and a series of radio programs allowing members of AARP/NRTA to pursue independent study at their own pace in their own fields of interest. Contact AARP, (202) 872-4700.

American Association of Community and Junior Colleges, No. 1 Dupont Circle, Suite 410, Washington, DC 20036, (202) 293-7050.

Adult Education Association: Aging Section. Publishes a quarterly newsletter, *Education and Aging News.* The association conducts seminars and has published Old Gold, a guide to financing in adult education. Contact Adult Education Association: Aging Section, Brookdale Center on Aging, Hunter College, 129 E. 79th Street, New York, NY 10021.

Organizations

The International Association of Laryngectomees, 219 E. 42nd Street, New York, NY 10017.

The American Cancer Society provides varied information and resources for the laryngectomee; frequently it also sponsors local Lost Chord clubs for laryngectomees.

To attend local Stroke Club meetings, write Stroke Club Coordinator, c/o American Heart Association, Texas Affiliate, Inc, PO Box 15186, Austin, TX 78761.

Publication

Resource Materials for Communicative Problems of Older Persons (1975) is available from the American Speech and Hearing Association, 9020 Old Georgetown Road, Washington, DC 20014 (cost: $4.95 [31 pages]).

REFERENCES

Bartol M: Dialogue with dementia: nonverbal communication in patients with Alzheimer's disease, *J Gerontol Nurs* 5:21, 1979.

Butler RN, Lewis MI, Sunderland T: *Aging and mental health: positive psychosocial and biomedical approaches,* ed 4, New York, 1991, Macmillan.

Clark F: Learning thrives when seniors take responsibility for their own program, *The Older Learner* 4(1):1, 1995-1996.

Gerontological Society of America: Fact sheet: low health literacy skills increase annual health care expenditures by $73 billion, *Gerontol News* 26(4):9, 1999.

Lee MH, Itoh M: General concepts of geriatric rehabilitation. In Abrams WB, Berkow R, editors: *Merck manual of geriatrics,* Rahway, NJ, 1990, Merck, Sharp & Dohme Research Laboratories.

Nagley S: *Personal communication,* CWRU, 1988, Cleveland.

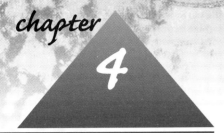

chapter 4

Cultural Considerations in Communication

▶ LEARNING OBJECTIVES

Upon completion of this chapter, the reader will be able to:

- Explain the prominent health care belief systems.
- Discuss approaches that facilitate an appreciation of diverse cultural and ethnic experiences.
- Identify factors contributing to personal ethnic and cultural sensitivity.
- Identify nursing care interventions appropriate for ethnic elders.
- Formulate a care plan incorporating ethnically sensitive interventions.

▶ GLOSSARY

Assimilation The merging of cultural traits into those of another or dominant culture, which does not include uniting biologically.

Ethnicity Belonging to or deriving from the culture, racial, religious, or linguistic traditions of a people or country.

Ethnocentrism The belief in inherent superiority of one's group and culture accompanied by devaluation of other groups or cultures.

Ethno-geriatrics The medical science dealing with disease, disabilities, and care of ethnic elders.

Folk medicine Curing methods originating among the people of culture and transmitted through the people of that culture.

Humoral Pertaining to body fluid or fluids.

Interpreter A person who explains the meaning of what is said in another language; often reads between the lines, what is implied. (Sometimes interchanged with translator but technically different.)

Translator A person who turns the spoken (or written) word of one language into another language; communicator, explainer.

▶ THE LIVED EXPERIENCE

I feel so out of place here. If my children weren't so busy, I suppose I could live with them, but they seemed so relieved when this retirement home would accept me. I wonder if they knew I was the only Chinese person in this place. A sweet young Chinese student tried to talk with me, but she only spoke Mandarin and that not very well. She had never lived in China. I want so much to talk to someone my age who lived in China.

Shin Lu, a 75-year-old woman

I thought I knew Chinese; after all, Grandma lived with us for so many years before she died and she taught me some. I felt so sad for Shin Lu and also for myself. I didn't talk enough to Grandma when she was alive, and I would like to have heard more from Shin Lu about how China was when she was a child. I wish I knew more about being Chinese.

Jenny Chen

BASIC CONSIDERATIONS OF CULTURAL CARE

Communication is achieved through verbal and non-verbal exchanges, such as facial and body expressions, postures, gestures, and touching. How these transmissions are interpreted is influenced by culture and ethnicity. To be an effective communicator and care provider, the nurse must be able to communicate in a culturally sensitive and competent manner. Clients have needs that require attention regardless of their cultural or ethnic origins. To be able to skillfully assess and intervene, nurses must first develop cultural sensitivity and competence by expanding their horizons about ethnicity, culture, language, and health belief systems, as well as their awareness of their own ethnocentricities.

Immigration in Late Life

During the early part of the twentieth century a wave of European immigration occurred, which was composed of youth and families. In the past 20 years the influx to the western states of Asians, Filipinos, and other individuals from the Pacific Rim has been significant. The composition of this immigration, from Asia and the Pacific islands, is often the elders who have come to the United States to join their adult children, who were concerned about their parents' welfare. These adult children wanted to watch over and care for them. This relocation to a new culture and language in late life has not been thoughtfully examined in the literature, but from anecdotal information the relocation seems to impinge on the sense of personal continuity and security. Available resources are underused, and the transplanted individual may lack the social and cultural nourishment necessary for satisfaction even though survival needs may be met at a higher level than in the mother country. It is not uncommon for elderly immigrants to feel isolated and depressed because of the discontinuity of their life-style and relationships.

Language

Seldom do we think of language as the foundation of self-concept, but the self is continuously constructed and inextricably bound up with the linguistic categories available in a given culture (Berman, 1991). We can conceive of ourselves only within the language we know. To make each contact with the elderly fully meaningful, shared communication is essential. Communication with persons of a different culture, ethnic group, or geographic region is an issue not only of language but also of idiom, style, and jargon. Even if it were possible for a nurse to learn all the deviations, it would likely not be useful. It would be similar to entering a family and using all the pet names and phrases treasured by the family. In most cases the artificiality and intrusive nature of such an action would be irritating. Asking the individual about a phrase can be illuminating. In turn, we must remember that as health professionals our jargon and idiomatic expressions may be perceived as frightening or threatening and will most certainly increase the social distance between the provider and the client.

Never assume you know what an aged person means. Ask him or her. If the person speaks a foreign language, every effort should be made to find a translator/interpreter. In old age, people find comfort in their mother tongue. However, when family members are used as translators/interpreters, they may be unable to aid a care provider because of role conflicts or inability to use medical terms appropriately. Often messages to the client and the provider are based on the interpreter's perception of the situation, and vital information may be withheld or omitted to shield the client or family from embarrassment.

In working with these elders, nurses must recognize the importance of their identification with past patterns and relationships. They are often living on the edge of anonymity. The most significant intervention is to find someone who speaks their language and can discuss their previous life-style. (See Box 4-1 regarding the use of interpreters.) Senior centers designed specifically for the elder's cultural needs may bring enjoyment. Churches may be another important source of other elders of the same ethnic background. Families need to understand that, no matter how pleasant the surroundings, the displaced individuals long for the old ways and are experiencing a grief process. If the elder can be encouraged to talk about the losses, he or she may experience the relief that comes with ventilation in the presence of a concerned listener. Ethnic elders often neglect health care because they may not know what is available to them; language is a barrier to information and expression of health needs. In addition, they may be frightened by the health care system.

Ethnicity

Ethnicity is a complex phenomenon. It is a social differentiation based on cultural criteria. Most important,

Box 4-1   HINTS TO WORKING WITH INTERPRETERS

Before an interview or session with a client, try to meet with the interpreter to explain the purpose of the session.

Encourage the interpreter to meet with the client before the session to identify the educational level and attitudes toward health and health care and to determine the depth and type of information and explanation needed.

Look and speak directly to the client, not the interpreter.

Be patient. Interpreted interviews take more time because long explanatory phrases often are needed.

Use short units of speech. Long, involved sentences or complex discussions create confusion.

Use simple language. Avoid technical terms, professional jargon, slang, abbreviations, abstractions, metaphors, or idiomatic expressions.

Encourage translation of the client's own words rather than paraphrased professional jargon to get a better sense of the client's ideas and emotional state.

Encourage the translator to avoid inserting his or her own ideas or interpretations or omitting information.

Listen to the client and watch nonverbal communication (facial expression, voice intonation, body movement) to learn about emotions to a specific topic.

Clarify the client's understanding and the accuracy of the translation by asking the client to tell you in his or her own words what he or she understands, facilitated by the interpreter.

Modified from Lipson JG, Dibble SL, Minarik PA, editors: *Culture and nursing care: a pocket guide,* San Francisco, Calif, 1996, UCSF School of Nursing Press.

there is a shared identity. Although culture and ethnicity frequently are used interchangeably, in reality a distinct difference exists in meanings (Giger, Davidhizar, 1991; Gunter, 1991; Spector, 2000).

An ethnic group may share common geographic origins, migratory status, race, language, and dialect. Religious factors (ties that transcend kinship, neighborhoods, and community boundaries) also are important in ethnicity. Traditions, values, symbols, literature, folklore, and diverse food preferences should be considered a part of ethnicity too. Settlement and employment patterns, special interests or politics in the homeland and in the United States, as well as an internal sense of distinctiveness or perception of external distinctiveness are additional facets of ethnicity that must be considered (Giger, Davidhizer, 1991; Gunter, 1991; Spector, 2000). The components *culture, social status,* and *support systems* shape ethnicity and influence the way people feel about themselves and how they interact with their environment (Hooyman, Kiyak, 1996).

Writers often focus on nutritional patterns, folk medicine, death rituals, and specific cultural beliefs of ethnic groups. These generalities may not meet individual needs and may serve only to stereotype a person into artificial boundaries. Our obligation is not to seek out minutiae of rituals and folkways and differences in habits of living but, rather, to respect those important to the individual. When we insist on regimented care, we infringe on an individual's ability to maintain his or her own cultural orientation. The concept of heritage consistency of an individual is shown in Fig. 4-1.

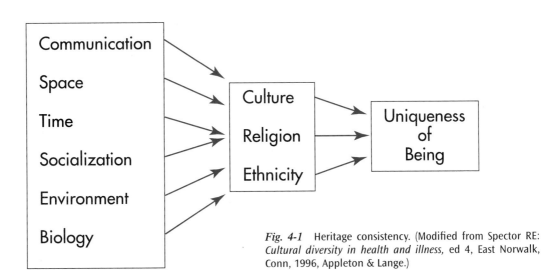

Fig. 4-1 Heritage consistency. (Modified from Spector RE: *Cultural diversity in health and illness,* ed 4, East Norwalk, Conn, 1996, Appleton & Lange.)

Ethnic elders prefer programs and services where the staff reflect the ethnic background and speak the language of the elderly clientele. Adequate and quality health care for the minority elders of today and tomorrow revolves around the issues of appropriate programs for them and cultural relativism. One of the most pervasive barriers to improving services has been the failure of caregivers to recognize race as a critical factor in the provision of such services. Others have noted that effective service delivery to ethnic elders requires a conscious effort to be responsive to the cultural uniqueness of these elderly populations. An example of just what cultural relativism in a senior center can do is described by Ochoco and Shimamoto (1987). They found that by introducing ethnic-related activities at a senior center in Hawaii they were able to increase patient self-esteem, independence, and satisfaction. Many of the participants had been passive, dependent, and depressed. Two thirds of the participants were widowed women who had originally emigrated from Japan. Because a language barrier existed, some of the widows lived with children and deferred to their wishes to the neglect of their own self-esteem and self-concept. The community health nurse who activated the group wished to strengthen the sense of self in group members through a focus on cultural heritage. In addition to health teaching sessions and education about the aging process, the nurse used reminiscence and construction of a collective oral history to stimulate interaction and the sense of accomplishment. This model is adaptable to many community and institutional settings.

CULTURAL AND HEALTH BELIEF SYSTEMS AND PRACTICES

Nurses who are familiar with health belief systems will be able to communicate more objectively with their elder clientele. Three of a number of health belief systems are widely and actively practiced today as they have been in the past. These are the biomedical or Western system, the personalistic or magicoreligious system, and the naturalistic or holistic system. The diversity of the population has brought the strong potential for a clash of health belief systems, language, and attitudes about health and illness between the care provider and the client. Many of the beliefs and practices do not fit into the traditional format of health care as most care providers know it or practice it.

Biomedical System

The Western medical or scientific belief system embraces disease as the result of abnormalities in structure and function of body organs and systems. It is still a dominant belief that permeates the thinking of those educated in Western health care. The objective term *disease* is used by care providers, and *illness* is a subjective term to describe symptoms of discomfort or sickness. A personal state of illness has distinct social dimensions. Assessment and diagnosis are directed at identifying the pathogen or process causing the abnormality and removing or destroying the cause or at least repairing or modifying the problem through treatment. Highly skilled clinicians use the scientific method and sophisticated laboratory and other procedures to stem the disease or disease process. Prevention in this belief system is to avoid pathogens, chemicals, activities, and dietary agents known to cause malfunction.

Personalistic or Magicoreligious System

Those who follow the beliefs of the personalistic or magicoreligious system accept that illness is caused by active, purposeful intervention of agents of the supernatural, such as gods, deities, or non–human beings. Ghosts, ancestors, evil spirits, or humans in the form of witches or sorcerers are responsible for sickness. The individual is considered a victim, an object of aggression or punishment. Someone may be put under a spell by a disgruntled neighbor so that he or she cannot eat or sleep. A dead relative may be angry that his or her wishes were not followed and send an animal to bite the person, cause a growth, or cause a woman to be infertile. Identifying the agent behind these events and rendering it harmless, lifting a spell, or reversing the method used by the agent is the aim of treatment. Once the agent is known, the curer or person can take steps to resolve the situation. Physical symptoms are secondary to finding the initial cause of the dilemma. Making sure that social networks with their fellow humans are in good working order is the essence of prevention in this health belief system. Therefore it is important to them that they avoid angering family, friends, neighbors, ancestors, and gods, for example, and that they adhere to and correctly perform rituals. Etiologies of the personalistic beliefs may be intertwined with religious beliefs. Entities that cause illness may be expanded to explain that the deities and ghosts, for example, are the cause of such events as crop failures, accidents, and financial reversals. The origins of this system are attributed to groups that were relatively small, isolated, and illiterate and lacked contact with ancient high civilizations (Jackson, 1993).

Naturalistic or Holistic Health System

Sickness is considered an impersonal, systemic term. Health is the result of the equilibrium of the elements of the body for balance and harmony. When this is not so, illness is present. The current naturalistic beliefs stem from the ancient civilizations of China, India, and Greece (Jackson, 1993).

Traditional Chinese medicine is the basis for the health belief system and practices today of such countries as Japan, Vietnam, Korea, Taiwan, Singapore, Hong Kong, and China. In India and some of its neighboring countries, Ayurvedic medicine, which arose in ancient India, is still practiced. Humoral pathology, practiced by the ancient Greeks, was disseminated both east and west and was embraced by the Moslem culture and Spanish and Italian explorers. Variations of humoral pathology can be found in the medical systems of rural and some urban people in Latin America and the Philippines and some low-income blacks and whites in the southern United States. These beliefs are found also in sophisticated and unsophisticated populations in Iran, Pakistan, Malaysia, and Java (Jackson, 1993). In the United States or countries that are steeped in the biomedical system, the aforementioned beliefs are considered "folk medicine."

Although the origins of naturalistic beliefs are different, they all consider illness the result of an excess of heat or cold that enters the body and causes an imbalance. Hot and cold is generally metaphoric, although at times temperature is an aspect. Various foods, medicines, environmental conditions, emotions, and bodily conditions such as menstruation and pregnancy may possess the characteristics of either hot or cold (Jackson, 1993; Spector, 2000).

Diagnosis is concerned with identifying the cause of the disease as either hot or cold in origin. Remedies are divided into hot and cold. Treatment then is focused on using the opposite element; if the disease is the result of excess hot, treatment will be with something that has cold properties, and vice versa. The treatments may take the form of herbs, food, dietary restrictions, or medications from Western medicine that have hot and cold properties such as antibiotics, massage, poultices, and other therapies. Naturalistic curers are physicians or herbalists who specialize in symptomatic treatment

and know which medicines will restore the body's equilibrium. Prevention is directed at protecting oneself from extremes of heat and cold in both the literal and metaphoric sense.

One may recognize a melding of the various health system beliefs in oneself and others. Therefore it behooves care providers to become sensitive to and versed in these systems to better understand, not necessarily agree with, persons for whom they are providing care, while recognizing their own ethnocentric tendencies. Table 4-1 illustrates variations in illness beliefs between the biomedical and other ethnically based models.

HEALTH PRACTICES

Elders who grew up in remote areas of any country, including the United States, where traditional health services were scarce or unavailable, developed a number of unusual health practices. Some are physiologically sound, and others may have been beneficial because of the placebo effects. Folk remedies abound among the various ethnic elders and among the dominant culture. The dominant cultural group also embraces many of the beliefs brought in from other countries and welcomes the relief from the mechanistic approaches of our Western, technology-dominated culture.

Even though the client may not admit to presently using any historic folk remedies or unusual practices, awareness of the possibility is important and should be included in the health assessment. Encourage and incorporate these practices unless the practice is clearly detrimental. We know belief and hope have therapeutic benefits. Alternative healers must also be discussed and encouraged if the client believes they are important. Many questions have been raised about the advisability of using indigenous health care providers and agency personnel to serve the elderly of ethnic minorities. We believe this is ideal but not always possible. A sensitive nurse needs to become aware of her own cultural roots, embrace and enjoy them, but keep them in proper perspective in the nurse-client relationship. As with clients of all backgrounds, one nursing function of great importance is to support the ties with family or reference group that maintain the aged person's sense of solidarity. Encourage family members to prepare specially enjoyed foods and perform significant rituals. Locate priests, monks, rabbis, or ministers who may comfort the aged person. When alternative healing methods are used, respect them as judiciously as the traditional. A

Table 4-1

Explanation of Illness: Biomedical and Behavioral

	Biomedical model	Behaviorally ethnic model
ETIOLOGIC BELIEFS		
Social causes of illness	Usually limited to the stress model or attributed to paranoia.	Many social indiscretions can cause illness. Blaming oneself or others for symptoms is common.
Environmental causes of illness	Exposure to known pathogens, toxins, and social stress may cause symptoms.	Dietary indiscretion can cause hot-cold imbalance in the body. Drafts may cause symptoms.
Blood conditions as causes of illness	Limited to specific hematologic disorders or hypertension.	Many conditions of the blood (too thick, thin, high, low, or stagnant) can cause illness.
SYMPTOM PRESENTATION AND INTERPRETATION		
Altered states of consciousness (trance, visions)	Likely to be considered abnormal.	Often considered to be normal or desirable.
Attitudes toward pain	Stoicism expected unless complaints are congruent with clear organic pathology.	Either total stoicism or emotional expression of pain is healthy and expected.
Focus on physical symptoms	May be considered a psychiatric syndrome.	Expected, proper way of showing distress.
TREATMENT EXPECTATIONS		
Who is the patient?	Individual is focus of decision making and care.	The family must be involved in decision making.
Beliefs about self-medication and alternative practitioners	Considered potentially dangerous or undesirable.	Self-medication and consulting with traditional healers are common.

Modified from Johnson TH, Hardt EJ, Kleinman A: Cultural factors in the medical interview. In Lipkin M Jr, Putnam SM, Lazare A, editors: *The medical interview,* New York, 1994, Springer-Verlag.

Box 4-2   GUIDELINES TO NURSING INTERVENTIONS FOR ETHNIC ELDERS

Respect the cultural preferences in food, music, and religion.
Design teaching to the vocabulary and attitude of the individual.
Listen attentively to complaints because these may be the clues to health problems.
In people of color, the signs of some disorders may be masked by color (pallor, cyanosis, ecchymosis); buccal cavity coloration is significant.
Base physical assessment on norms for the ethnic group:
    Adequate light is especially important in skin assessment for turgor, blemishes, and cyanosis; eye lens, nail beds, palms of hands, and soles of feet can be revealing.
Listen for signs of depression, often in the form of hypochondriasis and apathy.
Inquire about losses and the individual's adaptation to them.
Gather information about life-style preferences, and incorporate into care plans.
Inquire about health practices the individual finds effective.
Identify spiritual resources and incorporate in care plan; contact minister and church friends.

sense of caring is conveyed in these gestures of personal recognition. Caring can surmount cultural differences.

We must also become acutely aware of the influence of our own values, beliefs, and prejudices before we can hope to understand another's. If we do not become sensitive to the influence of values and beliefs on health, we will be unable to provide effective care. Scientific problem solving, the foundation of nursing care planning, is necessary but not inclusive. Intuition, superstition, belief, faith, and hope are necessarily woven into effective care packages. Jackson (1993), Grossman (1994), and Spector (1996) believe provider self-awareness is fundamental to this process. A number of measures suggested by Spector (1996) will assist the nurses to deal sensitively with people from other cultures (Box 4-2).

The nurse and the health care system have strong ethnocentric tendencies. That is, the individual's or the group's (the health care system) beliefs and ways of providing care are considered the most desirable when dealing with illness or health care. In essence, Western medicine and nursing care are considered superior to others. This latter statement is ethnocentrism (Leininger, 1978; Gunter, 1991; Grossman, 1994; Spector, 2000). To combat this and provide sensitively designed care, many components of the individual's life system must be considered (Box 4-3).

CULTURAL COMPETENCE AND SENSITIVITY

Cultural competence and sensitivity are being aware of the issues related to culture, race, gender, sexual orientation, social class, economic situations, and many other factors (Meleis et al, 1995) through knowledge and the ability to intervene appropriately and effectively. In sum, cultural competence encompasses a complex combination of knowledge, attitudes, mutual respect, skill, and negotiation (Chrisman, 1992). Attitudes are affected by experience, flexibility, empathy, and language facility. Skill includes cross-cultural communications, cultural interpretation, assessment, cultural interpretation of the assessment, and intervention (Lipson, 1996).

Knowledge is what the nurse learns and knows about the client, family, and community and their behaviors. Essential is knowledge of the person's way of life, ways of thinking, believing, and acting—knowledge obtained through personal experiences. Over time, the nurse builds up a reservoir of information about the beliefs of his or her clients and how they behave. An additional reservoir of knowledge comes from the clients and their families. Often nurses turn to these sources for information about ways they cope with chronic conditions and past health problems. Members of the health community who come from specific cultural backgrounds can also offer valuable data. A final source of knowledge comes from the literature. Books, pamphlets, articles, and journals can be significant sources of information about cultures different from that of the nurse. This knowledge should be related to professional principles of nursing care. A common example of this is when a client adheres to his or her food customs, which are contrary to the therapeutic regimen. The nurse must weigh the nutritional value of the customs to recommend a reasonable substitute that will conform to the client's health state.

Box 4-3	**CULTURALLY SENSITIVE HEALTH CARE**

Ethnic studies are essential in the curricula required of health care providers. Students may be required to interview aged individuals of other cultures. Guest speakers from representative cultures may be invited to classes.

Health care providers must be sensitized to their own perceptions and practices related to health and illness. Consciousness-raising exercises include interviewing family about health beliefs and health practices that have been or are part of the family heritage.

Health care providers should become aware of the complex issues of health care from the client's viewpoint: cost, religious beliefs, interpretation of services, inequality of treatment, and many others of which even the client may be unaware.

More minority persons must be recruited into health care professions. Support services for students entering professional education programs must be made readily available to compensate for deficits experienced in early education and language differences.

Health services must be accessible to ethnic minorities and delivered with respect to cultural beliefs and practices. Neighborhood health centers with indigenous providers are most effective for entry into the health care system and appropriate guidance and referral.

Summarized from Spector RE: *Cultural diversity in health and illness,* East Norwalk, Conn, 1985, Appleton & Lange.

Mutual respect is closely allied with knowledge. It is working "with" the client rather than "on" the client. Knowledge allows the nurse to recognize and react more positively to seemingly strange and even bizarre health beliefs and practices. A nonjudgmental reaction because of knowledge about the ethnic group can signal to a client that the nurse trusts and respects the individual. Mutual respect is fundamental to culture-sensitive care because it opens opportunities for innovative planning of care that depends on trust between client and nurse (Chrisman, 1992).

Negotiation should attempt to preserve helpful beliefs and practices, accommodate beliefs that are neither helpful nor harmful from the viewpoint of Western medicine, or repattern harmful beliefs or practices (Jackson, 1993). When repatterning is necessary, it is important to make the change without compromising underlying belief systems. When an impasse occurs between client and nurse, with each person perceiving the issue as nonnegotiable, the foundation of knowledge and trust or mutual respect that has been achieved will be helpful in seeking a goal that will optimize health outcomes beneficial to the client and still support the nurse's technical and ethical concerns.

A summary of Grossman's (1994) and Spector's (1996) suggestions of the steps to cultural sensitivity and competence appears in Box 4-4.

If nurses are unfamiliar with a particular ethnic group, churches or associations (e.g., Polish American Alliance, Celtic League, Jewish Family and Children's Society, Slovak League of America) can be helpful in identifying interpreters or persons who can serve as a cultural resource. Consulates for various countries may provide a list of organizations specific to a cultural group. Schools of nursing have recently started to address cultural aspects in their curriculum. Nurses who graduated before this time and who are working find the need individually to seek these experiences. Suggestions for upgrading knowledge about the minority aged include the following:

1. Develop interest in and commitment to the needs of minority groups.
2. Become involved in experiences with diverse ethnic and cultural groups.
3. Learn about historical and cultural roots of ethnic variations.
4. Respond to the diverse needs within your community.

Brislin and Pederson (1982) suggest caregivers be trained in self-awareness and sensitivity rather than focused on eating habits, religious customs, interpersonal etiquette, and decision-making styles of ethnic minori-

---

Box 4-4   STEPS TO CULTURAL SENSITIVITY AND COMPETENCE

- Know yourself: examine your own values, attitudes, beliefs, and prejudices and your cultural heritage and identity.
- Confront biases and stereotypes.
- Do not judge: do not measure others' behavior against your beliefs and values.
- Keep an open mind: attempt to look at the world through other cultures' perspectives.
- Respect differences among people: each group has strengths and weaknesses.
- Appreciate inherent worth of diverse cultures, value them equally, and do not consider them inferior to one's own.
- Listen! Develop the ability to hear things that transcend language, and foster understanding of the client and his or her cultural heritage and the resilience that supports family and community that comes from within the culture.
- Be willing to learn: this requires interest in people's beliefs, values, and practices.
- Travel, read, and attend local ethnic and cultural events in the community.
- Develop an awareness and understanding for the complexities of the health care delivery system—its philosophy, problems, biases, and stereotypes—and become keenly aware of the socialization process that brings the care provider into this complex system.
- Be resourceful and creative: there are many ways to accomplish the same thing.
- Adapt your nursing interventions to suit different cultures and individuals.

Data from Grossman D: Enhancing your cultural competence, *Am J Nurs* 94(7):58, 1994; Spector RE: *Cultural diversity in health and illness,* ed 4, East Norwalk, Conn, 1996, Appleton & Lange.

---

ties. It is wise for health care providers who encounter clients from different cultural backgrounds with varied levels of assimilation into the host culture to use this approach; to gain insight into one's own values and assumptions encourages a perspective that respects the validity and tenacity of others' values and assumptions.

ASSESSMENT AND INTERVENTIONS

A cultural history is one way to develop communication, understand where the aged adult's health beliefs

Box 4-5	CULTURAL ASSESSMENT RELATED TO CLIENT'S HEALTH PROBLEM

The clinician may need to identify others who can facilitate the discussion of the client's problem(s).

1. How would you describe the problem that has brought you here? (What do you call your problem; does it have a name?)
   A. Who in the community and your family helps you with your problem?
2. How long have you had this problem?
   A. When do you think it started?
   B. What do you think started it?
   C. Do you know anyone else with it?
   D. Tell me what happened to them when dealing with this problem.
3. What do you think is wrong with you?
   A. What does your sickness do to you?
   B. How severe is it?
   C. What might other people think is wrong with you?
   D. Tell me about people who don't get this problem.
4. Why do you think this happened to you?
   A. Why has it happened to the involved part?
   B. Why do you get sick and not someone else?
   C. Will it have a long or short course?
   D. What do you fear most about your sickness?
5. What are the chief problems your sickness has caused you?
6. What do you think will help clear up this problem? (What treatment should you receive; what are the most important results you hope to receive?)
   A. If specific tests, medications are listed, ask what they are and do.
7. Apart from me, who else do you think can make you feel better?
   A. Are there therapies that make you feel better that I don't know? (May be in another discipline.)

Modified from Kleinman A: *Patient and healers in the context of culture: an exploration of the borderland between anthropology, medicine, and psychiatry,* Berkeley, 1980, University of California Press; Pfeifferling JH: A cultural prescription for mediocentrism. In Eisenberg L, Kleinman A, editors: *The relevance of social science for medicine,* Boston, 1981, Reidel.

lie, and provide quality care to ethnic elders. Given the necessary data, the nurse is then able to use this information to negotiate a clear understanding of problems and solutions with the client or the individual who is the appropriate support figure in the client's life. One must remember that great generational cohort and cultural differences may exist between practitioner and client. A comprehensive cultural assessment takes time. It is clear that not all situations allow for this, but even if it must be done bit by bit over time, it will be valuable to the caregiver in better understanding how to work with and within the culture of the client. Few tools or instruments can assist the nurse to elicit health care beliefs and at the same time identify to the nurse his or her own perceptions of the beliefs. Two such tools are offered here.

The Exploratory Models developed by Kleinman (1980) and Pfeifferling (1981) have helped caregivers obtain needed information in a culturally sensitive manner. An adaptation of these models for use in obtaining a meaningful cultural health assessment appears in Box 4-5. Evans and Cunningham (1996) offer specific assessment topics and items to be assessed in Table 4-2.

Generally, information obtained about minority elders concerns rituals, medications, and the types of practitioners they use, but activities of daily living, which are vital to and in the care of the aged, receive little attention (Gunter, 1991). To plan for immediate and long-term care, Gunter (1991) offers an assessment of personal care practices of ethnic elders. These are shown in Table 4-3. Some of these orientations literally cannot be expressed in another language and cannot be fully understood outside the culture.

CARING FOR THE ETHNIC ELDERLY

The term *ethno-geriatrics* has entered the vernacular of health care professionals; it is a specialty in which we hope to work sensitively with ethnic elders. The prediction of a significant increase in ethnic elders suggests that they will have considerable impact on service needs and delivery. It is expected that 41% of elders in California will be non-Euro-American by the year 2020. Other states will also experience this upsurge in non-Euro-American elders. In light of this, it will be impossible to think of ethnic elders as incidental to the elderly population as a whole.

When we speak of traditional versus nontraditional medicine, we must clarify these terms. Mitchell (1989) believed popular versus professional is more accurate. In most parts of the world there is a formal system of health care and the informal system of "folk medicine" or "popular medicine." Euro-Americans are no excep-

Table 4-2

Nursing Care for the Ethnic Elder

	Assessment	Interventions
Ethnicity	Number of years living in United States. Age at immigration (immigrant vs refugee). Degree of affiliation with ethnic group or assimilation to U.S. culture.	Be sensitive to historical events that influence elders' perception of self and authority of health care providers. Demonstrate respect for elder by using surname and providing care in a manner sensitive to cultural norms. Use of translator for exchange of health information.
Communication	English as primary or secondary language. Level of fluency. Barriers to communication such as sensory deficits, lack of privacy, distractions. Meaning of nonverbal gestures.	Document system for communicating basic needs between patient and staff. Provide patient access to sensory aids (glasses, hearing aids, pocket talkers). Eliminate background noise, and provide optimum lighting. Smile, offer gestures of assistance with basic needs (warm blanket, glass of water).
Health perception	Perception of health problem, causes, and prognosis. Response to pain, illness, and death.	Educate patient/family about disease process and medical treatments. Identify and document reasons for behavior. Develop system for identifying and rating pain.
Folk practices	Use of cultural healers, herbal medicines, alternative health practices and beliefs.	Obtain order for use of folk remedies as indicated. Educate patient regarding contraindications for folk remedy and discourage use if dangerous.
Health care system	Previous hospitalization experiences. Current hospitalization planned or emergency?	Encourage patient to express fears regarding hospitalization and treatments. Keep patient/family informed of patient's progress.
Religion	Spiritual practices and beliefs. Level of incorporation of spiritual practices into healing/dying process.	Allow privacy and space for religious articles and practices. Arrange for visit from spiritual leader. Refer patients to hospital chaplain. Document beliefs about death and burial.
Food	Beliefs regarding food and healing. Use of hot/cold system. Specific food preferences.	Obtain consultation with dietician. Incorporate food preferences into menu selection. Ask family to supply familiar foods. Document use of hot/cold practices as they relate to nursing care.
Social support	Current living situation. Support of family and/or community.	Encourage family participation in care. Encourage visits or phone calls with peers.
Decision making	Primary decision maker for health care. How does the patient make decisions? Who is needed for decisions?	Involve family when providing patient with health care information. Arrange for family conference if disparity exists between goals of patient, family, and/or health care team.
Discharge planning	Expectations for care after hospitalization and during future years of aging. Financial status that affects discharge planning and long-term health status. Ability of patient/family to support discharge needs.	Involve family in discharge planning. Obtain consult for social services. Refer patient to community resources for legal advice, transportation, meals, shopping, and emotional support.

From Evans CA, Cunningham BA: Caring for the ethnic elder, *Geriatr Nurs* 17(3):105, 1996.

Table 4-3

Areas of Assessment of Personal Care Practices of Minority Elderly

Activities of daily living	Coping strategies	Environment	Family or significant support	Attitudes toward caregivers/ professionals
Eating	Problem solving	Home	Availability	Preferences
Feeding	Stress	Housekeeping	Acceptance	Rejections
Nutrition	Pain/discomfort	Safety and support/		
Bathing	Loneliness	reassurance		
Dressing	Religion, prayer,	Institution		
Toileting	meditation	arrangements		
Continence		Artifacts		
Mobility/disability				

From Gunter LM: Cultural diversity among older Americans. In Baines EM, editor: *Perspectives on gerontological nursing,* Newbury Park, Calif, 1991, Sage.
This form may be used as a comparative assessment of minority elders.

tion. We quickly adopt one fad after another that we think may preserve health. The difference between our "popular medicine" and that of many ethnic elders is that theirs is steeped in tradition and ritual. Theirs is truly traditional, and ours is not. In all of health care, from whatever culture, we must recognize the power of the mind in healing and incorporate the significant beliefs and rituals in the pattern of health care if we hope to be successful. And we often discover scientifically that the folk remedies were indeed beneficial.

The basis for much folk medicine is and was purely making the most of whatever was available. We speak in the past tense because most ethnic elders have now incorporated Western medicine into their care and rarely rely totally on their traditional cures. However, they do often cling to some of these and supplement their professional care as they see fit. Separation of cultural beliefs from economic resources and educational background is exceedingly difficult, and additional "education" related to health care rarely changes individual habits and rituals (Chavira, 1989).

Some guidelines for dealing with ethnic elders who are using a mixture of Western and traditional methods to cure their ills are offered by Mitchell (1989) in Box 4-6.

Scott and Polacca (1995-1996) note that a definition of pathologic condition and diagnosis in one culture may be different in another culture. For example, mental illness may be seen as dysfunctional in one culture but normal or a spiritual phenomenon in another culture.

As consumers of health care, the minority elders increasingly are being cared for in the home, and providers must adapt strategies to the beliefs and culture of the individual if they hope to be useful. Nursing concerns must focus on their overall health care by assisting them to gain access to needed services. This is done by ascertaining affordability, efficacy, accessibility, and availability of information, client satisfaction, respect for their health beliefs, illness perspective, and informal support systems.

For many ethnic elders, life is viewed as a balance of energy and forces; intrusion into body systems and drawing off vital fluids are viewed with alarm. Also, the family and environment are intrinsic to the energy systems and must be considered. Thus we can understand how hospitals, diagnostic procedures, and other noxious elements that disturb the peace can be interpreted as producing more harm than good.

It is interesting that some racial differences are identified in drug metabolism (Zhou et al, 1989). For instance, blacks with hypertension do not respond to beta-blockers, and Chinese men are twice as sensitive to them as are whites. Studies have focused on hypertension because it is easy to measure.

Isoniazid rapidly inactivates in Native Americans, Asians, and blacks, but inactivation can be slowed to some degree by adding pyridoxine (vitamin B_6). It has been suggested that there are many other metabolic differences in ethnic groups that are not as easily identified (Goldstein, 1989; Giger, Davidhizar, 1991).

Box 4-6 GUIDELINES FOR IDENTIFYING A MIX OF WESTERN AND TRADITIONAL METHODS OF TREATMENT

- Realize that many ethnic elders do not have a concept of chronic illness that cannot be cured and will continually search for a method to alleviate the problem experienced.
- Determine what the problem is from the client's perspective: what does he or she think is wrong?
- What does the client think caused the problem?
- Does the client understand the treatment plan and how it relates to symptoms?
- Try to find out if the elder is supplementing prescriptions and what is the expected result.
- Alert the individual to signs of adverse reactions to treatment.
- Always try to discover the underlying logic of the client's belief.
- Incorporate folk medicine beliefs if they are not harmful.

Data from Mitchell F: *Folk beliefs and health practices of ethnic elders. Traditional and nontraditional medication use among ethnic elders.* Conference sponsored by Stanford Geriatric Education Center, San Jose, Calif, April 28, 1989.

Mexicans are prone to diabetes and blacks to hypertension. These conditions are usually considered to be fundamentally dietary problems, but they may not be. In other words, much is still unknown. As we work with ethnic elders, we are learning with them and about them. We are not the experts with all the answers.

Nurses should not attempt to change the client's beliefs. It is difficult if not impossible and usually is counterproductive. Negotiating options with the client is helpful. The nurse should attempt to preserve helpful beliefs and practices, accommodate beliefs that are neither helpful nor harmful from the point of Western medicine, or repattern harmful beliefs or practices (Jackson, 1993). If the nurse has little or no knowledge of a belief or practice, the nurse should study and evaluate it to determine its helpfulness or its potential harm. The nurse should also keep an open mind, learn about practices, encourage their use, and be flexible, creative, and persistent. In this way beliefs and practices can be preserved. Respectfully explaining concern about harmful client practices with the offer of possible alternatives may show the client that the nurse is considering the client's beliefs and practices. The client is less likely to be dissatisfied and not return for future care (Chrisman, 1992; Grossman, 1994).

Self-Care

Ethnic groups differ in their preferential methods of self-care and the extent to which they use medical care versus traditional healing methods and alternative health practices. Crisis lines/health advice lines to serve specific ethnic populations have proved effective when publicized well within the select group.

Coulton (1988) presented preliminary evidence regarding the use of medical care among blacks, Hispanics, and Eastern European immigrants. Osteoarthritis is present in 85% of individuals between 75 and 79 years of age and thus becomes a focus of self-care practices for many. Coulton found that Hispanics, although poorest and least educated, were most likely to use medical care and prescription drugs for joint symptoms. They also had more chronic health conditions and generally rated their health poorer than blacks or Eastern Europeans.

Implications of Ethnicity in Long-Term Care

Jones and van Amelsvoort Jones (1986) studied the interactions of nursing staff with groups of elderly persons in a long-term care facility to determine the nature of verbal interactions. Immigrants, Canadian-born elders, and American-born elders were included in the study. Although the study used only a sample of 41 elders, it is significant to alert us that we may unwittingly be influenced by subliminal stereotypes and discriminatory feelings. Tape recorders were discreetly placed to determine the nature of verbal content: commands, words, statements, and questions. Most of the verbalization (42%) was in the form of commands. The Canadian group was communicated with most frequently, the ethnic Europeans the least, and the American-born in between. Men were spoken to less frequently than women and more frequently were given commands. Relating to ethnic elders in long-term care may be more difficult than has been thought. The most important finding of this study was that during the entire 72 hours in which it was conducted, only a total of 850 words were spoken to all of the subjects—an average of 20 words per person! It appears that elders in this long-term care facility, of whatever ethnic background, were severely deprived of communication. For more meaningful care and communication Jones and van Amelsvoort Jones (1986) suggest the following to improve long-term care of ethnic elders:

1. Develop transcultural programs in facilities by incorporating existing community culture-specific activities, groups, and clubs.
2. Select roommates with careful consideration of individuals' needs and preferences.
3. Establish hiring policies whereby the ethnic roots of staff reflect the resident ethnic population as closely as possible.
4. Construct monocultural facilities where population demographics warrant.

Ethnicity may be one of the major elements of self-concept, and when age and institutionalization make one vulnerable, ethnic heritage becomes even more important. To the Chinese, achieving old age is a blessing and the elderly are held in high esteem. The old are respected and sought for advice. The family unit is expected to take care of its elder members, and thus there may be a reluctance to utilize long-term care even when badly needed.

Originally, the Japanese did not consider nursing home placement for elderly parents, but the modern nisei (second generation) and sansei (third generation) face the same dilemmas as others when caring for their elderly parents, despite issei (first generation) expectations of oya koko or "care for parents." Thus nursing home placement is becoming more common. Nursing homes specifically for the aged Japanese are rare. One does exist near Los Angeles, California, in which familiar traditions are maintained by Japanese staff.

The ethnic-cultural systemic framework of Orque et al (1983) uses the concepts of Maslow. Orque's system is holistic and comprehensive in scope and can be used to understand elders in any culture. The core of the system contains the basic human needs, around which revolve eight components—religion, art and history, value orientation, social groups and interactive patterns, language and communication process, healing beliefs and practices, family life processes, and diet. These are cyclic in nature because people are continually adapting to their environment. The extent to which each aspect of culture is reflected in meeting these needs depends on the individual's ethnic/cultural system. Although all the components are universal, the nuances of the components indicate the diversity that exists among groups or individuals.

Cultural diversity of physicians and nurses who are choosing geriatrics and long-term care is increasing. These providers of geriatric care are an increasingly heterogeneous cultural group. The countries from which these providers come vary from one part of the United States to another. Some large groups have come from the Philippines, Haiti, and India (Yeo, 1996-1997). The positive aspects of this trend are that they (1) may bring respect for the elder, found in other cultures and less in the youth-driven society of the American and (2) may have the language skills and understanding to better care for the elders and families of their own cultural background. The concerns are (1) the complexities of cross-cultural communications and decision making when second languages are used and (2) the use of cultural norms not well understood by each other.

The study of the uniqueness and individuality of each surviving elder is one of the most complex and intriguing opportunities of our day. Realistically it is almost impossible to become familiar with the whole range of clinically relevant cultural differences of older adults one may encounter, but to attempt to serve them holistically and sensitively is the most challenging opportunity.

INTEGRATING CONCEPTS

Family, religion, community, and history are important reference points for self-worth and identity for any ethnic group. Familial supports are variable among groups, social classes, and subcultures, yet the nuclear or extended family is the chief avenue of transmitting cultural values, beliefs, customs, and practices. The family provides orientation, stability, and sanctuary. In a simplistic sense we may say that Asians value familial piety; Hispanics, the extended family (compadres translates to co-parents); blacks, extended or fictive kin supports; and Native Americans, a system of kinship and line of descent.

Church or religiosity plays a major role in defining many cultures. Religion may function as a consistent experience that affords psychic support in the individual's life. In the black community, religion is a pervasive force and the place to instill self-determination toward change (Moriwaki, Kobata, 1983; Walls, 1992). The issei seek religious tradition in the face of aging and death (Kitano, 1969). Padilla and Ruiz (1976) note that Hispanics tend to seek Spanish-speaking clergy rather than mental health professionals when they have emotional problems.

The ethnic community (barrios, Nihonmachi, and Chinatown) serves as a buffer and a means of strengthening cohesiveness for elders and others of various cultural groups. Within the community, members are protected from discrimination and strange language and customs of the dominant society.

Changes are threatening the historic role of the aged and the traditional family. Economic independence and mobility of the younger members of the family are chipping away at the insulation afforded by the community. Intergenerational discontinuities of assimilation create a communication gap between the young and the old. Often the elderly are not proficient in the language of the dominant culture, and the younger members tend not to retain the language of their parents. This may cause isolation and estrangement between the oldest and youngest generations. Members of ethnic minorities are extremely vulnerable in old age. They may be devalued because of age and ethnicity. Attitudes and economic inequality contribute to their problems.

▶ **KEY CONCEPTS**

- Population diversity will continue to increase rapidly for many years. This suggests that nurses will be caring for a greater number of ethnic elders than in the past.
- Culture is a complex concept reflecting the interrelationship of many components.
- Culture, social status, and support systems are essential within cultural groups.

NANDA and Wellness Diagnoses

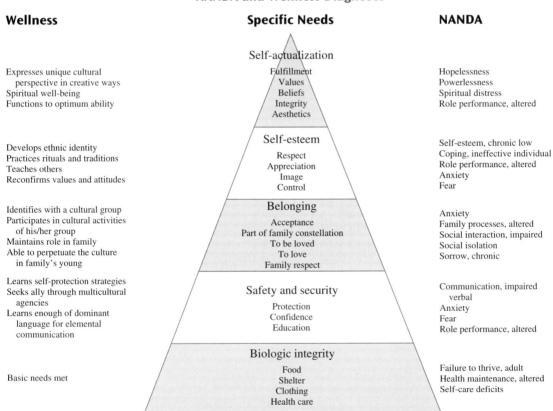

Wellness	Specific Needs	NANDA
	Self-actualization	
Expresses unique cultural perspective in creative ways	Fulfillment	Hopelessness
Spiritual well-being	Values	Powerlessness
Functions to optimum ability	Beliefs	Spiritual distress
	Integrity	Role performance, altered
	Aesthetics	
	Self-esteem	
Develops ethnic identity		Self-esteem, chronic low
Practices rituals and traditions	Respect	Coping, ineffective individual
Teaches others	Appreciation	Role performance, altered
Reconfirms values and attitudes	Image	Anxiety
	Control	Fear
Identifies with a cultural group	**Belonging**	
Participates in cultural activities of his/her group	Acceptance	Anxiety
Maintains role in family	Part of family constellation	Family processes, altered
Able to perpetuate the culture in family's young	To be loved	Social interaction, impaired
	To love	Social isolation
	Family respect	Sorrow, chronic
Learns self-protection strategies	**Safety and security**	
Seeks ally through multicultural agencies	Protection	Communication, impaired verbal
Learns enough of dominant language for elemental communication	Confidence	Anxiety
	Education	Fear
		Role performance, altered
	Biologic integrity	
	Food	Failure to thrive, adult
Basic needs met	Shelter	Health maintenance, altered
	Clothing	Self-care deficits
	Health care	

These are not all of the possible wellness or NANDA diagnoses that may be identified. The above are frequent examples of nursing diagnoses that should be considered when planning care for the older adult in whatever setting.

- Stereotyping negates the fact that significant heterogeneity exists within cultural groups.
- Family history, religion, and community are at the core of ethnic elders' self-worth.
- Health beliefs of various groups emerge from three general belief systems: biomedical, personalistic, and naturalistic.
- Nurses caring for ethnic elders must let go of their ethnocentrism before they can give effective care.
- Programs staffed by persons who reflect ethnic elders' background and speak their language are preferred by the elder.

▶ Activities and Discussion Questions

1. Discuss the various health care beliefs.
2. Explain the types of questions that would be helpful in assessing an elder's health problem(s).
3. What strategies would be helpful in planning care for ethnic elders?
4. List the elements that enable the nurse to develop cultural sensitivity and competency.
5. Formulate a nursing care plan utilizing wellness and NANDA diagnoses.

RESOURCES

Films

A Portrait of Older Minorities. AARP Fulfillment, 1909 K Street NW, Washington, DC 20049

Toto Le Hero. Triton Pictures (obtainable at local video stores). The reconstruction of an old man looking back on his life. Told primarily in flashbacks, the movie follows the key character from childhood through old age (90 minutes, color).

Responsive Health Care for Minority Elderly. A series of actual interviews demonstrates the need for health professionals working with elderly minority patients to expand the traditional concepts of assessment to include psychosocial, cultural, educational, economic, and environmental factors. Emphasized is the importance of integrating the patient's health care system, patient education, and preventive medicine. From Video Press, University of Maryland at Baltimore, School of Medicine, Suite 133, 100 Penn Street, Baltimore, MD 21201, (800) 328-7450, (410) 328-5497, or (410) 328-8471.

Triple Jeopardy (The Hispanic Elderly in the United States). Videocassette, 3/4 or 1/2 inch, $50; filmstrip version with cue signaled cassette, $30. Asociación Nacional Por Personas Mayores, National Association for Hispanic Elderly, 3325 Wilshire Boulevard, Suite 800, Los Angeles, CA 90010.

Barriers (Service Delivery to the Hispanic Elderly of United States). Videocassette, 3/4 or 1/2 inch, $50; filmstrip in either Spanish or English, $30. Asociación Nacional Por Personas Mayores, National Association for Hispanic Elderly, 3325 Wilshire Boulevard, Suite 800, Los Angeles, CA 90010.

Publication

A home care training manual, *Taking Care of Others: A Personal Guidebook for Home Care Workers.* Published by Chicago Coalition of Limited English Speaking Elderly (CLESE) in Arabic, Chinese, English, Korean, Polish, and Spanish. For information, contact CLESE, "Taking Care" Guidebooks, 327 S. LaSalle Street, Suite 920, Chicago, IL 60604. Development of the guides was funded by the Retirement Research Foundation.

Organizations

National Center on Black Aged (NCBA)
    1730 M Street NW, Suite 811
    Washington, DC 20020
National Asian Pacific Center on Aging
    Melbourn Tower, Suite 914
    1151 Third Avenue
    Seattle, WA 98101
    (800) 33-NACPA
National Hispanic Council on Aging
    2713 Ontario Road NW
    Washington, DC 20009
National Indian Council on Aging (NICOA)
    PO Box 2088
    Albuquerque, NM 87103

REFERENCES

Berman HJ: From the pages of my life, *Generations* 15(2):33, 1991.

Brislin RS, Pederson P: *Cross-culture orientation programs,* New York, 1982, Cardier.

Chavira J: *Common remedies used by Mexican-American elders: their source and use: traditional and nontraditional medication use among ethnic elders.* Conference sponsored by the Stanford Geriatric Education Center, San Jose, Calif, April 28, 1989.

Chrisman NJ: Culture-sensitive nursing care. In Patrick et al: *Medical-surgical nursing,* Philadelphia, 1992, Lippincott.

Coulton C: *Ethnicity, self-care and use of medical care among the elderly with joint symptoms.* Paper presented at the Veterans Hospital and Medical Center Gerontology Resource and Educational Center, Cleveland, Ohio, Oct 1988.

Evans CA, Cunningham BA: Caring for the ethnic elder, *Geriatr Nurs* 17(3):105, 1996.

Giger JN, Davidhizar RE: *Transcultural nursing,* St Louis, 1991, Mosby.

Goldstein M: *Overview of geriatrics and medications: traditional and nontraditional medication use among ethnic elders.* Conference sponsored by Stanford Geriatric Education Center, San Jose, Calif, April 28, 1989.

Grossman D: Enhancing your cultural competence, *Am J Nurs* 94(7):58, 1994.

Gunter LM: Cultural diversity among older Americans. In Bains EM, editor: *Perspectives on gerontological nursing,* Newbury Park, Calif, 1991, Sage.

Hooyman N, Kiyak HA: *Social gerontology,* Boston, 1996, Allyn & Bacon.

Jackson LE: Understanding, eliciting, and negotiating clients' multicultural health beliefs, *Nurse Pract* 18(4):30, 1993.

Jones D, van Amelsvoort Jones GM: Communication patterns between nursing staff and the ethnic elderly in long-term care facility, *J Adv Nurs* 11:265, 1986.

Kitano H: *Japanese Americans,* Englewood Cliffs, NJ, 1969, Prentice-Hall.

Kleinman A: *Patients and healers in the context of culture: an exploration of the borderland between anthropology, medicine, and psychiatry,* Berkeley, Calif, 1980, University of California Press.

Leininger M: *Transcultural nursing concepts: theories and practice,* New York, 1978, John Wiley & Sons.

Lipson JG: Cultural competent nursing care. In Lipson JG, Dibble SL, Minarik PA, editors: *Culture and nursing care: a pocket guide,* San Francisco, Calif, 1996, UCSF School of Nursing Press.

Meleis A et al: *Diversity, marginalization and culturally competent health care: issues in knowledge development,* Washington, DC, 1995, Academy of Nursing.

Mitchell F: *Folk beliefs and health practices of ethnic elders: traditional and nontraditional medication use among ethnic elders.* Conference sponsored by Stanford Geriatric Education Center, San Jose, Calif, April 28, 1989.

Moriwaki S, Kobata F: Ethnic minority aging. In Woodruff R, Birrin J, editors: *Aging,* ed 2, Monterey, Calif, 1983, Brooks/Cole.

Ochoco L, Shimamoto Y: Group work with the frail ethnic elderly, *Geriatr Nurs* 8:185, 1987.

Orque MS, Block B, Monrroy LSA: *Ethnic nursing care: a multicultural approach,* St. Louis, 1983, Mosby.

Padilla A, Ruiz R: Prejudice and discrimination. In Hernández CA, Haug MJ, Wagner NN, editors: *Chicanos: social and psychological perspectives,* ed 2, St Louis, 1976, Mosby.

Pfeifferling JH: A cultural prescription for medicentrism. In Eisenberg L, Kleinman A, editors: *The relevance of social science for medicine,* Boston, 1981, Reidel.

Scott RW, Polacca M: Staying in balance on the fourth hill of life: mental health and elderly Native Americans, *Dimensions* 2(4):1, 1995-1996.

Spector RE: *Cultural diversity in health and illness,* ed 4, East Norwalk, Conn, 1996, Appleton & Lange.

Spector RE: *Cultural diversity in health and illness,* ed 5, Upper Saddle River, NJ, 2000, Prentice Hall Health.

Walls CT: The role of church and family support in the lives of older African Americans, *Generations* 17(3):33, 1992.

Yeo G: Ethnogeriatrics: cross-cultural care of the older adult. In Geriatrics: a clinical care update, *Generations* 20(4):72, 1996-1997.

Zhou HH et al: Racial differences in drug response: altered sensitivity to and clearance of propranolol in men of Chinese decent as compared with American whites, *N Engl J Med* 320:565, 1989.

5

Developing the Life History

▶ **LEARNING OBJECTIVES**

Upon completion of this chapter, the reader will be able to:

- Relate the significance of the life story of an elder.
- Discuss the development of wisdom.
- Define the concept of life review.
- Specify the difference between *life story* and *life review*.
- Identify several possible legacies and discuss the importance to elders.

▶ **GLOSSARY**

Circumstantiality A speech pattern in which a person has difficulty separating relevant from irrelevant information while describing an event.
Eclectic Selecting the best from various sources.
Ideologic A body of ideas characteristic of an individual, group, or culture.

Life review A progressive return to consciousness of past troubling experiences.
Perseveration An involuntary persistence of the same verbal responses.

▶ **THE LIVED EXPERIENCE**

What a life I have had! I can remember when we thought the old Model T Ford was absolutely unbelievable, and that silly John tried driving it 35 miles an hour! And Maude almost broke her arm cranking hers one morning. Sometimes I think I should write it all down, but somehow I never get at it.

Lydia, age 90

Sometimes when Lydia begins talking about the old days, I get pretty bored hearing the same old stories again and again. I think I'll get one of those books about the century and take it to her the next time I see her. Maybe she will think of something else to talk about except the same old boring stories.

Jennifer, a home health care provider

THE LIFE STORY

The life story as constructed through reminiscing, journaling, psychotherapy, or guided autobiography has held great fascination for gerontologists in the last quarter century. The universal appeal of the life story as a vehicle of culture, a demonstration of caring and generational continuity, and an easily stimulated activity has held allure for many professionals. Each nurse who is allowed the privilege of hearing the life story of an el-

der is being given an incredible gift. Every life story is unique and whole within itself, and by virtue of these features, the most credible research investigations have followed somewhat of a Hiedeggarian hermeneutic phenomenologic (the detailed description and interpretation of the experience of existence in whatever way it has been lived, to describe, dissect, and attribute meaning) model. Chaudbury (1996) expresses this as the "container of lived experience."

The literature is vast, and some especially good sources for further study are cited in the Bibliography at the end of this chapter. The work of Haight and Webster (1995) is among the most comprehensive emanating from the nursing profession. Cole (1992) and Birren and Deutchman (1991) have also been active in seeking the life stories of elders.

Life History

An old person is a living history book, but unlike written history, the story remains flexible and changeable, similar to a kaleidoscope—each shift, however minor, in the person's self-esteem or interaction brings forth another pattern and colorful image. The most exciting aspect of working with the aged is being a part of the emergence of the life story: the shifting and blending patterns. Impatience with the early garrulous or tentative process may reduce the possibility of resolution in the resident and inspiration for the nurse. A memory is a gift to the nurse, a sharing of a part of oneself when one may have little else to give. The more personal memories are saved for persons who will patiently wait for their unveiling and who will treasure them.

Nurses should encourage details and elaboration, particularly when a story becomes repetitious. Of course, a lengthy recitation of a person's life history may be a boring affair. When the nurse finds boredom setting in, it may be helpful to confirm the feeling: "It sounds like life became pretty monotonous for you at that time," or "The small details of life may keep one from thinking of larger problems."

Creating a Life History

Becoming whole requires that one integrate all of life's remembered experience into a self-concept that sustains or enhances self-esteem and gives meaning to life as lived. Numerous geriatric nurses have used reminiscence, individually and in groups, as a therapeutic strategy to achieve these goals. Because it is such a natural function of many elders, it is one of the simplest and most enriching for elder and nurse. Working with the aged in the most mutually satisfying manner, regardless of the problems, requires some knowledge of the individual's life history. One's life history is a product of multiple histories and roles, intermingled with the life stories of intimates, friends, and acquaintances (Elder, 1974).

Development of a Life Line

Back and Bourque (1970) found it useful to have clients graphically represent life in terms of highs, lows, and plateaus experienced at various ages. Development of a life line in which each decade is marked and important events are placed at appropriate times and places is also useful; noting the feelings and impact of these events may create new understanding. The nurse may then match the client's life history against the graphic representation to gain a clearer understanding of events, patterns, and the impact of experiences. Development is facilitated by examining the peaks and valleys in one's life and recognizing patterns.

Geographic Memories

Geographic memories of places once lived, sketching or drawing these places, reexperiencing the effect of events attached to places—all are significant to stability of self (Rubinstein, 1996b). The social and physical settings of remembered episodes are potent. Developing a residential life history may have unexpected benefits in revealing surroundings significant to individuality and feelings of attachment and loss. During these activities the awareness of self is continually growing. This may also give a sense of the environmental supports that are particularly meaningful to the elder during translocation experiences.

Collective Histories

The use of a life history and reminiscence for older learners in group and classroom settings is useful in many ways. Often the collective memories are compiled into booklets that convey the experiences of a particular era or place. The reminiscing of elders attending classes in adult education or community college programs may reveal common connections between early life and present interests.

A group in Mill Valley, California, enrolled in a course for persons 60 years or older, "Tales Told From Memory," sponsored by the College of Marin's Emeritus College Program (Steinberg, 1996). There are many similar programs throughout the country.

Creation of Self Through Journaling

The central activity of human beings is creating meaning. Through the personal journal one can, in thoughtful reflection, discover meaning and patterns in daily events. The self becomes a coherent story with successive revisions as old events are reread and perceived in new contexts. "The self is not fixed, but rather is continuously reconstructed over time" (Berman, 1991, p. 38). This simply means that the thoughts one has at a given time reflect the present situation, as well as the past, and therefore are subject to change in content, as well as meaning, at later times.

The journals of certain elders provide rich descriptions of the interior lives of the authors. May Sarton (1984) and Florida Scott-Maxwell (1968) are two of the most well known. The study of their journals, as well as those of less well known and less articulate elders, assists nurses in understanding the inner experience of the aged and, perhaps, their own.

Seeking Wisdom

Pondering the life story touches not only the mind, but also the imagination and the unconscious depths in a person. As the life story comes to the surface of consciousness, new insights develop (Luke, 1982). The wisdom of old age develops from the ability to elicit new meanings from prior experience. Unlike ordinary knowledge, wisdom leads to an appreciation of reality in its grandest sense. The wisdom of old age involves a crisis of explanation in which the ordinary structures of thought are shaken and the meaning of life is reexamined. It may include the wisdom of questioning assumptions in the search for meaning. This is the rich, self-actualized experience that Maslow identifies as the highest level of human need.

REMINISCING

Reminiscing is an umbrella term that can include any recall of the past. Therapeutic reminiscing is the sharing of one's memories to achieve resolution, satisfaction, self-esteem, ego integrity, and clarification of identity issues. In this portion of the chapter the focus is primarily on the therapeutic aspects of reminiscence, life review, and legacy development.

Although it occurs from childhood onward, particularly at life's junctures and transitions, reminiscing has been viewed as a particularly adaptive activity during the last stage of life. Reminiscing cultivates a sense of security through recounting of comforting memories, belonging through sharing, and self-esteem through confirmation of uniqueness. Box 5-1 lists several ways that memories and reminiscences can be used effectively for the enrichment of the aging process. For the nurse, reminiscing is a tool of assessment and understanding.

There are many uses of reminiscence in addition to cognitive stimulation, reduction of depression, and psychologic restitution. The nurse can learn much about a resident's history, communication style, relationships,

---

Box 5-1	**SUGGESTED APPLICATIONS OF MEMORIES**

Life story recording for family
Legacy identification
   Products
   Contributions
   Qualities of character
   Talents
Scrapbooks
Photo albums
Establishment of rituals of security and comfort
Work history
Life's turning points—can be mapped out as a road
   map
Fantasy trips—follow the alternate road
Grief resolution
History of homes
Mapping of life geographically
Historic events—cohort identification
Life history of significant persons—why significant
Sensory stimulation
Development of memory chains
Inventory of significant items—why significant
   To whom would he or she like to give them?
Dietary history—significant foods of the past may
   stimulate appetite
Resolution of disappointment
Entertainment

---

coping mechanisms, strengths, fears, affect, and adaptive capacity by listening thoughtfully as the life story is constructed.

Caring nurses will want to protect themselves and others from boredom. The resident must learn how to relate in a manner that does not drive people away. On occasion the garrulous chatter is a warm-up for a life review. In those cases the nurse can facilitate meaning by directing the resident toward critical life passages; for example, the nurse might ask, "Mrs. J., tell me what it was like for you when you began school"; "Mrs. J., do you remember your first date?" or "Mrs. J., who was with you when your first child was born?"

The concept of reminiscence fits well with mechanisms of crisis and grief resolution and is a fitting tool to use to accomplish some of the work in these situations (see Chapters 25 and 26). Goals of reminiscing are related to enhancing one's identity, socialization skills, sense of continuity, and coping. There are many ways that the tendency to reminisce can be applied therapeutically: in socialization, remotivation, integration, and assessment and as part of reality orienta-tion (see Chapter 3 for discussion of groups). It is fairly well accepted that reminiscence is important to personal development and is also a very accessible ac-tivity with therapeutic implications, as can be seen in Box 5-2.

Life Review

Robert Butler (1963) first noted and brought to public attention the review process that normally occurs in the aged as the realization of one's approaching dissolu-tion and death creates a resurgence of unresolved con-flicts. Butler (1963) called this process *life review*. Psy-chotherapeutic reminiscence is akin to psychoanalysis and forms the conceptual basis for life review. Life re-view involves the review of remote memories (self-revelation), the expression of related feelings (cathar-sis), the recognition of conflicts (insight), and the relinquishment of viewpoints that are self-inhibiting (decathexis). Sometimes it increases depression. Parker (1995) found that life review occurs most fre-quently as an internal review of memories—an in-tensely private, soul-searching activity. It often occurs sporadically in a long-term trusted relationship. It oc-curs quite naturally for many persons during periods of crisis and transition. Butler and Lewis (1983) provide the following guidelines for the use of life-review therapy:

1. Be aware that mastery of the past is the basis for adaptation to the present.
2. Encourage any evidence of spontaneous life review.
3. Support the search for meaning, problem solving, and emotional gratification.
4. Use an eclectic approach.

> **Box 5-2 REMINISCENCE AS A DEVELOPMENTAL AND THERAPEUTIC STRATEGY**
>
> Maintain continuity.
> Extract meaning.
> Define and develop personal philosophy.
> Identify cycles and themes.
> Recapitulate learning and growth.
> Evolve identity.
> Provide insight and growth.
> Integrate and accept regrets and disappointments.
> Perceive universality.

5. Confront conflicts and anxieties regarding death, guilt, and dependency.
6. As a therapist, maintain the stance of a dependable confidant.

The psychologically disturbed elder may be reluc-tant or unable to reminisce fluently in dyadic or group situations. Self-view is often distorted, distressed, or suppressed. Some nurses are reluctant to stir the mem-ories of older persons who seem psychologically vul-nerable. We would not advocate confrontation or inter-pretation but, rather, exploration of the meanings and feelings relevant to the situation being shared. It is im-portant to determine how those feelings affect the per-son at present, as in the following situations:

- A particularly aggressive woman was the youngest of five sisters, and her anecdotes about her childhood help one to understand her sometimes abrasive ac-tions in the present.
- Another, as a small child in a drab, barren apartment, was sternly reprimanded for "playing with her food" while trying to express her artistic nature. She has difficulty now eating unless all foods on her plate are carefully separated.
- At 86 years old, one woman still remembers that she could never scrub the floor well enough to please her mother. She now frequently complains that the floors in her assisted living apartment are not clean enough.

When life review occurs during group reminiscing, it often produces anxiety or agitation in the individual. In that situation we would verbally validate the dis-comfort and move the focus to another group member by saying, "I can see this was a very difficult experience for you. When the group is over, I would like to spend a few minutes with you." Table 5-1 provides some guid-ance in dealing with difficult situations when using reminiscence in groups.

An effective life review would resolve (at least par-tially) some past disappointments in a manner that would hold significance for the present and future. For instance, a group of elders might indicate some regret about insufficient planning for retirement. Ideally, the group would remember the other, more pressing needs that at the time prevented them from making those plans. The goal would be for them to arrive at an ac-ceptance of their needs and motives then and now. When working with the elderly in a life-review process, it is important to have a clear understanding of goals:

1. Is the person reviewing the life course preparatory to letting go? If so, the main goal will be acceptance of what has been.

Table 5-1

Suggestions for Reminiscence Group Strategies

Patient selection	No more than five members Age cohorts Both sexes
Structure	Consistent place and time Frequent 30-minute meetings Co-leaders
Process	Connect specific events, things, and places common to group
Goals	Stimulate memory Enhance identity Raise self-esteem Increase socialization skills
Nurse's function	1. Provide a comfortable, mildly stimulating environment. 2. Select props that will stimulate memories. 3. Assist members by giving specific information, reminders, and clues. 4. Give praise and recognition for any participation.

2. Is the individual facing a major crisis in self-esteem or need? The goal will be to identify past coping strategies and, from those, gather strategies that will be currently effective. Evaluating times when one was effective will sustain confidence in future effectiveness.

3. Is the individual bound in a morass of regret? The goal will be to reenergize the person for present and future functioning by developing alternative views of past failures.

4. Is the individual suffering the effects of institutionalization? The goal will be to stimulate clear memories of what one has been and has accomplished to reaffirm uniqueness and individuality.

5. Has the person held long-standing grievances against significant others? The goal will be to explore the complexity of those relationships and provide opportunities for interpersonal resolution with the individuals involved.

When involved in life review, a person may get "stuck" and begin to sound very repetitious. Questions that may guide the individual away from perseveration and circumstantiality are as follows:

• What was most fearful (or difficult) about that experience?
• How would you have handled that event differently, knowing what you do now?

• If you could change your past, what would you do?
• What is the greatest lesson life has taught you?
• Who was most influential in your life? How did that person help you?
• If you could choose a time and place to live your life, when and where would it be?
• What were the major disappointments in your life?

These and many other exploratory statements will facilitate the life review. Do not ask if you are not prepared to listen carefully and without judgment or advice. It is usually helpful to begin with descriptions of events, since those are less threatening than sharing fears, failures, and feelings. During any interview it is important to comment on increasing evidence of anxiety and tension and ask if the interviewee wishes to continue, to sit quietly, or to be left alone. Guidelines for life-review therapy are provided in Box 5-3. Robert Butler (1995, p. xxi) says, "As one's life nears an end, the opportunity to confront lifetime conflicts and acts of omission and commission, which warrant guilt as well as opportunities for atonement, resolution, and reconciliation, is precious because this is the last opportunity one has."

Psychodrama and Life Review

Life review and reminiscence can be effectively implemented using the techniques of psychodrama (Stepath, Martin, 1987). Psychodrama emphasizes the reenact-

Box 5-3	GUIDELINES FOR LIFE-REVIEW THERAPY

1. Alert aged persons to the characteristics and normality of the life-review process.
2. Provide opportunities for aged persons to recapitulate events in their lives (e.g., "What has most influenced the course of your life?" "Who has most influenced the course of your life?").
3. Assist aged persons to view their life experiences in a broader or different context (e.g., "As you explain your regrets, can you think of other factors that contributed to those events?" "How would you have changed your life then?" "What factors influenced your course of action?" "What would you do differently now?").
4. Facilitate connections between past hopes, present events, and future expectations.
5. Be aware that the process may be carried out sporadically over several months. It is a painful examination of the past and is sometimes avoided.

Box 5-4	SPECIAL CHARACTERISTICS OF OLDER ADULTS

- Desire to leave a legacy provides a sense of continuity.
- "Elder" function is a natural propensity of the old to share with the young accumulated knowledge and experience.
- Attachment to familiar objects gives a sense of continuity; aids the memory; and provides comfort, security, and satisfaction.
- Change in the sense of time experienced as a sense of immediacy, of here and now, of living in the moment.
- Personal sense of the entire life cycle.
- Creativity, curiosity, and surprise may promote active and productive lives in the absence of disease and social problems.
- Feeling of consummation or fulfillment in life that brings "serenity" and "wisdom."

ment of troublesome memories that are consuming psychic energy and producing incongruence in an individual's self-concept.

Dreams and Life Review

Vignettes and fragments of unresolved issues embedded in the unconscious emerge not only in life review, but also in dreams. At times, one can clearly discern the resolution that is occurring in the dream process. In my early work with elders I (P.E.) observed that dreams, fantasies, and realities tended to overlap as one ages and that the boundaries blur in the telling of one's memories. Elders weave them into a whole. l am increasingly convinced that many dreams are natural healing mental processes. This may be a fruitful area to explore with an elder.

LEGACIES

A legacy is one's tangible and intangible assets that are transferred to another and that may survive the bequeather's mortality. Both giver and receiver are part of the concept of legacy; a recipient, individually or collectively, is essential (Kivnick, 1996; Frolik, 1996). Doers leave their products and live through them. Powerful figures are remembered in fame and infamy. The quiet, unobtrusive person survives in the memory of intimates and in family anecdotes. The intangible, nonmaterial legacy of our elders is embodied in the courage, wisdom, and insights that they show. The search for immortality seems to be the basic motivation for leaving a legacy. Characteristics of older adults significant to legacy development are seen in Box 5-4.

Throughout life, shared experiences provide satisfaction, but in the last years the identification of a legacy allows one to gain a clearer perspective on how one's existence has had enduring meaning. Old people must be encouraged to identify that which they would like to leave and whom they wish the recipients to be. This process has interpersonal significance and prepares one to leave the world with a sense of having truly lived. It can provide a transcendent feeling of continuation and ties with survivors. If transfers of significant items are made before death, the individual has the joy of seeing another appreciate treasured objects (Tobin, 1996). However, many families are reluctant to discuss the transfer of cherished belongings, as it brings one into direct awareness of the death of the elder.

Childless individuals are becoming more prevalent with each passing generation, and they must find a way to outlive the self through a legacy. Many choose a "social" legacy (Rubinstein, 1996a). Florence Nightingale would be one such person. The legacy of her thinking and accomplishments has influenced and will influence nurses for generations to come (Macrae, 1995).

Legacies are diverse and may range from memories that will live on in the minds of others to bequeathed

Box 5-5	EXAMPLES OF LEGACIES

Oral histories
Autobiographies
Shared memories
Taught skills
Works of art and music
Publications
Human organ donations
Endowments
Objects of significance
Written histories
Tangible or intangible assets
Personal characteristics such as courage or integrity
Bestowed talents
Traditions and myths perpetuated
Philanthropic causes
Progeny: children and grandchildren
Methods of coping
Unique thought: Darwin, Einstein, Freud, and others

fortunes. Box 5-5 is a partial list of legacies. The list is as diverse as individual contributions to humanity. Legacies are both generative and integrative. The activity involved in legacy identification reinforces integrity and life satisfaction. Certain questions, such as the following, may stimulate thoughts and discussions of legacies:

- Have you thought of writing your autobiography?
- What would you like to leave the younger generation?
- What contributions have you made in your life that make you particularly pleased?

Autobiographies/Oral Histories

Oral histories are gathered to pass traditions, significant episodes, and cultural history from one generation to the next. Oral histories are an organized approach to collecting the life stories of individuals who have been significant in some historic or important development. These often form special collections in particular libraries. Oral histories are influenced by gender, culture, history, social class and context, race, and ethnicity (Harrienger, 1996; Schuster, 1996). All come together to form a unique, never-to-be-reproduced individual or collective legend. An oral history from a grandparent will bring to life historical periods that have previously seemed sterile (Kivnick, 1996). Reaching out to the following generations in this way decreases self-

absorption and releases the "grand-generativity" that demonstrates the elder's care for the present and concern for the future (Kivnick, 1993).

Autobiographies may be a mix of letters, journals, and retrospective musings—generally part of an individual legacy. Everyone has a story to tell. Autobiographies and recorded memoirs can serve a transcendent purpose for those who are alone—and for many who are not. Nurses can encourage older people to write, talk, record, or express in other ways the story of their lives. Dying patients, too depleted to write, can express and order their memories through audiotapes that are then bequeathed to families according to the desires of the aged person. As long as one's story is captured, one remains alive in the minds of others. Sharing one's personal story creates bonds of empathy, illustrates a point, conveys some of the deep wisdom that we all contain, and connects us with our deepest human consciousness.

Collective Legacies

Each person is a link in the chain of generations (Erikson, 1963) and as such may identify with generational accomplishments. An old man may consider himself a significant part of a generation that survived the Great Depression. A middle-age man may identify with the generation that walked on the moon. The years of youthful idealism are impressed in one's memory by the political or ideologic climate of the time. That is the stage when one searches for a fit in the larger society. National and world events form part of one's generational identity. These events of importance affect the individual's satisfaction or dissatisfaction with the world passed on to the next generation. The nurse may ask, "Who were the great men of your time? Which ones were important to you? What events of your generation changed the world? What were the most important events you experienced?" Sometimes it is helpful to mention certain historic events and ask about the individual's reactions.

Legacies Expressed Through Others

There are many ways that one's legacy is expressed through the development of others: in a teaching/ learning situation or through mentorships, patronage, shared talents, and organ donations. Some examples may illustrate this type of legacy:

- An aged man cried as he talked of his grandson's great talent as a violinist. They shared their love for the violin, and the grandfather believed that he had genetically and personally contributed to his grandson's development as a musician.

* An older woman worried about preserving the environment for future generations, so she took young children on nature walks to stimulate their interest in birds, plants, and animals. She also donated land for a natural park.

Some creative works and research studies are evolving legacies, left to successive generations for continued modification and growth (Philip, 1995). In other words, one's legacy may be a product of his or her own thought, brought to fruition through someone else who may become an intermediary in the further development of the product or thought. A professor emeritus spoke of visiting his son in a distant state and hearing him expound ideas that had been partially developed by his father, the professor, before him. Thus people and generations are tied in sequential development.

People who amass a fortune and allocate certain funds for the endowment of artists, scientific projects, and intellectual exploration are counting on others to complete their legacy.

Developing a Legacy

The following are suggestions for assisting elders in identifying and developing their legacy:

1. Find out the older person's lifelong interests.
2. Establish a method of recording.
3. Identify recipients—either generally or specifically.
4. Record the person's legacy.
5. Distribute as planned.
6. Provide for systematic feedback of results to the person.

It is gratifying to the elderly if a legacy can be converted into some tangible form, ensuring that it will not be readily dismissed or forgotten. The following vehicles often serve that function:

Published summation of life work
Photograph albums, scrapbooks
Written memoirs
Taped memoirs (video or audio)
Artistic representations
Memory gardens
Mementos
Genealogies
Recorded pilgrimages

• • •

The greatest privilege a nurse has is to accompany an aged individual in the final journey of life (Cole, 1992). As each person confronts individual mortality, there is a need to integrate events and to then transcend the self. The human experience, the person's contributions, and the poignant anecdotes within the life story bind generations together, validate the uniqueness of each brief journey in this level of awareness, and provide the assurance that one will not be forgotten.

▶ KEY CONCEPTS

* In a rapidly changing society the shared life histories of elders provide a sense of continuity between the generations.
* The life history of an individual is a story to be developed and treasured. This is particularly important toward the end of life.
* Personal integration of life events through reminiscing facilitates acceptance of life as lived.
* Wisdom is achieved through integration, revision, and reconsideration of experiences and knowledge.
* Life review is the spontaneous recollection of guilt and disappointments and can be a growth experience when nonjudgmental, supportive persons are available.
* Establishing a legacy allows the individual to develop a sense of immortality and is a significant late-life task.

▶ Activities and Discussion Questions

1. Discuss the significance of the life story of one of your aged relatives, and talk about the significance to you and to the elder.
2. Discuss with your peer group the concept of wisdom and how it is shown.
3. Discuss the elements of life review that are different from ordinary remembering.
4. How would you encourage someone to record his or her life story?
5. Discuss your ideas about legacy, and define a legacy that you would like to leave to others.
6. Discuss your earliest memories and how they may or may not have shaped your life.

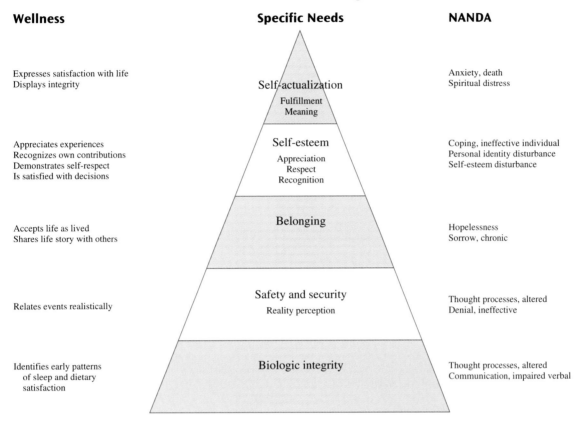

NANDA and Wellness Diagnoses

Wellness	Specific Needs	NANDA
Expresses satisfaction with life Displays integrity	Self-actualization Fulfillment Meaning	Anxiety, death Spiritual distress
Appreciates experiences Recognizes own contributions Demonstrates self-respect Is satisfied with decisions	Self-esteem Appreciation Respect Recognition	Coping, ineffective individual Personal identity disturbance Self-esteem disturbance
Accepts life as lived Shares life story with others	Belonging	Hopelessness Sorrow, chronic
Relates events realistically	Safety and security Reality perception	Thought processes, altered Denial, ineffective
Identifies early patterns of sleep and dietary satisfaction	Biologic integrity	Thought processes, altered Communication, impaired verbal

These are not all of the possible wellness or NANDA diagnoses that may be identified. The above are frequent examples of nursing diagnoses that should be considered when planning care for the older adult in whatever setting.

RESOURCES

Emil and Fifi: The Story of My Grandfather. An image of aging videotaped by a grandson of Emil Synek—a Czech playwright, journalist, and statesman—and Emil's constant companion, Fifi, a poodle (50 minutes). J. Rowe, Filmmakers Library, New York.

Giants of Time. Celebrates elders whose lives have already spanned two centuries and who are approaching their third (57 minutes). J. Rowe, Filmmakers Library, New York.

The Power of Memories: Creative Uses of Reminiscence (D14930). *Reminiscence: Reaching Back, Moving Forward* (D13186). Free from American Association of Retired Persons (AARP), PO Box 51040, Station R, Washington, DC 20091.

Fulfillment Reminiscence: Finding Meaning in Memories— Training Kit (D13403). Kit includes video, trainer's guide, and resource materials. Available for $30 from American As-

sociation of Retired Persons Program Resources Department, PO Box 51040, Station R, Washington, DC 20091.

Reminiscing: The game for people over 30
TDC Games Item 1110
1456 Norwood Drive
Itaska, IL 60143
(800) 292-7676

International Society for Reminiscence and Life Review
John Kunz, Program Manager
Center for Continuing Education/Extension
University of Wisconsin—Superior
Belknap & Catlin, PO Box 2000
Superior, WI 54880-4500
(715) 394-8469; (715) 394-8381 (fax)
e-mail: jkunz
http://staff.uwsuper.edu/reminisc/

REFERENCES

Back C, Bourque L: Life graphs: aging and cohort effects, *J Gerontol* 25:249, 1970.

Berman HJ: From the pages of my life, *Generations* 15(2):33, 1991.

Birren JE, Deutchman DE: *Guiding autobiography groups for older adults: exploring the fabric of life,* Baltimore, 1991, Johns Hopkins University Press.

Butler RN: The life review: an interpretation of reminiscence in the aged, *Psychiatry* 26:65-76, 1963.

Butler RN: Foreword. In *The art and science of reminiscing: theory, research, methods and applications,* Washington, DC, 1995, Taylor & Francis.

Butler R, Lewis M: *Aging and mental health: positive psychosocial approaches,* ed 3, St Louis, 1983, Mosby.

Chaudhury H: *Self and reminiscence of place: toward a theory of re-discovering selfhood in place-based reminiscence for people with dementia.* Paper presented at the meeting of the Gerontological Society of America, Washington, DC, Nov 19, 1996.

Cole TR: *The journey of life: a cultural history of aging in America,* Cambridge, UK, 1992, Cambridge University Press.

Elder G: *Children of the depression: social change in life experience,* Chicago, 1974, University of Chicago Press.

Erikson EH: *Childhood and society,* ed 2, New York, 1963, Norton.

Frolik LA: Legacies of possessions: passing property at death, *Generations* 20(3):9, 1996.

Haight B, Webster J: *The art and science of reminiscing: theory, research, methods and applications,* Washington, DC, 1995, Taylor & Francis.

Harrienger M: *Writing a life: the composing of grace.* Paper presented at the meeting of the Gerontological Society of America, Washington, DC, Nov 19, 1996.

Kivnick HQ: Everyday mental health: a guide to assessing life strengths, *Generations* 17(1):13, 1993.

Kivnick HQ: Remembering and being remembered: the reciprocity of psychosocial legacy, *Generations* 20(3):49, 1996.

Luke H: *The inner story,* New York, 1982, Crossroad.

Macrae J: Nightingale's spiritual philosophy and its significance for modern nursing, *Image J Nurs Sch* 27(1):8, 1995.

Parker RG: Reminiscence: a continuity theory framework, *Gerontologist* 35(4):515, 1995.

Philip CE: Lifelines, *J Aging Stud* 9(4):265, 1995.

Rubinstein RL: Childlessness, legacy and generativity, *Generations* 20(3):58-61, 1996a.

Rubinstein RL: *Feelings for the past: reminiscences about former residences.* Paper presented at the meeting of the Gerontological Society of America, Washington, DC, Nov 19, 1996b.

Sarton M: *At seventy: a journal,* New York, 1984, Norton.

Schuster E: *Transformative functions of life writing.* Paper presented at the meeting of the Gerontological Society of America, Washington, DC, Nov 19, 1996.

Scott-Maxwell F: *The measure of my days,* New York, 1968, Knopf.

Steinberg D: More than theater—an intergenerational connection, *Aging Today* 17(6):19, 1996.

Stepath S, Martin R: Psychodrama and life-review for the geriatric psychiatric patient (abstract). In *Proceedings of the third congress of the International Psychogeriatric Association* 3:107, Chicago, 1987.

Tobin S: Cherished possessions: the meaning of things, *Generations* 20(3):46, 1996.

BIBLIOGRAPHY

Bender M, Bauchham P, Norris A: *The therapeutic purpose of reminiscence,* Thousand Oaks, Calif, 1999, Sage.

Disch R: *Twenty-five years of the life review: theoretical and practical considerations,* New York, 1988, Haworth Press.

Edelman GM: *The remembered present: a biological theory of consciousness,* New York, 1989, Basic Books.

Haight B, Webster J: *The art and science of reminiscing: theory, research, methods and applications,* Washington, DC, 1995, Taylor & Francis.

Kaminsky M: *The uses of reminiscence: new ways of working with older adults,* New York, 1984, Haworth Press.

Kenyon GM, Randall WL: *Restorying our lives: personal growth through autobiographical reflection,* Westport, Conn, 1997, Praeger.

Moloney MF: A Heideggerian hermeneutic analysis of older women's stories of being strong, *Image J Nurs Sch* 27(2):104, 1995.

chapter 6

Communication Through Documentation

▶LEARNING OBJECTIVES

Upon completion of this chapter, the reader will be able to:

- Relate the purpose of the MDS 2.0.
- Specify several problems of data transfers from one facility to another.
- Describe advance directives and the nurse's role in dealing with them.
- Name the components of the Patient Self-Determination Act.
- Explain the reasons why documentation is critical to patient care.

▶GLOSSARY

Advance directives A legal declaration by a patient of the particulars of care desired during terminal illness. Must be signed, witnessed, and notarized.

Documentation As used in this chapter, written or electronically produced material specifying particulars of patient status, assessment, and plans of care.

Ombudsman A person who investigates and mediates patients' problems and complaints in relation to a hospital's services.

Protocol A written plan specifying procedures in a particular examination, in conduction of research, or in treatment of a particular condition.

Taxonomy As used in this chapter, the orderly classification of diagnoses based on categoric relationships.

▶THE LIVED EXPERIENCE

I can't remember when I didn't want to be a nurse, and what am I doing? Spending all my time at the computer or looking at and writing in charts! It seems like I spend more time documenting what I have done than I spend actually doing it. All this paperwork is a waste of my time.

Jane, Director of Nursing at Sweet Haven Nursing Home

Well, I don't know how we are going to manage financially if I can't accurately document the acuity of these residents. Jane doesn't seem to take it very seriously and sort of rushes through it. I guess I'll have to speak to her about it and impress its importance on her.

Harvey, Administrator of Sweet Haven Nursing Home

DOCUMENTATION

Communication through documentation is one of the most important issues in the present health care system. The economic survival of an agency, hospital, or health provider complex is directly dependent on the clarity and accuracy of documentation. Reimbursement levels are tied to recorded levels of patient acuity and progress. The concentrated efforts to obtain adequate funding for services provided have become more and more intense as pressures from every direction are focused on the need to subdue the galloping health care budget and control the excesses that have arisen in the last 40 years. I (P.E.) still remember my chagrin when as a young nurse I recorded that a patient "ate his dinner with relish." These flourishes were not appreciated then and are absolutely forbidden now. Student nurses are asked to report the progress of their patients but often are not allowed to chart, as they are inclined to be optimistic and indicate more progress in patient recovery than is realistic. This optimism may result in reduced reimbursement for the care of that patient. More and more, our data entries are circumscribed, leaving little latitude for incidental data that may be personally relevant in the care of one individual.

Economics and Influence of Medicare

Medicare regulations for reimbursement are stringent. The Health Care Financing Administration (HCFA) publishes regulations periodically for the operation of any Medicare-certified agency. Nurses in any organization are strongly advised to review the regulations applicable to the type of facility in which they are employed. These will outline the clinical documentation parameters for reimbursement, as well as criteria for coverage of services.

Home Care Restrictions

The providers (usually family) of the stable, chronically ill patient in the home can expect no reimbursement for their care and service (Rice, 1996). Reimbursement in home care depends on the individual being "home-bound, in the process of recovering from an illness or injury, unable to get about without assistance of supportive devices or another person" (Rice, 1996) (Box 6-1). To be covered, the services must be reasonable and require skilled nursing care.

Emergency Room Transfers

One of the most troublesome transfers of information is between the home or nursing home setting and the emergency room. Crises and quick decisions often result in inadequate or no information accompanying the elder to the emergency room. As soon as possible following a transfer, nurses involved in the transfer should make a concerted effort to call and provide information about the elder's prior status and needs. When individuals are admitted from the home, it is imperative that emergency room staff be informed of the elder's routine, capabilities, medications, and functional abilities before hospitalization. The home care nurse provider should discuss this with the family early on, particularly regarding conditions that may flare up and tend to require periodic hospitalizations. The family should be aware of trigger events that indicate the need for hospitalization. These should be written and given to the family or elder. Nurses are the holistic health care providers and are likely to have the most comprehensive information significant to an elder's needs. It is neglectful not to communicate this information.

Box 6-1   GUIDELINES FOR DOCUMENTING HOMEBOUND STATUS

Be as specific as possible. Indications of homebound status include:

1. Restricted mobility from disease process, such as unsteady gait, draining wounds, depressed immunity, or pain
2. Poor cardiac reserve, shortness of breath, or activity intolerance secondary to unstable or exacerbated disease process
3. Bed- or wheelchair-bound patients who require physical assistance to move any distance
4. Patients who require caregiver help with assistive devices such as a cane, walker, wheelchair, or other special device to leave home
5. Failure to thrive, low-birth-weight infants
6. A tracheostomy, abdominal drains, Foley catheter, or nasogastric tube that restricts ambulation
7. Home ventilator dependence or a patient who is unable to ambulate with portable oxygen
8. Psychotic ideation, confusion, or impaired mental status that restricts functional abilities outside of the home
9. A new colostomy or ileostomy that complicates ambulation
10. Fluctuating blood pressures or blood glucose levels that predispose patients to syncope or dizziness
11. Patients who cannot ambulate stairs or uneven surfaces without assistance of a caregiver
12. Five days or less postoperative eye surgery where the physician has restricted patient activity
13. Patients who are legally blind or cannot drive
14. Natural disasters or geographic barriers such as dirt roads or islands that restrict patient activity or make it a taxing effort for the patient to leave

From Rice R: *Home health nursing practice: concepts and application,* ed 2, St Louis, 1996, Mosby.

Protection of Patient Privacy

Computerization in documentation has introduced new problems into the communication of patient data. Each step forward in working toward consistency throughout the system of electronic recording is likely to be a step backward in protecting patient privacy. Although access may be protected by codes and passwords, one frequently sees a monitor with an array of confidential information visible as one walks through any hospital unit. Although we may not be able to solve some of the monumental problems of computer access, we can individually take responsibility for never leaving a monitor operational that is showing confidential data.

NURSING NEEDS ASSESSMENT INSTRUMENTS

The North American Nursing Diagnosis Association (NANDA) diagnoses, the Uniform Needs Assessment Instrument (UNAI), the Nursing Needs Assessment Instrument (NNAI), and the Minimum Data Set (MDS) are all designed to define a particular set of nursing behaviors that when applied will ensure that an individual is receiving appropriate nursing care.

Nursing Needs Assessment Instrument

The NNAI, derived from the UNAI, is a nursing needs assessment tool for adult hospitalized patients designed to identify on admission the data necessary for individuals to be returned to community care, a nursing home, or other provider (Holland et al, 1998). This tool is a significant step toward providing the continuity of care that we believe is critical to appropriate care (Table 6-1). Use of the NNAI has been found to contribute to efficient assessment and communication of discharge planning needs while conserving staff time. Uniformly transferring valid information to subsequent care providers is an overriding goal in the existing health care system as individuals are transferred from one setting to another more and more rapidly.

North American Nursing Diagnosis Association and Nursing Interventions Classification

The most usual taxonomy for nurses is derived from NANDA and the Nursing Interventions Classification (NIC). These have been used to categorize and delineate nursing interventions. They also form the basis for

---

Table 6-1

Domains and Subcategories of the Nursing Continuing Care Needs Assessment Form

COGNITIVE/BEHAVIORAL/EMOTIONAL STATUS

Anticipated level of consciousness on discharge
Cognition
Comprehension
Expression
Usual mode of communication
Emotional/behavioral factors

HEALTH STATUS

Perception of prognosis
Current health problems
Risk factors

FUNCTIONAL STATUS

Activities of daily living
Instrumental activities of daily living

FINANCES

Resources

ENVIRONMENTAL FACTORS IN POSTDISCHARGE CARE

Barriers
Need for assistive devices

ANTICIPATED SKILLED CARE REQUIREMENTS FOR DISCHARGE

Skin: pressure ulcer
Skin: wound care
Nutrition
Hydration
Respiratory
Cardiovascular
Elimination
Neuromusculoskeletal
Speech and language
Counseling
Patient/family education
Administration of medications
Coordination of care needed

MEETING CONTINUING CARE NEEDS

Summary of continuing care needs
Resource availability
Resource provider

From Holland DE et al: Continuity of care: a nursing needs assessment instrument, *Geriatr Nurs* 19(6):331, 1998.

specialized nursing practice. Because of the myriad care delivery models emerging, it has become exceedingly important to describe the practice parameters in various settings.

Developing a Taxonomy

A taxonomy is a classification system that clarifies natural relationships. The NANDA and NIC frameworks provide a basis for determining the taxonomy of specialized nursing practice. For example, Weis and Schank (2000) used these tools to order and classify the most frequent nursing diagnoses in parish nursing practice. In parish nursing it was found that health-seeking behavior, social isolation, grief, and pain were the most frequent diagnoses. These then provide fundamental bases for hospice nurses to begin planning basic care characteristic of this specialty. Developing a taxonomy for nursing specialties thus provides at the outset some knowledge of needs related to special situations. Clear definitions of purposes and a statement of mission may help develop a taxonomy appropriate for a particular agency or service model.

Standardized Protocols

Increasingly, standardized protocols are being developed and used to ensure thoughtfulness and consistency in decisions about complex problems. Many of these protocols provide suggestions for consideration at each step in the formulation of a nursing care plan. The NICHE project funded by the John A Hartford Foundation has developed a number of these (Abraham et al, 1999). These "best practice" protocols include sleep disturbances, nutritional problems, urinary incontinence, cognitive disturbances, fall prevention, pain management, and many others. (See the example of a sleep disturbance protocol in Box 6-2.) The intent is to make available a series of protocols that can be used nationwide to include components consistent with best practice. Many of these are suitable for computerization and ease of recording.

A protocol for enteral feeding was developed by nurses at the Providence Extended Care Center in Anchorage, Alaska. The implementation of the protocol enhanced staff collaboration and demonstrated ease of application. The critical elements in success of the protocol as identified by this group were clarity, measurable activities, and minimal documentation requirements that were tied to visible outcomes (Towner, Brown, 1996). This group concluded that they were able to set aside traditional habits as the protocol enhanced their practice and patient response. The move to use standardized protocols and decision-making trees can be a time-saver and, if used properly, can ensure

---

Box 6-2   NURSING STANDARD OF PRACTICE PROTOCOL: SLEEP DISTURBANCE IN ELDERLY PATIENTS

Assessment

Sleep-wake patterns:
- Inquire about usual times for retiring and rising, time for falling asleep; frequency and duration of nighttime awakenings; frequency and duration of daytime naps; daytime physical and social activity.
- Have person provide a subjective evaluation of the quality of sleep.

Bedtime routine/ritual:
- Inquire about activities performed by the individual before bedtime (e.g., personal hygiene, prayer, reading, watching TV, listening to music, snacks).

Intervention

Maintain normal sleep pattern:
- Maintain usual bedtime.
- Schedule nighttime activities to provide uninterrupted periods of sleep of at least 2-3 hours.
- Balance daytime activity and rest.
- Discourage daytime naps.
- Promote social interaction.

Support bedtime routines/rituals:
- Offer a bedtime snack or beverage.
- Enable bedtime reading or listening to music.
- Assist with aspects of personal hygiene at bedtime (e.g., a bath).
- Encourage prayer or meditation.

Evaluation

Objective evidence:
- Time required to fall asleep; should fall asleep within 30-45 minutes
- Time for awakening, at usual reported time
- Duration of sleep; patient should remain asleep for at least 4-hour intervals

Subjective evidence:
- Verbalizations about the quality and quantity of sleep (e.g., statements of difficulty falling asleep, frequent awakenings; having slept well, feeling well rested/refreshed; having an increased sense of well-being)

From Abraham I et al: *Geriatric nursing protocols for best practice,* New York, 1999, Springer.

Assessment	Intervention	Evaluation
Medications: • Obtain information relative to all prescribed and self-selected over-the-counter medications used by person, especially sleep-aids, diuretics, laxatives. • Determine types of medications and length of time used by person.	Avoid/minimize drugs that negatively influence sleep: • Pharmacologic treatment of sleep disturbances is treatment of last resort. • Discontinue or adjust the dose or dosing schedule of any/all offending medications. • Consider drug-drug potentiation. • Administer medications to promote sleep; give diuretics at least 4 hours before bedtime.	Objective evidence: • Time required to fall asleep; should fall asleep within 30-45 minutes • Time for awakening, at usual reported time • Duration of sleep; patient should remain asleep for at least 4-hour intervals
Diet effects: • Obtain information about the consumption of caffeinated and alcoholic beverages.	Minimize/avoid foods that negatively influence sleep: • Discourage use of beverages containing stimulants (e.g., coffee, tea, sodas) in afternoon and evening. • Encourage use of warm milk. • Provide snacks according to patient preference. • Generally discourage use of alcoholic beverages. • Decrease fluid intake 2-4 hours before bedtime.	Subjective evidence: • Verbalizations about the quality and quantity of sleep (e.g., statements of difficulty falling asleep, frequent awakenings; having slept well, feeling well rested/refreshed; having an increased sense of well-being)
Environmental factors: • Evaluate noise, light, temperature, ventilation, bedding.	Create optimal environment for sleep: • Keep noise to an absolute minimum. • Set room temperature according to patient preference. • Provide blankets as requested. • Use night-light as desired. • Provide soft music or white noise to mask the noise of hospital activity.	
Physiologic factors: • Evaluate breathing pattern with sleep, with attention to pauses. • Observe for periodic movement or jerking during sleep. • Inquire about usual position and the number of pillows used with sleep. • Note diagnoses of sleep disorders (e.g., sleep apnea or narcolepsy). • Note diagnoses of specific health problems that adversely affect sleep (e.g., congestive heart failure).	Promote physiologic stability: • Elevate head of bed as required. • Provide extra pillows per patient preference. • Administer bronchodilators, if prescribed, before bedtime. • Use medical therapeutics (e.g., continuous positive airway pressure machine) as prescribed.	
Illness factors: • Inquire about pain, affective disturbances (e.g., depression, anxiety, worry, fatigue, and discomfort).	Promote comfort: • Provide analgesia as needed 30 minutes before bedtime. • Massage back or foot to help patient relax. • Apply warm or cool compresses to painful areas as indicated. • Assist with progressive relaxation or guided imagery. • Encourage patient to urinate before going to bed. • Keep path to bathroom clear or provide bedside commode.	

consistent approaches to practice. Advanced nurse practitioners often work with protocols that involve sophisticated decision trees. These identify the numerous complexities that may arise in a given condition. Fig. 6-1 shows a model of a decision tree regarding urinary incontinence.

Minimum Data Set Version 2

Arising from the 1986 Institute of Medicine report highlighting deficiencies in long-term care, the nursing home reform law was put into place by the Omnibus Budget Reconciliation Act (OBRA) of 1987. Since that time, there have been many modifications, continual revisions, and updates of requirements in long-term care. These are intended to protect clients and staff and to

provide more accurate qualitative information and comprehensive assessment of clients. To accomplish this goal, the Omnibus Budget Reconciliation Act (OBRA) constructed the Minimum Data Set (MDS), which is to be completed within the first 24 hours after admission to a long-term care facility. The presently used Minimum Data Set version 2 (MDS 2.0) was developed, including the Resident Assessment Instrument (RAI), in 1993 to serve as an instrument to assess and measure needs and to ensure quality of care provided in a humane manner.

If the MDS is used as intended, the more exacting diagnoses, wholistic care plans, and emphasis on routine and periodic training of the hands-on providers (primarily nurse aides) result in individualized and

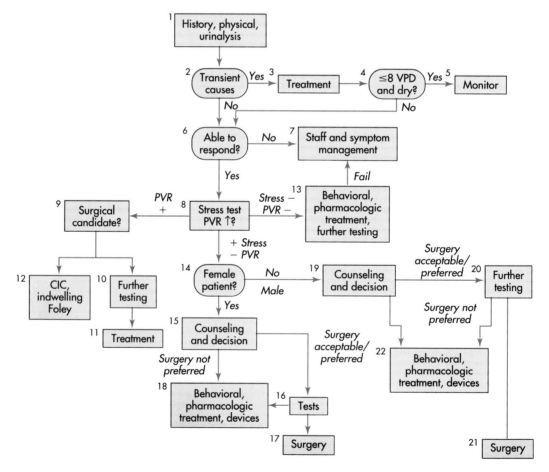

Fig. 6-1   Urinary incontinence in adults. *VPD,* Voids per day: *PVR,* post-void residual; *CIC,* clean intermittent catheterization. (From Urinary Incontinence Guideline Panel: *Urinary incontinence in adults,* Clinical Practice Guideline, AHCPR Pub No 92-0038, Rockville, Md, March 1992, US Department of Health and Human Services, Public Health Service, Agency for Health Care Policy and Research.)

comprehensive care. In addition, OBRA places emphasis on patients' rights and freedom from chemical and physical restraints. Requirements through the Occupational Safety and Health Agency (OSHA) for protection from tuberculosis, hepatitis, and human immunodeficiency virus (HIV) infection also benefit staff and patients. The consistency throughout the nation, made necessary by the OBRA requirements for the use of the MDS 2.0 in long-term care, has resulted in a marked improvement in care.

Resource utilization groups. The reimbursement mechanism is based on resource utilization groups (RUGs) that are generated when completing the MDS. These result in a fairly clear picture of patient acuity and the time needed for proper care. It is essential for providers to comply if they wish to have adequate reimbursement for the services they provide. Therefore nursing observations and especially those of nurse aides are extremely important. In all cases, unless it is recorded, it is assumed not to have been done.

In 1998 further impetus was added to the motivation for use of this instrument as retrospective reimbursement was entirely based on the RUG within which the elder's needs would place him or her (Morris et al, 1995). Although it has required an all-out effort of administration and line staff to institute the use of the MDS RUGs, it has been accomplished with great benefit to residents and administration alike. It is required that an initial RUG be established within the first 24 hours after resident admission and that a full MDS be in place for each resident within 2 weeks of admission. The major categories and measures are provided in Table 6-2. The importance of having these done in a timely manner cannot be overstated.

Resident assessment protocols. Resident assessment protocols (RAPs), a part of the MDS 2.0, are meant to guide an interdisciplinary team toward a comprehensive assessment of a resident's functional status and of the need for further assessment and planning related to functional status (Morris et al, 1995). This differs from clinical or medical status. The total situation of an individual is examined with the intent of helping the person to reach the highest practicable level of well-being—a driving goal of our entire textbook and desire for elders (Fig. 6-2).

Even though acute care is much less regulated than subacute and long-term care, the hope is that documentation of acute care will include all of the elements needed for the MDS 2.0 required in long-term care. Elements of the MDS are seen in the Condensed Minimum Data Set in Fig. 6-2. Interdisciplinary collabora-

tive sessions and a holistic approach to the patient are incorporated in the MDS, as indicated in the following:

1. Individualize care.
2. Learn who the patient was.
3. Recognize strengths.
4. Foster a sense of control.
5. Provide environmental cues for orientation.
6. Maintain patient's home schedule.
7. Adapt schedule of diagnostic procedures to patient's needs.
8. Communicate.
9. Time the giving of information.
10. Maintain consistency in staff-patient interactions.
11. Maintain activities of daily living (ADLs) using patient's coping resources and social supports.

Some contend that the MDS does not afford enough information, but the HCFA determined it best to compromise to some extent in the interest of having better participation. There are numerous software packages marketed by the major providers to help those in individual facilities to meet the requirements. Although there are probably some disadvantages to these mass-market approaches, the consistency in records from state to state and from one facility to another is most helpful. Efforts to establish more uniformity in records from the various levels of care are badly needed.

As elders move through the system more and more rapidly, it is imperative that documentation nationwide include similar components. The ideal would be for each elder, or responsible other, to have his or her own health care record and file copies in each appropriate venue. The MDS, if used to assess individuals throughout the continuum of care, would achieve consistency of care across care settings.

LEGALITIES

Not only is the economic survival of health care institutions dependent on accurate documentation, but the wishes of individuals regarding their care is often dependent on readily available documentation of their wishes regarding life extension, autopsy, cardiopulmonary resuscitation (CPR), organ donation, the agent of record (the individual who has power of attorney for health care), and disposition of the body in case of death.

Documentation involves the nurse in legalities that become particularly important as elders become incompetent or contrive to design a death with dignity. Proper recording of decisions regarding life-prolonging procedures is particularly important. Self-determination is at

Table 6-2

Minimum Data Set (MDS) Version 2.0 (Condensed) for Nursing Home Resident Assessment and Care Screening

Identification Information	Name, gender, birthday, Social Security and Medicare numbers, provider number, reasons for assessment
Background Information	Assessment reference date, date of entry, marital status, payment sources, responsible person, advance directives
Demographic Information	Date of entry, situation prior to admission, occupation, education, language, mental health history and conditions related to MR/DD status
Customary Routine	Usual cycle of daily events, eating patterns, functional ability in activities of daily living, social involvement
Cognitive Patterns	Consciousness, memory, recall ability, decision-making skills, delirium, disordered thinking, changes in cognitive status
Communication/Hearing Patterns	Hearing, communication devices/techniques, modes of expression, speech clarity, ability to understand, changes in communication or hearing
Vision Patterns	Vision, specific limitations/difficulties, visual appliances
Mood and Behavior Patterns	Indicators of depression, anxiety, sad mood, mood persistence, mood changes, behavioral symptoms, changes in behavioral symptoms
Psychosocial Well-Being	Sense of initiative/involvement, unsettled relationships, past roles
Physical Functioning and Structural Problems	Activities of daily living (ADL) self-performance: bed mobility, transfer, walking/locomotion, dressing, eating, toileting, personal hygiene, bathing, range of motion, modes of transfers, modes of locomotion, functional and rehabilitation potential, changes in ADL function
Continence in Last 14 Days	Self-control categories, bowel continence, bladder continence, bowel elimination pattern, appliances and programs, changes in urinary continence
Disease Diagnoses	Diseases, infections, other diagnoses
Health Conditions	Problem conditions, pain symptoms, pain site, accidents, stability of conditions
Oral/Nutritional Status	Oral problems, height and weight, weight changes, nutritional problems, nutritional approaches, parenteral or enteral intake
Oral/Dental Status	Oral status and disease prevention, tooth decay, disintegration; buccal cavity exam; dentures, bridges, missing teeth
Skin Condition	Ulcers, type of ulcers, history of unresolved ulcers, other skin problems or lesions, skin treatments, foot problems and care
Activity Pursuit Patterns	Time awake, time involved in activities, preferred activity settings, general activity preferences, prefers change in daily routines
Medications	Number of medications, new medications, injections, days received the following medications (antipsychotic, antianxiety, antidepressant, hypnotic, diuretic)
Special Treatments And Procedures	Treatments, procedures and programs; intervention programs for mood, behavior, cognitive loss, nursing rehabilitation/restorative care, devices and restraints, hospital stays, emergency room visits, physician visits, physician orders, abnormal lab values
Discharge Potential And Overall Status	Discharge potential, overall change in care needs
Resident Participation In Assessment	Resident, family members, significant other

the core of protecting patients within the medical system. Some physicians are unaware of or ignore patients' advance directives, and families often refuse to discuss these issues with the elder. Nurses are likely to be the best informed regarding patients' wishes. Nurses are in the role of patient advocate.

Advance Directives

The Patient Self-Determination Act (PSDA), under which the durable power of attorney (DPA) for health care (DPAHC), the living will (LW), and the directive to the physician (DTP) are subsumed, is an all-important law. All agencies that receive Medicare and Medicaid funds are mandated to disseminate PDSA information to their clients (Mezey et al, 1994; Berrio, Levesque, 1996; Mezey, 1996). Hospitals and long-term care facilities are responsible for providing written information at the time

of admission about the individual's rights under law to refuse medical and surgical care and to initiate this in a written advance directive. Health maintenance organizations (HMOs) and home health care agencies are required to do the same at the time of membership enrollment or before the patient comes under the care of the agency. Hospices are obliged to inform patients of their self-determination rights on the initial visit (Berrio, Levesque, 1996; Mezey, 1996; Parkman, 1996). An advance directive protocol is provided in Box 6-3, pp. 80-81.

Durable Power of Attorney

A DPA enables an individual to appoint a trusted person as "attorney in fact." It gives the person named the power to represent the elder in all legal matters. This should be carefully considered in later life, and it should be entered into with complete understanding of the risks and benefits (MacKay, 1992). In 1979 the

Text continued on p. 81.

PROCEDURES FOR COMPLETING THE RESIDENT ASSESSMENT PROTOCOLS (RAPs)

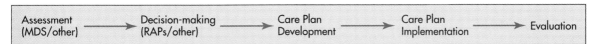

Assessment (MDS/other) → Decision-making (RAPs/other) → Care Plan Development → Care Plan Implementation → Evaluation

The Resident Assessment Protocols (RAPs) are used to assess conditions identified by the Minimum Data Set (MDS) triggering mechanism. The goal of the RAPs is to guide the interdisciplinary team through a structured comprehensive assessment of a resident's functional status. Functional status differs from medical or clinical status in that the whole of a person's life is reviewed with the intent of assisting that person to function at his or her highest practicable level of well-being. Going through the RAI process will help staff set resident-specific objectives in order to meet the physical, mental and psychosocial needs of residents.

4.1 What are the Resident Assessment Protocols (RAPs)?

The MDS alone does not provide a comprehensive assessment. Rather, the MDS is used for preliminary screening to identify potential resident problems, strengths, and preferences. The RAPs are problem-oriented frameworks for additional assessment based on problem identification items (triggered conditions). They form a critical link to decisions about care planning. The RAP Guidelines provide guidance on how to synthesize assessment information within a comprehensive assessment. The Triggers target conditions for additional assessment and review, as warranted by MDS item responses; the RAP Guidelines help facility staff evaluate "triggered" conditions.

There are 18 RAPs in Version 2.0 of the RAI. The RAPs in the RAI cover the majority of areas that are addressed in a typical nursing home resident's care plan. The RAPs were created by clinical experts in each of the RAP areas.

The care delivery system in a facility is complex yet critical to successful resident care outcomes. It is guided by both professional standards of practice and regulatory requirements. The basis of care delivery is the process of assessment and care planning. Documentation of this process (to ensure continuity of care) is also necessary.

The RAI (MDS and RAPs) is an integral part of this process. It ensures that facility staff collect minimum, standardized assessment data for each resident at regular intervals. The main intent is to drive the development of an individualized plan of care based on the identified needs, strengths and preferences of the resident.

Fig. 6-2 Resident assessment protocols. (Modified from *Minimum Data Set [MDS] Version 2.0 for Nursing Home Resident Assessment and Care Screening,* Form 1728HH, Des Moines, Iowa, 1995, Briggs Corporation.)

Continued

RESIDENT ASSESSMENT PROTOCOL TRIGGER LEGEND FOR REVISED RAPS (FOR MDS VERSION 2.0)

Resident _____   Numeric Identifier _____

Key:
- ● = One item required to trigger
- ❷ = Two items required to trigger
- ★ = One of these three items (Psychotropic Drug Use), plus at least one other item required to trigger
- ●★ = Psychotropic Drug Use triggered only when at least one of the three items (O4a, O4b, O4c) identified by ★ apply
- (a) = When both ADL triggers present, maintenance takes precedence

Proceed to RAP Review once triggered

Column legend (1–18):

1. Delirium
2. Cognitive Loss/Dementia
3. Visual Function
4. Communication
5A. ADL-Rehabilitation
5B. ADL-Maintenance Trigger A (a) / ADL-Maintenance Trigger B (a)
6. Urinary Incontinence and Indwelling Catheter
7. Psychosocial Well-Being
8. Mood State
9. Behavioral Symptoms
10A. Activities Trigger A (Revise)
10B. Activities Trigger B (Review)
11. Falls
12. Nutritional Status
13. Feeding Tubes
14. Dehydration/Fluid Maintenance
15. Dental Care
16. Pressure Ulcers
17. Psychotropic Drug Use
18. Physical Restraints

MDS 2.0 ITEM AND DESCRIPTION		CODE	1	2	3	4	5A	5B	6	7	8	9	10A	10B	11	12	13	14	15	16	17	18	ITEM
B2a	Short term memory	1		●																			B2a
B2b	Long term memory	1		●																			B2b
B4	Decision making	1,2		●																			B4
B4	Decision making	3		●		●																	B4
B5a-B5f	Indicators of delirium	2	●																		●★		B5a-B5f
B6	Change in cognitive status	2	●																		●★		B6
C1	Hearing	1,2,3				●																	C1
C4	Understood by others	1,2,3				●																	C4
C6	Understand others	1,2,3		●		●																	C6
C7	Change in communication	2																			●★		C7
D1	Vision	1,2,3			●																		D1
D2a	Side vision problem	√			●																		D2a
E1a-E1p	Indicators of depression, anxiety, sad mood	1,2									●												E1a-E1p
E1n	Repetitive movement	1,2																			●★		E1n
E1o	Withdrawal from activities	1,2								●													E1o
E2	Mood persistence	1,2									●												E2
E3	Change in mood	2	●																		●★		E3
E4aA	Wandering	1,2,3										●			●								E4aA
E4bA-E4dA	Behavioral symptoms	1,2,3										●											E4bA-E4dA
E5	Change in behavioral symptoms	1										●											E5
E5	Change in behavioral symptoms	2	●																		●★		E5
F1d	Establishes own goals	√								●													F1d
F2a-F2d	Unsettled relationships	√								●													F2a-F2d
F3a	Strong id, past roles	√								●													F3a
F3b	Lost roles	√								●													F3b
F3c	Daily routine different	√								●													F3c
G1aA	Bed mobility	1					●																G1aA
G1aA	Bed mobility	2,3,4					●													●			G1aA
G1aA	Bed mobility	8					●													●			G1aA
G1bA-G1jA	ADL self-performance	1,2,3,4					●																G1bA-G1jA
G2a	Bathing	1,2,3,4					●																G2a
G3b	Balance while sitting	1,2,3																			●★		G3b
G6a	Bedfast	√																		●			G6a
G8a,b	Resident, staff believe capable	√					●																G8a,b
H1a	Bowel incontinence	1,2,3,4																		●			H1a
H1b	Bladder incontinence	2,3,4							●														H1b
H2b	Constipation	√																			●★		H2b
H2d	Fecal impaction	√																			●★		H2d
H3c,d,e	Catheter use	√							●														H3c,d,e
H3g	Use of pads/briefs	√							●														H3g
I1i	Hypotension	√																			●★		I1i
I1j	Peripheral vascular disease	√																		●			I1j
I1ee	Depression	√																			●★		I1ee
I1jj	Cataracts	√			●																		I1jj
I1ll	Glaucoma	√			●																		I1ll
I2j	UTI	√																●					I2j
MDS 2.0 ITEM AND DESCRIPTION		CODE	1	2	3	4	5A	5B	6	7	8	9	10A	10B	11	12	13	14	15	16	17	18	ITEM

Form 1729HH BRIGGS, Des Moines, IA 50306 (800) 247-2343 PRINTED IN U.S.A.

MDS 2.0 RAP TRIGGER LEGEND
MDS 2.0 10/18/94N

Fig. 6-2, cont'd   See legend on p. 77.

Resident's Name:	Medical Record No.:

1. Check if RAP is triggered.
2. For each triggered RAP, use the RAP guidelines to identify areas needing further assessment. Document relevant assessment information regarding the resident's status.
   - Describe:
     - Nature of the condition (may include presence or lack of objective data and subjective complaints).
     - Complications and risk factors that affect your decision to proceed to care planning.
     - Factors that must be considered in developing individualized care plan interventions.
     - Need for referrals/further evaluation by appropriate health professionals.
   - Documentation should support your decision-making regarding whether to proceed with a care plan for a triggered RAP and the type(s) of care plan interventions that are appropriate for a particular resident.
   - Documentation may appear anywhere in the clinical record (e.g., progress notes, consults, flowsheets, etc.).
3. Indicate under the *Location of RAP Assessment Documentation,* column where information related to the RAP assessment can be found.
4. For each triggered RAP, indicate whether a new care plan, care plan revision, or continuation of current care plan is necessary to address the problem(s) identified in your assessment. The Care Planning Decision column must be completed within 7 days of completing the RAI (MDS and RAPs).

A. RAP Problem Area	(a) Check if Triggered	Location and Date of RAP Assessment Documentation	(b) Care Planning Decision—check if addressed in care plan
1. DELIRIUM			
2. COGNITIVE LOSS			
3. VISUAL FUNCTION			
4. COMMUNICATION			
5. ADL FUNCTIONAL/ REHABILITATION POTENTIAL			
6. URINARY INCONTINENCE AND INDWELLING CATHETER			
7. PSYCHOSOCIAL WELL-BEING			
8. MOOD STATE			
9. BEHAVIORAL SYMPTOMS			
10. ACTIVITIES			
11. FALLS			
12. NUTRITIONAL STATUS			
13. FEEDING TUBES			
14. DEHYDRATION/FLUID MAINTENANCE			
15. ORAL/DENTAL CARE			
16. PRESSURE ULCERS			
17. PSYCHOTROPIC DRUG USE			
18. PHYSICAL RESTRAINTS			

B. _____

1. Signature of RN Coordinator for RAP Assessment Process

2. ☐☐ – ☐☐ – ☐☐☐☐
   Month   Day   Year

3. Signature of Person Completing Care Planning Decision

4. ☐☐ – ☐☐ – ☐☐☐☐
   Month   Day   Year

TRIGGER LEGEND

1 - Delirium	7 - Psychosocial Well-Being	13 - Feeding Tubes
2 - Cognitive Loss/Dementia	8 - Mood State	14 - Dehydration/Fluid Maintenance
3 - Visual Function	9 - Behavioral Symptoms	15 - Dental Care
4 - Communication	10A - Activities (Revise)	16 - Pressure Ulcers
5A - ADL-Rehabilitation	10B - Activities (Review)	17 - Psychotropic Drug Use
5B - ADL-Maintenance	11 - Falls	18 - Physical Restraints
6 - Urinary Incontinence and Indwelling Catheter	12 - Nutritional Status	

Fig. 6-2, cont'd   See legend on p. 77.

| Box 6-3 | GERIATRIC NURSING STANDARD OF PRACTICE |

I. Background
  A. Decisions about stopping treatment are more prevalent among the elderly. The elderly compose 73% of deaths each year. Health care professionals can improve the end-of-life decision making for elderly patients by encouraging the use of advance directives.
  Advance directives have three functions:
    1. To allow individuals to provide directions about the kind of medical care they do or do not want if they become unable to make decisions or communicate their wishes.
    2. To provide guidance for health care professionals and families as to how to make health care decisions that reflect the person's wishes should that person be unable to make decisions.
    3. To provide immunity for health care professionals and families from civil and criminal liability when health care professionals follow the advance directive in good faith and respect the applicable state statute regarding advance directives.
  B. Advance directives are of two types: durable power of attorney for health care (also called a health care proxy) and living will.
    1. A *durable power of attorney* allows an individual to appoint someone, called a health care proxy, agent, or surrogate, to make health care decisions for him or her should he or she lose the ability to make decisions or communicate his or her wishes.
    2. A *living will* provides specific instructions to health care providers about particular kinds of health care treatment an individual would or would not want to prolong life. Living wills are often used to declare a wish to refuse, limit, or withhold life-sustaining treatment when an individual is unable to communicate.
  C. Nurses can make a difference in whether a patient completes an advance directive:
    1. Patients uniformly state that they want more information about advance directives.
    2. Patients want nurses (and doctors) to approach them about advance directives.
    3. Fewer than 20% of Americans have completed an advance directive.
    4. Patients who are non-white, have less education, or are from lower income levels are less likely to have executed an advance directive. These patients are also the most likely to state that they were not approached to discuss end-of-life decisions.
II. Assessment parameters
  A. All patients (with the exception of patients with PVS, severe dementia, or coma) should be approached soon after their admission to determine if they have a living will or if they have designated a proxy.
  B. All patients, regardless of their demographic characteristics such as age, gender, religion, socioeconomic status, diagnosis, or prognosis should be approached to discuss advance directives.
  C. Discussions about advance directives should be translated into the patient's preferred language to enable all patients to get information about advance directives.
  D. Patients who have been determined to lack capacity to make other decisions may still have the capacity to designate a proxy or make health care decisions. Decision-making capacity should be determined for each individual based on whether the patient has the ability to make the specific decision in question.
  E. If a living will or proxy has *not* been executed:
    1. Give the patient written information about advance directives.
    2. Have a conversation with the patient about advance directives.
    3. Help the patient to execute an advance directive if requested.
    4. Place a completed document in the patient's chart and make it available to the attending physician/nurse and health care proxy.
  F. If a living will has been completed or proxy *has* been designated:
    1. Is that document easily available on the patient's chart and located near the patient (i.e., not in the records department)?
    2. Does the attending physician/nurse know of its existence and have a copy? Did the attending physician/nurse review the document to ascertain if the stated wishes still reflect the patient's wishes?
    3. Does the designated health care proxy have a copy of the document?
    4. Has the document been recently reviewed by the patient, attending physician/nurse and the proxy?
  G. Oral advance directives (verbal directives) are allowed in some states if there is clear and convincing evidence of the patient's wishes. Clear and convincing evidence can include evidence that the patient has a significant relationship with the health care provider or the wish was repeated over time. Legal rules surrounding oral advance directives vary by state.

From Mezey M, Bottrell MM, Ramsey G: Advance directives protocol: nurses helping to protect patients rights, *Geriatr Nurs* 17(5):204-210, 1996.
PVS, Persistent vegetative state.

| Box 6-3 | GERIATRIC NURSING STANDARD OF PRACTICE—cont'd |

III. Care strategies
  A. Open the discussion about advance directives with patients and families. Nurses can assist patients and families trying to deal with end-of-life care issues.
  B. Patients who may be reluctant to discuss their own mortality or accept their current health situation may be willing to discuss these issues with a nurse if not a doctor.
  C. Assess each patient's need for and ability to cope with the information provided. Patients from other cultures may not subscribe to Western notions of autonomy, but that does not mean that these patients do not want this information or that they would not have conversations with their families if the issue was discussed by their nurse.
  D. Be sensitive to race, culture, ethnicity, and religion when discussing end-of-life care issues. A patient's feelings about these issues can substantially influence decisions to complete an advance directive.
  E. Race, culture, ethnicity, and religion may impact the health care decision-making process, and nurses should be mindful of these but always treat the patient as an individual, not as a class of persons.
  F. Be sensitive to each patient's fears about his or her own mortality and involve other professionals, including clergy, if desired by the patient in discussions about advance directives.
  G. Respect each person's right not to complete an advance directive.
  H. Inform patients that you will not abandon them or provide substandard care if they elect to formulate an advance directive.
  I. Know the hospital's method of resolving conflicts between family members and the patient or patient/family and care providers. This may include consultation from social work or the patient advocate or bringing the issue to the hospital ethics committee.
  J. Notify the appropriate persons if you are unable to provide care should the patient's wishes conflict with your beliefs.
IV. Evaluation of expected outcomes
  To determine if practice regarding discussions of advance directive has changed, note whether:
  A. The percentage of patients asked about advance directives in the hospital increased.
  B. All charts note whether the patient does not have an advance directive.
  C. When a patient has an advance directive, the advance directive is included in the patient's chart.
  D. The number of nurses and other staff who are comfortable and satisfied with the role of advance directives in patient care decisions increased.
  E. More staff were asked to assist patients in executing advance directives.

Commissioners on Uniform State Law (a federally appointed commission) adopted the Uniform Durable Power of Attorney that will survive a person's incapacity (Cohen, 1987). The DPA can be drawn up to include specific legal capacities within a specified period of time, or it may be broad and have no time limits. The principal may also express the intent to have the power of attorney survive the incompetency or incapacity of the principal. One can also draft a DPA that does not take effect until the principal becomes incapacitated. Such durable powers are called *spring powers* (Gilfix, 1987). The DPA can be regarded as a substitute for a funded revocable trust or as an alternative to court-oriented procedures such as conservatorship and guardianship (Cohen, 1987). A few states give the "attorney in fact" the power to make health care decisions through a document known as the *durable power of attorney for health care (DPAHC).*

Durable Power of Attorney for Health Care

The DPAHC, or health care proxy, is a legal, notarized, or witnessed document by which an individual can express his or her wishes regarding care in acute illness and in dying. The proxy authorizes someone of the individual's choosing (a proxy) to make medical decisions for him or her in case he or she is unable to do so. The proxy may be next of kin, friend, significant other, or in some cases a conservator appointed by the court (Delong, 1995; Berrio, Levesque, 1996; Mezey, 1996; Weenolsen, 1996). Many states have their own forms for the execution of a DPAHC. The forms are available from many agencies, including the state medical association and personal physicians. A resource list of agencies is provided under Resources at the end of this chapter. An example of one state's DPAHC, or health care proxy, appears in Fig. 6-3.

MY MEDICAL DIRECTIVE	SITUATION A	SITUATION B	SITUATION C
This Medical Directive shall stand as a guide to my wishes regarding medical treatments in the event that illness should make me unable to communicate them directly. I make this Directive, being 18 years or more of age, of sound mind, and appreciating the consequences of my decisions.	If I am in a coma or a persistent vegetative state and, in the opinion of my physician and two consultants, have no known hope of regaining awareness and higher mental functions no matter what is done, then my goals and specific wishes—if medically reasonable—for this and any additional illnesses would be:	If I am near death and in a coma, and, in the opinion of my physician and two consultants, have a small but uncertain chance of regaining higher mental functions, a somewhat greater chance of surviving with permanent mental and physical disability, and a much greater chance of not recovering at all, then my goals and specific wishes—if medically reasonable—for this and any additional illness would be:	If I have a terminal illness with weeks to live, and my mind is not working well enough to make decisions for myself, but I am sometimes awake and seem to have feelings, then my goals and specific wishes—if medically reasonable—for this and any additional illness would be:

*In this state, prior wishes need to be balanced with a best guess about your current feelings. The proxy and physician have to make this judgment for you. |

SITUATION A
☐ Prolong life; treat everything
☐ Attempt to cure, but reevaluate often
☐ Limit to less invasive and less burdensome interventions
☐ Provide comfort care only
☐ Other *(please specify):*

SITUATION B
☐ Prolong life; treat everything
☐ Attempt to cure, but reevaluate often
☐ Limit to less invasive and less burdensome interventions
☐ Provide comfort care only
☐ Other *(please specify):*

SITUATION C
☐ Prolong life; treat everything
☐ Attempt to cure, but reevaluate often
☐ Limit to less invasive and less burdensome interventions
☐ Provide comfort care only
☐ Other *(please specify):*

Please check appropriate boxes:

Each situation (A, B, C) has columns: I want. | I want treatment tried. If no clear improvement, stop. | I am undecided. | I do not want.

1. **Cardiopulmonary resuscitation** (chest compressions, drugs, electric shocks, and artificial breathing aimed at reviving a person who is on the point of dying). — *Not applicable* (A, B, C)

2. **Major surgery** (for example, removing the gallbladder or part of the colon). — *Not applicable* (A, B, C)

3. **Mechanical breathing** (respiration by machine, through a tube in the throat).

4. **Dialysis** (cleaning the blood by machine or by fluid passed through the belly).

5. **Blood transfusions or** blood products. — *Not applicable* (A, B, C)

6. **Artificial nutrition and hydration** (given through a tube in a vein or in the stomach).

7. **Simple diagnostic tests** (for example, blood tests or x-rays). — *Not applicable* (A, B, C)

8. **Antibiotics** (drugs used to fight infection). — *Not applicable* (A, B, C)

9. **Pain medications,** even if they dull consciousness and indirectly shorten my life. — *Not applicable* (A, B, C)

Fig. 6-3 Durable power of attorney for health care. (Copyright © 1995, Linda L. Emanuel and Ezekiel J. Emanuel.)

Autopsy in an Advance Directive

Advance directives may include the individual's wishes regarding autopsy. For some this is an insignificant consideration, but for others it may be very important. Individuals are rarely approached regarding autopsy, and more than 50% of the time it is not mentioned to the family after the death of a loved one. There is little to be gained by the physician in promoting autopsies, and the number done consistently decreases.

The informed and sensitive nurse will discuss it with the client and advocate for the client's wishes in this respect. Some elders consider this to be a final

SITUATION D

If I have brain damage or some brain disease that in the opinion of my physician and two consultants cannot be reversed and that makes me unable to think or have feelings, *but I have no terminal illness,* then my goals and specific wishes—if medically reasonable—for this and any additional illness would be:

☐ Prolong life; treat everything
☐ Attempt to cure, but reevaluate often
☐ Limit to less invasive and less burdensome interventions
☐ Provide comfort care only
☐ Other *(please specify)*:
_____

SITUATION E

If I ...
(Describe a situation that is important to you and/or your doctor believes you should consider in view of your current medical situation):

☐ Prolong life; treat everything
☐ Attempt to cure, but reevaluate often
☐ Limit to less invasive and less burdensome interventions
☐ Provide comfort care only
☐ Other *(please specify)*:
_____

SITUATION F

If I am in my current state of health (describe briefly):_____
_____
_____

and then have an illness that, in the opinion of my physician and two consultants, is life threatening but reversible, and I am temporarily unable to make decisions, then my goals and specfic wishes—if medically reasonable—would be:

☐ Prolong life; treat everything
☐ Attempt to cure, but reevaluate often
☐ Limit to less invasive and less burdensome interventions
☐ Provide comfort care only
☐ Other *(please specify)*:
_____

I want.	I want treatment tried. If no clear improve- ment, stop.	I am undecided.	I do not want.
	Not applicable		
	Not applicable		
	Not applicable		
	Not applicable		
	Not applicable		
	Not applicable		

I want.	I want treatment tried. If no clear improve- ment, stop.	I am undecided.	I do not want.
	Not applicable		
	Not applicable		
	Not applicable		
	Not applicable		
	Not applicable		
	Not applicable		

I want.	I want treatment tried. If no clear improve- ment, stop.	I am undecided.	I do not want.
	Not applicable		
	Not applicable		
	Not applicable		
	Not applicable		
	Not applicable		
	Not applicable		

Fig. 6-3, cont'd See legend on opposite page.

contribution that they can make to the knowledge about a certain disease or condition. An important consideration is that autopsy is also a method of quality control that ensures that misdiagnosis is recognized. Interestingly, even with all of the sophisticated diagnostic technologies we now have, autopsy confirms about a 10% error rate, which has remained constant for over 40 years.

Nurse's Role and Advance Directives
Mezey (1996) discusses barriers that hinder elders from dictating desires regarding control of their medical care

(Box 6-4). The nurse serves as the most accessible re-source when a person needs knowledge and under-standing of the PSDA. The question often arises re-garding the wishes of the cognitively impaired. In a small study of older patients who were diagnosed as de-mented by standard tests, 30% were found to possess the mental ability to understand the nature of a health care proxy and designate a relative as their decision maker. Twenty-seven percent of the group were able to express their preference for or against a do-not-resuscitate (DNR) option; 21% could do both a DNR and health care proxy (Schmitt, 1996). Although this is a limited study, the implication is that even impaired el-ders should not be excluded from making their wishes known in executing an advance directive.

The nurse must also ascertain proper disposition of the advance directive when it is completed. For the pa-tient who enters a facility with a directive, the nurse needs to determine that it is current and contains direc-tives reflective of the person's present choices. The doc-ument must be readily available to caregivers.

<table>
<tr><td>**Box 6-4**</td><td>**BARRIERS TO COMPLETION OF ADVANCE DIRECTIVES FOR THE ELDERLY**</td></tr>
</table>

Inability to speak English
Religious/ethnic affiliation
Memory
Inability to concentrate
Eyesight
Hearing
Print size of document/reading material
Family structure and support
Procrastination
Dependence on family to make decisions
Lack of knowledge about directives
Difficult topic to discuss
Waiting for physician to initiate discussion
Physician waiting for patient to initiate dis-
    cussion
Belief that a lawyer is needed for completion
    of forms
Fatalism or the acceptance of "will of God"
Fear of signing away life
Fear of being untreated

Modified from Mezey M: Advance directives protocol: nurse's helping to protect patient's rights, *Geriatr Nurs* 17(5), 1996; and Berrio MW, Levesque ME: Advance directives: most patients don't have one. Do yours? *Am J Nurs* 96(8):25, 1996.

The nurse needs to be aware of the types of direc-tives that are legally recognized in the state in which the nurse practices and the form used by the organiza-tion in which he or she is employed. Terminology asso-ciated with directives must also be investigated; for example, the term *surrogate* is not necessarily inter-changeable with *proxy* or *agent* (Weenolsen, 1996). In addition, the nurse must know how a directive is ac-complished. Elders in long-term care facilities usually need two witnesses for their directive, one witness be-ing the ombudsman from the department of aging, who serves as a patient advocate.

It is not unusual that necessity requires the timing of executing an advance directive to be concurrent with hospitalization, which sometimes interferes with judg-ment. Ideally, a values assessment will be made at a comfortable time for the elder—indicating what the el-der holds important in his or her life and how this re-lates to his or her desires for health care and quality of life. Does the elder want measures to be taken to pro-long life at all costs, or does the elder wish for a natural death if the alternative may mean prolonged mainte-nance on machines? Are there any persons the elder feels comfortable with who can act as a proxy to ensure that the elder's wishes will be carried out? Answers to these questions are helpful when the elder's wishes are being discussed. The discussion should include the family and perhaps the clergy and friends, before a di-rective is completed, to identify if those who are to be involved are comfortable with the decisions and will adhere to the directive. The nurse can help the elder un-derstand treatments that are available to sustain life and the implications of such interventions as resuscitation efforts (CPR), intubation, and artificial nutrition, as well as the technical terms associated with them.

Organ Donation

In several states professionals are required by law to discuss organ donation with dying individuals or their family members, and documents must reflect that the discussion has taken place. Because this is a recent re-quirement and one of which many professionals are un-aware, nurses are often in a dilemma. Educational ef-forts about organ procurement have traditionally been aimed at nurses, and the extraordinarily high levels of support among nurses imply the considerable success of these efforts. In many settings there are organ pro-curement specialists available who are specially trained to discuss the issues with individuals and families. When this is done with respect and sensitivity, families often feel some comfort in knowing that something of their loved one will go on and that there is some small gain in their loss.

Consent for Research

Consent for research leads to another set of issues regarding consent, particularly since Alzheimer's disease is one of researchers' major interests in the geriatric patient. Ideally, a living will or advance directive for health care would designate the willingness of an individual to participate in research, but realistically this is rarely the case. Patients with a diagnosis of senile dementia or psychosis may be incompetent in some respects but not in all (Sansone, Schmitt, 1996). Specific alterations of the consent process to obtain the patient's consent are suggested:

1. Make the material more readable.
2. Tailor the information to the needs of the patient.
3. Allow patients to review the material for a longer time than usual before determining competence to consent.
4. Use teaching, review, and testing regarding the patient's ability to understand material.
5. Develop rapport with the patient and encourage questions.
6. Involve the patient's family in the consent process. They may use language more familiar to the patient and make the material more understandable to the patient.

Almost two decades ago, the National Institute on Aging (NIA) established a task force to design a set of guidelines that might be helpful in the review of research protocols concerning senile dementia of the Alzheimer type (SDAT). When these were established, Melnick et al (1984) specifically addressed the fifth guideline, the determination of a subject's capacity for understanding a specific protocol. These authors state that consent should not be based on overall competency, because an individual may retain the capacity to consent but lack the capacity to manage his or her affairs in some other respects. This has been confirmed in studies by Sansone and Schmitt (1996).

Rights of Patients

Patients' rights in institutions of all types are mandated by federal and state laws and the Constitution, as are the rights of the general population. Legal rights vary according to the setting and individual competency. Rights in institutions are to be posted in a place visible to all and are to be reviewed with the individual soon after admission to a facility. In some settings, because of the difficulty of enforcement, rights are often not respected or protected.

Nursing responsibilities are (1) to ensure that the patient has seen, read, and/or understands the rights; (2) to document explicitly when and why any rights may be temporarily suspended; (3) to observe and record observations attesting to the individual's ability or inability to manage daily affairs; and (4) to be sure the patient's status is reviewed at appropriate time intervals (these vary from one state to another) and that he or she obtains legal assistance in presenting his or her defense. The rights of patients are enforced largely because of the integrity of nurses and our willingness to act as patient advocates.

Role of Ombudsman

Advocacy organizations for nursing home residents began flourishing between 1975 and 1979. Their various activities include complaint resolution, confrontation, and/or negotiation with nursing homes, community education, legal intervention, and legislative reform. *Ombudsman* as the term is used today most commonly denotes the nursing home advocate who is prepared to deal squarely but sensitively with the realities of a nursing home resident's life. An ombudsman must view the resident's problem as impartially as possible and act as advocate but not in an adversarial role with the nursing home administration.

In addition to acting as advocate, the ombudsman often locates appropriate resources and links residents with them, trains friendly visitors, provides a clearinghouse for problems or complaints, gives legislative updates, and provides assistance in conducting family councils and resident councils. The ombudsman must also assist families in transferring or discharging patients from a nursing home to another setting. The ombudsman is concerned about maintaining good relationships with nursing home personnel.

Ways that a nursing home can ensure a more collaborative long-term care ombudsman program are mandated by the Older Americans Act (OAA). Each state must have an Office of the State Ombudsman to which all substate programs report. Models may vary to reflect the needs and conditions within the state. Nursing home and board-and-care residents must have direct and immediate access to an ombudsman when needed for protection and advocacy. Netting et al (1992) studied and reported the type of complaints registered nationwide through state agency offices in 1990. The largest number (38,100) were about care issues such as abuse, neglect, poor care, poorly trained staff, and poorly dressed patients. The second largest area of complaint was against administration for understaffing, inadequate laundry procedures, roommate conflicts, and other items (21,500). The third area of complaint was for denial of rights, violation of privacy, and lack of grievance procedures (18,700). Given these patient concerns, it is clear that professional nurses must remain alert to their advocacy role in institutions. Nurses need to be aware of the procedure for filing a complaint against a nursing home. Some may wish to do so and will need the support of the legal system and other nurses in the advocacy of humane care for clients.

1. A complaint about practices, procedures, physical conditions, or quality of care in a nursing home is initially a request to the state health department to inspect a particular home and determine if a violation exists. Any person may file such a request simply by writing a letter. The letter should specifically detail the incidents of concern. However, even vague complaints such as lack of attention will be investigated. Numbers to call can be found in the telephone book.
2. Copies of licensing surveys are available to the public through the facilities licensing section of each state. They will show the violations that have been noted.
3. Copies of regulations are available through the state publications office. These will provide a basis for measuring violations.

Nursing Roles and Legalities

A relatively new role as legal nurse consultant emerged in the 1980s. In the past 5 to 7 years it has developed considerably. The American Association of Legal Nurse Consultants (AALNC) was organized in 1989 and has grown to include 1400 members with 23 local chapters. The organization supports, provides education, and markets the role. National conferences include current legal issues and updates on medical research, practice, and procedures (Mason, 1994).

Legal nurse consultants function in a variety of ways in independent consulting practice or are hired as expert witnesses in their clinical specialty. They may provide summaries related to allegations; identify standards of care in issues related to causation and damage; or collaborate with an attorney in preparing legal pleadings, trial briefs, and depositions. As this role is further developed, the profession will more fully realize the significance of documentation as more and more records are subjected to a detailed analysis by nurse experts.

• • •

Documentation begins whenever a client enters the health care system, sometimes even before the client is seen. Done correctly, this begins the process of discharge planning. It is not something that can be adequately patched together on the day of discharge from one level of care or a particular facility. Most important, in the case of elders, is a baseline functional assessment before the present incident and a thorough assessment of progress or decline after the current episode (Kresevic, Mezey, 1997). Continuity of care means that any individual in whatever providing institution will have an accountable team that will coordinate efforts, preplanned discharge goals, and a transfer of information that allows for continuation of care without interruption of important elements. Although this seldom exists at present, it is an abiding goal and is the model in which nursing has the most influence. Communication through accurate documentation that follows an individual's path through the health care system will do much to improve the care of our elders. In summary, communication through documentation has become critical to ensure patients' rights, adequate care, and the economic survival of providers.

> ## KEY CONCEPTS

- Documenting patient status and needs accurately in a format usable from one care facility to another is critical to good patient care.
- Standardized protocols for patient evaluation are integral to consistent determination of patient acuity and appropriate reimbursement.
- A nursing diagnosis taxonomy increases attention to holistic patient care.
- Advance directives are critical protection of patient rights and dictate wishes for end-of-life care.
- Electronic documentation of patient information raises questions regarding privacy.

▶ Activities and Discussion Questions

1. Discuss the origins and purpose of the MDS 2.0.
2. Discuss problems you have experienced with incomplete data or poor documentation in a health facility.
3. Discuss the elements that would be important to you when determining your own advance directives.
4. Discuss the components of the Patient Self-Determination Act.
5. Explain the reasons why documentation is critical to patient care.

RESOURCES

Health Care Advance Directives PFS302 (795) D15803. Available from the American Association of Retired Persons, 601 E Street NW, Washington, DC 20049.

American Bar Association
Commission on Legal Problems of the Elderly
1155 E. 69th Street
Chicago, IL 60673
(202) 662-8690

Mathy Mezey, Institute Director
John A. Hartford Foundation, Geriatric Nursing Education Center
New York University, School of Education, Division of Nursing
429 Shimkin Hall, 50 W. 4th Street
New York, NY 10012
(212) 998-5337; 212-995-4770 (fax)

MDS 2.0; *The Long Term Care Facility Resident Assessment Instrument (RAI) User's Manual.* Obtain copies from Briggs Health Care Products, Customer Service Department, (800) 247-2343.

MDS Coordinator
Center on Long Term Care
Health Standards and Quality Bureau
Health Care Financing Administration
7500 Security Boulevard
Baltimore, MD 21244-1850

REFERENCES

Abraham I et al: *Geriatric nursing protocols for best practice,* New York, 1999, Springer.

Berrio MW, Levesque ME: Advance directives: most patients don't have one. Do yours? *Am J Nurs* 96(8):25, 1996.

Cohen E: Durable powers of attorney: an overview, *Aging Connection* 8(2):8, 1987.

Delong MF: Caring for the elderly. V. Managing end of life issues, *NurseWeek* 8(9), 1995.

Gilfix IM: Legal planning is essential for Alzheimer's victims, *Senior Spectrum* 6(12):5, 1987.

Holland DE et al: Continuity of care: a nursing needs assessment instrument, *Geriatr Nurs* 19(6):331, 1998.

Kresevic DM, Mezey M: Assessment of function: critically important to acute care of elders, *Geriatr Nurs* 18(5):1216-221, 1997.

MacKay S: Durable power of attorney for health care: is DPAHC the best advance directive for patients residing in long-term care facilities? *Geriatr Nurs* 13(2):99, 1992.

Mason M: Nurse on the case, *Adv Pract Nurse,* p 2, spring/summer 1994.

Melnick V, Dubler N, Weisbard A: Clinical research in senile dementia of the Alzheimer type: suggested guidelines addressing the ethical and legal issues, *J Am Geriatr Soc* 32(7):531, 1984.

Mezey M: Geriatric nursing standard of practice protocol: advance directives—nurses helping to protect patient rights, *Geriatr Nurs* 17(5):208, 1996.

Mezey M, Ramsey GC, Mitty E: Making the PSDA work for the elderly, *Generations* 18(4):13, 1994.

Morris JN, Murphy K, Nonemaker S: *Long term care facility resident assessment instrument (RAI) user's manual,* Des Moines, 1995, Briggs Health Care Products.

Netting FE, Paton RN, Huber R: The long-term care ombudsman program: what does the complaint reporting system tell us? *Gerontologist* 32(6):843, 1992.

Parkman C: Using advance directives: part 2, *NurseWeek* 9(12):10, 1996.

Rice R: *Home health nursing practice: concepts and application,* ed 2, St Louis, 1996, Mosby.

Sansone P, Schmitt RL: *Elderly with dementia can decide own treatment at end of their lives.* Unpublished study conducted at Frances Schervier Home and Hospital in the Bronx, New York, under the auspices of the Bureau of Long Term Care Services of the New York State Department of Health (news release, April 17, 1996).

Schmitt RL: *The right to choose: capacity study of demented residents in nursing homes,* executive summary, 1996, Franciscan Sisters of the Poor, Hospital Systems Inc, Brooklyn, NY.

Towner LC, Brown AJB: Standardizing enteral feeding practice: an approach to achieve consistent practice with reduced documentation for long term care nurses, *Geriatr Nurs* (5):211-216, 1996.

Weenolsen P: *The art of dying,* New York, 1996, St Martin's Press.

Weis D, Schank MJ: Use of a taxonomy to describe parish nursing practice with older adults, *Geriatr Nurs* 21(3):125–131, 2000.

7

Physical Changes of Aging

Upon completion of this chapter, the reader will be able to:

- Identify normal age changes.
- Establish selected diagnoses for the changes that occur with age.
- Make a plan of care for the older adult that reflects prevention and maintenance associated with some of the changes with age.

▶ GLOSSARY

Drusen spots Collagenous outgrowths in the inner layer of the choroid of the eye, usually due to age.

Ectropion Eversion or turning outward of the margin of the eyelid.

Entropion Inversion or turning inward of the margin of the eyelid.

Glomerular filtration rate (GFR) The filtering rate of the kidney glomeruli.

Hyperopia Vision for far objects is better than for near objects; farsightedness.

Kinesthetic The sense by which position, weight, and movement are perceived.

Lipofuscin Fatty pigment formed by the solution of a pigment in fat.

Myopia Vision for near objects is better than for far objects; nearsightedness.

Nonstochastic Predetermined biologic changes as explored in the theories of aging.

Presbycusis Progressive, bilaterally symmetric perceptive hearing loss occurring with age.

Presbyopia Diminished accommodation of the lens of the eye occurring normally with age, usually resulting in farsightedness.

Ptosis Drooping of the upper eyelid.

Somesthetic Consciousness or awareness of the body.

Stochastic Skillful assumption about biologic changes, as in the development of theories of aging.

*P*hysiologic changes have a cumulative effect in the continuum of biologic, psychologic, social, and environmental processes of aging. Aging is not a disease, nor is it a condition that is correctable by medical or surgical intervention. Aging is a series of complex changes that occur in all living organisms. Goldman (1979) indicates four characteristics of physiologic aging: it is universal, progressive, decremental, and intrinsic. The universality of aging places it outside the realm of pathologic study. Stehler (1992) suggests that physical aging includes the following:

1. Universal changes occur in all people. However, just because a disease or condition occurs predominantly in older adults, it should not be concluded that the disease or condition is a consequence of aging.

2. Intrinsic changes are processes that occur exclusively within the body and do not result from an external factor or factors.

3. Progressive changes are processes, not events. Their onset is both gradual and cumulative.

4. Deleterious changes are processes or phenomena that are negative. These changes decrease the organism's capacity to survive.

Normal age changes have usually been studied with pathologic or disease conditions, which has led to the misconception that age changes indicate illness or disease. Progressive and decremental alterations of the whole body often interfere with an aged individual's ability to interact successfully with the environment and increase the risk of death. Age changes of the body as a whole are a matter of daily observation and have been happening for thousands of years. Most of these changes are intrinsic, whereas other alterations are a result of extrinsic influences specific to one's way of life. Extrinsic factors that affect intrinsic factors are discussed with the biologic theories of aging later in this chapter.

It is important for the nurse to understand that what is normal in an older adult may be abnormal in an adult of a younger age with the same condition. Also, the approach to the care of the younger adult and older adult with the same condition may be considerably different. This may be due to the biopsychosocial changes that accompany aging.

Interesting approaches to the aging process and age-related changes have been offered by Sloane (1992) and Lakatta (1995). Sloane suggests the "rule of thirds," which suggests that one third of age-related changes occur as a result of functional decline due to disease, one third are due to inactivity or disuse, and one third are caused by aging itself. Lakatta places age-related changes into two categories: usual (average) aging and successful (pure) aging. *Usual aging* refers to the "combined effect of the aging process, disease, and adverse environmental and lifestyle factors" (p. 422). *Successful aging* refers to "changes due solely to the aging

process uncomplicated by damage from environment, lifestyle, or disease" (p. 422).

To illustrate this, oxygen consumption by sedentary elderly persons is usually low (usual aging); however, take the sedentary elder and place him or her in a regular aerobic exercise regimen, and he or she can achieve oxygen levels equal to those of sedentary young adults (successful aging). In essence, normal (usual) age-dependent reductions in biofunction reduce compensatory reserve, but with successful aging the age-related changes may not result in clinical symptoms or disease.

Individual variations are enormous at every age and in every part of the body. For many years most research studies of physical and biologic age changes have based conclusions on the comparison of different age-groups in random samples rather than on groups using the longitudinal study approach. This presents an inherent error because the groups used may represent changes as a result of environmental differences (Goldman, 1979). The Baltimore Longitudinal Study (1984), which began in 1958, continues to follow a group of 1000 men as they age, with the objective of identifying normal changes of aging not associated with disease. The Baltimore Longitudinal Study of women began in the 1980s. Fig. 7-1 provides a summary of selected

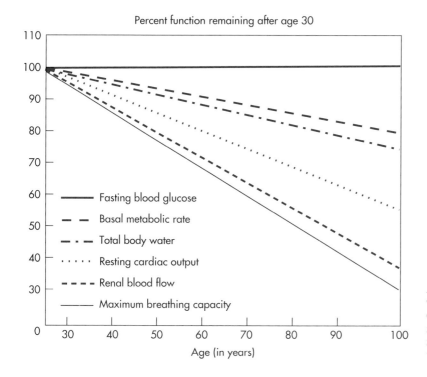

Fig. 7-1 Changes in biologic function with age. (Modified from Shock NW. In Carlston LA, editor: *Nutrition in old age: tenth symposium of the Swedish Nutrition Federation,* Uppsala, Sweden, 1972, Almquistand Wilksell.)

anatomic and physiologic changes with aging of healthy adults.

Changes in body structure and function are lifelong alterations that begin to take on significance internally and externally in the fourth and fifth decades of life. External signs are the clues by which most people judge aging. However, these signs can be deceptive. Skin can become deeply wrinkled or hair can become gray early in adult life, even though these features are considered signs of aging. Today individuals have at their disposal cosmetic surgery, hair coloring, makeup, and clothing choices that can make a person look younger than his or her chronologic age.

Common denominators emerge when one looks at age-related changes. Many changes are effected by a decrease in blood supply to tissues because of the natural deposition of fat and calcium in the vessel intima. Reduced circulation perfusion is also thought to produce the diminished endocrine secretion commonly noted in old age (Costa, Andres, 1986). Finally, lifelong use and abuse of the body through accidents, athletic injuries, and other physical trauma are responsible for some of the changes thought of as wear and tear. When one is young, it is difficult to realize that neglect of skin, teeth, or nutrition will not necessarily produce visible or significant changes until one moves into old age and compensatory reserve becomes limited. At that time the effects of earlier laxness become more apparent and important to a person's health.

Significant changes in structure, function, and biochemistry, as well as genetic endowment, are responsible for the alterations in tissue elasticity, subcutaneous fat, gastrointestinal function and motility, muscle, bone, immunity, and the sensorium. These changes are not mutually exclusive but, rather, are synergistic and contribute to alterations in each system and to the general evidence of advanced age. No system truly escapes age changes. Some changes are external and visible and therefore easy to recognize and address; others are internal and harder to realize that assistance is needed.

STRUCTURE AND POSTURE

Obvious manifestations, influenced by many factors such as age, sex, race, and environment, occur in the fifth decade of life. With age, height diminishes by $1^1/_2$ to 2 inches, and the trunk shortens as a result of dehydration of the vertebral disks (Jacobs, 1981; Cunningham, Brookbank, 1988; Lamb, 1996). Long bones take on the appearance of disproportionate size (long arms and legs) because stature decreases. Vertebral disks become thin as a result of dehydration, causing a shortening of the trunk. Many aged persons assume a stooped, forward-bent posture, with the hips and knees somewhat flexed and the arms bent at the elbows, raising the level of the arms. To maintain eye contact, the head is tilted backward, which makes it appear that the elderly individual is jutting forward. Degeneration of underlying cartilage appears to decrease intervertebral distance. The forward-leaning posture is attributed to muscle shrinkage. The decrease in abdominal length gives the overall picture of a disproportionate individual who needs to be stretched out a bit.

Posture and structural changes occur primarily because of calcium loss from bone and as a result of atrophic processes of cartilage and muscle. Bone mass is constantly undergoing cyclic resorption and renewal. Disequilibrium of this process with greater resorption and less calcium deposition is characteristic of aging bone. Excessive leaching of calcium from the bone matrix creates the condition called *osteoporosis*. This type of degeneration is four times more prevalent in women (Lindsay, 1985), becoming apparent as estrogen declines in older women. Men who develop osteoporosis do so from lack of exercise, smoking, and lack of calcium in the diet, as well as from many other causes associated with the condition regardless of gender. Kyphosis and osteoporosis are two factors that contribute to the shorter stature of the aged. Osteoporosis, however, is not a normal age change but a disease process. Resorption of the bone leads to poor-fitting dentures and painful sensations when chewing or biting (Coni et al, 1984). Bone demineralization affects the jaw or alveolar bone of the lower jaw, especially in individuals who are edentulous.

Skeletal Muscles

Skeletal muscle atrophy occurs because of physical inactivity, a decreased ratio of neurons to muscle cells, and endocrine factors and is greater in the lower extremities, in much the same manner as that which occurs in long-term muscle inactivity. Abdominal muscles decrease in size and number of fibers, in part because of disuse. Muscle tone or tension of particular muscle groups decreases steadily after 30 years of age. Possible causes are attributed to neuron loss and the loss of sensory and motor elements of spinal nerves of the muscles. Nerve cells in the spinal cord are lost after 80 years of age (Cunningham, Brookbank, 1988; Bartz, 1995).

Strength and stamina decrease to 65% to 85% of the maximum strength an individual had at 25 years of age.

Ligaments, Tendons, and Joints

Ligaments, tendons, and joints, over time, become hardened, more rigid, and less flexible in movement, which predisposes these structures to tears. Worn-down cartilage around joints produced by continuous flexing over the years coupled with stray pieces of cartilage and diminished lubricating fluid in the joints can lead to slower and painful movement.

SKIN, HAIR, AND NAILS

Epidermal cell renewal time increases by one third after 50 years of age, requiring 30 or more days for new epithelial replacement. Therefore wound healing is approximately 50% slower than at 35 years of age (Leyden et al, 1978) and may deplete the limited physiologic reserve that the older adult still possesses. Collagen decreases approximately 1% per year, causing the skin to "give" less under stress and tear more easily (Richey et al, 1988). The dermis becomes thinner in the absence of subcutaneous fat (Grove, Kingman, 1983).

Fewer melanocytes are identifiable in the epidermis as skin ages. However, melanin synthesis is increased in some areas of aged skin, resulting in pigment spots (freckles and nevi) that enlarge and can become more numerous when there is increased exposure to natural and artificial light. Vascular hyperplasia results in more pronounced varicosities, benign cherry angiomas, and venous stars.

Subcutaneous tissue plays a significant role in the body's adjustment to temperature change. The natural insulation that subcutaneous fat affords is lost, and it is not uncommon to hear aged people mention that they are cold; nor is it unusual to see them wearing a sweater or sitting with a lap blanket. All of these changes involve multiple developmental factors: skeletal, muscular, subcutaneous tissue, fat, and dermal changes. Landmarks become more prominent, and muscle contours are easily identified. Skinfold thickness, a measure of subcutaneous fat content, is markedly reduced in the forearm with age. Women over 45 years of age begin to see the skinfolds on the back of their hands rapidly diminish, even if there is a substantial weight gain. Such areas as the pubis, umbilicus, and waist do not change appreciably.

Regardless of sex, 50% of the population over 50 years of age have gray or partly gray scalp hair because of a decrease in melanin production in hair follicles. Body and facial hair becomes gray later. Overall scalp and body hair diminishes with advanced age. Hair loss is prominent in men, beginning in the second decade for some. By age 40, hair patterns have reached their maximum and begin to recede. Women have less pronounced hair loss.

Hair Distribution

Race, sex, sex-linked genes, and hormonal influences determine the maximum amount of hair that one has and the changes that will occur with it throughout life. In both sexes, hair distribution becomes more sparse; hair on the head thins, and leg hair frequently is lacking. This latter finding is often interpreted as a sign of peripheral vascular disease; however, other, more conclusive signs and symptoms should be observed to validate the diagnosis of abnormal hair loss on the legs. Asians and blacks are less hairy than whites, and American Indians have little or no hair on their bodies (Rossman, 1986). Dark, thick, abundant hair becomes lighter, gray, thinner, and less full. At times, hair color may turn shades of yellow or yellow-green. Axillary and pubic hair diminishes in quantity and thickness of the hair fibers.

Fingernails and Toenails

Fingernails and toenails grow at a slower rate than in younger adults and develop longitudinal striations. Toenails grow at an even slower rate than fingernails in the aged (Jacobs, 1981; Cornell, 1986). The nail plate may thicken and give the nail a yellow appearance. With aging, the cuticle becomes less thick and wide. Vigorous manipulation of the cuticle may lead to retardation of the already-slowed nail growth.

FACIAL CHANGES

Facial changes occur as a result of altered subcutaneous fat, dermal thickness, decreased elasticity, and lateral surface compression of underlying muscle contractions. Loss of mandibular bone mass accentuates the size of the upper mouth, nose, and forehead. An indented "loss of lip" appearance of the mouth occurs with tooth loss when uncorrected by dentures or other oral prostheses. Eyelids appear swollen as a result of the redistribution of fat deposits. The fat layer around the orbit of the eye disappears, creating a sunken appearance of the eyes.

LOSS OF TISSUE ELASTICITY

Tissue elasticity is most easily observed in skin integrity and reflects the progressive, universal, and intrinsic nature of age changes. The aged skin loses resilience and moisture, taking on a characteristic dryness. The face and neck wrinkles reflect life patterns of muscle activity in facial expressions, the pull of gravity on tissue, and diminished elasticity in general. Loss of elasticity accentuates jowls and elongated ears and contributes to the formation of a "double" chin. Sun exposure accelerates skin tissue changes by hastening collagen fiber alterations. Breasts that were full and firm begin to sag and become pendulous as the glandular envelope of fat atrophies and the skin elasticity weakens. Nipples may also invert because of the shrinkage and fibrotic changes.

Elasticity affects blood vessel integrity, particularly the arteries. Elastic fibers fray, split, straighten, and fragment. Calcium that leaves the bone is deposited in the vessels. This chemical and anatomic alteration decreases vessel lumen size and causes an alteration in blood supply to various organs. Change in flow to the coronary arteries and the brain is minimal, but perfusion of the liver and kidneys shows significant changes in the amount of blood brought to these two organs (Wardell, 1979; Cunningham, Brookbank, 1988; Malasanos et al, 1989). Advanced age increases peripheral resistance in the vessels, which results in a rise in both the systolic and diastolic pressures. This is a reflection of the elastic changes and calcium deposits. Lung elasticity declines, causing a rigidity in lung tissue. This alone is not responsible for the decrease in oxygen capacity, but it is a contributing factor (Tichy, Malasanos, 1979).

BODY COMPOSITION

Body weight changes because of a decline in lean body mass and a loss of body water (Kenney, 1982) (see Fig. 7-1). By 70 years of age, fat content of the body has increased by 16% and cellular sodium by 20%. Cellular solids and bone mass decline; extracellular water, however, remains relatively constant. However, there is a need to increase the proportion of protein, calcium, and vitamin D nutritional intake (Gugoz, Munro, 1985; Lakatta, 1995). The intercellular matrix (collagen and elastin) becomes more rigid, reducing resilience. Intracellular concentrations of structural proteins, enzymes, and chromosomal components, including deoxyribonu-

cleic acid (DNA) and ribonucleic acid (RNA), change. The aging pigment (lipofuscin) increases in the nervous system and other nonrenewing tissues, such as the heart.

CARDIOVASCULAR CHANGES

Cardiovascular disease is a major cause of death worldwide in people age 60 and over. In the United States, one half of all cardiovascular disease occurs in those 65 years of age and older (Health After 50, 1994). One of every two persons age 60 and over may have some severe narrowing of the coronary arteries, but only about 50% of those have clinical signs of coronary artery dysfunction. Screening for this occult manifestation can now be done with magnetic resonance imaging (MRI) (Health After 50, 1994). It is difficult to know whether widespread disease exaggerates functional decline presently considered to be a result of age-related change.

Health professionals are accustomed to caring for aged persons with cardiac-related conditions such as congestive heart failure and hypertension and may be inclined to assume that all aged individuals have enlarged hearts. Studies suggest that the left ventricle wall thickens as much as 30% by 80 years of age because of the increase in myocyte size, but the size remains relatively unchanged in healthy adults. The left atrium also increases in size—an adaptation that enhances ventricular filling. In healthy aged persons a fourth heart sound may be audible as a result of this atrial enlargement (Lakatta, 1993). A radiologic silhouette of cardiac size shows a slight increase, but the size remains within a clinically normal range (Gersteinblith et al, 1977; Gardin et al, 1979; Lakatta, 1995).

By age 60, the maximum coronary artery blood flow provides the cardiovascular system with 35% less blood than in earlier years. The decline in work response of the left ventricle at rest is a reflection of decreased stroke volume and cardiac output and a delay in heart muscle irritability and contractile recovery. Contraction of the older heart is prolonged, most likely because of the slow release of calcium into the myoplasm during systole. Reduced efficiency and contractile strength of the heart muscle are reflected in (1) a reduced cardiac output that decreases by 1% per year from the average baseline of 5 L/min and (2) a stroke volume decline of 0.7% per year (Jacobs, 1981; Kenney, 1982) (see Fig. 7-1).

Under normal, nonstressful conditions the smaller cardiac output of the aged heart is able to sustain adequate function to maintain an average active life, since the mechanisms that determine cardiovascular function depend on the interaction of intrinsic cell performance, heart rate, coronary flow, cardiac filling (preload), and cardiac afterload. These functions are governed by autonomic tone and a negative feedback system. Decreased overall energy demands and a moderate degree of body atrophy place less demand on cardiac function. Diminished cardiac output becomes significant when the aged person is physically or mentally stressed by illness, worry, or excitement. Sudden demands for more oxygen and energy brought on by various physiologic, psychologic, social, and environmental stress result in poor response of heart function attributed to the limited cardiac reserve, or presbycardia. It takes longer for the heart to accelerate to meet the demands placed on it and to return to a normal level. Tachycardia is not as great in the older person, but when it occurs, the heart requires a longer time to return to its baseline rate. The expected increase in the pulse rate when the patient is anxious, is in pain, hemorrhages, or demonstrates the presence of an infectious process is not as evident in the aged as in the young. Box 7-1 lists the risk factors that can exert added demand on the heart. An average circulation time of 27 seconds was found to be normal for men in the seventh decade of life (Diettert, 1963). No data have been established for women.

Heart valves may thicken and stiffen as a result of lipid deposits, collagen degeneration, and fibrosis. Valvular conditions in the aged are considered residual effects of earlier rheumatic infections and arteriosclerosis. Aortic and mitral valves are most commonly affected and result in slight to moderate regurgitation of blood. Valvular disease in the aged is often misdiagnosed because it is assumed that murmurs are a result of the arteriosclerotic process. Some aged do have aortic and mitral murmurs that were chronicled from childhood; others are from the stiffening of the valve leaflets. Generally, those murmurs are not as prominent as murmurs that occur in later life. At least 50% of elders have a systolic ejection type of murmur that is a grade 1 or 2 without radiation. Murmurs that are diastolic, however, should always be considered significant, since these indicate important alteration in cardiac hemodynamics (Lakatta, 1990).

Alteration in the excitation and contraction mechanism is an adaptive rather than a degenerative change because it maintains contractile function of the aged heart. A sinus rate of less than 50 beats/min is common in the elderly and does not necessarily indicate sinoatrial (SA) node disease. Sinus rhythm is the expected

Box 7-1 GENERAL RISK FACTORS THAT CAN STRESS THE HEART OR AGGRAVATE EXISTING CONDITIONS

Stressors
Continued high intake of dietary animal fat, salt, and calories
Obesity and excessive weight
Long-term cigarette smoking
Lack of regular exercise
Internalization of emotions
Air pollution

Extra Demand or Aggravating Events
Existing chronic conditions
Infection
Anemia
Pneumonia
Cardiac dysrhythmias
Surgery
Fever
Diarrhea
Hypoglycemia
Malnutrition
Avitaminosis
Circulatory overload
Drug-induced condition
Renal disease
Prostatic obstruction

norm of the aged person's heartbeat. During the third and fourth decade of life, pacemaker cells decrease in number as myocardial fat, collagen, and elastin fibers increase and then accelerate through the sixth decade. Similarly, the atrioventricular (AV) node and the bundle of His lose a number of conductive cells into the fourth decade and in the left bundle between the fifth and seventh decades (Fujino et al, 1982; Miller, 1990). Significant interference with the blood flow either by occlusion or by narrowed arteriosclerotic vessels to the SA node can produce dysrhythmias.

Dysrhythmias may be primary or secondary, but the majority of rate irregularities in the aged are attributed to myocardial damage either by interference with the coronary circulation or by valvular insufficiency and concomitant interference of the neurologic mechanisms essential to heart action.

Stiffening of the arteries and reduced cardiovascular responsiveness to adrenergic stimulation is responsible for a decline in baroreceptor sensitivity and an inability to respond adequately to hypertensive or hypotensive stimuli.

The intima of both arteries and veins becomes fibrotic, and endothelial cell variation increases. Smooth muscle and elastin diminish as collagen and fibrotic tissue take over. The result is loss of flexibility and recoil, an increase in systemic peripheral resistance, and a reduced perfusion to tissues and organs. This stiffer and more rigid structure of the vascular system may lead to an elevation of blood pressure in addition to influencing cardiac and renal changes. Loss of vein elasticity causes pooling of blood and increases the venous pressure, diminishing the effectiveness of peripheral valves and creating tortuous varicosities (Beare, Myers, 1998).

Decreased elasticity of arteries and arterioles produces changes that affect blood flow to body organs such as the heart, liver, kidneys, and pituitary gland. Dilation and elongation of the aorta occur as a result of collagen and elastin changes and calcium deposition from degenerating elastin (Lakatta, 1995). Increased resistance to peripheral blood flow occurs at a rate of about 1% per year, with a moderate decrease in circulation to the coronary arteries. Weakness of vessel walls and varicosities can lead to abnormal swelling of the lower extremities when the vessel walls and varicosities are subjected to increased pressure. Some atherosclerosis is normal with aging, but it can be exacerbated to a pathologic state by a diet high in saturated fat.

In the past, the accepted upper limits of normal blood pressure for the aged adult was 160/90. However, The Fifth Report of the Joint National Committee on Detection, Evaluation, and Treatment of High Blood Pressure (1993) states that both the young and the old have similar blood pressure. This report defines *hypertension* as systolic pressure at or above 140 mm Hg and diastolic pressure at or above 90 mm Hg. It is estimated that 50% of persons over age 65 in industrialized society have blood pressure at or greater than 140/90 mm Hg (Frohlich, 1995). Common in older adults is isolated systolic hypertension (ISH), in which the diastolic pressure is normal but the systolic pressure is elevated. Both hypertension and ISH increase during the eight and ninth decades of life.

The National Health and Nutrition Examination Survey (NHANES III) conducted during 1988 and 1991 confirms that hypertension rates for black men and black women over the age of 60 increased to over 60% for black men and 80% for black women (Health After 50, 1996).

Even though the death rate from heart and vascular disease is declining, the aged today remain a product of their previous health practices. Modifying behavior may lessen some of the resultant damage.

RESPIRATORY CHANGES

Changes in respiratory and pulmonary performance occur gradually, allowing the elderly to continue to breathe effortlessly in the absence of pathologic states. When the elderly are confronted with a little exertion or stress, however, dyspnea and other symptoms usually appear.

It is unclear if respiratory system changes are due to environmental toxins or the progressive subclinical exhaustion of internal respiratory reserve and repair caused by aging itself (Tockman, 1995). Respiratory changes that do occur in structure and function with superimposed consequences of acute illness and chronicity can be sufficiently debilitating to limit life enjoyment.

The prominent effect of age-related changes on the respiratory system is reduced efficiency in ventilation and gas exchange. It is accepted that exercise tolerance declines and that breathlessness leads to varying degrees of fatigue, but under usual or resting conditions the aged have little difficulty accomplishing and participating in customary life activities. However, when the aged are confronted with unusual and stressful circumstances, the demand for oxygen surpasses the available supply and establishes a significant respiratory deficit, which must be resolved. Stable respiratory function is also affected by a lower resistance to infection engendered by a diminished immune system response and less effective self-cleansing action of the respiratory cilia.

Calcification stiffens the tracheal and laryngeal cartilage. Cilia line the trachea and are less effective because of their decreased number, resulting in less respiratory epithelium and increased bronchial mucous gland hypertrophy (Schumann, 1995). The impact of this is difficulty moving mucus, debris, and dust into the pharynx. Tockman (1995) suggests that the importance of age and mucociliary transport is not fully established but that it may be clinically significant for the recurrence of respiratory infections.

The chest wall and lungs grow in proportion to the body and correlate with height when one is young (Tockmann, 1995). Around age 55, respiratory muscles begin to weaken, chest wall compliance begins to decrease, and a loss of elastic recoil that affects ventilation and gas exchange occurs. Normal physiologic changes can resemble pathologic entities. Several researchers state that the lungs of "healthy" older people who are nonsmokers show evidence of small, scattered areas of lung destruction similar to the manifestations identified in emphysema (Campbell, Lefrak, 1978; Lillington, 1979; Timaris, 1994). This is a critical factor to consider in determining normality or pathologic conditions (Kenney, 1989).

Ossification of the costal cartilage and the downward slant of the ribs limit chest expansion. Intercostal and accessory muscles and the diaphragm become "floppier" as a consequence of muscle weakness. The potential for greater lung expansion exists but cannot be realized because of structural limitations that develop in the thoracic walls. Skeletal defects such as kyphosis and scoliosis and the generally stooped posture of the aged also contribute to restricting chest expansion by further reducing the size of the chest cavity area in which the lungs can expand. The outcomes of these changes are increased dead space, decreased vital capacity, and decreased expiratory flow.

Lung size remains the same, but the lungs do become flabbier (Krumpe et al, 1985). The elastin and collagen changes due to cross-linkage and deterioration result in a decrease of outward movement and inward pull, with the end result being slightly smaller total lung capacity, increased residual capacity and residual volume, and early airway closure.

The alveoli progressively enlarge and structurally resemble air sac changes associated with emphysema. The elastin fibers in the alveolar walls are bound to the respiratory and terminal bronchioles, which help to maintain the small airway patency at low lung volumes. The loss of the elastin attachment causes collapse of the small airways and uneven alveolar ventilation, trapping air and increasing dead space (Schumann, 1995; Tockman, 1995). The alveolar dilation with loss of alveolar attachments and an increase in the number of collapsed small airways is referred to as *senile lung* and is seen in some individuals over age 60 (Tockman, 1995). Campbell and Lefrak (1978) referred to this physiologic change as *ductectasis* and considered it a normal aging phenomenon, not to be confused with the pathologic findings of emphysema.

Total lung capacity is not significantly altered but, rather, is redistributed. The residual capacity increase that occurs with the diminished inspiratory and expiratory thoracic muscle strength results in hyperinflation of the lung apices and underinflation of the lung bases (see Fig. 7-1). The changes that occur in the anatomic structures of the chest and the altered muscle strength do not lend themselves to the forcefulness needed to expel material that accumulates or causes an obstruction in the airway (Krumpe et al, 1985). Therefore the less effective cough response or cough reflex is a problem for elders. However, if other clearing mechanisms are intact, the cough reflex is not essential for respiratory clearance. With impairments such as dysphagia or decreased esophageal motility, an intact cough reflex is a necessity (Tockmann, 1995). The lack of basilar inflation, ineffective cough response, and a less efficient immune system pose potential problems for the aged who are sedentary, bedridden, or limited in activity.

Premature airway closure and loss of elastic recoil affect the blood oxygen (Po_2) level. The aged blood oxygen level is approximately 75 mm Hg, whereas that of younger adults ranges from 90 to 95 mm Hg (Timaris, 1994). The absolute lowest normal Po_2 level for an elder is 70 mm Hg. Pierson (1992) suggests that Po_2 falls 4 mm Hg per decade. The blood carbon dioxide (Pco_2) level remains constant for both the young and older adult. The blood oxygen (Po_2) tension also remains constant, but the distribution of inspired air to dependent parts of the lung is less sufficient (Timaris, 1988; 1994). There is a decline in the transmural gradient that holds airways open. Airway collapse limits the ability of the lungs to empty and decreases the exhalation of Pco_2. This places a greater demand on cardiac function to increase cardiac output to compensate for less oxygen delivery to body tissues. Diminished elastic recoil of the lungs makes gaseous exchange across alveolar membranes more difficult. Aged individuals with Po_2 levels as low as 40 mm Hg have little or no immediate compensatory response in cardiac function. Younger persons with the same blood gas level show a marked increase in cardiac rate as an attempt to compensate and deliver more oxygen to body tissues.

Chemoreceptor function is altered or blunted at the peripheral and central chemoreceptor sites or in the integrating central nervous system pathways. In healthy men ages 64 to 73, the response to hypoxia and hypercapnia is half that of younger adults. This response is independent of mechanical lung changes and is attributed to the neuromuscular drive to breathe.

The absence of reliable pulmonary function values with which to evaluate the respiratory status of the aged requires that the nurse use other methods to assess the aged person's respiratory ability and needs.

RENAL CHANGES

The kidney loses as many as 50% of the millions of nephrons (each kidney has at least 1 million) with little change in the body's ability to regulate the chemical composition of body fluids and the ability to maintain adequate fluid homeostasis in old age. The age-related decrease in size and function occurs primarily in the kidney cortex, begins in the fourth decade, and becomes significant by the eighth decade. Contour remains relatively smooth, and the decline in size parallels the general decrease in size and weight of other body organs.

By the eighth decade, 30% of the glomeruli are lost and there is evidence of age-related glomerular sclerosis. The cause of sclerosis of the glomeruli is unclear, but it is thought that a high-protein diet or glomerular ischemia may be responsible (Rowe, 1995). In general, these changes pose little threat to the well-being of the aged unless there is an abrupt reduction in nephron function caused by an acquired renal disease (Richard, 1995; Rowe, 1995).

The large renal vessels also show evidence of sclerosis with age but do not narrow the vessel lumen. Smaller vessels do not show this change. Only 15% of elders who are normotensive have sclerotic changes in the renal arterioles.

Changes in the arterioglomerular units affect the cortical area (hyalinization and collapse of the glomerular tufts), with the preglomerular arterioles becoming obliterated, reducing the blood flow. The medullary area of the kidney shows sclerosis and loss of the glomeruli and shrinking between the afferent and efferent arterioles; however, the arteriolae rectae verae preserve blood flow to the medullary area. Age does not decrease the number of arterioles in this area.

Blood flow through the kidney decreases from 1200 ml/min in young adults to 600 ml/min by the age of 80 as a result of the vascular and fixed anatomic and structural changes described above. Fig. 7-1 illustrates the altered renal blood flow. In view of these changes, the glomerular filtration rate (GFR), which is dependent on the number of glomeruli, steadily declines.

The GFR is measured by the creatinine clearance, which also changes with age. It is directly related to muscle mass and is a product of muscle metabolism. By age 80, the creatinine clearance is decreased to 100 ml/min. Urine creatinine, secondary to loss of muscle mass, alters the expected relationship of serum creatinine to the creatinine clearance. Approximately one third of elders do not show a decline in GFR (Lindeman et al, 1985), suggesting that factors other than age-related change may be responsible for altered renal function. Plasma creatinine clearance is constant throughout life. The urine creatinine declines in the older adult; therefore the urine creatinine clearance is an important indicator for appropriate drug therapy in the aged. The following formula for calculating the urine creatinine clearance provides a means for the nurse to determine this value and note the potential for toxicity from a medication regimen. The calculation for elderly women uses the same formula but multiplies the answer (CrCl) by 0.85. Clearance for a well elder is 70 ml/min.

$$CrCl = \frac{140 - Age \ (Weight \ in \ Kg)}{72 \times Serum \ creatinine}$$

Lower renin levels are associated with a parallel reduction of the same proportions in aldosterone. This decreases the kidneys' ability to conserve sodium and delay the response of the acid/base loading. A reduced ability to concentrate urine and conserve water resulting from medullary loss makes the collecting ducts less responsive to antidiuretic hormone (ADH). The importance of the age-related kidney changes is that elders are more susceptible to fluid and electrolyte imbalance and renal damage from medications and contrast media of diagnostic tests. Under normal circumstances, kidney function is sufficient to meet the regulation and excretion demands of the body. However, with the stress of disease, surgery, or fever, the kidneys have little capacity to respond.

ENDOCRINE CHANGES

Hormones are responsible for and control reproduction, growth and development, maintenance of homeostasis, and energy production. Two principles must be kept in mind when considering hormonal control and effects: (1) a particular hormone may have an effect on many body systems and functions, and (2) one body function may require the coordinated action of many hormones (Bartz, 1995). It is suggested here that backup and fine-tuning mechanism adjustments are made to maintain homeostasis or close-to-normal limits. Changes may produce hypoactivity from disease or physiologic down-regulating. Serum hormone levels are reflective of changes. Most glands atrophy and decrease their rate of secretion. There is no uniform direction of change;

some are less active, slightly active, or not active at all (Solomon, 1995).

Insulin secretion from the beta cells and glucose metabolism throughout life change little. The age-related change is in the tissue sensitivity to insulin and is thought to be due to a change in the molecular makeup of insulin (Bartz, 1995). In addition, higher levels of circulating proinsulin are found in older adults than in younger adults. Alteration of insulin receptor sites by the aging process is also considered to render insulin less effective (MacLennan, Peden, 1989). When the pancreas is stressed with sudden concentrations of glucose, blood levels are higher and prolonged (see Fig. 7-1). Because of this intolerance, increased levels of glucose in the blood make it difficult for physicians to determine if the condition is a physiologic decline or a genetic trait for which a treatment is needed.

Thyroid function remains adequate with age, as do the secretions of thyroid-stimulating hormone (TSH) and the serum concentration of thyroxine (T_4) (Bartz, 1995; Solomon, 1995). However, a significant decline in triiodothyronine (T_3) occurs with age, which is thought to reflect reduced conversion of T_4 to T_3 in extrathyroidal locations. Collective signs, such as a slowed basal metabolic rate, thinning of the hair, and dry skin are characteristic of hypothyroidism in the young but are normal manifestations in the aged who have no history of thyroid deficiencies. Some of the aged do develop hypothyroidism and should be evaluated. Based on these symptoms alone, it is difficult to establish the presence or absence of disease.

Cortisol is an important glucocorticoid of the adrenal cortex but does not seem to have an adverse effect on the aging body. Likewise, the effect of decreased adrenocorticotropic hormone production has not been elucidated. Epinephrine, norepinephrine, and dopamine produced by the adrenal medulla decrease with age, but again the significance is unclear.

The pituitary gland, with its diverse functions and central role in the complex hormone feedback system, decreases in volume. The significance of this change is unclear in light of the maintenance of adequate hormonal secretions.

Adrenogenic, estrogenic, and gonadotropic hormones undergo secretory and stimulatory changes. Diminished hormone levels lead to atrophy of the ovaries, uterus, and vaginal tissue in aged women. Aged men develop firmer testes and a tendency for prostatic hypertrophy, which is a benign condition in most instances. Libido remains present in both sexes. Sexual capacity may diminish as the tissues change and physical and mental health changes, but although intercourse may be less frequent and take longer to accomplish, this does not mean that it is less satisfying to the couple involved.

GASTROINTESTINAL CHANGES

The primary function of digestion and absorption by the digestive system handles age-related changes better than most systems of the body. Changes in other organ systems affect gastrointestinal structure and function. Studies have determined that extraintestinal causes, such as diabetes and vascular and neurologic changes, previously may have been mistaken for age-related changes in the gastrointestinal system.

Dentition, an important adjunct to the gastrointestinal system, can affect digestive activity if the food entering the mouth is not prepared by mastication and if saliva, which contains ptyalin to break down starch, is diminished. Normally, saliva production is unchanged with age (Schuster, 1995), but because of systemic disorders or their treatment, saliva may decrease. Unfortunately, many of the aged today continue to be edentulous or dependent on dentures. A number of the aged who have dentures choose not to wear them; others are unable to afford them.

Decreased esophageal peristalsis is a result of diminished muscle strength and motility. The esophagus increases the number of muscle movements but does not effectively propel its contents. The inadequate peristaltic action and the relaxation of the lower esophageal sphincter slow the emptying of the esophagus. The sluggish emptying of the esophagus (presbyesophagus) also forces the lower end to dilate, sustaining greater stress in this area and causing digestive discomfort to the aged. Improperly masticated food antagonizes this situation and in part is responsible for the forceful, emphatic, propulsive contractions that propel the food on its way to further digestion. Hiatal hernias are a common occurrence among more than half of those over age 70.

The reduction of hydrochloric acid (HCl) in the stomach occurs at about age 60, with a decline of pepsin starting in about the fourth decade and continuing in a sharp decline to the sixth decade. At that time the pepsin level evens out and remains at a constant low. Increased stomach pH interferes with the protective alkaline viscous mucus, causing the aged to be more susceptible to gastric irritation. Loss of smooth muscle in the stomach delays emptying time and also exposes the epithelial lining to extended contact with gastric contents. This can increase or delay the absorption time of nutrients and medications affected by the stomach pH.

The glandular secretions of the digestive system from the liver, gallbladder, and pancreas are altered with age. The liver continues to function throughout life even with a decrease in volume and weight (mass) (Bay, 1995; Schenker, 1995). This brings with it a concomitant 35% decrease in liver blood flow. Liver regeneration, although slow, is not greatly impaired, and liver function tests remain unaltered with age.

The gallbladder, which stores the bile manufactured by the liver, does not seem to change, but those 70 years of age and older account for one third of gallbladder surgeries (Tompkins, 1995; Welch, 1995). It is thought that this may be due to the increased lipogenic composition of bile from biliary cholesterol or to an age-related decline in pancreatic secretions and enzyme output, which decreases the tolerance for fatty foods. A decrease in bile salt synthesis is also thought to increase the incidence of cholelithiasis and cholycystitis (Altman, 1990; Cassmeyer, Blevin, 1993).

Smooth muscle, Peyer patches, and lymphatic follicles of the small intestine decrease with age. Changes in motility, epithelial membranes, vascular perfusion, and gastrointestinal membrane transport may affect absorption of lipids, amino acids, glucose, calcium, and iron. Calcium use is affected by lack of adequate gastric acid and slow active transport in the body. The tendency toward vitamin and mineral deficiency is caused partly by the faulty absorption of vitamins B_1 and B_{12}, calcium, and iron and by inadequate dietary intake of the aged. Vitamins K, B_1, and B_{12} and minerals such as iron and calcium are the ones in which the aged are most frequently deficient.

It is difficult to determine changes in the large intestine even though there is structural atrophy of the layers and glands and a decrease in mucous secretions. The internal sphincter of the large intestine loses its muscle tone, which can create problems in bowel evacuation. Weakness of the intestinal walls may also lead to outpouching of small segments of the colon (diverticula), which may or may not be symptomatic. The external sphincter, which retains much of its original tone, cannot by itself control the bowels. Slower transmission of neural impulses lessens the awareness of sensations of a forthcoming bowel evacuation. The outcome of this may be either fecal incontinence or constipation.

NERVOUS SYSTEM CHANGES

Lipofuscin, an aging pigment, is deposited in nerve cells, and amyloid deposition occurs in the blood vessels and cells. Senile plaque and, less frequently, neurofibrillary tangles are also found. The latter are usually associated with Alzheimer's disease, but they also appear in the brain of elders without evidence of dementia (Joynt, 1995).

Changes in the dopaminergic and cholinergic neurotransmitter systems occur with decreasing levels of choline acetylase, serotonin, and catecholamines. Other enzymes such as monoamine oxidase (MAO) increase. Redundancy of brain cells may forestall some changes, but the exact number of cells required for certain functions is not clear.

Nerve cell loss is minimal in the brainstem but more profound in the hippocampus. By the ninth decade, the cerebral ventricles have enlarged three to four times. The brain has the ability to compensate for areas of injury or destruction, with compensation more effective in the higher centers. The spinal cord is less able to do so. Peripheral nerves remain relatively unchanged and can regenerate slowly; however, conduction time of the peripheral nerves decreases in the aged.

As nerve cells gradually deteriorate and die, there is a compensatory lengthening of and an increase in the number of dendrites of the remaining nerve cells. The new connections in the dendrite tree may make up for the lower number of cells. This phenomenon is a normal age change, even though it may be seen to occur with Alzheimer's disease also.

Intellectual performance of the elder without brain dysfunction remains constant into and beyond 80 years of age; however, the performance of tasks may take longer, which is an indication that central processing is slowed. Verbal skills continue well into the 70s and beyond. Other subtle changes occur in mentation, such as difficulty learning language and benign forgetfulness. Both positive and negative factors or medical or psychologic stress may result in confusion, delirium, or depression in the elder.

SENSORY CHANGES

A number of sensory changes occur with age as a result of the intrinsic aging process in sensory organs and their association with the nervous system. Other changes are extrinsic and linked to the environment.

One does not totally escape diminution of taste, smell, sight, sound, and touch.

Eye and Vision Changes

A decline in visual acuity is a progressive change that occurs in the optic compartment (cornea, lens, pupil, aqueous and vitreous humor, retina) of the eye. All persons will eventually experience some decline in visual capacity with age.

Extraocular Changes

Eyelids droop (senile ptosis) as a result of the loss of elasticity, and skin atrophy can interfere with vision if the lids sag far enough over the lower lid margin. A decrease in the orbicular muscle strength of the eyes may result in ectropion or entropion. Ectropion may cause the lower lid to roll outward, exposing the palpebral conjunctiva. This may result in nonclosure of the lids with sleep and lead to corneal dryness. Spasms of the orbicular muscle may cause the eyelashes, particularly of the lower lid, to turn inward (entropion), irritating the eyeball with each blink (Kupfer, 1995).

The conjunctiva is the thin membrane over the sclera with goblet cells that provide mucin, which is essential for eye lubrication and movement. Mucin slows the evaporation of tear film. The number of goblet cells decreases, resulting in a deficiency of lubrication for the eye. Lack of tear secretions or nonspecific causes contribute to dry eye syndrome (Kupfer, 1995).

Ocular Changes

The cornea, which is responsible for refraction of light, is among the first eye structures to be affected by aging. A flatter, less smooth, and thicker cornea is noticeable by its lackluster appearance or loss of sparkling transparency, and it leaves the aged individual more susceptible to astigmatism. A gray-white ring or partial ring, known as *arcus senilis,* forms 1 mm to 2 mm inside the limbus. It does not affect vision and is composed of deposits of calcium and cholesterol salts. Almost everyone over the age of 65 will exhibit some degree of arcus senilis, which gives credence to an age correlation of this specific change.

Two sets of iris muscles regulate pupil size, affecting the amount of light that reaches the retina and limiting the efficiency of pupillary constriction and dilation. Pupil size is smaller in older adults, creating the problem of being dazzled in bright light because of the sluggishness of the pupil to constrict. Slowness to dilate in the dark creates moments when elders cannot see where they are going. Because of the slow ability of the pupils to accommodate to changes in light, glare is a major problem for the aged. Glare is a problem created not only by sunlight outdoors, but also by the reflection of light on any shiny object, especially light striking polished or linoleum floors.

The inability of the eyes to accommodate to close and detailed work (presbyopia) begins in the fourth decade and continues throughout the rest of one's life. Presbyopia occurs earlier in individuals who live in warm climates and later in individuals who are nearsighted (myopic). Suspensory ligaments, ciliary muscles, and parasympathetic nerves contribute to the decreased accommodation that occurs.

Pupil diameter is also decreased, along with the speed at which direct and consensual responses happen. If the pupil response is sluggish or absent, it may be that medication to dilate or constrict the pupils is being taken. Older people require three times as much light to see things as they did when they were in their 20s. There is a need for more light for all visual perception. It is more effective to place high-intensity light on the object or surface that is involved than to increase the intensity of the light in the entire area or room. For example, it would be more effective to focus a light directly on the newspaper a person was reading than to try to increase the light in the whole room.

The extent of the visual field begins to wane, affecting the breadth of vision that is possible. No longer can the aged view things panoramically; rather, the fringes are not as discrete and may be missed (Kupfer, 1995). The decreased ability to respond to rapid movement in front of the eyes presents problems for the aged. Rapid blinking or flickering lights or motion cannot be adequately accommodated as in youth.

The anterior chamber of the eye decreases because of the thickness of the lens. The iris becomes paler in color as a result of pigment loss and increases in the density of collagen fibers. Resorption of the intraocular fluid becomes less efficient with age and may lead to eventual breakdown in the absorption process. This creates the potential for the pathologic condition known as *glaucoma.*

The constant compression of lens fibers with age, the yellowing effect, and the efficiency of the aqueous humor, which provides the lens with nutrition, all have a role in altered lens transparency. Lens cells continue to grow but at a slower rate than previously. The cells on the periphery of the lens regenerate very slowly, whereas those toward the center are more active. Nearly everyone between ages 40 and 45 begins to discover the need for assistive lenses for reading and accommodation. Those who are nearsighted (myopic) tend to experience reading and accommodation difficulties later—in their 50s and 60s.

Lens opacity or cataracts begin to develop around the fifth decade of life. The origins are not fully understood, although ultraviolet rays of the sun contribute to the problem, with cross-linkage of collagen creating a more rigid and thickened lens structure.

Intraocular Changes

The vitreous humor, which gives the eye globe its shape and support, loses some of its water and fibrous skeletal support with age. Opacities other than cataracts can be lines, webs, spots, or clusters of dots moving rapidly across the visual field with each movement of the eye. These opacities, known as *floaters,* are bits of coalesced vitreous that have broken off from the peripheral or central part of the retina. Mostly they are harmless and annoying until they dissipate or one gets used to them. If, however, the person says that he or she sees a shower of these and a flash of light, this requires immediate medical attention, as it might indicate retinal problems (Kupfer, 1995).

The retina has less distinct margins and is duller in appearance than in younger adults. Fidelity of color is less accurate with blues, violets, and greens of the spectrum; light colors such as reds, oranges, and yellows are more easily seen. Color clarity diminishes by 25% in the sixth decade and by 59% in the eighth decade. Some of this difficulty is linked to the yellowing of the lens and impaired transmission of light through the retina. The macula also may not have as bright fovea reflective light. Drusen (yellow-white) spots may appear in the macular area. As long as these changes are not accompanied by distortion of objects or a decrease in vision, some pigment deposition is not clinically significant.

Arteries may show atherosclerosis and slight narrowing. Veins may show indentations (nicking) at the arteriovenous crossings.

The lubrication and cleansing actions of the lacrimal secretions diminish. Eyes take on a dull appearance, and there is a sensation of dryness, scratchiness, or tightness. Depending on the severity of discomfort, artificial tears are an available lubricant.

Auditory Changes

External Ear Changes

The auricle, or pinna, loses flexibility and becomes longer and wider as a result of diminished elasticity. The lobule sags, elongates, and develops wrinkles. To-

gether these changes make the ear appear larger. The periphery of the auricle develops coarse, wiry, stiff hair in men. The tragus also becomes larger in men.

The auditory canal narrows, causing inward collapsing. Stiffer and coarser hair lines the ear canal. Cerumen glands atrophy, causing thicker and dryer cerumen, which is more difficult to remove and a substantial cause for hearing impairment.

Middle Ear Changes

The tympanic membrane becomes dull, less flexible, retracted, and gray in appearance. The ossicle joints between the malleus and the stapes develop calcification, causing joint fixation or reduced vibration of these bones and reducing transmitted sound.

Inner Ear Changes

There is a decrease in vestibular sensitivity as a result of degeneration of the organ of Corti in the cochlea and otic nerve loss. Changes in the efficiency of the cochlea and hair cells of the organ of Corti are responsible for the impaired transmission of sound waves along the nerve pathways of the brain and are considered to be the most common cause of presbycusis. Atrophy of the organ of Corti begins in middle age and causes sensory hearing loss. Loss of cochlear neurons occurs in late life (even with the preservation of the organ of Corti), is a neural hearing loss, and is considered to be related to genetic factors. Familial tendencies in middle life associated with electrophysiologic function of the organ of Corti are the basis of metabolic hearing loss (Gulya, 1995). Altered motion of the cochlear ducts occurs in middle age and is considered cochlear conductive hearing loss. The role of basilar membrane stiffening as a possible cause of this type of hearing loss is not proved. All of these types of loss are presbycusis. Many elders have a combination of causes for their hearing deficit.

Constant or recurring high-pitched tinnitus (clicking, buzzing, roaring, ringing, or other sounds in the ear) is usually caused by impairment of the otic nerve accompanying the aging process, although it may be caused by medications, infection, cerumen accumulation, or a blow to the head (Gulya, 1995). Tinnitus may be unilateral or bilateral and becomes most acute at night or in quiet surroundings. It is a nuisance that is difficult to combat or treat. The most helpful strategy is to use "masking" techniques that introduce another, competing sound. "White noise" (soft static between FM radio stations) on low volume can be soothing.

Auditory changes occur subtly. Normal decrements in hearing acuity, speech intelligibility, level of auditory threshold, and discrimination of pitch, especially in the speech frequencies, are referred to as *presbycusis,* the "hearing loss of aging." Presbycusis is the type of loss, not the cause of the loss, and can be classified according to the structural source of impairment. Further discussion of vision and hearing is addressed in Chapter 9.

Changes in Somesthetic or Tactile Perception

Somesthetics, or tactile sensitivity, decreases with age because of skin changes and the loss of a large number of nerve endings. This is particularly striking in the fingertips, palms of the hands, and lower extremities (Whanger, Wang, 1974; Kenshalo, 1979; Verillo, 1980).

Changes in Kinesthetic Sense

The kinesthetic sense, or proprioception (one's position in space), is altered with age because of the changes in the central nervous system and muscles. Elders have more difficulty orienting their body in space when externally induced changes in body position are made. Slowed movements and altered position in space can lead to considerable difficulty with balance and spatial orientation. The aged cannot avoid obstacles as quickly in ordinary situations such as those that occur on a crowded street, nor are the aged as able as they once were to prevent an accident from happening to themselves or to others when fast movement might be essential. The automatic response to protect and brace oneself when falling is slower, and one can observe the aged making more precise and deliberate movements, such as placement of the feet when walking. Conditions such as arthritis, stroke, some cardiac disorders, or damage to the structures of the inner ear may affect peripheral and central mechanisms of mobility. Further discussion of sensory alterations appears in Chapter 10.

IMMUNOLOGIC CHANGES

Immune senescence, the lapse of time between exposure and rechallenge of pathogens, decreases as does the strength of response with advanced age (Miller, 1990; Hirsh, 1995; Yehuda, 1995). Old age brings a decrease in T-cell function that is due to a decrease in cell-mediated immunity, humoral immunity, and self-tolerance. The response to foreign antigens decreases, but the immunoglobulins increase. This creates an autoimmune response not associated with autoimmune

disease, which usually occurs before middle age (Miller, 1990). The loss of functional capacity of the cell-mediated system is demonstrated by a decreased hypersensitivity response to such skin tests as the tuberculin test. The implications are that aged persons are more susceptible to reactivation of latent herpes zoster and mycobacterium. Appendix 7-A presents the age-related changes and gives examples of functional effects and possible nursing interventions.

BIOLOGIC THEORIES OF AGING

Major causes of aging have been categorized as follows:
1. Aging results from external causes; that is, the life span would be indefinite were it not for environmental insults such as pollution, food, toxins, radiation, bacteria, and viruses.
2. Aging results from internal causes based on a finite life span that is determined through specific programming of body systems.
3. Aging results from internal and external cellular and molecular causes that singularly or together produce changes in fluidity, permeability, or transport; wear and tear; cross-linkages or free radical activity; or DNA damage, catastrophic RNA errors, or mutations, to mention a few.

Various biologic theories of aging have been more persuasive than others at various times. No unifying theory exists that explains the mechanics and causes underlying the biologic phenomenon of aging. Theories of aging can be addressed from a molecular, cellular, or systems level point of view. As one studies these theories, it will become apparent that some theories emerge from others and that one or more theories could be superimposed on others. Each theory in its own right provides a clue to the aging process. However, many unanswered questions remain. Scientists in their continual search for truth persist in piecing together the puzzle of aging. New and exciting data concerning biologic theories of aging have emerged recently through the application of more sophisticated methods of unlocking the secrets of the cell. We are beginning to confirm some of the previous suppositions and to develop a more thorough understanding of the genetic, molecular, and biochemical basis of cellular changes of aging. In time, the student will begin to discriminate and develop an eclectic approach to theories of aging as he or she becomes familiar with the many facets of the aging process.

Table 7-1

Summary of Biologic Theories of Aging

Theories	Dynamics	Retardants
STOCHASTIC THEORIES		
Error theory	Faulty synthesis of DNA and/or RNA; faulty protein or enzyme activity causes defective structure or function; transcription or translation failure between cells	
Free radical theory	Oxidation of fats, proteins, carbohydrates, and elements creates free electrons that attach to other molecules, altering cellular function	Improve environmental monitoring; decrease intake of free radical-stimulating foods; increase vitamin A, C, and E intake; use coenzyme Q10
Cross-link theory	Lipids, proteins, carbohydrates, and nucleic acid react with chemicals or radiation to form bonds that cause an increase in cell rigidity and instability	Caloric restriction, lathyrogen-antilink agents
Wear-and-tear theory	Repeated injury and overuse of cells, tissues, organs, or systems	
NONSTOCHASTIC THEORIES		
Programmed theory	Biologic clock triggers specific cell behavior at specific time; specific number of cell divisions dictates specific life span	Hypothermia and low-calorie diet can delay cell division but not the number of cell divisions
Neuroendocrine theory	Control mechanism (pituitary and hypothalamus) regulates interplay between organs and tissues; efficiency of signals between mechanisms is altered or lost	Treatment with potent hormones such as dehydroepiandrosterone (DHEA) and RU486
Immunologic theory	Alteration of B and T cells leads to loss of capacity for self-regulation; normal or age-related cells are recognized as foreign matter; system reacts by forming antibodies to destroy these cells	Immunoengineering, selective alteration, and replacement or rejuvenation of immune system

DNA, Deoxyribonucleic acid; *RNA,* ribonucleic acid.

Stochastic and Nonstochastic Theories

Stochastic theories suggest that aging events occur randomly and accumulate with time. These theories are molecular and cellular in nature and include such theories as the gene theory, the error theory, the somatic mutation theory, the free radical theory, the cross-link theory, the clinker theory, and the wear-and-tear theory.

Nonstochastic theories suggest that aging is genetically programmed for the specific life span of an organism and include programmed senescence, which implies aging of the entire organism. This category of theories is considered systems level and includes the intrinsic pacemaker, immune, and neuroendocrine theories.

A summary of these theories appears in Table 7-1.

▶ KEY CONCEPTS

- Age-related changes are the observable, measurable, or felt changes that occur in one's being over time and are chiefly focused on physiologic and biologic changes.
- Physiologic aging is universal, progressive, decremental, intrinsic, and unavoidable.
- There are enormous individual variations in the rate of aging of body systems and functions.
- The changes in the cardiovascular system are most likely to progress toward a disease state in late life.
- Careful assessment of individual aging changes, life-style, and desires is fundamental to good nursing care of the old.

NANDA and Wellness Diagnoses

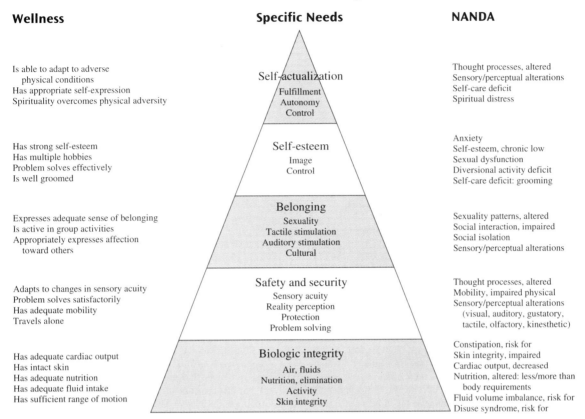

Wellness

Is able to adapt to adverse
    physical conditions
Has appropriate self-expression
Spirituality overcomes physical adversity

Has strong self-esteem
Has multiple hobbies
Problem solves effectively
Is well groomed

Expresses adequate sense of belonging
Is active in group activities
Appropriately expresses affection
    toward others

Adapts to changes in sensory acuity
Problem solves satisfactorily
Has adequate mobility
Travels alone

Has adequate cardiac output
Has intact skin
Has adequate nutrition
Has adequate fluid intake
Has sufficient range of motion

Specific Needs

Self-actualization
Fulfillment
Autonomy
Control

Self-esteem
Image
Control

Belonging
Sexuality
Tactile stimulation
Auditory stimulation
Cultural

Safety and security
Sensory acuity
Reality perception
Protection
Problem solving

Biologic integrity
Air, fluids
Nutrition, elimination
Activity
Skin integrity

NANDA

Thought processes, altered
Sensory/perceptual alterations
Self-care deficit
Spiritual distress

Anxiety
Self-esteem, chronic low
Sexual dysfunction
Diversional activity deficit
Self-care deficit: grooming

Sexuality patterns, altered
Social interaction, impaired
Social isolation
Sensory/perceptual alterations

Thought processes, altered
Mobility, impaired physical
Sensory/perceptual alterations
    (visual, auditory, gustatory,
    tactile, olfactory, kinesthetic)

Constipation, risk for
Skin integrity, impaired
Cardiac output, decreased
Nutrition, altered: less/more than
    body requirements
Fluid volume imbalance, risk for
Disuse syndrome, risk for

These are not all of the possible wellness or NANDA diagnoses that may be identified. The above are frequent examples of nursing diagnoses that should be considered when planning care for the older adult in whatever setting.

▶ **Activities and Discussion Questions**

1. Identify at least two normal and two abnormal physical/physiologic changes with age for each body system.
2. Discuss the age changes you would find most difficult to accept.
3. Obtain the creatinine level and prescribed medication from the chart of several aged persons. Calculate the urine creatinine levels to identify the GFR and to determine if there is a danger of drug toxicity from the medication(s) being taken.

4. Develop a nursing care plan using wellness and NANDA diagnoses.

REFERENCES

Altman DF: Changes in gastrointestinal, pancreatic, biliary, and hepatic function with aging, *Gastroenterol Clin North Am* 19(2):227, 1990.

Baltimore Longitudinal Study of Aging, National Institutes of Health No 84-2450, Washington, DC, 1984, US Government Printing Office.

Bartz B: Mechanisms of endocrine control and metabolism. In Copstead LEC: *Perspectives on pathophysiology,* Philadelphia, 1995, Saunders.

Bay MK: The aging liver. In Abrams WB, Beers MH, Berkow R, editors: *The Merck manual of geriatrics,* ed 2, Whitehouse Station, NJ, 1995, Merck Research Laboratories.

Beare P, Myers J: *Adult health nursing,* ed 3, St Louis, 1998, Mosby.

Campbell EJ, Lefrak SS: How aging affects the structure and function of the respiratory system, *Geriatrics* 33:68, 1978.

Cassmeyer VL, Blevin DB: The patient with biliary and pancreatic problems. In Long BC, Phipps WJ, Cassmeyer VL, editors: *Medical-surgical nursing: a nursing process approach,* ed 3, St Louis, 1993, Mosby.

Coni N, Davison W, Webster S: *Aging: the facts,* New York, 1984, Oxford University Press.

Cornell RC: Aging and the skin: what is normal aging? *Geriatr Med Today* 20(5):24, 1986.

Costa PT, Andres R: Patterns of age changes. In Rossman I, editor: *Clinical geriatrics,* ed 3, Philadelphia, 1986, Lippincott.

Cunningham WR, Brookbank JW: *Gerontology: the psychology, biology, and sociology of aging,* New York, 1988, Harper & Row.

Diettert G: Circulation time in the aged, *JAMA* 183:1037, 1963.

Fifth report of the Joint National Committee on Detection, Evaluation, and Treatment of High Blood Pressure, *Arch Intern Med* 153(2):154, 1993.

Frohlich EV: Hypertension. In Abrams WB, Beers MH, Berkow R, editors: *The Merck manual of geriatrics,* ed 2, Whitehouse Station, NJ, 1995, Merck Research Laboratories.

Fujino M, Okada R, Arakawa K: The relationship of aging to histologic changes in the conduction system of the normal heart, *Jpn Heart J* 24:13, 1982.

Gardin JM et al: Echocardiographic measurements in normal subjects: evaluation of the adult population without apparent heart disease, *J Clin Ultrasound* 7:85, 1979.

Gersteinblith G et al: Echocardiographic assessment of a normal adult population, *Circulation* 56(2):273, 1977.

Goldman R: Decline in organic function with age. In Rossman I, editor: *Clinical geriatrics,* ed 2, Philadelphia, 1979, Lippincott.

Grove GL, Kingman AM: Age associated changes in human epidermal cell renewal, *J Gerontol* 38:137, 1983.

Gugoz Y, Munro HN: Nutrition and aging. In Finch CE, Schneider EL, editors: *Handbook of the biology of aging,* ed 2, New York, 1985, Van Nostrand Reinhold Co.

Gulya AJ: Ear disorders. In Abrams WB, Beers MH, Berkow R, editors: *The Merck manual of geriatrics,* ed 2, Whitehouse Station, NJ, 1995, Merck Research Laboratories.

Health after 50: the next five years: our experts look ahead, *Johns Hopkins Med Lett* 6(1):1, 1996.

Health after 50: important new advice for treating hypertension, *Johns Hopkins Med Lett* 8(2):7, 1994.

Hirsh B: Normal changes in host defenses. In Abrams WB, Beers MH, Berkow R, editors: *The Merck manual of geriatrics,* ed 2, Whitehouse Station, NJ, 1995, Merck Research Laboratories.

Jacobs R: Physical changes in the aged. In Deveraux MO et al, editors: *Elder care: a guide to clinical geriatrics,* New York, 1981, Grune & Stratton.

Joynt RJ: Normal aging and patterns of neurologic disease. In Abrams WB, Beers MH, Berkow R, editors: *The Merck manual of geriatrics,* ed 2, Whitehouse Station, NJ, 1995, Merck Research Laboratories.

Kenney RA: *Physiology of aging: a synopsis,* New York, 1982, Mosby.

Kenney RA: *Physiologic aging,* ed 2, New York, 1989, Mosby.

Kenshalo DR: Changes in vestibular and kinesthetic systems as a function of age. In Ordey JM, Brizzee KR, editors: *Sensory systems and communication in the elderly,* New York, 1979, Raven Press.

Krumpe P et al: The aging respiratory system, *Clin Geriatr Med* 1:143, 1985.

Kupfer C: Ophthalmologic disorders. In Abrams WB, Beers MH, Berkow R, editors: *The Merck manual of geriatrics,* ed 2, Whitehouse Station, NJ, 1995, Merck Research Laboratories.

Lakatta EG: Normal age changes. In Abrams WB, Berkow R, editors: *The Merck manual of geriatrics,* Rahway, NJ, 1990, Merck Research Laboratories.

Lakatta EG: Cardiovascular regulatory mechanisms in advanced age, *Physiol Rev* 73(2):413, 1993.

Lakatta EG: Normal age changes. In Abrams WB, Beers MH, Berkow R, editors: *The Merck manual of geriatrics,* ed 2, Whitehouse Station, NJ, 1995, Merck Research Laboratories.

Lamb KV: Musculoskeletal function. In Lueckenotte A, editor: *Gerontologic nursing,* St Louis, 1996, Mosby.

Leyden JJ, Grove GL, Ginley JK: Age-related differences in the rate of desquamation of skin surface in the aging process. In Adelman R, Roberts J, Christofalo VJ, editors: *Pharmacological interventions in the aging process,* New York, 1978, Plenum.

Lillington GA: *Diagnosis and arrangement of pulmonary problems in the elderly.* Presentation at Eldercare workshop, The National Institute of Care of the Elderly, University of Nevada, Reno, October 1979.

Lindemann RD, Tobin JD, Shock NW: Longitudinal studies on the rate of decline in renal function with age, *J Am Geriatr Soc* 33(4):278, 1985.

Lindsay R: The aging skeleton. In Haug M, Ford A, Sheafor D, editors: *Physical and mental health of aged women,* New York, 1985, Springer.

MacLennan W, Peden N: *Metabolic and endocrine problems in the elderly,* New York, 1989, Springer-Verlag.

Malasanos L, Barkauskas V, Stoltenberg-Allen K: *Health assessment,* ed 4, St Louis, 1989, Mosby.

Miller RA: Aging and the immune response. In Schneider EL, Rowe JW, editors: *Handbook of biology of aging,* ed 3, San Diego, 1990, Academic Press.

Pierson DJ: Effects of aging on the respiratory system. In Pierson DJ, Kacmarek RM, editors: *Foundations of respiratory care,* New York, 1992, Churchill Livingstone.

Richard C: Renal function. In Copstead LEC, editor: *Perspectives on pathophysiology,* Philadelphia, 1995, Saunders.

Richey ML, Richey HK, Fenske NA: Age-related skin changes: development and clinical meaning, *Geriatrics* 43:49, 1988.

Rossman I, editor: *Clinical geriatrics,* ed 3, Philadelphia, 1986, Lippincott.

Rowe JW: Aging process: renal changes and disorders. In Abrams WB, Beers MH, Berkow R, editors: *The Merck manual of geriatrics,* ed 2, Whitehouse Station, NJ, 1995, Merck Research Laboratories.

Schenker S: The aging liver. In Abrams WB, Beers MH, Berkow R, editors: *The Merck manual of geriatrics,* ed 2, Whitehouse Station, NJ, 1995, Merck Research Laboratories.

Schumann L: Alterations in respiratory function. In Copstead LEC, editor: *Perspectives on pathophysiology,* Philadelphia, 1995, Saunders.

Schuster MM: Effects of aging on the GI system. In Abrams WB, Beers MH, Berkow R, editors: *The Merck manual of geriatrics,* ed 2, Whitehouse Station, NJ, 1995, Merck Research Laboratories.

Sloane PD: Normal aging. In Ham RJ, Sloane PD, editors: *Primary care geriatrics: a case based approach,* ed 2, St Louis, 1992, Mosby.

Solomon DH: Age-related endocrine and metabolic changes: normal and diseased thyroid gland. In Abrams WB, Beers MH, Berkow R, editors: *The Merck manual of geriatrics,* ed 2, Whitehouse Station, NJ, 1995, Merck Research Laboratories.

Stehler B: Physical changes. In Porterfield JD, St. Pierre R, editors: *Healthy aging,* Sluice Dock, Guilford, Conn, 1992, Dushkin Publishing Group.

Tichy AN, Malasanos LJ: Physiologic parameters of aging, *J Gerontol Nurs* 5:42, Jan/Feb 1979; 5:38, April/May 1979.

Timaris PS: *Physiologic basis of geriatrics,* New York, 1988, Macmillan.

Timaris PS: *Physiologic basis of aging and geriatrics,* ed 2, New York, 1994, CRC Press.

Tockman MS: The effects of aging on the lungs: lung cancer. In Abrams WB, Beers MH, Berkow R, editors: *The Merck manual of geriatrics,* ed 2, Whitehouse Station, NJ, 1995, Merck Research Laboratories.

Tompkins RG: Surgery: preoperative evaluation and interoperative and postoperative care: surgery of the gastrointestinal tract. In Abrams WB, Beers MH, Berkow R, editors: *The Merck manual of geriatrics,* ed 2, Whitehouse Station, NJ, 1995, Merck Research Laboratories.

Verillo RT: Age-related changes in sensitivity and vibration, *J Gerontol* 135:185, 1980.

Wardell S: *Acute intervention: nursing process throughout the life span,* Reston, Va, 1979, Reston.

Welch CE: Surgery: preoperative evaluation and intraoperative and postoperative care: surgery of the gastrointestinal tract. In Abrams WB, Beers MH, Berkow R, editors: *The Merck manual of geriatrics,* ed 2, Whitehouse Station, NJ, 1995, Merck Research Laboratories.

Whanger AD, Wang HS: Clinical correlates of the vibratory sense in elderly psychiatric patients, *J Gerontol* 29:39, 1974.

Yehuda AB: Normal change in host defense. In Abrams WB, Beers MH, Berkow R, editors: *The Merck manual of geriatrics,* ed 2, Whitehouse Station, NJ, 1995, Merck Research Laboratories.

appendix 7-a   Physiologic Changes and Functional Effects With Age: Implications and Interventions

System	Physiologic Changes	Functional Effect	Nursing Implications*	Possible Interventions*
Integument	Skin loses elasticity: wrinkles, folds, sagging, dryness	Easy tearing; itching Incisions, cuts, bruises heal more slowly than in younger adults	Introduction of organisms leading to infections Bath or shower water temperature should be between 95° and 105° F	Nurse should keep own nails short; handle skin with care; limit bathing to every other day; lubricate skin with perineal area daily; lubricate skin with lotion at least once daily
	Spotty pigmentation in sun-exposed areas; face paler (even without presence of anemia)			Apply sunscreen before going outside; wear a hat and sunglasses
	Atrophy of epidermal arterioles		Prone to pressure ulcers; slow wound healing	Inspect skin when bathing; check pressure areas at least every 2 hours if patient is bedridden; if sitting in chair, as soon as medically possible; if ambulating, at least every few days; maintain immaculate aseptic technique
	Atrophy of oil, moisture, and sweat glands	Dryness Prone to hyperthermia	Life threatening	Hydrate; wear light, cool clothing; stay in cool area; apply ice to back of neck or head to keep cool
	Decreased subcutaneous fat; fat deposition mainly through trunk, less on extremities	Altered thermoregulation (hypothermia)	Life threatening	Maintain warm environment; use warm blankets; warm intravenous (IV) fluids postoperatively if necessary or if very chilled; in cold weather provide warm environment and maintain humidity at 60%; adequate warm clothing
	Hair thins on scalp, axillae, and pubic areas; decreases on upper and lower extremities; decreased facial hair in men; women may develop chin and upper lip hair			
	Nail growth slows	Nails prone to snagging, chipping, ragged edges, tearing	Intentional or unintentional scratching	Keep nails clipped short and filed; offer periodic basic manicure; buff nails or apply nail polish

Respiratory	Nose elongates Stiffer pharynx and larynx Decreased cilia Increased anterior-posterior chest diameter Rigidity of chest wall Fewer alveoli Airway resistance	Congestion Voice pitch higher Potential for upper respiratory tract infections	Place in upright position when eating, drinking, or having respiratory problems; limit exposure to airborne viruses, bacteria, pollutants; adequate ventilation; yearly flu immunization Establish exercise program (walking or stationary bike riding, etc.); pace activity; provide adequate rest periods Deep-breathing exercises; ascertain that patient has Pneumovac immunization (1 time after age 65); auscultate lungs; smoking cessation program
	Decreased cough reflex Decreased removal of mucus, dust, irritants Decreased vital capacity Decreased chest expansion reduces recoil Decreased endurance Hyperinflation of apices; underinflation of bases		
Cardiovascular	Thickening of walls of blood vessels Narrowing of vessel lumen Loss of vessel elasticity Lower cardiac output Decreased number of heart muscle fibers Decreased elasticity and calcification of heart valves Decreased baroreceptor sensitivity	Fatigue, shortness of breath Dependent edema Decreased cardiac output Dysrhythmias Murmurs Dizziness from too-rapid change of position	Pace activities; monitor blood pressure; establish aerobic exercise program; smoking cessation program Check for swelling and pitting edema; wear support hose; elevate feet periodically during day Auscultate heart and lungs; if on medication, ascertain that they are taken (given correctly); teach client about taking medications Overall teaching for heart-healthy diet: decrease intake of fat, sodium, sugar; control weight Instruct on proper way to get up after lying in bed, sitting for extended periods of time; how to bend over and get up
	Left ventricle hypertrophy (only in fiber size) Decrease in rate, rhythm, and tone (heart rate normal at rest)		
	Decreased efficiency of venous valves	Poor venous return	Venous pooling, stasis dermatitis; stasis ulcers; varicosities; dependent edema
			Inspect for color and swelling, beginnings of stasis dermatitis or ulcers; palpate for temperature; wear support hose; no crossing of legs at knees

Data from Ebersole P, Hess P: *Toward healthy aging: human needs and nursing response*, ed 5, St Louis, 1998, Mosby; Copstead LEC: *Perspectives on pathophysiology*, Philadelphia, 1995, Saunders; Stanley M, Beare PG: *Gerontological nursing*, Philadelphia, 1995, Davis; Abrams WB et al: *The Merck manual of geriatrics*, ed 2, Whitehouse Station, NJ, 1995, Merck Research Laboratories; and Saxon SV, Etten MJ: *Physical change and aging*, ed 3, New York, 1994, Tiresias Press.
*Provides examples of some implications and interventions.

Continued

appendix 7-a Physiologic Changes and Functional Effects With Age: Implications and Interventions—cont'd

System	Physiologic Changes	Functional Effect	Nursing Implications*	Possible Interventions*
Gastrointestinal	Periodontal disease; loss of teeth	Change in jaw/mouth contour; poor mastication	Changes in food intake; fetid breath; edentulousness	Appropriate oral hygiene regimen: brushing teeth 2-3 times daily, use of dental floss; minimum of yearly teeth cleaning and checkup (every 6 months is best) If dentures: clean daily; remove at night; keep in good repair
	Decrease in saliva production	Dry mouth	Breakdown of tissue integrity of oral mucosa	Chew gum to create moist environment; use artificial saliva; drink adequate fluids (minimum 1500 ml/day); monitor/instruct on chewing food slowly and thoroughly
	Decrease in secretion of digestive juices Pancreas less active—decrease in production of insulin Decreased smooth muscle Decreased esophageal peristalsis Decreased small intestinal peristalsis	Food intolerances; difficulty with digestion	Improper eating patterns; dependency on antacids	Assess for food intolerance; avoid offending foods
Musculoskeletal	Decreased muscle mass	Muscle strength diminishes	Unable to do tasks done when younger; danger of injury	Muscle-strengthening exercises (weight training)
	Skeletal changes Decalcification of bones	Brittle bones	Fractures; osteoporosis; thoracic-vertebral hump	Adequate calcium intake; flexibility exercises and weight-bearing exercises (walking)
	Degenerative joint changes	Stiffer joints; restricted movement; aches and pains with movement; femoral joint angle causes legs to turn outward	Limited mobility; arthritis; potential for gait changes, falls	Gentle exercise (water aerobics); use of acceptable analgesics as necessary (topical, systemic); application of heat, cold
	Dehydration of intervertebral disks	Decreased height	Shorter stature; flexed posture	

Neurologic	Nerve cell degeneration and atrophy (25%-40%) Decrease in neurotransmitters Decrease in rate of nerve cell conduction impulses	Some degree of recent memory loss (age associated—benign) Learning occurs as usual but more slowly	Forgetfulness; requires longer time for response Potential for dementing processes Client becomes frustrated Longer reaction time to questions and response to danger	Approach learning projects slowly Use memory aids (adhesive notes, calendars, word association, etc.) Assess mental status using clock drawing and Mini-Mental Status Examination as appropriate Assess environment for safety Use reminiscence as appropriate
Sensory (Refer to Appendix 9-A.)	Eyes: pupils decrease in size; less light enters eyes; lens yellows	Presbyopia: decreased accommodation to near/far; difficulty adjusting to light and dark Color distortion Glare Cataracts Decreased tear production	Difficulty reading small print, seeing objects in distance, dealing with fine detail of objects Poor accommodation to rapid light changes in environment Difficulty seeing colors at dark end of spectrum (greens, blues, violets, browns) Squinting or pain from bright light or sunshine Decreased ability to see Dry, scratchy eye	Adjust lighting to decrease glare Increase light intensity—direct light directly over area where client is working Use bright and contrasting colors; stay away from dark end of spectrum Provide magnifying glass or magnifying sheet for reading labels or small print; print information in larger type Slowly change light intensity from bright to dim and vice versa
	Ears: thickening of tympanic membrane; sclerosis of inner ear; ear wax buildup	Presbycusis: loss of high-frequency sounds; decreased mobility of ossicles; impaired hearing		
	Taste: may have fewer taste buds on tongue, mouth Smell: often diminished Touch: decreased skin receptors Proprioception: decreased awareness of body position in space	Correlation between taste and smell		

Continued

appendix 7-a Physiologic Changes and Functional Effects With Age: Implications and Interventions—cont'd

System	Physiologic Changes	Functional Effect	Nursing Implications*	Possible Interventions*
Genitourinary	Gradual loss of nephrons (30% to 50%)	Decreased absorption of tubules; decreased glomerular filtration rate (GFR)		Remove barriers to getting to toilet
	Decrease in renal blood flow	More time needed for filtration; urine may be more dilute		Answer call lights or bell as quickly as possible and provide assistance to toilet as needed
	Decreased bladder capacity Women: may develop lax sphincter	Need to urinate frequently; incontinence; decreased bladder tone		Assess pattern of voiding with continence log if incontinence is occurring; look at circumstances that might be responsible; establish a toileting plan
	Men: enlargement of prostate	Benign prostatic hypertrophy; potential for urinary retention		Use continence pads or pants as needed, but make sure they are checked and changed when wet Provide commode if toilet is too far away
				As a last resort, catheterize
Reproductive	Women: decreased estrogen production; ovaries degenerate; vagina atrophies; uterus and breasts atrophy	Lose ability to procreate; vaginal dryness; uncomfortable intercourse; menopause		Discuss types of hormone replacement therapy, from natural products to medical prescriptions
				Explore various vaginal lubricants for dryness
				Explain normal age changes that occur to both men and women
	Men: sperm count diminishes; testes smaller; less firm erections take longer to occur	Erectile dysfunction concerns		Discuss importance of using condoms if individuals are single (never married, widowed, divorced) or live an alternative life-style
				Dispel myths of loss of sexual drive
				Discuss impotence and need for professional consultation

System	Change	Effect	Clinical manifestation	Nursing intervention
Endocrine	Alteration in hormone regulation	Decrease in ability to respond to stress	Impaired physiologic and psychologic responses	Modulate environment to reduce physical, psychologic, and social stressors
Thyroid	Decreased thyroid hormone	Temperature intolerance; decreased target organ sensitivity	Feels too cold or too hot; possible depression or nervousness; weight gain or loss	Periodic thyroid-stimulating hormone (TSH) check
Thymus	Involution of thymus gland	Decrease cell-mediated immunity	More susceptible to infection	Good hand washing; ensure that flu and Pneumovac inoculations are updated; limit exposure to obvious pathogens; maintain aseptic technique in dressing changes and any invasive procedures
Cortisols/glucocorticoids	Increased antiinflammatory hormone	Slower ability to respond to inflammatory process	Decreased speed of tissue repair; slower ability to respond to inflammatory process	
Pancreas	Increased fibrosis; decreased secretions and enzymes	Effect on glucose metabolism	Potential for diabetes mellitus	Periodic blood glucose test

chapter 8

Psychologic, Cognitive, and Social Aspects of Aging

▶ LEARNING OBJECTIVES

Upon completion of this chapter, the reader will be able to:

- Explain the major cognitive, psychologic, and sociologic theories of aging.
- Understand several normal cognitive changes of aging.
- Recognize that culture and cohort affect psychologic and social adaptation.
- Identify several social roles that elder members of a society usually fulfill.
- Discuss several "buffers" that make transitions to new roles somewhat easier.
- Compare some of the differences you would expect between the retirement adjustment of women and men.
- Explain the major issues in adaptation to a major role change such as retirement or widowhood.

▶ GLOSSARY

Cognition The mental process characterized by knowing, thinking, learning and judging.

Cross-sectional A study design that includes several groups, assessing these subjects at different points in a process. An example of this would be cohort studies that involve several cohorts and survey their experience around a given event.

Depersonalization As used in this chapter, not a severe psychiatric disturbance but, rather, the loss of identity and sense of self that occurs when a person is treated as an object.

Longitudinal research A study design that studies a group of subjects over time, assessing their experiences at predetermined stages. The Harvard Nurses' Study is an example of this in that a large group of nurses have been assessed every few years for over 20 years.

Psychometrics The development, administration, and interpretation of psychologic and intelligence tests.

Psychosocial Pertaining to a combination of psychologic and social factors.

Regeneration Rebuilding of impaired or injured tissues.

Synaptogenesis To form a connection between neurons.

▶ THE LIVED EXPERIENCE

Somehow I always thought life would just go on as it has. I never expected to be old. Gradually I realize that people treat me differently at times and recognize that it is because they see me as old. I feel just as I did at 30, but I know there have been some changes in my reactions. I forget things oftener, especially names, and that worries me. I wonder if that is normal.

Jennie, age 70

Sometimes I think that I am not important to Jennie. If I were, she would surely remember my name. Just this week she asked me again, for the third time!

Laurie, age 30

*T*here are normal psychologic, cognitive, biologic, and social changes in the process of aging. The biologic changes are fully explained in Chapter 7. This chapter is meant to provide the reader with information on the psychosocial aspects of aging. The student can then identify normal cognitive, psychologic, and sociologic changes and begin to detect those that go beyond the normal changes and need attention. All of the psychosocial aspects of aging are less measurable than the biologic changes, and there is much to be learned about the aging process. Each individual has unique life experiences and because of this must be seen holistically, through the lens of his or her time, place, and personal history.

LIFE SPAN DEVELOPMENT THEORY

Life span development refers to an individual's progress through time and an expected pattern of change: biologic, sociologic, and psychologic.

Two theories form the basis for life span development theorists. One is the belief that over time, strong personality characteristics become exaggerated. The contrasting view is that living organisms tend to adapt and become more complex, but in time these changes become less organized. Regardless of which theory one believes, the course of behavior throughout the life span appears to have three major forces: hereditary, cultural, and individual choice (Birren, Cunningham, 1985). The close relationship between biologic, social, and psychologic development that exists through childhood and adolescence varies more in adulthood because of the greater variations in life experiences and demands as one matures.

Psychologic age is expressed through a person's ability and control of memory, learning capacity, skills, emotions, and judgment. Maturity and capacity will direct the manner in which one is able to adapt psychologically over time to the requirements of the physical and social environment. One must also consider life space; a healthy psychologic adaptation to a nursing home would be entirely different from psychologic adaptation to a penthouse apartment in New York City.

Social age may be quite different from chronologic age and is measured by age-graded behaviors that conform to an expected status and role within a particular culture or society. For example, seeking donor egg implants in order to bear a child is considered outside of expected normal behavior in a woman of 60 years or more.

From a biologic perspective, the influence of genetics on psychosocial aging is demonstrated in the Swedish Adoption/Twin Study of Aging. This ongoing longitudinal study includes a comparison of identical twins raised apart. The twins studied have later shown similar life experiences and personal inclinations that seem to have some genetic basis (Plomin, McClearn, 1990).

Buhler (1964) was one of the first humanistic psychologists who saw the uniqueness and potential in each phase of the life span. Lehman (1953) and Kuhlen (1968) added to the picture of the varied nature of adult development, and Jung (1971) considered the importance of different personality types as they develop. The idea is that individuals will develop in particular ways because of their heredity or social environment. A factor that is often ignored is gender differences. These are discussed throughout the text when there are important differences.

PSYCHOSOCIAL THEORIES OF AGING

The three major psychosocial theories of aging—disengagement, activity, and continuity—are important because they influence the expected behaviors of the aged.

Disengagement Theory

The disengagement theory states that "aging is an inevitable, mutual withdrawal or disengagement, resulting in decreased interaction between the aging person and others in the social system he belongs to" (Cumming, Henry, 1961, p. 2). This means that withdrawal from one's society and community is natural and acceptable for the aged and their society. The measures of disengagement are based on age, work, and decreased interest or investment in societal concerns.

Consider the example of Mary: Mary has been active most of her life in protecting the legal rights of children and has been very involved in important state legislation that has affected them. She has also been known for her marvelous parties, often entertaining the powerful people within the community. Shortly after her retirement she sold her huge home, moved to a rural area, and is now quite content taking care of her yard, flowers, and grandchildren. Mild arthritis sometimes interferes with her gardening pleasure. Occasionally someone from her working years will call for advice about an issue affecting the children in the state, but others have taken her place in those affairs. She was the mentor for several of the individuals who carry on her work.

Activity Theory

The activity theory is based on the belief that remaining as active as possible in the pursuits of middle age is the ideal in later life. Because of improved general health and wealth, this is more possible than it was 40 years ago when Maddox (1963) proposed this theory. Consider the example of Bill, an architect and a hiker. He loved discovering new trails, people, and places. They often inspired new architectural designs. He often traveled to Eastern Europe to study the intricate architecture. On retirement, he had sufficient health, wealth, and opportunity to continue his lifelong interests.

Continuity Theory

The continuity theory, proposed by Havighurst and co-workers (1968), explains that life satisfaction with engagement or disengagement depends on personality traits. Three ideas about personality (Neugarten et al, 1968) are important to understanding continuity theory:

1. In normal aging, personality traits remain quite stable as men and women age.
2. Personality influences role activity and one's level of interest in particular roles.
3. Personality influences life satisfaction regardless of role activity.

Consider the example of Jim, a Chicano, who had always felt a bit out of step with those around him. His parents were immigrants, spoke only Spanish, and maintained the traditions of their Guatemalan origins. Jim was a loner and a rather poor student. He had to begin working as a house painter when he was 17 years old. He did not expect life to be much more than hard work and a few pleasures along the way. Over the years he became an excellent painter and progressed to a foreman, but he was cautious by nature and never considered going into business for himself. His desire was to retire early and rest, which he did.

• • •

In all three of the psychosocial theories of aging, the importance of opportunity, ethnicity, gender, and social status is largely ignored. For example, Mary had many choices, a good education, and sufficient retirement resources. She also had lifelong interests in homemaking that provided continuity, although in many ways she was disengaged.

PSYCHOLOGIC ASPECTS OF AGING

The psychology of aging is the study of changes in behavior that characteristically occur after young adulthood. Healthy psychologic aging involves coping in ways that ensure one's psychologic integrity. The self-view must be maintained and appreciated.

Retaining dignity and self-respect in the face of the catastrophes accompanying aging is a poorly understood psychologic component of successful aging (Lenker, Polivka, 1996). Some individuals maintain a strong sense of self regardless of devastating changes. These are the psychologically "hardy" persons (Bowsher, Keep, 1995). The hardy ones are capable of enduring physical and emotional stressors because they maintain a sense of control and challenge. Each event is seen as an open door on new experience and one that allows for choice (Kobasa, 1979; Ebersole, 1996).

Self-Efficacy

Some older persons are *hardy* individuals who believe that their personal actions and decisions are effective (perceived self-efficacy [Bandura, 1977]). These individuals are able to manage well even in circumstances that overwhelm others. They are able to do so partially because they have developed strong social networks and adequate financial resources (McAvay et al, 1996). Hardiness involves control, competence, and challenge. Some also add a fourth characteristic—compassion. Indeed, it seems that those who manage best against all odds are those whose central concerns go beyond self to include others. This presupposes some underlying altruism and a sense of humor. Nurses can further self-efficacy by respecting elders' decisions, commenting on areas of competence, and asking about challenges. By listening thoughtfully, one hears the compassion and sense of humor that is often present.

Personality Styles and Phases

One's personality under ordinary conditions is assumed to remain quite stable across the adult life span. Such personality traits as interiority (tending toward introversion), extroversion (sociability), stability, creativity, sensitivity, and openness to experience do not seem to change when studied over time and during different life stages. Two of the most important of these for older adults are interiority and stability.

Interiority

The last half of life is often a time of inner discovery, quite different from the biologic and social issues that demand a great deal of outward attention during the first half of life (Jung, 1971). The last half of life, ideally, is less intensely demanding and allows more time for inner growth, self-awareness, and reflective activity. The development of the psyche and the inner person is accompanied by a search for personal meaning and the spiritual self. However, many older persons may not be released from the demands of daily living and have little time for such indulgences. Others do not value psychologic exploration and remain action oriented. Spirituality is an important aspect of development in later life and the means by which one becomes whole and develops the integrity described by Erikson. Wholeness may be achieved by doing, as well as reflecting. Seeing a valued activity toward completion may be a very enlightening experience.

Stability

Stability of personality over time is in itself a personality characteristic. Some persons act in very predictable ways throughout their life. These individuals will accept the demands of aging just as they do every other event in their lives. They are fairly predictable in their responses and thus may be easier to care for than those who are inconsistent in their life patterns and actions. Age does not in itself appear to affect personality traits in healthy, community residents. Some serious disease states, especially pathologic brain conditions, and institutional living may bring about major personality changes.

Psychologic Tasks of Aging

Theories are the organizing framework from which tasks quite naturally will arise. Box 8-1 summarizes some of the concepts, dynamics, issues, and tasks that have been formulated by various life span theorists over the years to explain human development. These, like the biologic theories of aging, all have some elements of truth but must be seen only as the particular theories that various groups ascribe to. Psychosocial theories of human development are much less clear than biologic theories because there are many variables—culture, cohort, and gender being the most significant. The most recognized theories are those of Jung and Erikson. Jung has not established tasks but, as explained previously,

sees a natural shift in concerns in the aging process. Erikson has provided the most useful framework for human development considerations.

Establishing Integrity

Erikson (1963) saw the last stage of life as a vantage point from which one could look back with integrity or despair on one's life. Erikson believed in a predetermined order of development that proceeded by critical steps, all dependent on timing and sequence. However, he also theorized that individuals return again and again to the stages that have been poorly resolved. It is assumed that certain inner biologic and outer sociologic conditions are required to achieve integrity in late life. Thus some elders will be struggling with much earlier developmental needs. In later years Erikson and his wife, Joan, reconsidered his seminal work from the perspective of their own aging (they were both octogenarians at the time). They reframed their presentation of the theoretic framework as achieving balance at each stage of life. Thus ego integrity is tinged with some regrets, wisdom is balanced with frivolity, and letting go is balanced with hanging on. The Eriksons define wisdom as "detached concern with life itself, in the face of death itself. It maintains and learns to convey the integrity of experience, in spite of the decline of bodily and mental functions" (Erikson et al, 1986, p. 38).

Peck (1968) identified discrete tasks of old age that must be addressed to establish integrity:

- *Ego differentiation versus work role preoccupation.* The individual can no longer be defined by his or her work.
- *Body transcendence versus body preoccupation.* The body is cared for but does not consume the interest and attention of the individual.
- *Ego transcendence versus ego preoccupation.* The self becomes less central, and one feels a part of the mass of humanity, their struggles, and their destiny.

It is clear that to achieve integrity by Peck's model, one must develop the ability to redefine self, to let go of occupational identity, to rise above body discomforts, and to establish meanings that go beyond the scope of self-centeredness. Although these are admirable and idealistic goals, they place a considerable burden on the aged individual. Not everyone may have the courage or energy to laugh in the face of adversity or surmount all of the assaults of old age. The wisdom of old age involves a crisis of understanding in which the ordinary structures are shaken and the meaning of life is reexamined. It may include the wisdom of questioning assumptions in the search for meaning in the last stage of life.

Box 8-1   SUMMARY OF THEORIES OF HUMAN DEVELOPMENT

I. Life stages model
   A. Jungian (popular)
     1. Anchored in psychoanalytic theory
       a. Mid-life shift—second stage of development
         (1) Anima—female; emergence of in men
         (2) Animus—male; emergence of in women
     2. Issues
       a. Masculinity-feminity
       b. Creativity-destructiveness
       c. Attachment-loss
   B. Eriksonian—psychosexual stages
     1. Organized in sequences of life structures and transitions (6- to 10-year average)
       a. Stability-disruption (1- to 3-year average)
       b. Equilibrium-imbalance
       c. Denial, rebirth (Kübler-Ross)
       d. Socially and personally motivated with genetic and chronologic influence
   C. Levinsonian—mentors (7 to 10 years older) to guide
     1. 35- to 45-year shift
       a. Guided by a dream
       b. Mid-life crises
       c. End of dream
       d. Death of youth
II. Adaptational model (Valliant)
   A. Basic premises
     1. Gradual shifting of self and understanding
     2. Incremental-decremental shifts
     3. Trade-offs
     4. Holding on and letting go—critical
   B. Examples
     1. Sensory decrease/quality of perception increase
     2. Excitement decrease/experience increase
     3. Physical decrease/wisdom increase
   C. Quantity versus quality
     1. What are you willing to let go of or diminish?
     2. What is not worth pursuing?
     3. What are your best assets?
     4. What is possible?
       a. Undiscovered self
       b. New births of self
     5. Stay with growing edge of self
     6. Bargaining is the essence
III. Life structure and transitions (Lowenthal) (based on organizational life cycles)
   A. Family life cycles
   B. Transitions
     1. College
     2. Marriage
     3. Retirement

   C. Premises
     1. Significant others may not be in the same sequence
     2. Evidence from clinical world
     3. Accelerated life structure transitions
       a. Toffler—*Future Shock*
     4. Choice—intolerance of change or creative change
IV. Dialectic/ecologic/systems (Riegel)
   A. Premises
     1. Based on social psychology
     2. No life span approach
     3. Intersection of events produces change by breaking equilibrium
       a. Triggering event
       b. Turning point
       c. Timing of events (Rossi)
     4. Discover self by reaction
     5. Perspective on development by looking backward
     6. Metaphoric conceptualizations
     7. Restoration of balance
     8. Essence in energy exchanges with impact
   B. Examples
     1. World events, trends, culture, milieu
       a. Geography
       b. Ideational
       c. Situational
       d. Micro and macro systems
       e. Health evolution
V. Fielding model—Roger Gould—psychoanalytic consultation
   A. Premises
     1. Become finest self
       a. Give up safety
       b. Creativity reaches beyond myth of safety
       c. Self-actualizing
         (1) Maslow
         (2) Bueler
       d. Past life, future self
       e. Autonomy/control/taking charge
       f. Pilgrimage of the self
         (1) Teleologic
         (2) Future oriented
         (3) Proactive
         (4) Goal oriented
         (5) Shaping one's own world
   B. Agenda for mature adulthood
     1. Individualization
     2. Recreation
     3. Undo the boring—trigger a transition, renewal
     4. Endings and beginnings—the essence of development

Cynthia Kelly (1990) identified the three *R*'s that define the tasks of aging as (1) accepting reality, (2) fulfilling responsibility, and (3) exercising rights. Realities have to do with accepting one's capacities in the health, social, and financial realms; responsibilities include planning for one's survivors and for making the best choices regarding the remainder of life; and rights include exercising the right to move at one's own pace, the right to privacy, the right to respect, the right to refuse what one does not desire, and the right to participate in plans and decisions related to one's own life. Developmental tasks, as defined by several theorists, are included in Fig. 8-1.

Maintaining Caring and Continuity

For many, caring remains focused on children and grandchildren. Reflecting on the successes of children confirms their own success as parents. The aspect of caring, so predominant during the generative stages in the adult years, is the quality that provides the greatest sense of continuity. As individuals nurture their young and watch their descendants nurture their young, they experience a connectedness with the repetitious cycles of life and at times an opportunity to redo their youth. Continuity and vicarious fulfillment are experienced as one sees qualities in grandchildren that were identified in the self or in the parents or grandparents of self. As many as six generations may be viewed in continuous progression. Others find caring and connectedness through ideas, creative works, mentoring, and contributing to progress in their fields of expertise.

COGNITION AND AGING

Cognition is both a biologic and psychologic factor that must be considered in caring for the older adult. The abnormal biologic aspects of brain function are dealt with in Chapter 21; normal functions are addressed in this chapter and in Chapter 7.

In general, cognitive performance in testing is poorer for the very old than for those 60 to 80 years old (Poon et al, 1992). Most tests were designed by adults

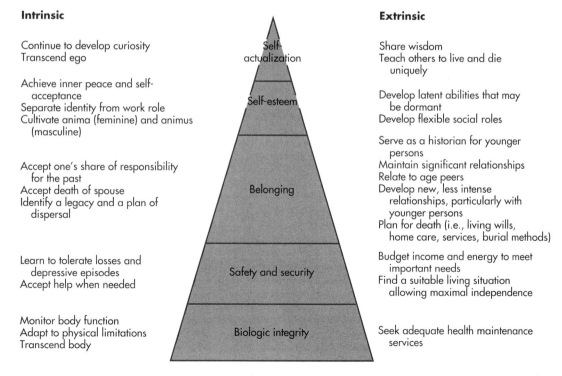

Intrinsic

Continue to develop curiosity
Transcend ego

Achieve inner peace and self-
  acceptance
Separate identity from work role
Cultivate anima (feminine) and animus
  (masculine)

Accept one's share of responsibility
  for the past
Accept death of spouse
Identify a legacy and a plan of
  dispersal

Learn to tolerate losses and
  depressive episodes
Accept help when needed

Monitor body function
Adapt to physical limitations
Transcend body

Extrinsic

Share wisdom
Teach others to live and die
  uniquely

Develop latent abilities that may
  be dormant
Develop flexible social roles

Serve as a historian for younger
  persons
Maintain significant relationships
Relate to age peers
Develop new, less intense
  relationships, particularly with
  younger persons
Plan for death (i.e., living wills,
  home care, services, burial methods)

Budget income and energy to meet
  important needs
Find a suitable living situation
  allowing maximal independence

Seek adequate health maintenance
  services

Pyramid levels (top to bottom): Self-actualization, Self-esteem, Belonging, Safety and security, Biologic integrity

Fig. 8-1 Developmental tasks of late life in hierarchic order. (Data from Peck R: Psychological developments in the second half of life. In Neugarten B, editor: *Middle age and aging*, Chicago, 1968, University of Chicago Press; and Havinghurst R: *Developmental tasks and education*, New York, 1972, McKay.)

to test children or young adults. These tests may have no relevance for daily function and are of little value.

Ecologic validity and context are important in testing normal cognitive capacities. That is, psychometric tests of intelligence must have relevance to the daily lives of older adults if they are to be useful.

However, cognitive development of the aged is often measured against the norms of young or middle-age people, which may not be appropriate to the distinctive characteristics of the aged. Intelligence in old age is dynamic, and certain abilities change and even improve with age (Fig. 8-2).

More and more theorists are now speculating about the possibility of the unique cognitive powers of old age, as did Plato. Reflective regression (intense reliving and reviewing of old memories) and life review seem to be a form of cognitive development characteristic of late life. Individuals become absorbed with memories and meanings.

Berry (1974) provides a good example in Old Jack, who sat in a rocking chair on the veranda of the general store, immersed in the span of his years and the meanings of events. He failed to see what was going on around him or recognize people, not because of cognitive decline but because of immersion in memories. It is doubtful that he would remember, if asked, what he ate for breakfast, or even if he ate breakfast. If we are not alert to the normal-

ity of this tendency, we will not understand the cognitive differences that occur in the process of aging.

Late adulthood is no longer seen as a period of growth cessation and arrested cognitive development; rather it is seen as a life stage programmed for plasticity and the development of unique capacities. Education, pulmonary health, general health, and activity levels all influence cognitive activity in later life. Other reasons have been advanced for the variations of intellectual performance of the older adult being tested (Box 8-2). Crowley (1996) says that if brain function becomes impaired in old age, it is a result of disease, not aging.

The Aging Brain

Because neurons in adult brains were believed not to replicate themselves and many older people do lose mental acuity, generations of people believed that the brain stopped growing early in childhood. We now understand the necessity of stimulation and that continued development requires appropriate levels of challenge throughout life. The brain is influenced by the environment, and even with the death of some neurons, there is potential for patterning and learning through stimulation of alternate cerebral cells to expand function. This is shown most remarkably in the retraining of individuals in speech and other functions following a stroke. With

Fig. 8-2 Life span cognitive developmental strengths. (Developed by Priscilla Ebersole.)

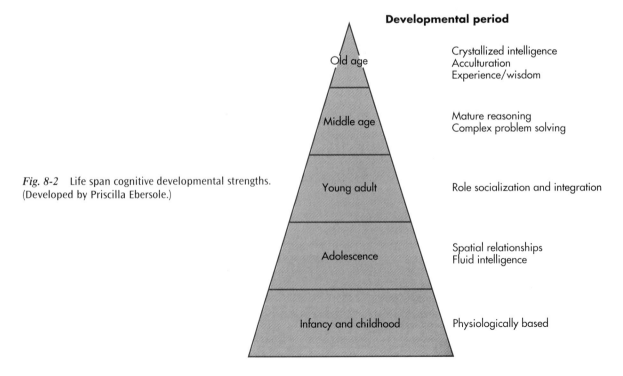

stimulation, the aging human brain has shown increases in neuron size and in the number of dendrites, or neuron branches, that transmit information to other cells. There is potential for regeneration of cerebral cells. Nerve cells are designed to receive stimuli and will very quickly shrink when in an unstimulated state. When neuronal input to a neuron or a group of neurons is lost, the nerve fibers from undamaged neurons may sprout and form new connections to replace the lost connections. This phenomenon is known as *axon sprouting*. A presently unidentified growth factor may stimulate regeneration, and some people may lose this growth factor more readily than others. By learning about the growth factor, it will be possible to determine whether the regrowth of brain tissue can be stimulated. This self-reparative process is known as *reactive synaptogenesis*.

Reactive synaptogenesis is now known to be part of a general process known as *synapse turnover*. This process of synapse turnover is a stimulus-induced loss and replacement and is not part of the normal growth and development processes. The stimulus may vary, and examples of documented cues are (1) an injury; (2) a metabolic insult; (3) a subtle modification in behavior, such as learning a new task; and (4) a physical or chemical stimulus (Cotman, 1990).

The regeneration and rebuilding of lost circuits in the brain have been termed *plasticity* and have been thought to be limited to the immature brains of children and adolescents. Cotman (1990) has shown that plasticity continues, with training, into very old age. He has even reported this regenerative process in the brains of some older adult victims of Alzheimer's disease. When brain cells die and the connections are lost, the healthy cells rebuild those connections.

Living in isolation or in institutional settings with little individually significant input is detrimental to brain function. When working with the older adult to improve cognitive functions, there must be regular input and "exercise" of the brain around ideas that are significant and interesting to the older person.

Memory Retrieval

Memory, according to the information processing (IP) model of adult cognition, is the process of storing and retrieving information. The computer is the metaphor for human cognition. Memory includes a number of capacities that make up the system enabling us to remember. The initial register on the senses maintains a literal copy of a stimulus for up to 2 seconds. Short-term memory (STM) requires attention and retention of information

---

Box 8-2   COMPLEXITIES OF ACCURATELY ASSESSING INTELLECT IN OLD AGE

- The old are most frequently compared with college students, whose chief occupation is proving their intellectual capacity.
- Young adults are in the habit of being tested and have developed test wisdom, a skill never developed by the elderly or one that has grown rusty with disuse.
- Test material may not be relevant to the world of the aged.
- The ability to concentrate is inversely related to anxiety.
- Intellectual function declines differentially. The old are assumed deficient in encoding during learning, storing information for retention, and/or speed of retrieving stored information.
- Adrenal or stress hormones may be responsible for some of the gradual changes in the brain during aging.
- A distinct relationship may exist between cognitive function and nutritional status.
- Older persons always perform more slowly than younger people in tasks involving neuromuscular learning because of slower reaction time and an increase in cautious behavior.
- Aged clients often perform poorly on test items because they are less likely to guess and more likely not to answer any items that seem ambiguous to them.

- Cautiousness has often been described as the reason why older adults do not perform as well as younger people in memory tasks. Other personality traits such as greater activity levels, less impulsiveness, and greater emotional stability also seem to influence how well older people perform on memory tests.
- Old people may have difficulty focusing attention and ignoring irrelevant stimuli.
- Subject attrition in longitudinal studies of the aged shows evidence of the survival of the intellectually superior.
- There is no evidence of general slowing of central nervous system activity in old age as had been commonly presumed and reported by researchers.
- Intellectual performance relying on verbal functions shows little or no decline with age, but speeded tests using nonverbal psychomotor functions show a great decline.
- Social cognition and social context are related in terms of elder function. The elderly who maintain the best cognitive function are also those with a high social interactional level.

from 30 seconds to 30 minutes, and long-term memory (LTM) stores and retains information for long periods.

The practicality of these distinctions in everyday life is that even though some older subjects show decrements in processing information, reaction time, perception, and attentional tasks, the majority of functioning remains intact and sufficient. Familiarity, previous learning, and life experience compensate for the minor loss of efficiency in the basic neurologic processes. In unfamiliar, stressful, or demanding situations these changes may be more marked.

Elders seem to learn best when new information or expectations can be related to familiar concepts and prior knowledge. Mood is extremely important in terms of what individuals (old and young) will recall. In other words, when we attempt to measure recall of events that may have occurred in a crisis situation or an anxiety state, recall will be impaired. This is significant for health care workers who give information to elders when the elders are ill or upset. They are very likely not to remember it.

Age-Associated Memory Impairment

The term *age-associated memory impairment (AAMI)* is used to describe recall deficiencies that occur with aging. This condition was previously termed "benign senescent forgetfulness" and is thought to be normal among the old. Some elders suffer AAMI even though they have no dementia. It is not yet understood what all of the factors are that produce AAMI, but it is known that anxiety and fear of memory loss will often result in memory impairment. If the memory loss is not affecting daily function in a negative way, then the elder simply needs to be reassured that it is common. Some find memory training programs very beneficial.

Mental Frailty

A problem similar to AAMI is mental frailty (Wolanin, 1997). The concept is rooted in the triad of change, stress, and lack of support. Mental frailty can be thought of as a decrease in mental flexibility, similar to the decreases in physical flexibility experienced by the very old. The elder has a sense of continuity of self that persists throughout life and that must be maintained to properly integrate events into the self-image. When undesired, unexpected, or overwhelming changes occur—sociologically, psychologically, or physiologically—an older person may become incapable of thinking clearly. The elder needs stress relief and familiar supports to restore the disturbed balance of self-perception. When these are not available at the appropriate time and degree to maintain the sense of continuity of the predictable self, the elder's mentation goes awry and various psychologic

and cognitive disturbances emerge. Nurses are in a position to restore the personal continuity of the elder by focusing on the familiar, obtaining the support of those within the individual's comfort zone, and immediately reversing (to the extent possible) the overwhelming changes and relieving stress. Maintaining familiar patterns and settings is critical. Many elders who are mentally frail function very well by following a set routine that has become habitual. Caregivers must avoid surprises and unexpected demands. Given assistance to restore the predictable, or careful orientation, encouragement, and time to adapt to new settings, the mentally frail can function very effectively.

SOCIOLOGIC AGING

Sociologic aging is composed of the performance of expected social roles appropriate to one's chronologic age, culture, and capacity. Terms that are associated with sociologic aging are *age norms, social time clocks, age grading,* and *social time.* All of these are descriptive of the place individuals should occupy in a society at any given time in their lives. The great diversity of individuals in the United States has made social aging complex and social norms virtually nonexistent. Social scientists are now focusing more attention on the interaction of age, origins, historic period, and cohort in attempts to study the social aspects of aging from a life course perspective.

Life Course

The life course is composed of elements that make up the overall structure and timing of events in one's life from cradle to grave. It must be examined and taken into account to understand an aged individual. This is the basis for longitudinal studies. Life structure is composed of roles (occupational, social, and family), relationships (intimate, personal, and professional), and inner structure (goals, values, motives, and memories). The progress of all these aspects of life can be considered a life course. Helping elders record and understand the story of their lives, as explained in Chapter 5, clarifies the life course and structure.

Life Transitions

The transitions throughout the life course include major shifts in social expectations and responsibilities due to age, role, occupation, family, and economics (Cunningham, Brookbank, 1988). Fig. 8-3 outlines the distribution of these transitions.

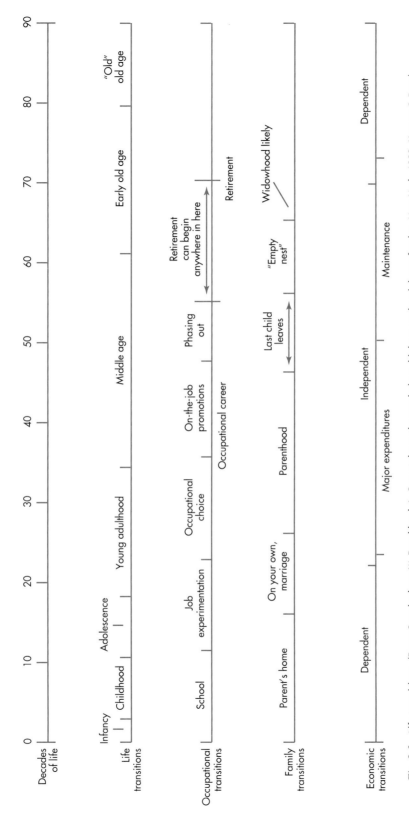

Fig. 8-3 Life transitions. (From Cunningham W, Brookbank J: *Gerontology: the psychology, biology, and sociology of aging.* New York, 1988, Harper & Row.)

Many of the major transitions in the lives of elders involve the loss of roles. In some cases there is role accumulation, such as that of grandparent. Shifts in the parental roles are gradual and do not require complete role deletion or role reversal. Those transitions that make use of past skills and adaptations are least stressful. Some shifts, such as from functional independence to functional dependence, are particularly difficult. A transition is socially recognized and entails a reorientation of perceptions and expectations of and by the individual and significant others. Cohort and gender differences are inherent in all of life's major transitions.

Age Norms

Norms are socially shared expectations of the "shoulds" and "oughts" of behavior. As mentioned earlier, norms are difficult to identify in a multicultural society. The large population of extremely old persons lacks predictable transitions, and thus after age 80 norms are virtually nonexistent.

Status and Role Changes

Status and role are the concepts around which norms, relationships, conformity and deviance, and stability and change are organized. The role of the aged in our society remains highly variable. The major issues to be considered are the number and significance of an elder's roles as personally defined and valued.

Social Support

Social support is derived from the assurance of love, esteem, and belonging to a network of individuals with common goals and mutual concerns. Social support has traditionally come from intimates, family, friends, and neighbors. In the age of electronic communication and travel ease, many elders receive a great deal of social support through less intense but frequent involvement with others, such as through e-mail, on-line chat groups, and Elderhostel travel groups.

Reciprocity

Many of our elders grew up feeling self-sufficient and highly independent. Yet in this nuclear age we are all aware that we must depend on others and be depended on if we are to survive individually and culturally. The concept of reciprocity in relationships and society is basic to survival. In old age, as people become physically and functionally dependent in various ways, their contribution often involves sharing their history and wisdom and demonstrating their survival capacities to younger persons. The aged become our teachers of life. Many also think of reciprocity in terms of payback time: elders spent much of their lives assisting the younger generations, and then it becomes time for the younger ones to assist the elders.

ROLES OF ELDERS

Numerous minor role changes occur in the aging process, but the transitions expected by most elders are related to the work role and the role of spouse or partner. From a life course perspective, the transitions and adaptations required produce both stability and change in individual preferences, capacities, expectations, and behavior. Age-related transitions are socially created, shared, and recognized. A transition is socially recognized and entails a reorientation of perceptions and expectations of and by the individual. Cohort and gender differences exist in all of life's major transitions.

Concepts Related to Role Transitions

To the degree that an event is perceived as expected and occurring at the right time, a role transition may be comfortable and even welcomed. Those persons who must retire "too early" or are widowed "too soon" will have more difficulty adapting than those who are of an age when these events are expected. The speed and intensity of a major change may make the difference between a transitional crisis or a gradual and comfortable adaptation. Role changes that produce crises are usually abrupt losses of familiar functions at a time when meaningful substitute functions are not available.

Anticipatory planning, awareness of potential problems, positive or negative attitudes, and a sense of control (by far, the most important) make role transitions easier.

During the transition from familiar roles to new ones, an individual needs the freedom to try various possibilities in an accepting atmosphere that encourages success, tolerates failure, and recognizes that progress is not accomplished by slow, even steps. In real life, progress follows a more wayward, uneven course. One is easily distracted and often falls back to the familiar. A nurse is most helpful in providing an accepting milieu that encourages independence and exploration, as well as the awareness that transitions all create some anxiety. Useful nursing interventions will assist the aging person in maintaining self-esteem and developing new and satisfying roles.

The most common roles of the aged are retiree, parent, grandparent, great-grandparent, spouse, homemaker, widow, kin, friend, citizen, volunteer, church member, club member, acquaintance, patient, and service recipient. In cases of role accumulation, such as that of grandparent, some previous development will be applicable, with modification, to the new role. Likewise, the shifts in parent-child relationships are gradual and do not require complete role deletion or role reversal. Those transitions that make use of past skills and adaptations may be least stressful.

Role Reversal

Developmental transitions in relationships have received insufficient attention. An interesting area of investigation would be that of the elder's experience of moving from caregiver to care recipient. Most attention has been given to the experience of the caregiver and little to that of elders and their adjustment to the need to be a care recipient. When a strong and independent elder retires because of failing health, the reaction to dependency and role reversal with the spouse may sap the patience and energies of both. Long-standing relationship dynamics may reverse in the illness of old age.

Sometimes a passive/dependent spouse may be unable to make the transition without considerable help. (See Chapter 23 for additional discussion of caretakers.) Assuming an unfamiliar role is difficult for both parties. The nurse should discuss with the couple particular activities that the couple can maintain that are symbolic of their previous roles. For example, perhaps the man always wrote the checks or the woman always determined the need for household supplies. The man may have organized outings and the woman decided on holiday activities. These routines can be sustained with some creative methods devised by nurses. The nurse should be alert to situations in which health care personnel may be able to provide the supports and resources that make it possible for an individual to sustain important habitual activities and assume new responsibilities without being totally overwhelmed.

When a spouse is ill and the mate needs to take over functions for both, it is essential that someone be available to give reinforcement, encouragement, and relief. A day care program, routine visits from a community health nurse, or periodic assistance from a home health aide or a housekeeper may make it possible for the couple to continue to live together. One important consideration is counseling the couple to maintain as much independent function as possible for both persons.

Gender Considerations in Role Transitions

Although women are thought to have greater continuity in their late lives, the roles of old women are generally judged less attractive than those of old men (Barer, 1993). Women are considered "old" earlier than men and are more often economically and vocationally disadvantaged when single, divorced, or widowed. However, throughout their lives women are confronted with more frequent and visible physical and social transitions and thus may become more adept at adapting to new roles. They have also generally developed a larger network of friends that is not necessarily work related, whereas men are more likely to have closest relationships with those with whom they have worked. These trends have changed somewhat and are expected to continue changing with the emergence of the "baby boomers" on the aging scene.

With few exceptions, all elders must adapt to two major changes that occur with aging: changes in the work role and in the role of spouse or partner.

Retirement

Retirement is no longer just a few years of rest from the rigors of work before death. It is a developmental stage that may occupy 30 years of one's life and involves many stages (Antonovsky, Sagy, 1990). Employers encourage early retirement of older, more expensive workers by offering attractive incentives. The goals of the government and industry are in conflict regarding the older workforce. The government cannot afford a large body of nonworking individuals, and industry cannot afford to keep those individuals in top-salaried positions. With pension security and portability, workers no longer feel forced to remain in a position.

Nursing concern must focus on the group of retirees who did not wish to retire but have been forced into an unplanned job termination as a result of illness or company "downsizing," a euphemism (a pleasant expression for something unpleasant) for cutting out jobs. These individuals are likely to suffer and be in need of counseling and assistance through the transition.

Others, given the opportunity to work past retirement age, must weigh the benefits. Clients should be advised to contact the Social Security office 6 months before their sixty-fifth birthday to qualify for Medicare and to find out exactly how earned income and Social Security will be computed and the net benefit they will garner by continued employment. Generally speaking, it is advisable to begin taking Social Security as soon as one qualifies. Earnings beyond the allowable amount will reduce benefit payments. These figures change each year and between ages 65 and 70. In addition, the age to receive full benefits is gradually increasing; therefore we suggest that anyone approaching retirement age should be advised to contact the Social Security office.

The adequacy of retirement income is dependent not only on work history but on marital history as well. The poverty rates of divorced older women, as seen in Fig. 8-4, are excessively high. Couples who have had previous marriages and divorces have significantly lower incomes than those in first marriages. However, among couples presently approaching retirement age, less than one half are in a first marriage (Holden, Hsiang-Hui, 1996). Policies have been based on the traditional lifelong marriage, and this is no longer appropriate. Traditionally, the variability of women's work histories, interrupted careers, the residuals of sexist pension polices, Social Security inequities, and low-paying jobs created hazards for adequacy of income in retirement. The large group of women living into their 90s quite literally outlive their fixed income. It is now illegal to base retirement calculations on gender and projected survival statistics, but until the early 1980s, women were allotted less pension income based purely on their expected longevity in comparison with men. Although this is no longer true, those who retired 15 to 20 years ago remain penalized because of gender.

Working After Retirement Age

The Regional Coordinating Council for Older Workers (RCC) has been established in all nine federal regions to develop older worker programs. One of these, Operation ABLE (in several regions), offers seminars to assist the older professional in a job search. Other, similar programs include Second Careers, Forty Plus, Experience Unlimited Job Club, The Los Angeles Council on Careers for Older Americans, and AARP Works. For further information see Resources at the end of this chapter.

Career transition programs have appeared in several universities across the United States. Senior Corps of Retired Executives (SCORE) has proved to be a dynamic organization using the talents of retired individuals. Many groups and communities have established job banks to match employers and older workers (see Resources).

Retirement Intentions

Decisions to retire are often based on attitude toward work, chronologic age, health, and self-perceptions of ability to adjust to retirement (Taylor, Shore, 1995). Retirement intentions are variable and include four types of "retirement": to retire from work, to change jobs, to partially retire, or to work for self (Ekerdt et al, 1996). It is important to know just what an individual means

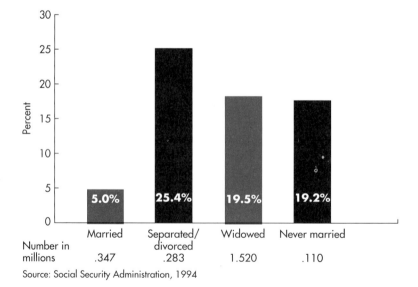

Source: Social Security Administration, 1994

Fig. 8-4 Poverty rates 1993—women Social Security beneficiaries by marital status. (Modified from *The path to poverty: an analysis of women's retirement income,* 1995 Mothers Day Report, Washington, DC, 1995, Older Women's League.)

when discussing retirement. Issues to consider are summarized in Box 8-3.

Working couples must plan together for retirement. Decisions will depend on their career goals, shared future interests, and the quality of their interpersonal relationship.

The following are some questions one must weigh when deciding to retire or continue working:

- What do I want to do?
- Who needs me, and what are my best opportunities?
- What am I best able to do?
- What is the meaning of my life?
- What should my life accomplish or contribute?
- Am I financially independent for the rest of my life if I live 30 more years?
- Am I in good physical condition, and do I enjoy spending time with my spouse?
- Can I afford to completely retire from paid work?

Individuals who are retiring in poor health, minority persons, and those in lower socioeconomic levels need specialized counseling. These groups are neglected in retirement planning programs. Retraining for more satisfying positions and part-time work may be essential.

Many older persons preparing for retirement are also caring for older adult parents. Increasingly, large corporations are developing employee assistance programs that provide support and resources in coping with the needs of these elders. Legislation now supports the right to unpaid leave from jobs for parental or spousal care; however, many persons cannot afford this.

Women are often called on to retire because of a spouse's illness or parents who need help rather than at the most expeditious time. The complexity of the issues includes differences between retirement patterns of single and married women. Single women are as likely as men to retire early, whereas married women, the larger portion of the female workforce, are unlikely to do so. Single and married women differ in the degree of dependency on their own benefits and work history. Pension coverage and health are useful predictors of retirement for men but not for women. The decision to retire for women is often based on the age and health of the spouse or the need to provide care for elder or younger dependents (Talage, Beehr, 1995). For single women, recent income is a more important factor in the decision to retire, and health is less often related to retirement decisions. For both women and men, the most significant factors in adaptation to retirement are health, income, and social involvement.

Retirement Planning for Domestic Partners

Those couples who have lived together for years and have jointly acquired assets may suffer undue discrimination in retirement and death benefit planning. Because automatic survivor benefits are not in place in many

---

Box 8-3   ISSUES IN RETIREMENT POTENTIAL

1. Financial need versus resources
2. Employability
3. Rewards derived from employment
   - Wages sufficient for needs and morale
   - Satisfaction level, possibility for resolution of job frustrations
   - Meaning of job, contact with friends, source of prestige
4. Psychosocial characteristics—attitudes toward retirement
   - Attitudes of significant others (advising? directing?)
   - Strength of work ethic
   - Effect of retirement on prestige
5. Personality factors
   - Time orientation (past, present, future)
   - Active versus passive in planning
   - Rationalism versus fatalism as life stance
   - Type-A versus type-B personality (hard-driving, easy-going)
   - Inner directed versus other directed (enjoyment of self or need for high level of external motivation)

6. Level of information about retirement
   - Planning programs on job, adult education, or community programs
   - Awareness of friends and family who have retired and how influenced by them
7. Pressures to retire
   - Compulsory, age discriminatory
   - Unemployment (how long?)
   - Job retrogression (being moved down the ladder)
   - Skill obsolescence (opportunities for developing other skills?)
   - Peer pressure, organized or informal
   - Employer pressure (reduced incentives to continue work, increased incentives to retire)
   - Family pressure (spouse's working status)
   - Health discomfort, or disability interfering with job performance and dependability

states, it is important to have specific insurance policies or arrangements made that ensure the economic viability of the survivor. Bartley (1996) offers these tips: (1) the financial planner selected should not be prejudiced regarding sexual orientation or preferences; (2) advice must be given that is protective of clients' interests regardless of sexual orientation; (3) it should be kept in mind that a partner may be of first concern to the client even before children; and (4) retirement planners are ethically obligated to be sure that clients have the necessary legal documents on file to provide a smooth transition in the event of premature death or incapacity. Nurses may introduce the topic simply by asking, "Do you have a will or living trust and advance directive on file and plans for your survivors?"

Retiring to a Community

More and more elders are retiring to senior communities. There have been numerous studies of these retirees because they form a collective group, in some ways homogeneous and fairly available. In most of these secluded communities the residents are protected from intrusions by solicitors or researchers. The most likely elders to move to these senior communities are those who are moderately affluent, live alone, and have no children involved in their daily lives. The move is often motivated not only by the social and amenity features but also by awareness of increasing frailty and the urging of family members.

Nurse's Role in Retirement Preparation

Questions a nurse may introduce to clients considering retirement include the following:

- Will retirement income be adequate to provide a lifestyle that includes items and activities that are currently most satisfying?
- Are peer or health pressures significant factors in the decision?
- Is the job depleting to health and energy?

Nurses counseling older adults might gather information and give anticipatory guidance related to retirement issues. The following are guidelines for nurses interested in developing retirement preparation programs:

1. Prepare proposals, documented with facts, for retirement programs.
2. Offer assistance to personnel departments with preretirement programs and encourage the development of programs where they do not exist. Large organizations are likely to be more receptive than smaller ones.
3. Develop and market a preretirement program suitable to individual or group participation. (Suggested topics for retirement education are listed in Box 8-4.)

Box 8-4	TOPICS FOR RETIREMENT EDUCATION

Family and couple concerns
Normal aging processes
Maintenance of physical and mental health in the later years
Financial planning: pensions, Social Security, investments, discounts, property tax rebates
Budgeting
Full- and part-time employment opportunities
Housing and relocation
Legal arrangements and estate planning
Management of real estate
Health care services; Medicare and Medicaid
Death and dying
Leisure and recreational pursuits
Community organizations for elderly
Government role in retirement

4. Support the development of community programs in a college or library for employees who do not have access to such services within their company.

On a more individual level, we would add the following considerations:

- What are the work-related satisfactions, and what might compensate for the loss of those?
- Are friendship networks tied to the person's job?
- How do spouse and family enter into the decision-making process?
- Is there an opportunity to test partial work status or nonworking status before actual retirement?
- Has sufficient information been available regarding retirement planning?
- Is the work situation more stressful than satisfying?
- How much of self is defined by job status?
- Is competitive activity an important source of satisfaction?

Support groups for retirees may be particularly beneficial in the first year following retirement. During the retirement transition, men who retire unwillingly are at risk. Issues that need to be addressed in group discussion are alcoholism, depression, and suicidal feelings. The group leader must be supportive and an empathetic listener and must provide resources and direct referrals when needed. (See Chapter 25 for further discussion of depression.) Encouraging the client to fully review the work experience and its meaning in order to gain closure, as well as inquiring about other stressors that may add to the chaotic feelings during transitions, is important.

Box 8-5 PATTERNS OF ADJUSTMENT TO WIDOWHOOD

Stage One: Reactionary (first few weeks)

Early responses of disbelief, anger, indecision, detachment, and inability to communicate in a logical, sustained manner are common. Searching for the mate, visions, hallucinations, and depersonalization may be experienced. INTERVENTION: Support, validate, be available, listen to talk about mate, reduce expectations.

Stage Two: Withdrawal (first few months)

Depression, apathy, physiologic vulnerability occur; movement and cognition are slowed; insomnia, unpredictable waves of grief, sighing, and anorexia occur. INTERVENTION: Protect against suicide and involve in support groups.

Stage Three: Recuperation (second 6 months)

Periods of depression are interspersed with characteristic capability. Feelings of personal control begin to return. INTERVENTION: Support accustomed life-style patterns that sustain and assist person in exploring possibilities.

Stage Four: Exploration (second year)

Individual begins new ventures, testing suitability of new roles; anniversaries or holidays, birthdays, and date of death may be especially difficult. INTERVENTION: Prepare individual for unexpected reactions during anniversaries. Encourage and support new trial roles.

Stage Five: Integration (fifth year)

Individual will feel fully integrated into new and satisfying roles if grief has been resolved in a healthy manner. INTERVENTION: Assist individual in recognizing and sharing own pattern of growth through the trauma of loss.

Widows and Widowers

By age 78, 63% of all women will be widows and 21% of men will be widowers (US Bureau of the Census, 1998). For those who have been married for many years, this is the most difficult adjustment one can face, aside from the loss of a child. Losing a partner when there has been a long, close, and satisfying relationship is essentially losing one's self and one's core. The mourning is as much for self as for the individual who has died. Part of oneself has died with the partner, and even with satisfactory grief resolution, that self will never return. Even those widows and widowers who reorganize their lives and invest in family, friends, and activities often find that many years later they still miss their "other half" profoundly. With the loss of the intimate partner several changes occur simultaneously that involve social status, economics, and self-image. Individuals who have been self-confident and competent seem to fare best.

Patterns of adjustment can be seen in Box 8-5. Knowing the stages of the transition to a new role as a widow or widower may be useful, although each individual is unique in this respect. Many studies have found that widowers adapt more slowly than widows to the loss of a spouse and often remarry quickly. Common bereavement reactions of widowers are listed in Box 8-6 and should be discussed with male clients.

Box 8-6 COMMON WIDOWER BEREAVEMENT REACTIONS

The search for the lost mate
The neglect of self
The inability to share grief
The loss of social contracts
The struggle to view women as other than wife
The erosion of self-confidence and sexuality
The protracted grief period

Widowhood or widowerhood is a stage in the life course that leads to a new identity. The transitional phase of grief, if handled appropriately, leads to the confirmation of a new identity. It is the end of one stage of life and the beginning of another. When the long-frozen winter is over, the woman or man emerges, shedding the intense grief and ready to cultivate strength and independence to the fullest. The self, previously "halving" identity with another, tries to emerge from the cocoon. This is not always done successfully, but those who do emerge gain a new identity.

Nurse's Role With Widows and Widowers
- Provide resources as needed, such as groups or grief therapists.
- Sponsor grief support groups in the community.
- Discuss intimacy needs.

- Assess the presence of severe depression and recommend therapy.
- Discuss the effects of depression on sexuality.
- Encourage churches to sponsor programs, groups, and outings.
- Especially for widowers:
  - Provide resources for homemaking courses and skills if needed.
  - Emphasize the need for maintaining male friendships.
  - Encourage delay in making female attachments.

During grief, individuals are vulnerable to inappropriate alliances and must recover before they can gain the energy to make a real investment. Nurses who are empathetic and responsive may find that a grieving man misunderstands their intentions.

Nurses working with the bereaved will need to peruse Chapter 26 for further information on grief. Supporting the grief requires an extension of self to reconnect the severed person with a world of warmth and caring. Each gesture crosses the void to bring the lost back to the land of the living. No one nurse or one family member can do this alone. Hundreds of small caring gestures build strength and confidence in one's ability and willingness to survive.

Divorce and the Elderly

Although 6% of men and 7.4% of women over 65 years old are divorced, this may be a cohort effect that is rapidly changing, because in the past 6 years the numbers of divorced elders have doubled since 1980 (US Bureau of the Census, 1998). There are large generational and individual differences in expectations from marriage, but older couples are becoming less likely to stay in an unsatisfactory marriage (Lanza, 1996).

As health care workers, our concern is with supporting a client's decision to seek a divorce and assisting him or her in the transition. A nurse should alert the client that a divorce will bring on a grieving process similar to that of the death of a spouse and a severe disruption in coping capacity until an adjustment to a new life is made. The grief may be more difficult to cope with because there are no socially sanctioned patterns as in widowhood. In addition, tax

---

Table 8-1

Nursing Care Plan to Deal With Loss of Spousal Role

Nursing diagnosis	Expected outcomes	Interventions
Loss of identity, spousal role, and balance in dependence and independence related to loss of spouse as evidenced by decreased self-concept and self-esteem		
Manifestations: feelings of uselessness, hopelessness; decreased pride in appearance; uninterested in developing new skills, hobbies, and social interactions; lacks initiative to take part in previous roles and activities; unable to manage own affairs	The survivor will: Verbalize feelings of self-worth and self-esteem Set realistic goals that are readily achievable Replace spousal role with self-role Actively participate in meaningful social relationships Begin to accept independent role	Emphasize positive aspects of behavior and appearance; ignore negative aspects. Encourage reminiscing if helpful. Assist in setting realistic, meaningful, attainable goals. Treat with respect and recognize as an individual of worth. Encourage volunteer work, hobbies, and crafts if desired. Assist in replacing lost roles with new ones. Encourage new relationships or the rekindling of old ones. Confirm that need for a sexual relationship is normal and healthy.

From Alexander J, Kiely J: Working with the bereaved, *Geriatr Nurs* 7(2):85, 1986.

and fiscal policies favor married couples, and many a divorced older adult woman is at a serious economic disadvantage in retirement (Holden, Hsiang-Hui, 1996).

A nursing care plan related to dealing with individuals who have lost the spousal role, whether through death or divorce, is provided in Table 8-1.

Grandparental Role

The emergence of grandparents as surrogate parents has become an important consideration for individuals and sociologists. Grandparents serving as parents is a major social phenomenon of the times.

Grandparenting requires a revival of certain elements of the parental role, but the shift in generational needs and expectations, as well as the reduced energy of the elder and, at times, the reduced economic resources and disposable income, is significant,

Personal developmental changes of the elder, as well as the rapidly shifting needs of children, add to the stress of adaptation to the new role. When grandparents believe, correctly or incorrectly, that their deficiencies in parenting are the cause of their adult children's inability to parent, there is often an element of grief and guilt. Full-time grandparenting requires reorganization of life-style, relationships, and patterns of behavior. Therapeutic support groups can be of enormous value. The wide range of involvement with grandchildren must be examined very individually to determine if the role of grandparent is actually transitional.

The following cases exemplify the extreme differences in the grandparental role:

- As a lifelong homemaker, Mary's primary identity, role, and life-style have changed little. She is healthy, has sufficient resources, and enjoys renewing the activities of parenthood. She says it makes her feel younger.
- On the other side, Mary's neighbor, Bob, is facing many changes because his 10-year-old grandson has moved in with him. Now he cannot afford to retire, has found it necessary to become involved in primary school activities again, has little time for old friends and golfing at his club, must be both mother and father to his grandson, and must find child care for his grandson whenever he is not available and the boy is not in school.

These cases exemplify some of the extremes in the continuum of grandparenting.

Volunteer Role

Many elders continue to be contributing members of society through volunteer activities. It is unknown how much they contribute in time, economic savings, and personal satisfaction. One of the predominant reasons for joining volunteer groups is the social contact with other volunteers (Musson et al, 1997). Nurses may explore the possibilities with elders and discuss latent interests and ways they can contribute to others from their vast store of life experience and creative endeavors. Some of the myriad ways they may be involved are seen in Box 8-7.

Box 8-7   VOLUNTEER COMMUNITY SERVICES

Perform in a choral group in nursing homes.
Sew for institutionalized children.
Help deprived persons obtain entitlements.
Provide widow-to-widow help.
Perform American Cancer Society clerical work.
Assist at nutrition programs.
Make dolls for hospitalized children.
Assist children in school remedial reading programs.
Organize food co-op, sell to elders at discount prices.
Raise money with bazaars, white elephant sales for nutrition programs.
Serve as musicians for senior dances.
Teach language classes in senior centers.
Become "fix it" men.
Prepare kits for Red Cross Blood Mobile.
Telephone for homebound.

Present puppet shows to schoolchildren, bringing history alive.
Serve coffee and act as language interpreters at geriatric centers.
Help residents settle into new living arrangements, nursing or retirement homes.
Assist with shopping, walking around.
Teach remedial math to schoolchildren.
Present slide shows as museum volunteers in churches and senior centers.
Assist in child care shelters.
Work with retarded—teach swimming, cooking, and activities of daily living.
Alert isolated elderly to services and Supplemental Security Income (SSI).

Interfaith Volunteers

Religious communities nationwide have organized interfaith volunteer services to provide in-home services for isolated frail elders. Some of the most successful have been organized and supported by the Robert Wood Johnson Foundation. The Interfaith Volunteer Caregivers Program (IVCP) demonstrates the commitment of religious congregations to serving the needs of elders in the community.

Health Care Volunteers

Elderly volunteers serving in hospitals act as foster grandparents, tutor ill children, and write letters for or visit with ailing elders. Johns Hopkins Hospital has had such a volunteer program for 60 years and finds the services of elders invaluable.

Nursing Home Volunteers

There is a meaningful role for senior citizens as workers in nursing homes. Older volunteers have been used extensively in nursing homes without pay. A newsletter from a long-term care facility posted in settings where senior citizens gather or reside, explaining various volunteer activities (such as for entertainers, office workers, transportation aides, cafeteria attendants, activity assistants, workshop assistants, boutique salespeople, gardeners, and friendly visitors) would be a useful method of recruiting volunteers. Having support groups for such volunteers is essential, because they may confront their own fears of decline and disability. Legislation that would train and pay older people who may wish to work in nursing homes would be desirable, since there is currently a great shortage of personnel in long-term care institutions.

Some other successful programs that include or require senior volunteers are the National Network on Aging (Nursing Home Ombudsman Program, National Nutrition Program), ACTION (Foster Grandparents [FGP], Retired Senior Volunteer Program [RSVP], Volunteers in Service to America [VISTA], Senior Companion, Peace Corps), Legal Service Corporation, Service Corps of Retired Executives (SCORE) (Small Business Administration), Department of Veterans Affairs, and National Volunteer School Program (teacher aides). Many of these volunteers are paid or are given other inducements to supplement low incomes. Although the work is considered volunteer activity, positions in all ACTION programs provide some minimal income.

Volunteer Training

Training programs, supervision, and ongoing support are critical to the success of volunteer programs. The

---

Box 8-8   STEPS IN DEVELOPMENT OF VOLUNTEER ROLE

1. Volunteer role uses skills from previous work or community experience. A gain in status, prestige, and community sanction is experienced.
2. Volunteer role improves interest in self and others. Dependence is reduced, and interdependence is created.
3. Feedback is gained from recipients of services. Self-view is improved, and resourcefulness is recognized.
4. Social and psychologic stimulation is found in volunteer settings. Personal growth and development occur as skills are refined.
5. Community rewards and recognition are awarded. New roles of social significance are internalized.

---

following considerations guide the development of successful volunteer programs:

- Administrative support of volunteers
- Clearly determined goals for the program
- A specific orientation program with printed support materials to give volunteers
- Buddy systems to orient and reinforce the volunteer role and expectations
- Periodic evaluations and modifications as needs are indicated by volunteer participants
- Determination of specific awards and rewards to sustain interest and involvement

Individuals should be encouraged to begin minimal participation in volunteer programs before discontinuing the work role. This can serve as a bridge of continuity. There are certain identifiable steps in the full development of a role as a volunteer. These can be seen in Box 8-8. Group involvement and group meetings will solidify and strengthen the identification with the volunteer role. Some, such as the Foster Grandparents program, are particularly fulfilling.

ALONENESS, ISOLATION, AND LONELINESS

The sociology of aging examines the integration of individuals into society, and when a great number of these individuals are alone, lonely, and isolated, the responsive society must address their special needs.

Living Alone

The United States has a large number of elders living alone. Forty-one percent of women and 17% of men over 65 years of age lived alone in 1997 (US Bureau of the Census, 1998). This reflects the affluence of our times, the likelihood of widowhood for women, the involvement of families willing to assist elders in maintaining an independent life-style, and the cultural value of individual independence that is highly treasured in parts of our society. Cultures vary significantly in this respect.

Living alone does not equate with loneliness. The size and quality of the social network and the life patterns of the elder are far more significant than whether the elder has a partner. Those elders who are alone but have supportive friendships may treasure their independence and times of solitude.

Men living alone or with someone other than their spouse are thought to be at a disadvantage in terms of survival, whereas the living situation seems to make less difference to women. Both sexes are affected by income, race, physical activity, and employment, but these are variables that are not necessarily related to being alone. To be alone is to be solitary, apart from others, and undisturbed. Many people have a strong need to be alone. Box 8-9 provides useful guidelines for assessing aloneness.

Isolation

Isolation is a response to conditions that inhibit the ability or opportunity to interact with others or is a result of the desire not to interact. At times, self-imposed isolation by individuals enhances creativity, individuality, and integrity, but when isolation is externally imposed by life situations, it is rarely satisfying.

The classic study by Berkman and Syme (1979) showed that socially isolated individuals were more prone to certain diseases such as ischemic heart disease, cancer, and cerebrovascular and circulatory disorders. They concluded that circumstances that create social isolation may have pervasive health consequences and that the lack of social involvement may influence host resistance and disease vulnerability. Other researchers have since replicated these findings. Isolation increases vulnerability to disease, suicide, and death. Yet there are many who are isolated from the mainstream by age, race, culture, frailty, poverty, geography, appearance, sexual orientation, or stereotypic thinking.

Social isolation has many causes and numerous defining characteristics: absence of supportive signifi-

Box 8-9   ALONENESS

Assessing the Need to Be Alone

Does the patient frequently close the door or turn toward the wall?
Does the patient wear earplugs or eyeshades?
Is the patient reluctant to engage in conversation?
Is there any time allowed for total privacy?
Does the patient seem absorbed in thought without agitation? Daydream?
Does the patient lie or sit with eyes closed frequently?

Interventions

Share your observations of behavior with the patient.
Ask about the meaning.
Assure the patient of certain times of privacy.
Attempt to assign a room with a quiet patient.
Minimize disturbances as much as possible.
Discuss the needs and perceptions of the patient in regard to being alone.

cant others; lack of purpose or challenges; aloneness imposed by others; or withdrawal because of hearing deficits, feelings of rejection, limited mobility, or visual impairment. Recognizable symptoms of the problem in individuals include personal withdrawal from interactions; institutionalization; sad, dull affect; preoccupation with own thoughts; insecurity in public; poor eye contact; being uncommunicative; and seeking to be alone (Lien-Gieschen, 1992). Self-isolation may occur because of shame and guilt or the inability to keep up appearances in public.

Social isolation and emotional isolation are not necessarily equivalent. Older adults are particularly susceptible to social isolation because of environmental strictures, loss of familiar friends, and inability to perform certain activities. In addition, they may voluntarily disengage from some activities and become more intensely involved in those that are more valued. This is characteristic of healthy adaptation, but enforced isolation is likely to have detrimental effects. Emotional isolation involves unfilled needs for affiliation and often results from the loss of significant others.

Biordi (1995) notes that there are four patterns of social isolation with varying consequences. In the first pattern the individual has been socially involved throughout life and will find isolation the most painful. In the second pattern the individual has spent much of adulthood in isolated pursuits and may desire more involvement with others in retirement but may not know how to effectively integrate into a social group. In the third pattern the individual has been actively involved and abruptly, voluntarily, withdraws in late life because of events that cause shame. Finally, in the fourth pattern the lifelong isolate may find the social limitations of old age tolerable, expecting little else.

Assessing elders for vulnerability to undesired social isolation and devising proactive measures to prevent or delay debilitating emotional isolation are nursing functions. Assessing vulnerability involves determination of the following: sensory status and decrements that interfere with communication and participation; absence of interactional opportunities; degree and intensity of losses experienced; and alterations to the sense of self. Interventions in general will involve compensating for sensory deficits, increasing opportunities for interaction with others, working through grief processes, and restoring self-esteem.

Care of the social isolate must be planned based on the source of the isolation, the level, the pattern, and the degree of vulnerability. Isolation conceptualized in levels of a hierarchy and life patterns provides a more accurate assessment of issues and possible interventions (Fig. 8-5 and Box 8-10).

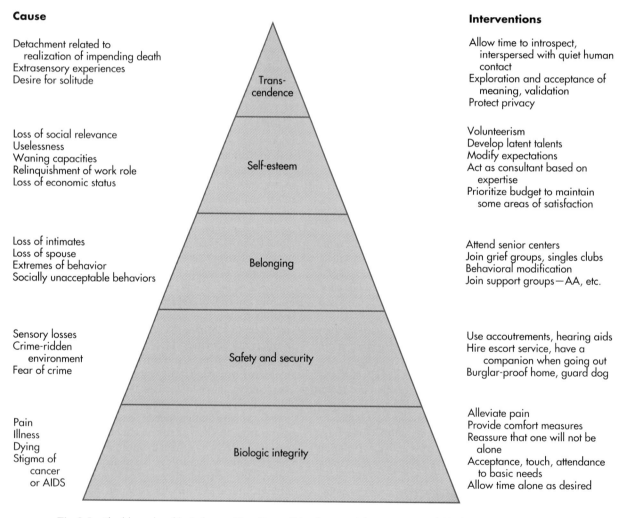

Cause

Detachment related to
   realization of impending death
Extrasensory experiences
Desire for solitude

Loss of social relevance
Uselessness
Waning capacities
Relinquishment of work role
Loss of economic status

Loss of intimates
Loss of spouse
Extremes of behavior
Socially unacceptable behaviors

Sensory losses
Crime-ridden
   environment
Fear of crime

Pain
Illness
Dying
Stigma of
   cancer
   or AIDS

Interventions

Allow time to introspect,
   interspersed with quiet human
   contact
Exploration and acceptance of
   meaning, validation
Protect privacy

Volunteerism
Develop latent talents
Modify expectations
Act as consultant based on
   expertise
Prioritize budget to maintain
   some areas of satisfaction

Attend senior centers
Join grief groups, singles clubs
Behavioral modification
Join support groups—AA, etc.

Use accoutrements, hearing aids
Hire escort service, have a
   companion when going out
Burglar-proof home, guard dog

Alleviate pain
Provide comfort measures
Reassure that one will not be
   alone
Acceptance, touch, attendance
   to basic needs
Allow time alone as desired

(Pyramid levels, top to bottom: Trans-cendence, Self-esteem, Belonging, Safety and security, Biologic integrity)

Fig. 8-5   The hierarchy of isolation and loneliness. (Idea from Ravish T: Prevent social isolation before it begins, *J Gerontol Nurs* 11[10]:10-13, 1985.)

Institutionalization

Despite varying reasons for institutional living, residents of institutions are alienated from the community at large, and their presence is not fully appreciated or understood by the larger community.

The old are usually institutionalized for care and protection. In addition to being isolated from the community by institutionalization, they are often isolated from significant personal interaction and validation within the setting. This isolation produces depersonalization or loss of significance and influence as a person. One becomes a nonentity. The collective identity and pride cultivated in some institutionalized groups are rarely found among the institutionalized aged.

Nursing homes, regardless of quality, carry stigma in the minds of the general population. People who work in institutions for the aged are tainted by the same exclusion and suffer some of the same stigma as the residents. Much of the stigma lingers from the poorhouse concepts of the early part of the century.

Considerable efforts have been made toward enhancement of the experience of institutional living for aged residents and to provide opportunities for meaningful lives within the setting and individual limitations. Many nursing homes today are truly restorative care centers. However, the individuals within them are usually ignored by the community at large and set aside from meaningful contributions. Even in the upscale "health care centers" of life care communities, numerous residents avoid going near the health care center as if the disabilities of the residents were contagious.

A variety of activities for dyads and small groups of interest to residents will increase spontaneous interactions and help develop friendships within the setting. This may address individual isolation, but much remains to be done to establish stronger ties between the long-term care institutions and communities.

Infusing nursing home life with companion animals, plants, gardens, and children allows residents richer opportunities to make connections and reactivate capacities for caring. Some remarkable examples of institutions providing such opportunities are the Benedictine Nursing Center in Mt. Angel, Oregon; Southland Lutheran Home in Los Angeles; and the more than 100 nursing homes involved in the Eden Alternative concept developed by Dr. William Thomas of Sherburne, New York.

Combating institutional isolation and depersonalization. Combating the effects of depersonalization in an institutional setting or community begins with the individual. Some suggestions for decreasing depersonalization include the following:

- Individuals may need assistance in developing a reciprocal relationship with at least one trusted person. Resources for "friendly visitors" and peer counselors can be found through suicide prevention centers, the mayor's office of the city, or senior centers. We seldom bring these resources into institutions, but they should be considered.
- In all situations, options should be made clear in small and large matters.
- Legal aid should be sought for those whose rights have been or are being ignored. Legal aid for the older adult is available, as well as appeals to the human rights commission.
- Every person must have some personal items of importance and his or her own money.
- Contact with pets, plants, natural settings, and children can be renewing.

Box 8-10   PATTERNS OF ISOLATION

Type 1: Lifelong extrovert isolated by condition or situation
- Ameliorate the situation to the greatest extent possible.
- Seek to bring in contact with individuals and groups through the Internet, distance learning.
- Help to identify like individuals who may enjoy frequent telephone contact.
- Establish pen-pal network.

Type 2: Retiree whose contacts were mostly through work and who is now bereft of socialization opportunities
- Seek ready-made groups with some shared interests, often similar to work skills and expertise.
- Interest person in volunteer activities that will use particular skills.
- Provide opportunities to express particular skills in arenas where others will appreciate abilities.

Type 3: Active extrovert who withdraws in late life because of events causing shame (e.g., divorce, alcoholism, poverty)
- Assist with grief resolution, suggest counseling, seek support, self-help group.
- Help find resources addressing specific alienating condition.

Type 4: Lifelong isolate
- Assist in finding resources to augment areas of interest, hobbies.
- Initiate dyadic interactions if individual is willing.

- Writing, taping, or telling one's life history can be a strong affirmation of identity.
- Aged persons should be given accurate information. Half-truths and concealment increase psychologic stress and confusion and refute individual worth.

Rural Isolates

Commonly reported stressors of rural older adults include loss, isolation, financial concerns, and decreased ability to manage (Johnson et al, 1993). In addition, one of every three rural-residing elders is a member of a racial or ethnic minority, compounding the problem of reaching these elders effectively. Nurse practitioners in Nevada, Arizona, Wyoming, and Montana have found that geographically isolated elders tend to demonstrate self-reliance, self-care, alcoholism, stoicism, and individualism (Johnson, 1996). Many of these fall into a category of lifelong semi-isolates, always having had a small network of affiliates that gradually shrinks even more as they age. They have a strong sense of pride and a need for privacy. These isolated elders are unlikely to accept social agency assistance even if it is available. They feel a strong need to reciprocate for any help they receive and may insist on paying or giving a gift even when depriving themselves.

One successful program reported by Boyd et al (1993) concerned the YES (Youth Exchanging with Seniors) program initiated in Texas with the cooperation of the Future Homemakers of America (FHA), Future Farmers of America (FFA), and 4-H clubs. These group members were uniquely suited to interact with isolated elders and, as grandchildren of neighbors and acquaintances, were not seen as intruders. More information regarding the YES project may be obtained from the Robert Wood Johnson Foundation.

Poverty as an Isolating Factor

Throughout the text it is made clear that very old, widowed women of color are among the most poverty-stricken individuals in our society. These elders are more likely to be isolated because of their lack of funds, as well as infirmities that hamper their ability to obtain the services they need. When thinking of ways to intervene with these neglected individuals, the nurse must seek supports that will not stigmatize the individual further by the appearance of poverty. These women rarely feel comfortable in senior centers, even when the centers are available to them. The most likely acceptable resource will be within the churches of their ethnic group and affiliation. Transportation is a high priority and one seldom easily found. Calls to the regional Office on Aging or local senior centers should apprise the nurse of resources that the elder may find acceptable.

Loneliness

Loneliness seems to increase in direct proportion with perceptions of physical incapacity for both men and women. Lonely persons visit the physician oftener, take more medications, and have lower energy levels and multiple psychosomatic illnesses.

Tornstam (1990) studied loneliness among Swedish people and identified four distinct variables of loneliness: intensity and quantity (how often and how painful), inner loneliness (personality introversion), and positive loneliness (isolation sought). Early developmental experiences and present situations remain important factors in the loneliness experienced by the aged. The important contribution of Tornstam's study is his attempt to show loneliness as a complex and multidimensional effect. It is not a categoric condition of the aged.

For nurses, this indicates the need to assess and discuss loneliness in depth rather than simply identify it as a possible factor in the existence of clients. Loneliness is a passive, possessive, and painful emotion, whereas aloneness, solitude, and isolation may be actively sought, enhancing, and creative. Nurses need to assess whether clients are lonely or like to be alone. Nursing care plans for the alone and those for the lonely will be distinctly different. To make an adequate assessment, one must understand loneliness as different from being alone:

- Loneliness is an affective state of longing, emptiness, and feeling bereft.
- Lonely people may be physically alone or surrounded by others.
- Self-growth comes from one's ability to recognize and cope with loneliness.
- Loneliness accompanies self-alienation and self-rejection.
- Loneliness is evidence of the capacity for love. The degree of attachment is directly correlated with the felt loss when detachment occurs.

The Geriatric Orphan

The "geriatric orphan" is an older adult person with no close friends or family members surviving or available to provide supports (Boyack, 1983). He or she has had significant others and lost them to death, distance, or fractured relationships. He or she has not desired to be alone. In the event that such individuals are the last surviving member of their clan, nurses may encourage them to talk about those they have lost. Some have serious "survivor's guilt" that they need to express, particularly if the individual is the eldest and last survivor of a large sibling group. They can be assured that this is an aspect of grief that is often experienced. The survivor may say, "I was always the sickly one. I never expected to live so long. Why me and not them?" The sensitive nurse will resist platitudes and will respond, "Tell me about them."

For some geriatric orphans it may be a relief to be among others in a congregate or institutional setting, whereas others may find it depressing and react much better to friendly visits from younger people. Nurses are urged to make a loneliness assessment with their clients and discuss with them ways in which they could establish contact with others.

Assessing Loneliness

Luggen and Rini (1995) found it useful to assess the social network of community elders to predict those at risk of isolation. Almost half of the sample were found (based on the Luggen Social Network Scale) to be at great risk of isolation and detrimental loneliness. The greatest risk factor was childlessness.

- Does the patient initiate contact?
- Is the patient anxious, withdrawn, apathetic, or hostile?
- Does the patient cling to others or attempt to detain them?
- Is the patient unable to articulate his or her own needs?
- Is the patient eager for visitors and distressed when they leave?
- Does the patient exhibit contempt for his or her condition or self?
- Has there been a major disruption in the number of contacts with the patient?
- How often does the patient feel lonely and under what circumstances?
- Does the patient provoke to gain attention?

Interventions

- Ask about loneliness.
- Spend time with the patient in silence or in conversation.
- Assist the patient in keeping contact with people important to the patient.
- Let the patient know when you will be available.
- Explore the nature of the loneliness with the patient, as well the phenomenon of loneliness.
- Guide the person in reviewing life experiences related to loneliness to gain insight (for the patient) and data (for you).
- See or call the client frequently for brief periods.

Combating Loneliness With Pets

The most common reason people want pets is to combat loneliness. In 1859 Florence Nightingale (reprint, 1992) wrote that pets were excellent companions for persons confined with long-term illnesses. Studies of the value of animals for the aged began to appear in 1980.

For stigmatized or isolated persons, pets may assume great importance because they are always available and nonjudgmental. The unquestioning, uncritical, and unconditional affection seldom found in human relationships may somewhat compensate for the lack of human contact. Touching and fondling a pet may provide a substitute for human touch. In addition, a dog may provide a sense of protection and safety. Individuals recovering from a major loss or those who are institutionalized seem to experienced beneficial effects from a pet (Erickson, 1985).

In organizing and operating a volunteer community-based pet placement program for the community-dwelling older adult, consideration should be given to ethics, legalities, and pragmatic issues, including the desired organizational structure of the service process, criteria for client and animal selection, organization liability in placing pets, facilitation of bonding, development of support services for the older adults and their animals, and evaluation of the success or failure of the placements.

A consideration in the selection of a pet may be potential longevity, because the loss of a pet can produce deep grief. Aged persons losing a pet often grieve intensely for a short period but may not find others responding to their grief. Recognizing the significance, nurses may inquire about pets and the attachment and validate the grief. At these times it is important to make every effort to assist the elder in finding a support system. It may be useful to consider establishing grief groups for individuals whose pets have died. We sometimes become so preoccupied with "serious" issues that we do not fully understand the meaning of the loss of a pet in the life of a lonely elder. These individuals need some sort of funeral or memorial for their pet.

GOVERNMENTAL POLICIES AND THE AGING EXPERIENCE

More than any other factor, the biopsychosocial aspects of aging have been influenced by the governmental policies related to aging. Research dollars influence the rate and substance of new knowledge,

Box 8-11   POLITICAL EVENTS INFLUENCING AGING

1935   Social Security Act signed by Franklin D. Roosevelt.

1937   National Institute of Health established first of the special institutes to study diseases common to older people.

1948   Hospital Construction and Facilities Act (Hill-Burton) provided funds for construction of long-term care facilities.

1950   First National Conference on Aging held in Washington, D.C.

1951   Federal Committee on Aging and Geriatrics created to coordinate federal programs for the aging.

1952   First Federal-State Conference on Aging held in Washington.

1956   Special Staff on Aging established within U.S. Department of Health, Education, and Welfare (HEW). Federal Council on Aging replaced Intradepartmental Working Group on Aging.

1959   Senate subcommittee authorized to consider problems of the aged and aging. Federal Council on Aging reconstituted at Cabinet level.

1960   First appropriation passed for Section 202, Housing Act of 1959, authorizing direct loans for housing for the elderly.

1961   First White House Conference on Aging held in Washington. Senate Special Committee on Aging established as advocate for older Americans. First Annual Conference of State Executives held in Washington.

1962   Federal Council on Aging became President's Council on Aging.

1963   John F. Kennedy sent Congress the First Presidential message on elderly citizens; designated May as Senior Citizens Month. Special Staff on Aging became Office of Aging in HEW's new Welfare Administration.

1965   President Johnson signed Older Americans Act, creating Administration on Aging (AOA). Amendments to the Social Security Act established Medicare program. Foster Grandparent Program initiated by Office of Economic Opportunity and Administration on Aging.

1967   Age Discrimination in Employment Act brightened job outlook for Americans 40 to 65 years old.

1970   Older Americans White House Forums held across the nation to identify problems and issues for upcoming White House Conference on Aging.

1971   Second White House Conference on Aging held in Washington. Cabinet-level Domestic Council Committee on Aging created. ACTION—the Federal volunteer agency—established and given responsibility for senior volunteer programs previously administered by AOA.

1972   New act passed establishing Nutrition Program for the Elderly to be administered by AOA.

1973   Amendments to Older Americans Act called for state agencies on aging to establish area agencies on aging to plan for comprehensive, coordinated service delivery systems for older people at the local level.

Establishment of a National Clearinghouse on Aging and a Federal Council on the Aging with members appointed by the President. Amendments included a separate Older Americans Community Employment Act with responsibility for administering given to Department of Labor.

Federal Aid Highway Act of 1973 provided funds for a demonstration program of public transportation in rural areas with an emphasis on the needs of the elderly and handicapped.

1974   Research on Aging Act established National Institute on Aging within National Institute of Health; Robert N. Butler appointed director. Amendments to Urban Mass Transportation Act of 1964 made funds available to nonprofit private organizations and corporations for transportation vehicles and equipment for the elderly and handicapped. National Mass Transportation Act mandated reduced fares for the elderly and handicapped on all public transportation systems assisted by the Act.

1975   House of Representatives Special Committee on Aging established. Amendments to the Older Americans Act established four new priority areas under Title IV:
a. Transportation
b. Home Services
c. Legal Services
d. Residential Repair and Renovation

1976   Title V of the Older Americans Act received an appropriation for the first time since inception of the Act in 1965. Five million dollars was appropriated "to pay part of the cost of acquisition, alteration, or renovation of community facilities that will serve as multipurpose Senior Centers."

1977   Title V re-funded at rate of $20 million annually.

1981   Third White House Conference on Aging held in Washington, D.C.
Mandatory retirement laws revised.

1982   T. Franklin Williams appointed director of National Institute of Aging.

Box 8-11   POLITICAL EVENTS INFLUENCING AGING—cont'd

1983	Diagnostic-related groups (DRGs) instituted by the Health Care Financing Administration to control costs of Medicare.
1984	Sexual discrimination in pension benefit payments outlawed by U.S. Supreme Court.
1988	Medicare Catastrophic Coverage Act.
1989	Medicare Catastrophic Coverage Act repealed.
1991	Fourth White House Conference on Aging stalled. AOA Funds cut drastically.
1992	Proposals from multiple sources for rescue of health care system.
1995	Fourth White House Conference on Aging. Focused on preservation of Medicare, Medicaid, Social Security, and the Older Americans Act (OAA).
1996	Majority of elders moved through Medicare changes to managed care systems.

Social Security and retirement policies influence income adequacy in later life, and health care policies have a major impact on the last years of life. Box 8-11 lists the events that have had a major impact on the psychosocial experience of the aged in the past 70 years. Nurses need some basic understanding of these major changes in the way the government has dealt with the aging population.

• • •

Throughout this chapter we have presented the various psychosocial theories and aspects of aging that may result in both inner satisfaction and distress. Nurses can provide the opening for elders to discuss the process of aging and its psychologic and social effects. In our highly biomedicalized approach to aging, it is imperative that we seek to know individuals beyond the problem that brings them to the attention of the health care team. Ask elders, "How has aging affected your inner life and outlook?" Listen and learn. We are all aging, and those we serve are our best teachers.

KEY CONCEPTS

- Normal aging involves a gradual process of biopsychosocial change over the course of time.
- Life span development theorists tend to study the total life course of cohort groups to determine the influence of major historic events on their development.
- The impact of gender, culture, and cohort must always be considered when discussing the validity of biopsychosocial theories.
- It is becoming more generally accepted that personality characteristics, as well as biologic characteristics, are to some degree inherent in the individual and that they remain relatively stable throughout life.
- Role transitions may be more difficult than in the past because there are fewer constant and relevant models in a rapidly changing society.
- Loneliness in old age is prevalent because of loss of longtime friends, companions, and family members.
- The most devastating aspect of institutionalization is the loss of personhood. Efforts must always be made to maintain the individuality of each resident.
- The totality of the aging experience is greatly influenced by the place, time, and general health of individuals as they reach the age of retirement.
- Governmental policies greatly impact the aging experience.

▶ Activities and Discussion Questions

1. Discuss some of the problems of adequately testing the cognitive function of elders.
2. Discuss the concept of mental frailty.
3. Identify and discuss the major flaws in the sociologic theories of aging.
4. Select one role that you might assume as an older person, and discuss pros and cons of this role.
5. What are some of the factors elders should consider when contemplating retirement?
6. Is retirement essentially different for older women than for older men and, if so, in what ways?
7. Discuss the variables that must constantly be considered when assessing the psychosocial aspects of the aging experience. Identify and discuss those that seem most significant.

NANDA and Wellness Diagnoses

| Wellness | Specific Needs | NANDA |

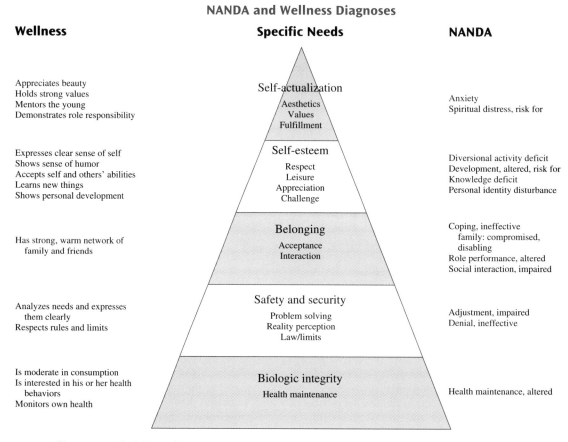

Wellness

Appreciates beauty
Holds strong values
Mentors the young
Demonstrates role responsibility

Expresses clear sense of self
Shows sense of humor
Accepts self and others' abilities
Learns new things
Shows personal development

Has strong, warm network of
    family and friends

Analyzes needs and expresses
    them clearly
Respects rules and limits

Is moderate in consumption
Is interested in his or her health
    behaviors
Monitors own health

Specific Needs

Self-actualization
Aesthetics
Values
Fulfillment

Self-esteem
Respect
Leisure
Appreciation
Challenge

Belonging
Acceptance
Interaction

Safety and security
Problem solving
Reality perception
Law/limits

Biologic integrity
Health maintenance

NANDA

Anxiety
Spiritual distress, risk for

Diversional activity deficit
Development, altered, risk for
Knowledge deficit
Personal identity disturbance

Coping, ineffective
    family: compromised,
    disabling
Role performance, altered
Social interaction, impaired

Adjustment, impaired
Denial, ineffective

Health maintenance, altered

These are not all of the possible wellness or NANDA diagnoses that may be identified. The above are frequent examples of nursing diagnoses that should be considered when planning care for the older adult in whatever setting.

RESOURCES

Social Security Administration
    (800) 772-1213
    www.ssa.gov
    Phone book lists local offices under the Government section.
American Association of Retired Persons (AARP)
    601 E Street NW
    Washington, DC 20049
    e-mail: member@aarp.org
    www.aarp.org
    AARP has numerous publications regarding consumer, economic, health, legal, and work issues. Most are available in English and Spanish.

REFERENCES

Antonovsky A, Sagy S: Confronting developmental tasks in the retirement transition, *Gerontologist* 30:362, 1990.
Bandura A: Self-efficacy: toward a unifying theory of behavioral change, *Psychol Rev* 84:191-215, 1977.
Barer BM: Men and women aging differently, *Int J Aging Hum Dev* 38(1):29, 1993.
Bartley SK: Retirement planning for nonheterosexuals, *Aging Today* 17(5):8, 1996.
Basu JL, Diamond MC: Challenging the myths of aging, *San Francisco Focus* 30:43, 1983.
Berger RM: *Gay and gray: the older homosexual man,* New York, 1996, Haworth.

Berkman LF, Syme L: Social networks, host resistance, and mortality: a nine-year follow-up study of Alameda County residents, *Am J Epidemiol* 109:186, 1979.

Berry W: *Memory of Old Jack,* New York, 1974, Harcourt Brace Jovanovich.

Biordi D: *Social isolation.* In Lubkin I, editor: *Chronic illness: impact and interventions,* Boston, 1995, Jones & Bartlett.

Birren J, Cunningham W: Research on the psychology of aging: principles, concepts, and theory. In Birren J, Schaie K, editors: *Handbook of the psychology of aging,* ed 2, New York, 1985, Van Nostrand Reinhold.

Bowsher JE, Keep D: Toward an understanding of three control constructs: personal control, self-efficacy, and hardiness, *Issues Mental Health Nurs* 16:33-50, 1995.

Boyack V: *The geriatric orphan: research and practice perspectives.* Paper presented at the annual convention of the Western Gerontological Society, Albuquerque, New Mexico, March 18, 1983.

Boyd SH, Stout BL, Volanty K: Youth exchanging with seniors: a rural Texas program, *Pride Institute J Long Term Home Health Care* 12(3):21, 1993.

Buhler C: The human course of life in its goal aspects, *J Hum Psychol* 4:1, 1964.

Cotman CW: Synaptic plasticity, neurotrophic factors, and transplantation in the aged brain. In Schneider EL, Rowe JW, editors: *Handbook of the biology of aging,* San Diego, 1990, Academic Press.

Crowley SL: Aging brain's staying power, *AARP Bull* 37(4):1, 1996.

Cumming E, Henry W: *Growing old,* New York, 1961, Basic Books.

Cunningham W, Brookbank J: *Gerontology: the physiology, biology and sociology of aging,* New York, 1988, Harper & Row.

Ebersole PR: May your goals never be fully accomplished, *Geriatr Nurs* 17(5):258-259, 1996.

Ekerdt DJ, DeViney S, Kosloski K: Profiling plans for retirement, *J Gerontol* 51(3):S140, 1996.

Erickson R: Companion animals and the older adult, *Geriatr Nurs* 6(2):92, 1985.

Erikson EH: *Childhood and society,* ed 2, New York, 1963, Norton.

Erikson EH, Erikson JM, Kivnick HQ: *Vital involvement in old age: the experience of old age in our time,* New York, 1986, Norton.

Havighurst RL, Neugarten BL, Tobin SS: Disengagement and patterns of aging. In Neugarten BL, editor: *Middle age and aging,* Chicago, 1968, University of Chicago Press.

Holden KC, Hsiang-Hui DK: Complex marital histories and economic well-being: the continuing legacy of divorce and widowhood as the HRS cohort approaches retirement, *Gerontologist* 36(3):383, 1996.

Johnson J: Social support and physical health in the rural older adult, *Appl Nurs Res* 9(2):61, 1996.

Johnson JE, Waldo M, Johnson RG: Stress and perceived health status in the rural older adult, *J Gerontol Nurs* 19(9):24, 1993.

Jung C: The stages of life. In Campbell J, editor: *The portable Jung,* New York, 1971, Viking Press (translated by RFC Hull).

Kelly C: Perspectives of gerontic nurse pioneers. In Ebersole P, Hess P, editors: *Toward healthy aging: human needs and nursing response,* ed 3, St Louis, 1990, Mosby.

Kobasa SC: Stressful life events, personality, and health: an inquiry into hardiness, *J Pers Soc Psychol* 37(1):1-11, 1979.

Kuhlen R: Developmental changes in motivation during the adult years. In Neugarten B, editor: *Middle age and aging,* Chicago, 1968, University of Chicago Press.

Lanza ML: Divorce experienced as an older woman, *Geriatr Nurs* 17(4):166, 1996.

Lehman H: *Age and achievement,* Princeton, NJ, 1953, Princeton University Press.

Lenker LT, Polivka L: Project rationale and history, *J Aging Identity* 1(1):3-6, 1996.

Lien-Gieschen T: *Nurse validation of social isolation related to maturational age,* master's thesis, Washington, DC, 1992, Georgetown University.

Luggen AS, Rini AG: Assessment of social networks and isolation in community based older adult men and women, *Geriatr Nurs* 16(4):179, 1995.

Maddox G: Activity and morale: a longitudinal study of selected older adult subjects, *Soc Forces* 42:195, 1963.

McAvay GJ, Seeman TE, Rodin J: A longitudinal study of change in domain-specific self-efficacy among older adults, *J Gerontol* 51B(5):243-253, 1996.

Musson ND, Frye GD, Nash M: Silver spoons: supervised volunteers provide feeding of patients, *Geriatr Nurs* 18(1):18, 1997.

Neugarten B, Havighurst R, Tobin S: Personality and patterns of aging. In Neugarten B, editor: *Middle age and aging,* Chicago, 1968, University of Chicago Press.

Nightingale F: *Notes on nursing,* Philadelphia, 1992, Lippincott (originally published in 1859).

Peck R: Psychological developments in the second half of life. In Neugarten B, editor: *Middle age and aging,* Chicago, 1968, University of Chicago Press.

Plomin R, McClearn GE: Human behavioral genetics of aging. In Birren J, Schaie K, editors: *Handbook of the psychology of aging,* ed 3, San Diego, 1990, Academic Press.

Poon LW et al: Biomarkers of aging, *Generations* 16(4):11-14, 1992.

Talage JA, Beehr TA: Are there gender differences in predicting retirement decisions? *J Appl Psychol* 80(1):16, 1995.

Taylor MA, Shore LM: Predictors of planned retirement age: an application of Beehr's model, *Psychol Aging* 10(1):76, 1995.

Tornstam L: Dimensions of loneliness, *Aging* 2(3):259, 1990.

US Bureau of the Census: *Statistical abstract of the United States: 1998,* ed 118, Washington, DC, 1998, US Government Printing Office.

Wolanin M: Mental frailty, Unpublished essay, 1997.

9 Sensory Changes of Aging

►LEARNING OBJECTIVES

Upon completion of this chapter, the reader will be able to:

- Identify sensory changes accompanying aging that alter the perceived world of the aged.
- Relate sensory changes to perceptual and environmental insecurity and behavioral disturbances.
- Describe nursing assessment and interventions that can be implemented to help elders with various decreased vision and hearing problems.

►GLOSSARY

Presbycusis Normal decrement in hearing acuity, speech intelligibility, auditory threshold, and pitch discrimination that occurs with aging.
Presbyopia Decreased ability of the lens of the eyes to accommodate for close and detailed work as one advances in age.

Sensory deprivation A condition in which there is insufficient stimuli to sensory apparatus to allow integrative perceptions to develop.
Sensory overload Bombardment of the sensory apparatus by environmental stimuli that reaches levels that are physically and psychologically overwhelming.

►THE LIVED EXPERIENCE

I was so embarrassed when I finally realized my eyesight was simply not as good as it was 15 years ago. I thought the headlights on my car were just not strong enough and the halo around the streetlights was some new kind of lighting. And, of course it really made me angry when the glare of oncoming cars almost blinded me. I thought that they simply weren't courteous enough to turn off their brights. And then, when my grandson told me about all the changes in vision that go with getting old, I was really upset. Well, now I don't think I will drive at night anymore.

George, age 70

Boy, was that a scary ride. I don't think Grandpa had any idea that he couldn't really see well enough for night driving. I sure hated telling him his eyes weren't so good. He has always been so proud of his driving ability. I don't know how I got the courage, except I was afraid he would have an accident and really hurt himself. I hate to think that someday I won't be able to drive well at night.

George III, age 20

APPRECIATION OF SENSORY CHANGES AND EXPERIENCES

All senses gradually loss their acuity with old age. The normal changes result from the accumulated atrophy of sensory receptors in the eye, ear, nose, buccal cavity, and peripheral afferent nerves, substantially reducing the vividness of environmental impressions. Events no longer alert the nervous system with such clarity as in youth. Habituation to certain sensations may also diminish their impact. The normal gradual diminution of the senses during the aging process is usually well accommodated by experience. When the experience remains within the boundaries of constancy and familiarity, normal sensory loss is not detrimental to function. It may in fact be desirable. An old person, because of lowered energy and concentration, may be more vulnerable to sensory overload than to sensory deprivation. We are all subject to alterations in our sensory experience, and with increasing age it is likely that these circumstances will occur more frequently and perhaps be more devastating.

The issues of concern to nurses include the following: devising methods to keep the organismic senses functional enough to negotiate the environment effectively by keeping the environment within reach; supplementing sensory loss with additional pleasures to the remaining senses; providing touch, color, and variety; and refraining from pushing and shoving the elements in haste and irreverence. The sensory environment is to be revered and cultivated. Therein lie many problems. Old age subjects one to decreased appreciation of the environment through drugs, machines, treatments, paresthesias, presbyopia, presbycusis, agnosia, etc. Life may be more cautiously sampled. Stored experiences often come to the rescue, and old people remember things they can no longer perceive.

When describing the capacities and changes in the various sensory apparatus, we must understand that they all work in consensus. Situations are experienced through sight, sound, smell, and touch simultaneously (Sacks, 1989). The senses are tightly interwoven in forming the perceptual base of our world. Possibly the "sixth sense" (intuition, or the power of perception that goes beyond that of the five senses) is really the consensus of all the senses in an acutely aware individual. In some cases a disorder of one of the senses may stimulate the others in a compensatory manner.

Age-related declines are variable and cannot be generalized to all sensory systems (Meeuwsen et al, 1992). Personal hardiness and an environment that conveys order and meaning contribute in ways yet unidentified to good perceptual processing and high-level functioning. It is not uncommon that elders are thought to be cognitively impaired when in fact attention to enhanced sensory function through an adapted environment and well-fitted accoutrements reveal much higher functional levels. General perceptual organization and efficiency are modified by health status, frailty of aging, illness, medications, fatigue, and stress and anxiety.

Alterations in sensory input may contribute to increased anxiety in the aged population. Caregivers of the aged are concerned about manipulating stimuli and enhancing sensory apparatus to induce an optimal functional level of perceptual adequacy. When the senses

are grossly underloaded or overloaded, perception and reactions are distorted. The world becomes an alien, confusing place. Fear and anxiety increase, or one withdraws into a fabricated world that provides security. Altered sensory experience will affect one's view of self and one's ability to relate to others. Isolation and loneliness may be the result. Emotional responses to altered sensory input include boredom, diminished concentration, incoherent thoughts, anxiety, fear, depression, lability of affect, and even hallucinations. Clear and sometimes repetitive data about the environment must be given when perceptions are impaired. Manipulating the environment to reduce demands and enhance sensory function should decrease these symptoms, although studies show that signs may persist for several days. Adequate input is essential to continued cognitive development. Box 9-1 lists circumstances affecting sensory experience.

Sensory Deprivation

There are at least three types of sensory deprivation: (1) reduced sensory capacities, (2) elimination of patterns and meaning from input, and (3) restrictive, monotonous environments. Certain effects thought to be "confusion" or "old age" may arise from sensory deprivation. Any situation lacking varied environmental stimuli deprives the senses of adequate material for per-

Box 9-1	**CIRCUMSTANCES AFFECTING SENSORY EXPERIENCE**

Environmental Alterations
Protective isolation
Experimental isolation
Environmental overload: size, frequency, intensity
Noxious agents: noise, glare, temperature

Organic Alterations
Pain and illness (e.g., ability to smell and taste altered by a cold)
Receptor changes of biologic origin
Receptor changes of chemical origin

Perceptual Alterations
Selective inattention
Habituation
Expectations derived from past experience
Conflicts and psychologic defenses

Box 9-2 **Box 9-2** **EFFECTS OF SENSORY DEPRIVATION**

- Sensory deprivation tends to amplify existing personality traits.
- Perceptual disorganization occurs in visual/motor coordination, color perception, apparent movement, tactile accuracy, ability to perceive size and shape, and spatial and time judgment.
- Sensory deprivation alters mechanisms of attention, consciousness, and reality testing (similar to brain anoxia).
- Marked changes of behavior occur, such as inability to think and solve problems, affectual disturbance, perceptual distortions, hallucinations and delusions, vivid imagination, poor task performance, increased anxiety and aggression, somatic complaints, temporal and spatial disorientation, emotional lability, and confusion of sleep and waking states.
- Monotony produces a disruption of the capacity to learn and the ability to think.
- In the absence of varied stimulation, brain function becomes less.
- Illness often increases the perceptual confusion, particularly in the aged.

ceptual integrity. Box 9-2 summarizes some effects of sensory deprivation.

Common contributors to sensory deprivation in the elderly, such as poor vision, decreased energy, poor hearing, extended periods in a supine position, debilitating illness and chronic disorders, few pleasant sounds, and limited meaningful contact with others, often result in disorientation. Late afternoon may aggravate the deprivation if daylight is diminished and there is inadequate indoor lighting. Simple nursing actions will alleviate this barren existence. Open drapes and the window a crack; the sights, sounds, and smells of outdoors and life can be enjoyable and reassuring. Turn on lights; raise the head of the bed, or assist the person to a chair bolstered comfortably with pillows; bring a flower to the room; sit down; speak; touch; and listen to the client's feelings and perceptions. Discuss the isolated person's interests; radio, television, computers, books, puzzles, and handicrafts may all amuse the solitary person. It is essential to plan with the elderly, not for them. When these efforts fail, it is because of inadequate assessment. If the individual is concerned about more fundamental issues such as maintaining biologic integrity, comfortable and nondemanding surroundings will be a priority.

When the ambiance is one of monotony, even a small stimulus may trigger a strong response. Knowing this makes it easier to understand the overreactions displayed when a routine is interrupted. People are more sensitive to change of any sort when there are so few and they feel deprived of control. There is a good response to gradual environmental enrichment. Rapid increases may produce emotional outbursts.

Meanings and patterns that throughout life have formed the basis of precepts, and on a preconscious level have sorted data in ways meaningful to the individual, may be shattered in crises, unnatural events, and catastrophes. The senses are no longer reliable.

Sensory Overload

A decrease in neuroexcitability and secretion of stimulating neurotransmitters occurs as one ages and can produce overarousal from abrupt, unexpected environmental change, such as that brought on by an accident or hospitalization. These are situations of sensory overload precipitated by actual or perceived environmental demands. Emergency reactions sustained for long periods exhaust the organism's physiologic adaptive mechanisms (Selye, 1956). An individual with marginal adaptation and cognitive decrements is particularly vulnerable. Sensory overload is a very individual matter, often related to cognitive capacity. It can be recognized by certain symptoms—thoughts may race, and attention scatters in many directions. People find it difficult to sit still. Aberrant thoughts or actions may occur. Evidence of anxiety is present. The amount of stimuli necessary for healthy function varies with each individual; the relevance and familiarity of stimuli may be more important than the amount. Biorhythms are another important consideration. Individuals may be more subject to environmental overload at one time than at another. Sensations are generally most acute in the late afternoon.

Sensory overload cannot always be avoided, but when one is extremely stressed and bombarded with adaptive demands, time must be arranged for peacefulness and frequent rest periods. It is often helpful to sit quietly with the person, saying very little, or engage him or her in a nondemanding repetitive activity that will help focus attention on something that provides security and reduces stress. Walking can be beneficial. One must, however, be cautious in arbitrarily attributing anxiety, agitation, mood swings, or disorientation to sensory overload.

VISION AND VISUAL IMPAIRMENT IN THE AGED

Visual acuity and accommodation normally decrease with age. These changes begin making themselves felt in the mid-40s for many people and are mainly an inconvenience rather than a problem. Major aging of the eye (presbyopia) occurs between 45 and 55 years of age; still, 80% of the aged have fair to adequate vision past 90 years of age. Much can be done to improve vision for the majority of elders, and compliance is high when vision is affected. The causes of visual impairment include macular degeneration, diabetic retinopathy, glaucoma, and cataracts.

It is estimated that about 3 million of those with low vision are so seriously impaired that they are unable to read (Schneider, 1996). For many of these individuals, the problem cannot be corrected by ordinary lenses, medical treatment, or surgery (Stuen, 1996). Approximately 2% of the aged are totally blind (Stuen, 1996). Women completely lose vision more frequently than men, and in both sexes it is common to have better vision in one eye than in the other. It is probable that the identification and treatment of depression are frequently neglected in the care of those with low or no vision. It seems clear that the psychosocial ramifications of various kinds of visual impairment are, at this time, poorly understood and treated.

Several ophthalmologic changes that occur with aging are not serious but may cause discomfort or alarm in the elder experiencing them. Headache accompanied by eye muscle pain can be caused by the tendency with aging for a gradual decrease in the tone of the medial rectus muscle, which turns the eye inward while focusing on close objects. This then creates exophoria (slight turning outward of the eye) and may result in headache when one is doing close work for an extended period. Headaches associated with this condition can be remedied by taking more rest breaks while doing close work, doing close work early in the day, and engaging in eye muscle exercises three times daily for 5 minutes each session. Symptomatic relief is usually achieved in 4 to 6 weeks.

A decrease in pupil size, which hinders light from reaching the retina, is a major factor in visual changes of aging. Small objects cannot be seen at a distance. Adaptation to darkness is also deficient in old age, with depletion of certain retinal functions.

Night vision decreases, which may become a source of great insecurity to those aged who must drive at night. In addition, individuals who have had surgical radial keratotomy to correct nearsightedness may develop impaired night vision related to scarring (Radial Kera-

totomy, 1995). Many limit themselves to daytime driving. Many safety factors are obviously attached to visual adequacy, although people with limitations often adapt remarkably well.

Vitreous floaters and occasional lightning flashes in the visual field may be alarming. As the vitreous undergoes liquefaction with eye movements, the vitreous attachment is placed under intermittent tension. This creates a mechanical stimulation of the peripheral retina that causes vertically oriented flashing lights unilaterally. In addition, other lines, spots, clusters of dots, and webs may move slowly across the visual field. Although none of these conditions are serious, explanation and client reassurance are essential because the threat of blindness is one of the most devastating thoughts one can entertain. Visual distortions that require immediate attention and may signal retinal detachment include any change that persists and is accompanied by a decrease in the visual field, a shower of opacities accompanied by flashing lights in the peripheral visual fields, or a feeling of a "veil over the eye."

Presbyopia

The problem with accommodation, or the ability to focus on objects at various distances, is noticeable by the mid-40s. This is when most people become aware of the need to hold objects farther away to properly focus their gaze. This change is presbyopia. For most individuals the reading lens must be increased in strength every 2 or 3 years between the ages of 45 and 65. Presbyopia tends to occur earlier in farsightedness (hyperopia) than in nearsightedness (myopia). As lens opacity increases, some refractive power increases at the same time that accommodation, or lens resilience, decreases. The result is a temporary shift toward myopia and improved close vision. Thus some individuals at 60 or 70 years of age develop "second sight" in which they can again read without glasses (Kupfer, 1995a). Increasingly, contact lenses to correct presbyopia are being used with varying degrees of acceptance and success (Back et al, 1989; Collins et al, 1989; Stein, 1991).

Glaucoma

The most common cause of blindness in Americans over age 65 is glaucoma, a chronic, progressive, degenerative disease involving increased intraocular pressure (IOP), usually bilaterally, that can lead to permanent damage of the optic nerve. Open-angle glaucoma accounts for about 80% of cases and is asymptomatic until very late in the disease, when there is a noticeable loss in visual fields (Kupfer, 1995a, 1995b). Glaucoma has been described as the "silent thief" because it will steal vision with no forewarning.

Age is the single most important predictor of glaucoma. Aged women are afflicted twice as frequently as aged men (Schappert, 1995). Blacks develop glaucoma at younger ages and with more frequency than whites. Asians, particularly the Chinese, are prone to develop glaucoma. Many drugs with anticholinergic properties or those that cause pupillary dilation will exacerbate glaucoma in the aged. The etiology is variable and often unknown; however, when the natural fluids of the eye are blocked by ciliary muscle rigidity and the buildup of pressure, damage to the optic nerve occurs. An acute attack of closed-angle glaucoma is characterized by a rapid rise in intraocular pressure accompanied by redness and pain in and around the eye, severe headache, nausea and vomiting, and blurring of vision.

Usually medication can control glaucoma, but when surgery is necessary, it is only successful if scar tissue does not later obstruct the drainage channel. Increased surgical success for glaucoma has been reported to occur when it is followed by injections of the antimetabolite drug 5-fluorouracil (National Institute on Aging, 1990b).

Glaucoma screening is an important way to identify this silent condition. A simple handheld noncontact method of tonometry that can be used to identify 90% of patients with IOPs greater than 22 mm Hg has been used since 1972 (Ralston et al, 1992). Ordinarily, a tonometry reading of 10 to 20 is considered acceptable, although there are many complicating factors. Persons with measurements of pressure over 21 mm Hg are "ocular hypertensives" and may not yet need treatment but will need visual field testing at 6-month intervals (Kupfer, 1995b). About one sixth of patients with diagnosed glaucoma do not have IOPs above those considered normal. These persons are considered to have "normal-tension glaucoma."

An ophthalmologic examination and tonometry are necessary to diagnose glaucoma. These procedures can be performed by a primary care provider, an optometrist, or a nurse practitioner, who will then refer the person to an ophthalmologist if glaucoma is suspected. Many elders may have undiagnosed glaucoma that has not been screened for or evaluated. It is recommended that individuals with any identified risk factors be evaluated annually and that those with medication-controlled glaucoma be examined at least every 6 months (Kupfer, 1995a).

Cataracts

A prevalent disorder among the aged, cataracts are caused by oxidative damage to lens protein and fatty deposits (lipofuscin) in the ocular lens. When lens opacity reduces visual acuity to 20/30 or less in central vision, it is considered a cataract. Cataracts are categorized according to their location within the lens. They are virtually universal in the very old but may be only minimally visible, particularly in individuals with pale irises. Cataracts are recognized by the clouding of the ordinarily clear ocular lens. They are normal in the aging process but may be worsened by diabetes, hypertension, kidney disease, and injuries or exposure to toxic situations. The cardinal sign of cataracts is the spraying of light and the blurriness around the edges of objects. Other common symptoms include blurring, seeing double moons, decreased perception of light and color, and sensitivity to glare. The hallmark of cataracts is painless, progressive loss of vision (Kupfer, 1995b). Cataracts are the second leading cause of blindness in the United States. Eighteen percent of people between 65 and 74 years of age have cataracts, and 46% of those ages 75 to 84 years have cataracts that impair their daily activities and ability to live independently (Bass et al, 1995).

Cataract surgery is considered whenever the visual disturbance becomes an impediment in the individual's daily life. Most often, cataract surgery involves removing the entire lens capsule and replacing it with an artificial lens. These are often slipped into place without the need for suturing. When necessary, cataract surgery has the potential to improve not only sight but quality of life as well. Studies have shown that patients undergoing first-eye cataract surgery achieved or surpassed their expected level of postoperative functioning (Tielsch et al, 1995) and that the rate of satisfaction for those who had surgery in both eyes was significantly higher (Javitt et al, 1995). Those with coexisting visual problems were less satisfied. Unfortunately, glaucoma and cataracts often occur simultaneously, which complicates the management of each. Individuals who have had cataract surgery are less likely to be surgically treated effectively for glaucoma. The nursing role is to prepare individuals for significant changes in vision and adaptation to light and to be sure they have received adequate counseling regarding realistic postsurgical expectations.

It is important for both the client and the care provider to be aware that current Medicare policies restrict payment for cataract surgery to those unable to function normally without the surgery or those whose problem cannot be corrected with eyeglasses. These restrictions have been put in place because of the enormous number of individuals having cataract surgery: 2 million individuals in 1994 at a cost of nearly $1.5 billion (US Department of Health and Human Services, 1995).

Diabetic Retinopathy

Some visual disabilities are acquired through the deleterious effects of elevated blood glucose levels due to diabetes, which creates microaneurysms in retinal capillaries, the source of diabetic retinopathy. Because of vascular and cellular changes accompanying diabetes, there is often rapid worsening of other visual pathologic conditions as well. Diabetic retinopathy accounts for 7% of the blindness in the United States, and the incidence curves upward abruptly with increasing age (Kupfer, 1995b). Constant, strict control of blood glucose and photocoagulation laser treatments can halt progression of the disease (National Institute on Aging, 1995).

Macular Degeneration

The macula is the central visual point of the retina and as such is the source of central visual clarity. Age-related macular degeneration (ARMD) results from systemic changes in circulation, accumulation of cellular waste products, tissue atrophy, and growth of abnormal blood vessels in the choroid layer beneath the retina. It is the most common visual impairment of individuals over age 50. It leads to permanent loss of central visual acuity, but not to blindness; peripheral vision is not affected. The National Eye Institute found that macular degeneration occurs in 36.8% of individuals over 75 years of age (Eastman, 1996).

The etiology is unknown. Early in the disease an Amsler grid is used to determine clarity of central vision. A perception of wavy lines is diagnostic of beginning macular degeneration, and the disease can be halted by laser treatment if diagnosed early (Macular Degeneration, 1990).

Virtanen and Laatikainen (1991) found that 91% of patients with ARMD were able to read newsprint with simple magnifiers or high-powered (5$\times$ to 9$\times$) reading glasses. Antioxidants, thalidomide, blocking of ultraviolet light rays, and laser photocoagulation are some of the treatments that are being used. Transplanting healthy retinal cells to replace degenerating ones is under investigation (Eastman, 1996).

Assessment of Vision

Although low vision is defined in terms of visual acuity and visual field, these parameters are insufficient to determine individual treatment and rehabilitation needs.

The National Eye Institute is developing a comprehensive Visual Function Questionnaire that will be used to assess levels of functional impairments such as mobility; near vision; and ability to read, drive, work, and manage independent living. It will also consider the influence of psychosocial factors such as stress, frustration, isolation, loss of privacy, and existing levels of social support (Kupfer, 1995a).

Nearly one fourth of nursing home residents were found to have visual impairment. Despite numerous other chronic impairments, low vision was the most significant predictor of functional dependency (Horowitz, 1994). In addition, it has been found that increased visual cues and aids reduced agitation and improved function of individuals with Alzheimer's disease (Koss, 1995). It seems evident that the complex effects of low vision on function are not yet fully understood. However, various problems with vision are common in aging, and nurses are most likely to make a preliminary assessment before referring the individual for further evaluation. Certain signs and behaviors of visual problems that should alert the nurse to action are noted in Box 9-3.

Box 9-3   SIGNS AND BEHAVIORS THAT MAY INDICATE VISION PROBLEMS

Client May Report
Pain in eyes
Difficulty seeing in darkened area
Double vision/distorted vision
Migraine headaches coupled with blurred vision
Flashes of light
Halos surrounding lights

Staff May Notice
Getting lost
Bumping into objects
Straining to read or no reading
Stumbling/falling
Spilling food on clothing
Social withdrawal
Less eye contact
Placid facial expression
TV viewing at close range
Decreased sense of balance
Mismatched clothes

Modified from McNeely E, Griffin-Shirley N, Hubbard A: Diminished vision in nursing homes, *Geriatr Nurs* 13(6):332, 1992.

Important systemic, circulatory, and vision information can be obtained by an ophthalmologic examination of the retina and optic nerve disc. However, pupillary constriction and clouding of the vitreous and lens often hamper the eyeground examination of an older person.

Infrared scanning of the retina and the laser scanning ophthalmoscope (SLO) are also providing safe and more sophisticated examination data. The SLO generates digital imaging, computerized projections that measure specific visual changes corresponding to retinal damage of various degrees and types (O'Connell, 1995). The retinal scanner will become commonplace in providing computer-generated exact replicas of the pattern of blood vessels in the retina.

Caring for the Elder With Visual Impairment

General principles in caring for the elder with visual impairment include the following: use warm incandescent lighting, control glare by using shades and blinds, suggest yellow or amber lenses to decrease glare, suggest sunglasses that block all ultraviolet light, select colors with good contrast and intensity, and recommend reading materials that have large, dark, evenly spaced printing (Stuen, 1996).

Environmental Lighting

The pupil of the aged eye admits less light to the retina. This normal condition is known as *senile miosis*. A simple and effective, yet often neglected, intervention is to provide increased environmental lighting (Kolanowski, 1992). Three variables—intensity, spectral power distribution (color), and temporal pattern of exposure (Kolanowski, 1992)—are important when considering improved lighting for an elder.

The intensity of illumination needs to be three times greater to produce the same visual capacity for the aged as for younger persons. Intensity must be tempered by appropriate diffusion to avoid glare. Sensitivity to glare increases markedly in the aged because of clouding of the lens and vitreous, resulting in the scattering of light as it passes through the lens. This may cause eyestrain, fatigue, tension, and actual pain. It is particularly noticeable with driving at night or in low levels of illumination when the pupil is slightly dilated (Kupfer, 1995b). Individuals are advised to avoid night driving and looking directly at oncoming headlights.

Fluorescent lighting may also have adverse effects on behavior because it contributes to sensory overload (Wolanin, Phillips, 1981). The quality of artificial light becomes exceedingly important for the aged, particularly those who are institutionalized, because they often spend a great deal of their time indoors. Although we often think of light in terms of visualization only, the characteristic color of a particular light source is an issue of concern. *Spectral power* refers to the radiant power emitted at each wavelength over the visible electromagnetic spectrum (Kolanowski, 1992). Some fluorescent lights filter out the red (longer wavelengths), and others filter out the blue (shorter wavelengths). Kolanowski found that a significant number of elders preferred broad-spectrum fluorescent lighting that simulates natural sunlight. There is some evidence that these types of lighting also produce calmness and relaxation.

Contrasting Colors

Color contrasts are used to facilitate location of items. Sharply contrasting colors assist the partially sighted. It is much easier to locate a bright towel than a white towel hanging on a beige wall. Box 9-4 offers ideas for communicating and caring for the visually impaired elder. Most visually impaired people have enough residual vision to use their eyesight with proper aids or training to read, write, and move around safely. Unfortunately, many older persons with serious visual impairments consider themselves blind and are usually treated as if they are. Adequate training in using residual vision can prevent partially sighted older persons from falling into unnecessarily dependent life-styles.

Low-Vision Assistive Devices

Technology advances in the last decade have produced some low-vision assistive devices that may be used successfully in the care of the visually impaired elder. An array of assistive devices are now available for these individuals, such as microspiral Galilean telescopes, telephoto microscopes, clear-image lenses, behind-the-lens telescopes, and low-vision enhancement systems. These last devices use tiny cameras to place an enlarged image on a video screen in front of the eyes. Worn as a headset, they can be used for distance viewing and reading (O'Connell, 1995). Persons with reduced visual acuity should be encouraged to consider some of these sophisticated aids because severe visual deficits may result in mobility restrictions in addition to creating cognitive, sensory, and behavioral disturbances.

Magnifying lenses are available in many forms in addition to those commonly found in spectacle frames. These can be recommended in relation to the use for which they are desired. The most complex of the low-

Box 9-4	SUGGESTIONS FOR COMMUNICATING WITH AND CARING FOR VISUALLY IMPAIRED ELDERS

Remember, there are many degrees of blindness; allow as much independence as possible.

- Assess your position in relation to the individual. One eye or ear may be better than the other.
- When in the presence of a blind person, speak promptly and clearly identify yourself and others with you. State when you are leaving to make sure the person is aware of your departure.
- Make sure you have the individual's attention before you start talking.
- Speak descriptively of your surroundings to familiarize the blind person, and state the position of the people who are in the room.
- Speak normally but not from a distance; do not raise or lower your voice, and continue to use gestures if that is natural to your communication. Do not alter your vocabulary; words such as *see* and *blind* are part of normal speech. When others are present, address the blind person by prefacing remarks with his or her name or a light touch on the arm.
- Try to minimize the number of distractions.
- Use the analogy of a clock face to help locate objects. Describe positions of food on the plate in relation to clock positions (e.g., 3 o'clock, 6 o'clock).

- Check to see that the best possible lighting is available.
- Try to keep the individual between you and the window; you will appear as a dark shadow.
- Whenever possible, choose bright clothing with bold contrasts.
- Do not change the room arrangement or arrangement of personal items without explanation.
- Speak before handing a blind person an object.
- Keep color and texture in mind when buying clothes.
- When walking with a blind person, offer your arm. Pause before stairs or curbs; mention them. In seating, place the person's hand on the back of the chair. Let him or her know the position in relation to objects.
- Blind people like to know the beauty that surrounds them. Describe flowers, scenery, colors, and textures. People who have been blind since birth cannot conceive of color, but it adds to their appreciation to hear full descriptions. Old people most frequently have been sighted and can enjoy memories of beauty stimulated by descriptive conversation.
- Use some means to identify residents who are known to be visually impaired.
- *Be careful about labeling a resident as confused.* He or she may be making mistakes as a result of poor vision.

vision devices are telescopes that can be focused at various distances, thus increasing the number of tasks that can be performed. In addition, closed-circuit television magnifying units are available that can enlarge written characters up to 45 times. Although these are currently expensive, the prices are rapidly dropping as they become more commonly available.

Another method of magnification is through the use of a standard copying machine that has magnifying capabilities. One need not buy one of these but only make use of those available to the public. By repeatedly magnifying printed words or images, even small print can be made as large as desired.

Eyeglasses, once heavy and bulky, are now cosmetically appealing. Many also incorporate prismatic lenses that expand the visual field. Sunglasses are designed to filter out ultraviolet rays that may be harmful to sensitive retinas. Some eyeglasses adjust to the light source and become darker in the sun. Magnifiers have been redesigned for ease of changing batteries and bulbs, positioning, and grasping. Telescopic lens eyeglasses are smaller, easier to focus, and have a greater range. It is

now possible to electronically magnify video- and computer-generated text. Some software converts text into artificial voice output. All of these resources must be considered when attempting to help the visually impaired elder achieve the visual activities that are important to his or her quality of life (Silverstone, 1988). Because individual needs are unique, it is recommended that before investing in any of these vision aids, the client be advised to consult with a low-vision center or low-vision specialist. For further information contact the organizations for the blind listed in the Resources at the end of this chapter.

Orientation Strategies for the Nonsighted

Methods to assist those individuals with total lack of sight are not generally included in nursing curricula. Methods in common use include the following: (1) the clock method, in which the individual is simply told where the food or item is as if it were on a clock face; (2) the sighted guide, in which a companion guides the visually impaired and enables safe mobility; (3) the cane sweep, which encounters obstacles; (4) sound signals (e.g., at street crossings); (5) varied-textured surfaces; and (6) guide dogs.

Sighted Guides

Ask the blind person if he or she would like a "sighted guide." A strong element of dependency and trust is necessary in this method, and many people would rather manage on their own. Initially, as a person is adjusting to blindness, it can be helpful. If assistance is accepted, offer your elbow or arm. Instruct the person to grasp your arm just above the elbow. If necessary, physically assist the person by guiding his or her hand to your arm or elbow.

Go a half step ahead and slightly to the side of the blind person. The shoulder of the person should be directly behind your shoulder. If the person is frail, place his or her hand on your forearm. With this modified grasp, the person will be positioned laterally to your body. Relax and walk at a comfortable pace. Tell the person when approaching doorways or a narrow space.

Cane Sweep

White canes, or "long canes," are used by about 109,000 persons in the United States to alert others to their presence as a nonsighted person and to signal the blind person of obstacles in the space ahead (American Foundation for the Blind, 1996). However, an architectural design that includes slanted beams and inverted pyramid designs can be deceiving.

Sound Signals

In some U.S. cities and most European and Japanese cities, intermittent sound signals alert the nonsighted when it is safe to cross the street—a simple solution, surprisingly not common in the United States.

Varied Textures

Those elders who have been blind for quite some time have developed hypersensitivity to textural variations. This sensitivity can be incorporated into the environment in numerous ways to assist the blind person.

Guide Dogs

There are 14 guide dog schools in the United States, and about 10,000 persons who use guide dogs to assist them in mobility. Trained guide dogs are matched to individuals' needs and personalities, and those elders who have guide dogs have had several during the course of their adult years (Schneider, 1996). Each dog becomes a companion, as well as a guide.

HEARING AND HEARING IMPAIRMENT IN THE AGED

It is estimated that 50% of persons over age 65 have a hearing problem; the occurrence is as much as 90% among the institutionalized aged (US Bureau of the Census, 1995). Reasons for this are not clear, because hearing impairment is not ordinarily a trigger to institutionalization. There are many others who have not been tested and/or whose hearing impairment has not been recognized or documented.

Presbycusis

Presbycusis is primarily an affliction of individuals over age 50, but it is not a universal change, and although age-related, it may really be more reflective of environmental conditions and life-style. It is a bilateral and symmetric sensorineural hearing loss associated with aging. Men seem to experience more severe presbycusis than women of the same age. Changes in the middle and inner ear make many elders intolerant of loud noises and incapable of distinguishing between some of the sibilant consonants, such as *z, s, sh, f, p, k, t,* and *g.* High frequency is not interfered with in understandable speech; however, the condition does begin to affect high-frequency sibilant consonant discrimination. Vowels that have a low pitch are more easily heard. Without consonants, the high-frequency-pitched language becomes disjointed and misunderstood. Consider the simple sentence "How are you today?" To the individual with presbycusis it might sound like "hOw arE yOU tOdAy?"

The condition progressively worsens with age. The influence of genetics, noise exposure, cardiovascular status, central processing capacity, systemic disease, smoking, diet, personality, and stress have all been implicated to varying degrees in the etiology of impaired hearing (National Institute on Aging, 1990a). Older adults often complain of difficulty understanding women and children, as well as conversations in large groups or when there is background noise in restaurants. Loud music and intercoms or pagers such as those used in hospitals or airports mask conversation with noise. Use of rapid speech when conversing with an older adult will make sounds garbled and unintelligible, and even though the problem is related to presbycusis, it is one that can be easily remedied. The common problem of cerumen in the ear canal, which is treatable, intensifies presbycusis.

Impaired hearing increases isolation and suspicion that sometimes progress to paranoia. Feeling cut off from others, a deaf individual may act angry even when someone attempts to break through the barrier to sound (Chen, 1994). There is normally a loss of speech, tone, and directional discrimination. Older persons are often unaware of hearing loss because of the gradual manner in which it usually develops. Some people are aware of a hearing loss and are disturbed by misperceptions and distortions, often imagining that derogatory remarks are being said about them. However, knowing that one has a hearing loss is not sufficient. Testing must be done to determine the nature of the loss, how much it interferes with communication, whether it is treatable (as may be the case with metabolic alterations or middle ear structural changes), and whether a hearing aid will be useful.

Elderly persons with presbycusis have more difficulty filtering out background noise unless the primary signal is 10 times louder than the noise factor (von Wedel et al, 1990). This has implications for institutional noise factors, intercoms, and general high levels of extraneous sounds. Hearing loss after 65 years of age varies according to the degree and type of loss being considered. Certain sounds and words are much more difficult to hear than others. Those less than 40 decibels and of frequencies over 1000 are particularly difficult.

Prelingual Deafness

Prelingual deafness in the aged is rarely addressed because it is assumed that individuals deaf since childhood have learned early on to communicate through the use of sign language. Until 50 years ago it was common for deaf children to be placed in a state school for the deaf to develop within a culture of their own; therefore many elders with prelingual deafness will have had an entirely different childhood than those with hearing. The prelingual deaf often learn audible speech very well. Those individuals who have been deaf most of their lives are said to share a collective identity that involves their own values; appreciation of certain types of art, drama, and literature; and American Sign Language (Vernon, Makowsky, 1961; Schein, 1991). They prefer to socialize with each other and typically choose a deaf spouse. In the event of later institutionalization they may indeed find it easier to adapt to a collective lifestyle reminiscent of childhood experiences.

In elders with prelingual deafness, reading and writing skills may be impaired even though their intelligence is normal (Andrews, Wilson, 1991). They may not have had the common educational opportunities of their cohort based on the idea that their early orientation was to signing and lipreading. For these individuals, signing is their first language and English their second. Subtleties of verbal communication may be lost to them, although they often compensate and become extremely alert to nonverbal cues and feelings. At times a certified interpreter, well enmeshed in the world of the deaf, will be needed. Communication can be extremely difficult for some elders, since some become dependent on vision for understanding speech at the same time that vision is becoming compromised (Thorn, Thorn, 1989).

Cerumen Impaction

Cerumen impaction is the most common and easily corrected of all interferences in the hearing of the aged. The reduction in the number of cerumen-producing glands and activity of the glands results in a tendency toward cerumen impaction in the aged.

Long-standing impactions become hard, dry, and dark brown. Many elderly persons admit to using foreign objects to clean their ears. Some have perforated the tympanic membrane in the process, resulting in severe hearing loss in the injured ear. Individuals at particular risk of impaction are old men with large amounts of ear canal hair that tends to become entangled with the cerumen, which prevents dislodgment.

Others who may develop excessive cerumen are those who habitually wear hearing aids, those with benign growths that narrow the external ear canal, and those who have a predilection to cerumen accumulation. This can be removed and must be before accurate audiometry can be done. Irrigation is contraindicated if the tympanic membrane has been perforated, because it may induce an infection. Cautions are also necessary for those with especially sticky cerumen, which can damage the mechanism of a hearing aid and involve costly repairs. The factory cost for placing a wax guard is approximately $100; however, adhesive covers and wire baskets are available for less than $10. A protocol for removal is described in Box 9-5.

Tinnitus

Tinnitus (ringing, buzzing, hissing, whistling, or swishing sounds arising in the ear) is a condition that afflicts many aged persons. In addition to being very irritating, it can interfere with hearing. It is estimated that nearly 50 million adults in the United States are afflicted, 12 million severely enough to seek medical help (American Tinnitus Association, 1996). The incidence of tinnitus peaks between ages 65 and 74 and then seems to decrease in men. About 11% of those in

Box 9-5   PROTOCOL FOR CERUMEN REMOVAL

- Assess for ear pain, traumas, abnormalities, drainage, surgeries, or perforations. These or any other unusual findings should be referred to an otolaryngologist.
- When aural examination reveals cerumen impaction with no other abnormalities, the nurse may irrigate for cerumen removal using the following techniques:
  1. Carefully clip and remove hairs in ear canal.
  2. Instill a softening agent, such as slightly warm mineral oil, 0.5 to 1 ml twice daily for several days until wax becomes softened.
  3. Protect clothing and linens from drainage of oil or wax by placing small cotton ball in each external ear canal.
  4. When irrigating the ear, use handheld bulb syringe, 2- to 4-ounce plastic syringe, or Water Pik with emesis basin under ear to catch drainage; tip head to side being drained.
  5. Use solution of 3 ounces 3% hydrogen peroxide in quart of water warmed to 98° to 100° F; if client is sensitive to hydrogen peroxide, use sterile normal saline.
  6. Place towels around neck; empty emesis basin frequently, observing for residue from ear; keep client dry and comfortable; do not inject air into client's ear or use high pressure when injecting fluid.
  7. If the cerumen is not successfully washed out, begin the process again of instilling a softening agent for several days.

Modified from Webber-Jones J: Doomed to deafness, *Am J Nurs* 92(11):37, 1992.

the 65- to 74-year-old age-group (more men than women) experience tinnitus, After age 75, women experience tinnitus far more frequently than men (US Bureau of the Census, 1995).

Tinnitus can be caused by loud noises, excessive cerumen or auditory canal obstruction, disorders of the cervical vertebrae or the temporomandibular joint, allergies, an underactive thyroid, cardiovascular disease, tumors, conductive hearing loss, anxiety, depression, degeneration of bones in the middle ear, infections, or trauma to the head or ear. In addition, more than 200 prescription and nonprescription drugs list tinnitus as a potential side effect, aspirin being the most common. (Gulya, 1995; American Tinnitus Association, 1996). Tinnitus has a significant impact on daily life even in those with normal or very mildly impaired hearing. It is exacerbated by noise and increases in severity over time in many elders.

Assessment

Tinnitus may be described as pulsatile (matching the beating of the heart) or nonpulsatile, and as unilateral, asymmetric, or symmetric. Tinnitus may be subjective (audible only to the person) or objective (audible to the examiner). Subjective tinnitus is more common. Objective tinnitus is rare and is frequently due to a vascular or neuromuscular condition (Ciocon et al, 1995). The mechanisms of tinnitus are unknown but have been thought to be like cross-talk on telephone wires, phantom limb pain, or transmission of vascular sounds such as bruits, and are sometimes hallucinatory.

A Tinnitus Handicap Questionnaire developed by Newman et al (1995) measures physical, emotional, and social consequences of tinnitus. It also can remeasure the changes that the individual experiences with treatment. Some sufferers of tinnitus never find the cause; for others the problem may arbitrarily disappear.

Nursing Management

Therapeutic modes of treating tinnitus include transtympanal electrostimulation, iontophoresis, biofeedback, tinnitus masking with alternative sound production, dental treatment, cochlear implants, and hearing aids (American Tinnitus Association, 1996). Interestingly, the benefits of a hearing aid prove helpful to some, but for others hearing aids increase the problem. Some have found hypnosis, acupuncture, chiropractic, naturopathic, allergy, and drug treatment effective. Lidocaine is helpful to a large number of persons but impractical because of the necessity of intravenous administration and the brevity of relief.

Nursing actions include discussions with the client regarding times when the noises are most irritating; having the person keep a diary may identify patterns. There is some evidence that caffeine, alcohol, cigarettes, stress, and fatigue may exacerbate the problem (Gulya, 1995). Assess medications for possible contribution to the problem. Discuss life-style changes and alternative methods that some have found effective. Also, refer clients to the American Tinnitus Association for research updates, education, and support groups.

Assessment of Those With Impaired Hearing

Assessment of a hearing disability may be done in a superficial manner by almost any observant health care professional. However, the responsibility for the initial identification of hearing problems usually falls on the nurses, and therefore rapid, reliable, effective screening methods must be available to them. Screening should

Box 9-6   ASSESSMENT AND INTERVENTIONS FOR HEARING-IMPAIRED ELDERS

Assessment

History

In the past 3 months, have you had discharge from your ears?

In the past 3 months, have you experienced dizziness (not related to sudden changes in position)?

In the past 3 months, have you had pain in your ears?

In the past 3 months, have you noticed a sudden or rapid change in your hearing?

Have you ever experienced tinnitus, vertigo, or sudden or gradual hearing loss?

In which situations do you have difficulty hearing?

In the past, have you experienced ear infections, surgery, treatment, or hearing aid use?

Is there a family history of hearing loss?

What drugs have you used or are you now using (note particularly toxic levels of streptomycin, neomycin, or aspirin)?

Observations by family and/or caregiver

Does the person often seem inattentive to others?

Does the person respond with inappropriate anger or irritation when spoken to?

Does the person believe people are talking about him or her?

Does he or she lack a movement response to sounds in the environment?

Does the person have difficulty following clear directions?

Is he or she withdrawn and alone much of the time?

Does the person frequently ask to have something repeated?

Does he or she tend to turn one ear toward a speaker?

Does the person have a monotonous or unusual voice quality?

Is speech unusually loud or soft?

Interventions

General

Face the individual, and stand or sit on the same level.

Gain the individual's attention before beginning to speak.

Speakers need to keep hands away from their mouth and project their voice by controlled diaphragmatic breathing.

Avoid conversations in which the speaker's face is in glare or darkness.

Enunciate carefully and speak in a normal cadence.

Careful articulation and moderate speed of speech are helpful.

Avoid eating, chewing, or smoking while speaking.

Facial and hand expressions used liberally facilitate understanding.

Pause between sentences or phrases to confirm understanding.

Restate with different words when you are not understood.

Some languages and some cultural levels of verbal expressiveness facilitate understanding more than others (romance languages and stoic, stolid individuals are more difficult to understand).

When changing topics, preface the change by stating the topic.

Provide visual cues to locate noise direction, since there appears to be an age-related deficit to picking up directional cues.

In most cases there is a better ear.

Reduce background noise.

If paranoia has developed, the individual may not respond well to touch. A handshake is a benign gesture and will signal acceptance or rejection of your efforts to communicate.

The hospitalized hearing impaired

Note on the intercom button and the patient's chart whether the patient is deaf.

Note the most effective way to communicate with the patient.

Never restrict movement in the arms of deaf patients who use sign language as the primary means of communication.

Use charts, pictures, or models to explain medications and procedures.

Adequate lighting is essential.

If the patient has a hearing aid, encourage its use.

Determine a means of readily identifying the hearing impaired.

Obtain a certified sign language interpreter for obtaining consent for any procedure. *It is essential that the patient understand possible risks and outcomes.*

---

include the use of the Hearing Handicap Inventory for the Elderly—Screening (HHIE-S), visual inspection of the ear, pure-tone screening, and the client's history.

It is important that nurses become aware of these considerations. The client's history and visual inspection require little time to administer and effectively identify subjects who need medical referral. Hearing handicap scales vary in their predictive accuracy. Pure-tone screening is highly reliable but is sometimes difficult to administer to elders. Each elder is entitled to a complete and thorough audiometric examination if there is any doubt about adequate hearing capacity. Early detection of hearing loss often depends on a nurse's observational assessment. Box 9-6 provides screening observations.

Before concluding that any of these signs are evidence of "senility" or other aberrant behaviors, consider the possibility of a hearing problem. When there is any doubt, referral should be made to an otologist or otolaryngologist to identify possible medical conditions and then to an audiologist or a speech-hearing clinic for an audiologic evaluation before contacting a hearing aid representative.

Nurses are reminded that the best judge of adequate hearing capacity will come from the aged individual's own evaluation. Clark et al (1991) found high levels of accuracy of self-reported hearing loss among old women if it hampered their daily life. However, older persons are often unaware of mild to moderate hearing loss because of the gradual manner in which it usually develops. Wearing hearing aids is problematic in the minds of many, whether because of cost or inconvenience, and unless hearing loss significantly impairs one's quality of life, it may be ignored.

Hearing Evaluation

Few elders have had audiometric testing although nearly half of elders over 75 years old have hearing impairment (US Bureau of the Census, 1995). Nursing service can and should provide initial assessment by investing in a tuning fork, an otoscope, and an audioscope and learning to use them appropriately. Otoscopic examination allows visualization of the ear canal and tympanic membrane for possible discovery of cerumen impaction or a perforated eardrum.

Assessment of hearing disorders is done with audiometric and nonaudiometric testing tools. Assessment of structural changes and gross evidence of hearing loss is part of a physical examination.

The Weber test, placement of a vibrating tuning fork on the forehead of the individual, will determine the presence of unilateral conductive hearing loss. This is a screening test and does not measure bilateral hearing loss. The Rinne test screens for difficulty in air and bone conduction. The audioscope (similar to the ear thermometer) is used to determine the frequency range of hearing. Human speech is usually heard below the 2000- to 3000-Hz range. Those who have used the audioscope find it a highly valid screening instrument. It is a simple, fast, and accurate method of screening for hearing loss. Audiometry is still needed for more precise information.

Because many elders are very sensitive about admitting losses, they may be reluctant to share such information. It can best be obtained by first establishing rapport with the elderly person and then proceeding to open interviewing with a comment such as "Many people have difficulty hearing in certain situations. Have you experienced any difficulty? Describe these situations for me." If friends and relatives have insisted that the older person needs a hearing evaluation, he or she may be doubly resistant.

Interventions for Those With Impaired Hearing

Physical examination, interview, self-assessment, relative or friend assessment, and audiometric findings are all necessary to arrive at a meaningful recommendation for the hearing-impaired aged person. Counseling includes specific information regarding the problem, encouragement that sensorineural loss (nerve deafness) can often be partially counteracted by a hearing aid, assistance in the adjustment phase of wearing a hearing aid, and work with family members to improve their communication techniques.

Hearing Aids

Many factors may influence an individual who refuses to wear a hearing aid. If the person has been taught to use an aid gradually and correctly and yet does not do so, the nurse should attempt to discover the reasons: the appearance of having an infirmity, the difficulty manipulating a small object, lack of energy, uncomfortable fit, forgetfulness, anger expressed through passive resistance, cost, or simply self-neglect. In this era of highly sophisticated, personalized, and computerized hearing aids, most individuals can obtain some hearing enhancement that is acceptable to them. Hearing aids have changed dramatically in recent years, both in effectiveness and appearance, but many individuals, having tried one a number of years ago, have decided against using them.

A hearing aid is a personal amplifying system that includes a microphone, an amplifier, and a loudspeaker. The appearance and effectiveness of hearing aids have greatly improved in recent years. Hearing aid miniaturization may present difficulties for the aged with visual deficits, loss of finger sensation, or arthritic hands. A recent advance has been the introduction of a remote control device that contains an on/off switch and volume device. There are approximately 50 different manufacturers of hearing aids, and thus the informed consumer has a broad selection from which to choose.

The law requires that audiologic testing be preceded by an examination by a physician to rule out ear, nose, and throat (ENT) disorders. Many ENT specialists have an audiologist and audiologic testing available in the office. Audiologists may favor certain models, and it is wise for a client to shop around for fit and sound regardless of what the physician and audiologist recommend. The investment in a good hearing aid is considerable, and a good fit is crucial.

Numerous hearing aids and assistive devices to improve hearing exist. The "behind-the-ear aid" looks like a shrimp and fits around behind the ear; it is less commonly used now than the small "in-the-ear aid," which fits in the concha of the ear. A larger one can be custom made to fit the entire external auricular cavity (Silverstein et al, 1992). Today the entire system can fit easily in the ear canal. The analog hearing aids are designed to be worn at all times; other devices are designed to solve specific problems (Wylde, 1998). Some products are designed to overcome the effects of noise and distance. These transform sound waves to a different energy spectrum, such as infrared or electromagnetic waves that are then transmitted from the microphone to the receiver and delivered as a clear signal directly in the person's ear.

Digitally programmed hearing aids that have more than a million different settings from which to select are becoming available. These are matched to the individual's hearing loss.

In the past 5 years a miniaturized computer with a memory chip has been integrated into a hearing aid that eliminates many major hearing aid problems, such as adjustment levels, background noise, and whistling. These aids automatically electronically separate incoming sound without the need to adjust the volume.

Because of the rapidly developing technology, it behooves the hearing-impaired individual to be thoroughly evaluated in an audiologic center that is not marketing specific hearing aids. Many hospitals and health centers have such services and may have dozens of models an individual can try until the most suitable one is found. Wylde gives the following guidelines for anyone who is thinking of purchasing a hearing aid:

- Have a complete hearing evaluation by a qualified audiologist.
- "Nerve deafness" is no longer a reason for not seeking a timely evaluation.
- Hearing aids of whatever type will require individual motivation to adapt and adjust to the aid.

Suggestions for using and caring for a hearing aid are given in Table 9-1. At least a 30-day trial should be given before a hearing aid is purchased. If problems occur during that time, the person should return to the audiologist for assistance. Recent federal regulations have influenced hearing aid manufacturers toward more careful marketing and fitting procedures.

Table 9-1

The Use and Care of Hearing Aids

Hearing aid use	Care of the hearing aid
Initially, wear aid 15 to 20 minutes daily.	Insert battery when hearing aid is turned off.
Gradually increase time until 10 to 12 hours.	Store hearing aid in a dry, safe place.
Hearing aid will initially make client uneasy.	Remove or disconnect battery when not in use.
Insert aid with canal portion pointing into ear; press and twist until snug.	Batteries last 1 week with daily wearing of 10 to 12 hours.
Turn aid slowly to $1/3$ or $1/2$ volume.	Clean cerumen from tip weekly with pipe cleaner.
A whistling sound indicates incorrect ear mold insertion.	Common problems include switch turned off, clogged ear mold, dislodged battery, twisted tubing between ear mold and aid.
Adjust volume to a level comfortable for talking at a distance of 1 yard.	Ear molds need replacement every 2 or 3 years.
Do not wear aid under heat lamps or hair dryer or in very wet, cold weather.	Check ear molds for rough spots that will irritate ear.
Do not wear aid while bathing or perspiring heavily.	Avoid exposing aid to excessive heat or cold.
Concentrate on conversation; request repeat if necessary.	Clean batteries occasionally to remove corrosion; use a sharpened pencil eraser and gently scrape.
Sit close to speaker in noisy situations.	
Continue to be observant of nonverbal cues.	
Be patient with self and realize the process of adaptation is difficult but ultimately will be rewarding.	

Currently before a hearing aid can be purchased, medical clearance consisting of a signed waiver from a physician is mandatory, stating that none of the following conditions exist:

1. Visible congenital or traumatic deformity of the ear
2. Active drainage from the ear in the last 90 days
3. Sudden or progressive hearing loss within the last 90 days
4. Acute or chronic dizziness
5. Unilateral sudden hearing loss within the last 90 days
6. Visible evidence of significant cerumen accumulation or a foreign body in the ear canal
7. Pain or discomfort in the ear
8. Audiometric air-bone gap equal to or greater than 15 dB

The first seven of these conditions can be detected by the nurse in a history and physical examination, and the nurse can advise clients to seek further counseling from an otolaryngologist. It is also important to advise clients that charges for hearing aids or routine hearing loss examinations are not paid for by Medicare, nor does insurance generally cover any of the cost of hearing aids (Health Care Financing Administration, 1995).

Sound Booster Hearing Accessory

Sound amplifiers that fit in a pocket and are inexpensive walkabout-style hearing boosters are readily available. They are similar to the common Walkman. These are particularly useful for individuals with conductive hearing loss and in situations where background noise is inevitable. The amplifying microphone can be attached to a television or telephone or clipped on a friend's collar. In situations where a primary sound source is desirable, these devices are ideal. Headsets with small or large earphones are available. Thus when amplification of desired sounds is necessary, hearing aids are not necessarily as effective as these amplifiers.

Cochlear Implants

Cochlear implants became available in the 1980s to profoundly deaf individuals with sensorineural hearing loss. Considerable refinement has since been achieved and has shown the most success for those elders who have not been deaf for long and have a strong desire to hear (Cochlear Implants, 1991). Unlike hearing aids that amplify sound, the cochlear implant converts sound waves into electrical impulses and transmits them to the inner ear. A cochlear implant is surgically implanted in the mastoid bone behind the ear and electrically stimulates the primary hearing organ, the cochlea, setting the cilia in motion and transmitting impulses along the auditory nerve to the brain's hearing center. Although these are not yet in common use, they offer hope to some and are forerunners of even more effective refinements to come in electronic hearing devices.

The National Institutes of Health (NIH) finds the implants most effective in those who receive the implant soon after the hearing loss and recommends use of the hearing device in adults who are not totally deaf but are not helped sufficiently by hearing aids (Newsline, 1995). The implant carries some risk because the surgery destroys any residual hearing that remains. Therefore cochlear implant users can never revert back to using a hearing aid.

Adaptive Devices and Other Interventions

Many devices have been developed to assist the hard of hearing. These include alarm clocks that shake the bed or activate a flashing light; television and telephone amplifiers; and sound lamps that respond with light to sounds such as doorbells, babies crying, telephones, or other noises. These can be purchased from hearing aid dealers, telephone companies, electronic and appliance shops, or catalogues.

Any facility that receives financial aid from Medicare is required by the Americans With Disabilities Act to provide equal access to public accommodations. Such facilities are required to have sign language interpreters, telecommunication devices (TDDs), flashing alarm systems, and telecaptioning devices on televisions for the deaf. Unfortunately, these are seldom seen.

Some very innovative people have developed ideas and products to enrich the lives of the hearing impaired. Music especially for the profoundly hearing impaired that is focused only in the low-frequency cycles (which are most easily heard) has been recorded.

Another program, Hearing Dogs for the Deaf, has gained recognition. Seventeen locations in the United States train hearing dogs. In some locations the Society for the Prevention of Cruelty to Animals (SPCA) trains "shelter dogs"; some dogs are especially bred and raised to be hearing dogs; and in some locations the individual's own dog is trained appropriately. Hearing dogs serve to warn the hearing impaired of impending danger, audible signals, phones ringing, fire and smoke alarms, emergencies, and intruders. Although there are other, electronic means of dealing with many of these problems, the hearing impaired consistently comment on the alleviation of the sense of isolation that so often accompanies hearing impairment. With a hearing dog companion, elders express renewed courage, confidence, and freedom.

Janken and Cullian (1990) suggest a redefinition of significant variables to consider in making a nursing diagnosis of sensory/perceptual alterations related to impaired hearing. In a study of acutely ill geriatric patients they found that psychosocial dysfunction is not a significant indication of sensory/perceptual alterations due to hearing impairment but must be considered in conjunction with other variables such as levels of depression, cognitive function, social contacts, self-reported hearing ability, and overall health status.

Extensive nursing care plans related to presbycusis can be found in many recent clinical manuals. We suggest that these plans, such as the ones provided by Hogstel (1992), be reviewed for routine management but carefully and thoughtfully modified in relation to the patient's unique needs. Box 9-6 suggests some interventions that can help the nurse make a significant difference in an elder's ability to hear.

• • •

When vision and hearing are diminished, the elder has lost major sensory input, which has a direct effect on his or her everyday life. Decreases in these senses can potentiate isolation, depression, withdrawal, and loss of self-esteem and raise personal safety issues. It is the role of the nurse to identify sensory problems and assist the individual in adapting and compensating for these losses.

Age-related vision and hearing sensory changes, along with outcomes and health prevention, promotion, and maintenance, appear in Appendix 9-A.

NANDA and Wellness Diagnoses

Wellness	Specific Needs	NANDA
	Self-actualization	Role performance, altered
Is fulfilled		
	Self-esteem Image Control	Self-esteem, situational low Diversional activity deficit
Is active in group activities	Belonging Auditory Visual	Social interaction, impaired Social isolation
Has adequate vision Has adequate hearing	Safety and security Sensory acuity	Injury, risk for Sensory/perceptual alterations, (visual/auditory)
	Biologic integrity	

These are not all of the possible wellness or NANDA diagnoses that may be identified. The above are frequent examples of nursing diagnoses that should be considered when planning care for the older adult in whatever setting.

▶ KEY CONCEPTS

- The loss of vision is greatly feared by many elders, although visual impairment is only one third as common as hearing loss; total vision loss is rare and is due to pathologic processes rather than aging per se.
- Those with hearing impairment often find it difficult to adjust to hearing aids.
- Elders with visual impairment usually greatly appreciate it when nurses announce their presence and provide vivid, detailed descriptions of the surroundings.
- Environments and environmental changes have major effects on sensory input available to elders.
- Environmental sensory deprivation may have seriously disorienting consequences for the elderly.

▶ Activities and Discussion Questions

1. Which of the various sensory/perceptual changes would you find the most difficult to cope with? Why?
2. What measures would you suggest to a person with changes in his or her visual perception?
3. Discuss the stigma of hearing loss and hearing aids.
4. Discuss why individuals do not wear their hearing aids. What suggestions would be helpful in adapting to the wearing of a hearing aid?
5. Use wellness and NANDA diagnoses to develop a nursing care plan(s) for an aged individual with sensory changes.

RESOURCES

Visual Impairment

Association for Macular Diseases, Inc.
210 E. 64th Street
New York, NY 10012
For information send a business-size self-addressed stamped envelope (SASE).
Better Vision Institute
1800 N. Kent Street, Suite 904
Rosalyn, VA 22209
The Lighthouse, Inc.
111 E. 59th Street
New York, NY 10022
(800) 334-5497
Send an SASE with 66 cents postage for low-vision information.

Hearing Impairment

American Association of the Deaf-Blind
814 Thayer Avenue, Room 300
Silver Spring, MD 20910
American Tinnitus Association
PO Box 5
Portland, OR 97207-0005
(503) 248-9985; (503) 248-0024 (fax)
Hearing Dog Program
San Francisco SPCA
2500 16th Street
San Francisco, CA 94103
(415) 554-3020 (voice); (415) 554-3022 (TDD)
National Information Center on Deafness
Gallaudet University
800 Florida Avenue NE
Washington, DC 20002
(202) 651-5051
Resound Corporation
Redwood City, CA
Self Help for Hard of Hearing People
7910 Woodmont Avenue, Suite 1200
Bethesda, MD 20814
(301) 657-2248

REFERENCES

American Foundation for the Blind: *Fact sheet: guide dogs for the blind,* New York, 1996, The Foundation.

American Tinnitus Association: *Information about tinnitus,* Portland, Ore, 1996, The Association.

Andrews JF, Wilson HF: The deaf in the nursing home, *Geriatr Nurs* 12(6):279, 1991.

Back AP, Holden BA, Hine NA: Correction of presbyopia with contact lenses—comparative success rates with 3 systems, *Optom Vis Sci* 66(8):518, 1989.

Bass E, Steinberg E, Luthra R: Do ophthalmologists, anesthesiologists, and internists agree about preoperative testing in healthy patients undergoing cataract surgery? *Arch Ophthalmol* 113:1248, 1995.

Chen H-L: Relation of hearing loss, loneliness, and self-esteem, *J Gerontol Nurs* 20(6):22, 1994.

Ciocon J et al: Tinnitus: a stepwise workup to quiet the noise within, *Geriatrics* 50(3):16, 1995.

Clark K et al: The accuracy of self reported hearing loss in women aged 60-85, *Am J Epidemiol* 134(7):704, 1991.

Cochlear implants: technological advances offer new worlds of sound, *Mayo Clin Health Lett* 9(11):4, 1991.

Collins MJ et al: Peripheral visual acuity with monovision and other contact lens corrections for presbyopia, *Optom Vis Sci* 66(6):370, 1989.

Eastman P: When the light fades . . . macular degeneration in the spotlight, *AARP Bull* 37(7):2, 1996.

Gulya AL: Ear disorders. In Abrams WB, Beers MH, Berkow R, editors: *The Merck manual of geriatrics,* ed 2, Whitehouse Station, NJ, 1995, Merck Research Laboratories.

Health Care Financing Administration: *1995 Guide to health insurance for people with Medicare,* Washington, DC, 1995, US Government Printing Office.

Hogstel MO: *Clinical manual of geriatric nursing,* St Louis, 1992, Mosby.

Horowitz A: Vision impairment and functional disability among nursing home residents, *Gerontologist* 34(3):316, 1994.

Janken JK, Cullian CL: Auditory sensory/perceptual alteration: suggested revision of defining characteristics, *Nurs Diag* 1(4):147, 1990.

Javitt J, Steinberg E, Sharkey P: Cataract surgery in one eye or both? *Ophthalmology* 102(11):1583, 1995.

Kolanowski AM: The clinical importance of environmental lighting to the elderly, *J Gerontol Nurs* 18(1):10, 1992.

Koss E: Increasing visual cues to reduce agitation in patients with Alzheimer's disease, *Res Rep Aging* 2(2):4, 1995.

Kupfer C: Measuring quality of life in low vision patients, *Aging Vision News* 7(2):5, 1995a.

Kupfer C: Ophthalmologic disorders. In Abrams WB, Beers MH, Berkow R, editors: *The Merck manual of geriatrics,* ed 2, Whitehouse Station, NJ, 1995b, Merck Research Laboratories.

Macular degeneration, *Mayo Clin Health Lett* 3(9):5, 1990.

Meeuwsen HJ, Tesi JM, Goggin NL: Psychophysics of arm movement and human aging, *Res Q Exerc Sport* 63(1):19, 1992.

National Institute on Aging: *Diabetic retinopathy and blood sugar management,* Bethesda, Md, 1995, National Institutes of Health.

National Institute on Aging: *Hearing problems common in older people studied,* National Institute of Deafness and Other Communication Disorders, 1990a, Baltimore, Md, National Institutes of Health, US Department of Health and Human Services.

National Institute on Aging: *Scientists study treatment for glaucoma,* National Eye Institute, Baltimore, Md, 1990b, National Institutes of Health, US Department of Health and Human Services.

Newman C, Wharton J, Jackson G: Retest stability of the tinnitus handicap questionnaire, *Ann Otol Rhinol Largyngol* 104(9, pt 1):718, 1995.

Newsline: FDA considers expanded use for cochlear implants, *NurseWeek* 8(11):30, 1995.

O'Connell WF: Low vision—new developments and future directions, *Aging Vision News* 7(2):3, 1995.

Radial keratotomy, *Mayo Clin Health Lett* 13(4):4, 1995.

Ralston ME et al: Glaucoma screening in primary care: the role of noncontact tonometry, *J Fam Pract* 34(1):73, 1992.

Sacks O: *Seeing voices: a journey into the world of the deaf,* Berkeley, 1989, University of California Press.

Schappert SM: Office visits for glaucoma: United States, 1991-1992, *Advance data from vital and health statistics,* No 262, Hyattsville, Md, 1995, National Center for Health Statistics.

Schein JD: The deaf community in the twenty-first century. In Garretson M, editor: A deaf American monograph, *Perspectives on Deafness* 41:131, 1991.

Schneider E: *Demographics update: blind persons who use guide dogs,* New York, 1996, American Foundation for the Blind.

Selye H: *The stress of life,* New York, 1956, McGraw-Hill.

Silverstein, H, Wolfson RJ, Rosenberg S: Diagnosis and management of hearing loss, *Clin Symp* 44(3):2, 1992.

Silverstone B: Technology and low-vision aids, *Aging Connection* 4(4):5, 1988.

Stein HA: Contact lenses in the management of presbyopia, *Int Ophthalmol Clin* 31(2):61, 1991.

Stuen C: Vision care and rehabilitation, *Focus Geriatr Care Rehabil* 10(1):1, 1996.

Thorn F, Thorn S: Speech reading with reduced vision: a problem of aging, *J Opt Soc Am A* 6(4):491, 1989.

Tielsch J, Steinberg E, Cassard S: Preoperative functional expectations and postoperative outcomes among patients undergoing first cataract surgery, *Arch Ophthalmol* 113:1312, 1995.

US Bureau of the Census: *Statistical abstract of the United States: 1995,* Washington, DC, 1995, Superintendent of Documents, US Government Printing Office.

US Department of Health and Human Services: *Medicare policy proposed for eye surgery,* HHS News press release, Oct 5, 1995.

Vernon M, Makowsky B: Deafness and minority group dynamics, *Deaf American* 21:3, 1961.

Virtanen P, Laatikainen L: Primary success with low vision–related macular degeneration, *Acta Ophthalmol* 69(4):484, 1991.

von Wedel H, von Wedel UC, Streppel M: Selective hearing in the aged with regard to speech perception in quiet and in noise, *Acta Otolaryngol* 476(suppl):13, 1990.

Wolanin MO, Phillips LRF: *Confusion: prevention and care,* St Louis, 1981, Mosby.

Wylde M: Technologies help compensate for hearing loss, *Aging Connection* 4(4):6, 1998.

Appendix 9-A Age-Related Vision and Hearing Changes; Outcomes; and Prevention, Health Promotion, and Maintenance Approaches

Age-related changes	Outcomes	Health prevention, promotion, and maintenance
VISION		
Lid elasticity diminishes	Pouches under the eyes	
Loss of orbital fat		
Decreased tears	Excessive dryness of eyes	Use isotonic eye drops as needed
Arcus senilis become visible		
Sclera yellows and becomes less elastic		
Yellowing and increased opacity of cornea	Lack of corneal luster	
Increased sclerosis and rigidity of iris		
Decrease in convergence ability	Presbyopia	Have eyes examined at least once a year
Decline in light accommodation response	Lessened acuity	Use magnifying glass and high-intensity light to read
Diminished pupillary size	Decline in depth perception	Increase light to prevent falls
Atrophy of ciliary muscle	Diminished recovery from glare	Clip-on sunglasses, visors, sun hat, nonglare coating on prescription glasses/sunglasses
Night vision diminishes	Night blindness	Don't drive at night
		Keep night-light in bathroom and hallway
		Paint first and last step of staircase and edge of each step in-between with a bright color or a reflective color
Yellowing of lens	Diminished color perception (blues, greens)	
Lens opacity	Cataracts	Surgical removal of lens (lens implants)
Increased intraocular pressure	Rainbows around lights	Have a yearly eye examination, including tonometer testing
	Altered peripheral vision	
Shrinkage of gelatinous substance in the vitreous		
Vitreous floaters appear		
Ability to gaze upward decreases		
Thinning and sclerosis of retinal blood vessels		
Atrophy of photoreceptor cells		
Degeneration of neurons in visual cortex		
HEARING		
Thinner, drier skin of external ear		
Longer and thicker hair in external ear canal (of men)		
Narrowing of auditory opening		
Increased cerumen	Impaired hearing	Check ears for wax or infection
Thickened and less resilient tympanic membrane	Difficulty hearing high-frequency sounds (presbycusis)	Formal hearing test
Decreased flexibility of basilar membrane		
Ossicular calcification	Gradual loss of sound	Consultation for proper hearing and speaking tone—shouting distorted
Diminished neuron, endolymph, hair cells, and blood supply to inner ear and auditory nerve		
Degeneration of spiral ganglion and arterial blood vessels		

chapter 10

Nutritional Needs of the Aged

▶ LEARNING OBJECTIVES

Upon completion of this chapter, the reader will be able to:

- Identify factors affecting the nutrition of the aged.
- Discuss interventions that can aid or provide better nutrition for the elder.
- Identify interventions to help the elder with dysphagia to eat.
- List the causes of constipation.
- Identify interventions that can reduce or alleviate constipation in the aged.

▶ GLOSSARY

Dysphagia Difficulty swallowing.
Gastroesophageal reflux disease (GERD) Backward flow of stomach contents into the esophagus.

Soul food Food possessing emotional significance and providing personal satisfaction; often has some cultural or traditional origins.

▶ THE LIVED EXPERIENCE

I just can't chew very well, and then when I try to swallow, it feels like there is a huge lump in my throat. Since I had the stroke, I can't even talk enough to tell them to slow down when they try to feed me. I think if I had just a little help, I could probably almost feed myself, but everyone is always in such a hurry.

Lorraine, a poststroke victim

Lord, another day with six feeders. How can I ever get everything done? Sue said they were going to have extra help at lunchtime, but no one came. There must be volunteers or family members somewhere who can help out. I'm definitely going to look into the possibility. It is just not fair to expect me to do so much, and I'm worried about Lorraine and several others who aren't really getting enough food.

Vivian, a nurse aide

*W*ell-being is influenced by the triad of aging, nutrition, and health. Proper nutrition means that all of the essential nutrients (carbohydrates, fat, protein, vitamins, minerals, and water) are adequately supplied and used to maintain optimal health and well-being. Proper nutrition provides the energy and building blocks necessary to maintain body structure and function. The variances in nutritional requirements throughout the life span are not well established for the aged. Increased amounts of calcium and vitamins A and C are needed in late life but tend to be deficient in the average diet of the aged or are affected by alterations in storage, use, and absorption.

Total caloric intake should decline in response to corresponding changes in metabolic rate and a general decrease in physical activity; however, a person's food choices and the amount of food they consume are mainly formed by economics and culture; both are components that make the person who he or she is (Peters, 1998).

FOOD GUIDE PYRAMID

The current guide to proper nutrition across the life span is the Food Guide Pyramid. The pyramid provides the

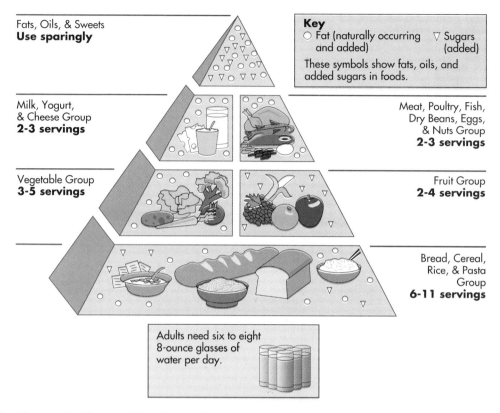

Key
○ Fat (naturally occurring and added)   ▽ Sugars (added)
These symbols show fats, oils, and added sugars in foods.

Fats, Oils, & Sweets
Use sparingly

Milk, Yogurt, & Cheese Group
2-3 servings

Meat, Poultry, Fish, Dry Beans, Eggs, & Nuts Group
2-3 servings

Vegetable Group
3-5 servings

Fruit Group
2-4 servings

Bread, Cereal, Rice, & Pasta Group
6-11 servings

Adults need six to eight 8-ounce glasses of water per day.

Fig. 10-1   Food guide pyramid for older adults. (Courtesy US Department of Agriculture, Washington, DC.)

types and amounts of foods that should be eaten in ascending order of dietary importance. This differs from previous guides that accorded all of the food groups equal importance and emphasized too much fat. The U.S. Department of Agriculture's basic food pyramid specifically for elders appears in Fig. 10-1. Note the addition of six to eight glasses of water; this is because fluids are so critical for elders. With proper instruction, the pyramid is an easy and systematic way for a person or caregiver to evaluate nutritional intake and make corrective adjustments. Pictures can be used to transcend cultural and speech barriers and educational limitations.

FACTORS AFFECTING FULFILLMENT OF NUTRITIONAL NEEDS

Fulfillment of the aged person's nutritional needs is affected by numerous factors, including lifelong eating habits, socialization, income, transportation, housing, and food knowledge.

Lifelong Eating Habits

The nutritional state of a person reflects the individual's dietary history and present food practices. Lifelong eating habits are developed out of tradition, ethnicity, and religion, all of which collectively can be called *culture.* Krebs-Smith et al (1995) found that food habits established since childhood influenced the intake of older adults.

Eating habits do not always coincide with fulfillment of nutritional needs. Rigidity of food habits increases with age as familiar food patterns are sought. Ethnicity determines if traditional foods are preserved, whereas religion affects the choice of foods possible. Throughout life, then, preferences for particular foods bring deep satisfaction and possess emotional significance. Such foods are called *soul food* or *comfort food.* Preferences for soul food influence food choices and affect nutrient intake. Foods prepared or served in a special way provide "soul" and are not unique to any one group but, rather, are found all over the world.

Lifelong habits of dieting or eating fad foods also echo through the later years. The aged, in particular, are taken in by food fads that profess to partially or completely cure various ailments or to make one look younger or feel more vital. Skipping meals is another practice that one finds with the aged. The quantity of food eaten diminishes, and the adequacy of nutrition becomes questionable. It is very difficult to reach an adequate nutritional intake if the total calories are fewer than 1200 per day. Individuals who are on self-imposed diets of 1000 calories or less per day are inviting malnutrition.

Food Use Patterns

Individuals establish their diets and eating patterns for various reasons. Five patterns were identified by Shifflett (1987). Three of these patterns reflect self-determination and individual control or self-responsibility. These patterns are described in Box 10-1. Usually active participation in dietary matters is a determinant in adherence or nonadherence to dietary regimens.

Socialization

The social essence ascribed to eating is sharing and providing a feeling of belonging. All of us use food as a means of giving and receiving love, friendship, or belonging. Many aged persons are forced to remain isolated from the mainstream of life because of impinging factors. When one eats alone, the outcome is often either overindulgence or depression (a common problem of aging and a significant inhibitor of appetite) and disinterest in food. Disinterest in food may also result from the effects of medication or disease processes.

Some aged persons spend much of their time in neighborhood bars, the center for social interaction. In seeking this type of fleeting social support, the aged spend money that is needed for adequate nutrition on alcohol. The perception that drinking is a sanctioned way to maintain social contact, which is preferable to not drinking and becoming isolated, is a very powerful consideration, particularly for men who are single-room occupants. Drinking alcohol depletes the body of necessary nutrients and often replaces meals, thus making an individual doubly prone to malnutrition.

There are more constructive means of maintaining social contact and nutritional status. Title VII of the Older Americans Act provides funding for strategically located outreach centers or nutrition sites whose purposes are to provide at least one nutritionally sound meal daily and to facilitate congregate dining to foster social contact and relationships. No one age 60 or over (all spouses are also included) can be denied participation in the nutrition program because of his or her economic situation. Those who are able to pay for their meal do so according to their ability.

Meals on Wheels, another community program, encourages both the attainment of good nutrition and human contact for those who are unable to prepare meals or go out to obtain them. Other group feeding programs exist through church and other community auspices, such as food cooperatives, home grocery delivery services, and chore services for shopping and meal preparation. In the past, the federal government has awarded grants to the Congregate Housing Services Project to provide meals to elderly residents who needed them to remain independent.

One objective for *Healthy People 2000* is to increase to at least 80% the receipt of home food services by people age 65 and older who have difficulty in preparing their own meals or are otherwise in need of home-delivered meals. Only 7% of those needing home food services are receiving them at this time (US Department of Health and Human Services, 1995).

Income

Inflation is constantly eroding the purchasing power of the aged, forcing them to buy foods that satiate hunger

---

Box 10-1	FOOD PATTERNS

Physician-prescribed/suggested. Treatment for or prevention of disease (such as reduction of sodium, fat, sugar, weight reduction).

Change in food use. Factors beyond individual's control (such as alteration in taste, isolation, income), all of which are linked to a decrease in food intake.

Self-prescribed diets. Implemented by the individual, not the physician. Similar to prescribed diet, but individual puts self on high-fiber, low-fat, etc., diet because of family history of disease (such as heart, diabetes mellitus, cancer).*

Overall reduction of food intake. Through a conscientious effort to maintain healthy body weight and decrease health problems.*

Maintenance of lifelong food use. Continuous conscious diet pattern has been incorporated into healthy dietary practices long before old age.*

*Self-determined.

but provide many empty calories. These foods may or may not be expensive. Some aged persons eat only once a day in an attempt to make their income last through the month. Aged individuals accustomed to eating meat, fish, and poultry as their main sources of protein have watched the cost climb to heights beyond their purchasing power. Inexpensive alternative protein sources such as tofu (soybean curd) are foreign to the diets of the aged in Western society today but have slowly been making their way into acceptance. At present the development of a taste for alternative protein sources and an understanding of what foods to mix to obtain complete dietary protein require some knowledge and practice to ensure adequate protein intake and to prevent monotony. If at all possible, the aged should be encouraged to use vegetable protein sources to meet daily needs. This is a more economical form of protein that may help the aged conserve their income for other necessities, unexpected bills, or special treats. Combinations such as milk or cheese with bread or pasta; cereal with milk; rice-and-cheese or rice-and-bean casseroles; wheat soy or corn soy bread; wheat bread with baked beans, beans, or pea curry; tortillas and beans; and legume soup with bread are sources of protein.

The food stamp program has the potential for increasing the purchasing power of the aged who qualify, but such programs are vulnerable to federal budget cutting. Many aged persons find that the amount of money required to purchase the food stamps is greater than they think they can afford, or they do not see the benefit to them. Transportation may be limited and the distance too far for the aged to travel to acquire the food stamps, which are sold only at designated locations in cities.

Free food programs, such as donated commodities, are also available at distribution centers (food banks) for those with limited incomes. Although this is another valuable option for the aged, use of such programs is not always entirely feasible. One takes a chance on the types of food available any particular day or week; quantities distributed are frequently too large for the single aged person or the aged couple to use or even carry from the distribution site; and the site may be too far away or difficult to reach. The time of distribution of the food may be inconvenient, too.

Some cafeterias and restaurants that provide special meal prices for the aged have had to increase their prices as food costs have risen; thus the previous advantages of eating out have diminished. Yet many single elders rely on them for most meals.

Transportation

Availability of transportation may be limited for the aged. Many small, long-standing neighborhood food stores have been closed in the wake of larger supermarkets, which are located in areas that serve a greater segment of the population. It may become difficult to walk to the market, to reach it by public transportation, or to carry a bag of groceries while using a cane. It is nearly impossible to do this with a walker. Fear is apparent in the elderly's consideration of transportation. They fear not being able to cross the street in the time it takes the traffic light to change and being knocked down or falling as they walk in crowded streets. Despite reduced senior citizen bus fares, the aged remain very fearful of attack when using public transportation. Transportation by taxicab for an individual on a limited income is unrealistic, but sharing a taxicab with others who also need to shop may enable the aged to go where food prices are cheaper and to take advantage of sale items. For the aged, convenience foods, devoid of many essential nutrients, are lighter to carry or pull along in a cart than fresh fruits and vegetables.

Senior citizen organizations in many parts of the country have been helpful in providing the elderly with van service to shopping areas. In housing complexes it may be possible to schedule group trips to the supermarket. Most communities have multiple sources of transportation available, but the aged may be unaware of them.

Housing

Poor and near-poor aged persons are likely to reside in substandard housing. Some who live in single rooms lack storage space for food, a means of refrigeration, and a stove for cooking. At certain times of the year some of the single-room dwellers use the window ledges and fire escapes to keep perishables cool for several days' use. It is difficult for the single-room occupant to prepare adequately nutritious meals unless the individual is aware of other alternatives.

Ideally, one meal that consists of protein (generally meat, fish, or poultry), potato, vegetable, salad, and dessert should be eaten out daily. Other meals can be prepared and eaten with a minimum of effort in the aged person's room. Pantry-type foods can be safely stored in a heavy cardboard or wooden box with a tight-fitting lid and in the driest, coolest place in the room. This box not only serves as a place of storage but can also be used as a table when one is not available. Cookies and crackers should be placed in plastic bags and then in airtight containers. Screw-top jars or coffee cans will accommodate dried fruit, beans, and sugar. Vacuum-packed foods do not require refrigeration, and a greater variety is available than in the past. Canned food should be purchased in the single-serving size so that there will not be any leftovers. Boxes of edibles should be carefully opened to ensure tight reclosure. Additional factors affecting dietary intake include living arrangements, the number of meals eaten daily, who cooks and shops, the presence of physical impediments affecting cooking and shopping, problems with chewing, use of dentures, alcohol use, medication use, and taste and smell. The individual's meal patterns and preferences are the foremost concern of the nurse in tailoring an acceptable diet.

Taste and Smell in Nutrition

The senses of taste and smell (chemosenses) are intertwined and can, when acute, provide great pleasure, as well as protection from harm.

Taste

Fine, subtle taste to discriminate between flavors is an olfactory function, whereas crude taste (such as sweet and sour) is dependent on the taste buds. It is thought that there is about a 40% decrement in smell and taste in old age (Wilson, 1995). The pleasure of eating comes more from masticating than from the taste buds or the hunger center in the lateral hypothalamus. This is important knowledge in preparing food for older people. Individuals have varied levels of taste sensitivity that seem predetermined by genetics and constitution, as well as age variation. Many denture wearers say they lose some of their satisfaction in food, possibly because texture is a very important element in food enjoyment. Difficulty in flavor appreciation comes from individual variables such as smoking, olfactory sensitivity, attitude toward food and eating, and the presence of moistening secretions. There are also aberrations in flavor sensation caused by certain medications. Refer to Appendix 7-A for age-related changes in taste.

Smell

Three causes are thought to explain most of the loss of the sense of smell: nasal sinus disease, repeated injury to olfactory receptors through viral infections, and head trauma that results in bleeding into the nasal mucosa. The last-mentioned cause is the least common.

The National Geographic Smell Survey found that exposure to medications and environmental agents affected chemosensation, especially in men and particularly those who have worked in factories and whose accumulated exposure to noxious agents has resulted in an impaired sense of smell (Corwin et al, 1995). Refer to Appendix 7A for age-related changes in smell.

PROBLEMS IN NUTRITION

Dentition, dysphagia, adequate fiber, constipation, and malnutrition are a few of the factors that affect or are affected by nutritional status and that the nurse will encounter in the care of the elderly. Adequate hydration, which is an influential factor in nutrition of the aged because of its importance, is discussed in Chapter 11.

Dentition

The ability to communicate, socialize, and maintain adequate nourishment depends on dental health. Tooth loss is not a natural part of the aging process but, rather, is a problem that accrues over time and is most evident in the aged. The lack of teeth affects the type and consistency of food chosen to eat. This often leads to limited and monotonous meals. Frequently food eaten by those who are edentulous is inadequate and deficient in nutritive value. Age-related changes in the buccal cavity are listed in Box 10-2. The major cause of tooth loss in the aged is periodontal disease. "Almost pandemic in

---

Box 10-2   AGE CHANGES OF THE BUCCAL CAVITY

Decrease in the cellular compartment
Loss of submucosal elastin in oral mucosa
Loss of connective tissue (collagen)
Increase in thickness of collagen fibers
Decrease in function of minor salivary glands
Decrease in number and quality of blood vessels and
   nerves
Attrition on occlusive contact surfaces
Enamel less permeable—teeth more brittle
Tooth color change
Excessive secondary dentin formation
Decrease in rate of cementin deposition
Decrease in size of pulp chamber and root canals
Decrease in size and volume of the tooth pulp
Increase in pulp stones and dystrophic mineralization

the older population, gingivitis may affect up to 80% of all teeth" (Feldman, 1986, p. 5).

The most prevalent cause of gingivitis, gum inflammation and disease, is inadequate removal of plaque and calculus. This may be exacerbated by partial dentures, overhanging ledges of fillings, and faulty bridges that allow plaque to accumulate between teeth. A predisposition to gingivitis may also occur when the mucous membranes are irritated by dryness of the mouth. Systemic problems such as endocrine dysfunction, chronic airway limitations, medications, and nutritional deficiencies may influence the development of the disease (Box 10-3).

The increased retention of teeth by today's elderly population is creating concern about the increase of periodontal conditions because they affect the tissue supporting the teeth, cementum, periodontal ligaments, alveolar bone, and gingiva. It is important for the nurse to assess for periodontal disease in the elderly and teach elders the signs to look for (Box 10-4).

Assessment

A brief dental history that includes questions about dental visits, frequency of brushing teeth, existence of oral conditions, and identifying risk factors for periodontal disease should be combined with inspection and palpation of the oral cavity (gums, tongue, natural teeth or dentures, and mucous membranes). This should be done at least every 6 to 12 months. The Brief Oral Health Status Exam (BOHSE), developed by Kayser-Jones et al (1995), is a useful tool that is usable by most health care providers to assess oral health of elders in community and institutional settings; however, the tool requires an in-service session from a dentist before it can be implemented.

Interventions

Impaired manual dexterity makes it difficult for elders to adequately maintain their dental routine and remove plaque adequately. The hand grip of manual toothbrushes is too small to grasp and manipulate easily, although enlarging the handle by adding a foam grip or wrapping it with gauze to increase handle size has been

---

Box 10-3	**CONTRIBUTING FACTORS IN PERIODONTAL PROBLEMS IN THE AGED**

Anatomic
Tooth malalignment
Thinning gingival mucosa

Bacterial
Plaque accumulation
Invasion of organisms at or below gum line
Food impaction

Drugs, Metallic Poisons
Allergic responses
Phenytoin
Cytotoxins
Heavy metals (lead, arsenic, mercury)

Emotional and Psychomotor
Bruxism (grinding of teeth)
Cerebrovascular accident
Mental impairment

Intrinsic (Systemic)
Endocrine
Metabolic
Altered immune system

Mechanical
Calculus
Retention of impacted food
Movable and spreading teeth
Ragged-edged fillings and crown overhangs
Poorly designed or poorly fitting dentures

Data compiled from Zach L, Trieger N. In Rossman I: Clinical geriatrics, ed 3, Philadelphia, 1986, Lippincott; Odslehage JC, Magilvey K: Geriatr Nurs 7:238, 1986; and Papas AS, Niessen LC, Chauncey HH: Geriatric dentistry: aging and oral health, St Louis, 1991, Mosby.

Box 10-4	**SIGNS OF PERIODONTAL DISEASE***

Gums bleeding when teeth are brushed (Even a little bleeding is not normal. If you have a "pink" toothbrush, see your dentist.)
Red, swollen, or tender gums
Detachment of the gums from the teeth
Pus that appears from the gum line when the gums are pressed
Teeth that have become loose or change position
Any change in the way your teeth fit together when you bite
Any change in the fit of partial dentures
Chronic bad breath or bad taste

*Not limited to elders alone.

effective in facilitating grasp. The ultrasonic toothbrush is an effective method for elders or those who must brush the teeth of elders to use. The base is large enough for easy grasp, and the ultrasonic movement of the bristles with the usual brushing movement is very effective in plaque removal (Whitmyer et al, 1998). The ultrasonic toothbrush is also valuable in dental care of those who are institutionalized or cognitively impaired (Pyle et al, 1998). Anyone who has a pacemaker should not use the ultrasonic toothbrush, because the transducer of the toothbrush affects pacemaker function.

For the homebound elder, daily oral care should be part of general hygiene. Having the proper equipment and using the appropriate technique greatly simplify the task and ensure better results. Box 10-5 provides directions for caregivers. Many elders believe that once they have dentures, there is no longer a need for oral care. Older adults with dentures should be taught the proper home care of their dentures and oral tissue to prevent odor, stain, and plaque buildup; home care should include removal of debris under dentures to prevent pressure on and shrinkage of underlying support structures. Dentures and other dental appliances such as bridges should be cleaned after each meal and any time they are removed (Box 10-6). Dentures should be worn constantly except at night (bedtime; to allow relief of the compression on the gums) and replaced in the mouth in the morning (Rounds, Papas, 1991).

Box 10-5   DENTAL CARE: INSTRUCTIONS FOR CAREGIVER

1. If the patient is in bed, elevate his or her head by raising the bed or propping it with pillows and have the patient turn his or her head to face you. Place a clean towel across the chest and under the chin, and place a basin under his or her chin.
2. If the patient is sitting in a stationary chair or wheelchair, stand behind the patient and stabilize his or her head by placing one hand under his or her chin and resting his or her head against your body. Place a towel across his or her chest and over the shoulders. (It may be helpful to secure it with a safety pin.) The basin can be kept handy in the patient's lap or on a table placed in front of or at the side of the patient. A wheelchair may be positioned in front of the sink.
3. If the patient's lips are dry or cracked, apply a light coating of petroleum jelly.
4. Brush and floss the patient's teeth as you have been instructed (sulcular brushing, if possible). It may be helpful to retract the patient's lips and cheek with a tongue blade or fingers in order to see the area that is being cleaned. Use a mouth prop as needed if the patient cannot hold his or her mouth open. If manual flossing is too difficult, use a floss holder or interproximal brush to clean the proximal surfaces between the teeth. Use a dentifrice containing fluoride.
5. Provide the conscious patient with fluoride rinses or other rinses as indicated by the dentist or hygienist.

From Papas AS, Niessen LC, Chauncey HH: *Geriatric dentistry: aging and oral health,* St Louis, 1991, Mosby.

Box 10-6   INSTRUCTIONS FOR DENTURE CLEANING

1. Rinse your denture or dentures after each meal to remove soft debris.
2. Once a day, preferably before retiring, brush your denture according to the method described below. Then place it in a denture-cleaning solution and allow it to soak overnight or for at least a few hours. (Acrylic denture material must be kept wet at all times to prevent cracking or warping.)
3. Remove your denture from the cleaning solution and brush it thoroughly.
   a. Although an ordinary *soft* toothbrush is adequate, a specially designed denture brush may clean more effectively. (CAUTION: Acrylic denture material is softer than natural teeth and may be damaged by being brushed with very firm bristles.)
   b. Brush your denture over a sink lined with a facecloth and half-filled with water. This will prevent breakage if the denture is dropped.
   c. Hold the denture *securely* in one hand, but do not squeeze. Hold the brush in the other hand. It is not essential to use a denture paste, particularly if dentures are soaked before being brushed to soften debris. Never use a commercial tooth powder, because it is abrasive and may damage the denture materials. Plain water, mild soap, or sodium bicarbonate may be used.
   d. When cleaning a *removable partial denture,* great care must be taken to remove plaque from the curved metal clasps that hook around the teeth. This can be done with a regular toothbrush or with a specially designed clasp brush.
4. After brushing, rinse your denture thoroughly and insert it into your mouth.

From Papas AS, Niessen LC, Chauncey HH: *Geriatric dentistry: aging and oral health,* St Louis, 1991, Mosby.

Box 10-7   HISTORY AND ASSESSMENT FOR DYSPHAGIA

History

Do solid foods or liquids cause your symptoms?

Is dysphagia constant or intermittent?

Is heartburn or indigestion associated with the dysphagia?

When did the dysphagia begin?

What other symptoms are present (such as chest pain, nocturnal symptoms)?

Has hoarseness, nasal regurgitation, or aspiration occurred?

Assessment

Ask the elder to place his or her tongue against the palate (this movement is necessary to push food into the throat).

Stroke the elder's tonsillar arch and soft palate with a moist cotton swab and ask if this can be felt (for swallowing to take place, some feeling is necessary in these areas).

With a moistened cotton swab dipped in ice-cold lemon water, stroke the tonsillar arch (elicits contraction of the pharyngeal muscles if normal).

Observe for weight loss.

Check for dehydration.

Modified from Castell DO: Esophageal disorders in the elderly, *Gastroenterol Clin North Am* 19:235, 1990; Maat MT, Tandy L: Impaired swallowing. In Maas M et al, editors: *Nursing diagnosis and interventions for the elderly,* Redwood City, Calif, 1991, Addison-Wesley; Knudsen SF: Gastrointestinal and metabolic problems in older adults. In Steffl BM, editor: *Handbook of gerontological nursing,* New York, 1984, Nostrand Reinhold; and Hufler DH: Helping your dysphagic patient eat, *RN* 50:36, 1987.

Box 10-8   GUIDE FOR DYSPHAGIC ELDERS

1. Sit upright with head positioned to facilitate passage of food.
2. Obtain suction equipment, and keep it on standby.
3. Place food on the tongue exactly as prescribed, when eating.
4. Drink plenty of liquids or include large amounts with food on a daily basis.
5. Weigh yourself on a regular basis, and report weight loss and/or lack of appetite to your health care provider.
6. Report a resurgence or worsening of symptoms to your health care provider.

Dysphagia

Dysphagia is associated with many conditions, the most common of which is gastroesophageal reflux (GERD). Incidences of dysphagia increase as one ages or experiences neurologic impairment. Weight loss, malnutrition, aspiration pneumonia, and even death are problems associated with dysphagia. It is the neurologically impaired elder who is most likely to be dysphagic. Dysphagia can be categorized as transfer dysphagia (difficulty moving the food from the mouth to the esophagus), transport dysphagia (difficulty passing the ingested food down the esophagus), or delivery dysphagia (the propulsion of a bolus of food to the stomach is difficult). These problems are attributed to motor abnormalities such as oropharyngeal paralysis following a stroke, when food may be misdirected—particularly liquids into the nose and respiratory passages. These types of events occur when the vagus and/or cranial nerves that innervate the oral and pharyngeal motor function are impaired, as in stroke patients and those with other neurologic problems. Mechanical, or structural, obstruction, such as stricture or tumor, results from long-standing reflux as a result of gastroesophageal incompetence. All or part of the esophagus may be affected by structural or neurologic abnormalities.

Assessment

It is important to obtain a careful history of the elder's response to dysphagia and to observe the person during mealtime (Box 10-7). The most important assessment is to identify if swallowing difficulty progresses from solids to liquids (most likely mechanical or organic) or from liquids to solids or progresses with both simultaneously (most likely motor in nature). This gives major direction in planning interventions.

Interventions

Aspiration is the most profound and dangerous problem for the elder. It is important to have in the home or in the institution, at the bedside or in the dining area, a suction machine available for use. It is also of the utmost importance for those with motor dysphagia to have an evaluation by a speech-language pathologist. Other interventions for dysphagia are described in Box 10-8, and Table 10-1 offers guidance by symptoms. Additional measures include administration of prescribed anticholinergics and long-acting nitroglycerin, control of gastric acidity with such medications as H_2 blockers,

Table 10-1

A Guide to Symptom Assessment and Interventions For Dysphagia

Signs and symptoms	Therapies	Positioning	Feeding devices
Poor lip closure, drooling, poor oral motor control	Tongue exercises, modified feeding, lip pursing	Head and torso upright at 90-degree angle	Feeding spoons
Intraoral and facial weakness with reduced sensitivity, reduced oral secretions	Use of hot and cold food, as well as liquids, to stimulate swallow; may need suction for oral secretions, chewing; strengthening and range-of-motion exercises; tongue and lip exercises (holding a tongue blade tautly between lips while trying to pull the tongue forward)	Place food on stronger or most sensitive side of mouth	Feeding devices may not be helpful
Inability to start and transport food posteriorly in mouth; poor lingual control (lingual pressure declines with age)	Tongue exercises; adjust size and composition of food bolus; have patient chew and place food on better side; multiple swallows	Tilt head to better side	Use of a palatal lift prosthesis
Leakage into nasal cavity; oral residue gets into larynx before swallowing (cough, choke)	Use thickened liquids and semi-solid foods; hold bolus in mouth long before swallowing	Hold head and chin down; tilt head to better side	Use of a palatal lift prosthesis
Aspiration before and during swallowing (delayed trigger of reflex in pharynx)	Thermal stimulation; thickened liquids; learn supraglottic swallow	Hold head and chin down	Use a chin support during feeding
"Wet" sound in voice (insufficient closure of vocal cords; larynx)	Thickened liquids and thin semi-solid food; Mendelsohn maneuver (larynx is manually raised and held up as patient swallows)	Upright position; turn head to either side	Feeding devices may not be helpful
Paresis on side or sides of pharynx; "wet" voice	Control size and consistency of bolus; start with liquids then semisolids; multiple swallows; supraglottic swallow	Turn and tilt head toward weaker side, then turn and tilt head toward stronger side	Feeding devices may not help
Aspiration after swallowing (esophagus does not open); difficulty swallowing (takes several attempts)	Limit amount and type of food; control size of bolus; liquids and thin semisolids; multiple swallows; supraglottic swallow	Turn head and trunk to either side	Feeding devices may not be helpful

Modified from Evans WB et al: Managing dysphagia, *Clinicians Rev* 8(8):59, 1998; Rasley A et al: Prevention of barium aspiration during videofluoroscopic swallowing studies: value of change in posture, *Am J Roentgenol* 160:1005, 1993.

acid pump inhibitors, and, as a last resort, promotility agents. Educating the elder to eat less at one time and to drink only small quantities of fluid with meals will help prevent overdistention of the stomach. The diet eaten should be relatively dry. If the individual smokes, smoking cessation should be attempted. The head of the bed should be elevated 4 to 8 inches on blocks. The elder should sleep with a support or pillow placed so that the shoulders are elevated at least 30 degrees if raising the head of the bed is not feasible. Tight garments should be avoided and a weight loss program implemented for the elder who is overweight or obese.

Malnutrition

The occurrence of malnutrition among the elderly has been documented in both institutionalized and community-living elderly persons. Older adults in institutional settings are often among the most frail elders. The estimate of malnutrition for this group ranges from 10% to 85%, thus making malnutrition a serious problem for caregivers (Peters, 1998). The term *malnutrition* encompasses more than pathologic states that result from a deficiency of essential nutrients and calories. It also refers to significant deviations in dietary patterns that may produce undesirable risk factors. Researchers concur that the intake of vitamins and select minerals, as well as calories, is below minimum requirements for urban and rural community elders, as well as for institutionalized elders (Lipski et al, 1993; Payette, Gray-Donald, 1994; Gaspar, 1996; van der Wielen et al, 1996). The mean daily intake of protein; vitamins A, D, and E; folate; calcium; magnesium; and zinc is below recommended levels for over 50% of individuals. Besides the age changes creating a decline in taste and smell among the older group, Yen (1996) lists a number of disorders and factors affecting taste and smell, including Alzheimer's disease; Parkinson disease; chronic renal failure; upper respiratory tract infections; smoking; bronchial asthma; diabetes mellitus; certain medications; and deficiencies of zinc, niacin, and vitamin B_{12}.

Protein calorie malnutrition (PCM) is a commonly misdiagnosed disorder of the elderly. PCM is the inadequate intake of calories and protein because of a high-carbohydrate, low-protein diet (Gupta et al, 1988; Cape, 1990). Symptoms include weight loss; pallor; dry, flaky skin; and loss of muscle mass. Biochemical analysis reveals low serum albumin levels if the malnutrition has been long term. Otherwise, there is no evidence of hypoproteinemia. Elderly clients institutionalized for 2 weeks or more are at high risk for this nutritional problem. PCM also occurs in the presence of poor nutritional intake due to socioeconomic status, loss of dentition, gastrointestinal malabsorption, and functional disorders. Generally, the elder complains of fatigue, weakness, dyspnea on exertion, and pedal edema. All of these complaints could be attributed to anemia and congestive heart failure when in reality the symptoms may be due to PCM. If PCM occurs in the presence of congestive heart failure, one must be concerned with the possibility of digitalis toxicity. The symptoms of anorexia, nausea, and vomiting associated with digitalis toxicity are also precipitators of PCM. Because PCM may coexist with other disorders, it is important to have a medical evaluation and imperative that a complete nutritional history be included.

Aged persons who are at high nutritional risk include those who have psychosocial and mechanical difficulty. Wolanin (1976), Cape (1990), Garofalo and Hynak-Hankinson (1995), and Gaspar (1996) identify situations that potentiate malnutrition in the aged (Box 10-9). One need not be ill or hospitalized to have or develop one or more mechanical or psychosocial nutritional risk factors. Nutritional deficiencies, according to Roe (1992), develop from diets that are monotonous, destructive, low in energy, and low in the ratio of nutrients to calories. Medications are also a significant factor in the development of malnutrition, either by interfering with absorption or by causing the excretion of vitamins and minerals.

Box 10-9 FACTORS POTENTIATING MALNUTRITION IN THE AGED

Psychosocial Risk Factors

Limited income
Abuse of alcohol and other central nervous system depressants
Bereavement, loneliness, or living alone
Removal from usual cultural patterns
Confusion, forgetfulness, or disorientation
Working toward intentional or subintentional death

Mechanical Risk Factors

Decreased or limited strength and mobility
Neurologic deficits, arthritis, handicap, impairment of hand-arm coordination, loss of tongue strength, and dysphagia
Decreased or diminished vision or blindness
Inability to feed self
Decubitus ulcers
Loss of teeth, poor-fitting dentures, or chewing problems
Difficult breathing
Polypharmacy
Surgery, nothing by mouth (NPO) for extended periods of time, or intravenous therapy only

Assessment

A nutritional assessment that provides the most conclusive data about a person's actual nutritional state consists of four steps: interview, physical examination, anthropometric measurements, and biochemical analysis. The collective results can provide the nurse with data needed to identify the immediate and potential nutritional problems of the client. The nurse can then begin to establish plans for supervision, assistance, and education in the attainment of adequate nutrition for the aged person.

The American Nurses Association's position statement on nutritional screening for the elderly (1992) acknowledges the numerous risks for nutritional deficiencies that are encountered by some older persons. Routine nutritional screening and assessment of elderly individuals on admission into the health care system are supported. Nurses are also urged to collaborate with other professionals in all settings to promote nutritional screening for older adults.

Unless inadequate diet has become an obvious problem, an intensive nutritional assessment is infrequently done. Weight alone is an inaccurate measurement of nutritional status, since it does not indicate the adequacy of the diet. One can meet the correct weight value for height, but the weight may be a result of fluid retention, edema, or ascites. The adequacy of muscle mass and body fat are the two measurements that can provide accurate information about body nutrition but are usually not assessed.

The Nutrition Screening Initiative of 1991 developed nutritional screening materials to promote routine nutritional care in America's health care system. The elderly population was its initial focus in hopes of improving their nutritional state. A basic checklist was developed that has two elements: a self-assessment protocol to help identify specific eating habits and lifestyles that might put the elder at nutritional risk and advice to provide basic education concerning nutritional risk factors and to remind the public and professionals of these risk factors (Fig. 10-2). A level I and level II screening tool that is more detailed is used by the professional when nutritional risks are identified. The Nutrition Screening Initiative also presents an algorithm for nutritional assessment and approaches.

Keeping a dietary record for 3 days is another assessment tool. A careful recording of when one ate, what was eaten, and the amounts eaten must be made. This approach works when the elder is dependable and cooperative. Computer analysis of the dietary records provides information on energy and on vitamin and mineral intake. Printouts can provide the elderly and the health care provider with a visual graph of their intake.

Interview. The interview provides background information and clues to the nutritional state and actual and potential problems of the elderly person. Questions about the individual's state of health, social activities, normal patterns, and changes that have occurred should be asked. The nurse must explore the individual's needs, the manner in which food is obtained, and the client's ability to prepare food. Information concerning the relationship of food to daily events will provide clues to the meaning and significance of food to that person. The aged who eat alone are considered candidates for marginal malnutrition. Information about occupation and daily activities will suggest the degree of energy expenditure and caloric intake most correct for the overall activity. One's economic state will have a direct bearing on nutrition. It is therefore important to explore the client's financial resources to establish the income available for food. Knowledge of medications taken should be included in the nutrition history. Additional medical information should include the presence or absence of mouth pain or discomfort, visual difficulty, and bowel and bladder function. Food intake patterns should be explored.

Frequently a 24-hour diet recall compared with the Food Guide Pyramid can present an estimate of nutritional adequacy. When the aged person cannot provide all of the information requested, it may be possible to obtain data from a family member or another source. There will be times, however, when information will not be as complete as one would like, or the aged person, too proud to admit that he or she is not eating, will furnish erroneous information. The nurse will still be able to obtain additional data from the other three areas of the nutritional assessment.

Physical examination. The second step of the nutritional assessment, the physical examination, furnishes clinically observable evidence of the existing state of nutrition. Data such as height and weight; vital signs; condition of the tongue, lips, and gums; and skin turgor, texture, and color are assessed, and the general overall appearance is scrutinized for evidence of wasting.

Use of the body mass index (BMI) has been shown to be more accurate than the standard height and weight charts. Weight, however, is not the only issue; fat distribution needs to be considered. Dr. William Castelli, head of the Framingham Heart Study, suggests the use

The Warning Signs of poor nutritional health are often overlooked. Use this checklist to find out if you or someone you know is at nutritional risk.

DETERMINE YOUR NUTRITIONAL HEALTH

Read the statements below. Circle the number in the yes column for those that apply to you or someone you know. For each yes answer, score the number in the box. Total your nutritional score.

	YES
I have an illness or condition that made me change the kind and/or amount of food I eat.	2
I eat fewer than 2 meals per day.	3
I eat few fruits or vegetables, or milk products.	2
I have 3 or more drinks of beer, liquor or wine almost everyday.	2
I have tooth or mouth problems that make it hard for me to eat.	2
I don't always have enough money to buy the food I need.	4
I eat alone most of the time.	1
I take 3 or more different prescribed or over-the-counter drugs a day.	1
Without wanting to, I have lost or gained 10 pounds in the last 6 months.	2
I am not always physically able to shop, cook and/or feed myself.	2
TOTAL	

Total Your Nutritional Score. If it's—

0–2   **Good!** Recheck your nutritional score in 6 months.

3–5   **You are at moderate nutritional risk.** See what can be done to improve your eating habits and lifestyle. Your office on aging, senior nutrition program, senior citizens center or health department can help. Recheck your nutritional score in 3 months.

6 or more   **You are at high nutritional risk.** Bring this checklist the next time you see your doctor, dietitian or other qualified health or social service professional. Talk with them about any problems you may have. Ask for help to improve your nutritional health.

These materials developed and distributed by the Nutrition Screening Initiative, a project of:

AMERICAN ACADEMY OF FAMILY PHYSICIANS

THE AMERICAN DIETETIC ASSOCIATION

NATIONAL COUNCIL ON THE AGING, INC.

Remember that warning signs suggest risk, but do not represent diagnosis of any condition.

Fig. 10-2   Warning signs of poor nutrition. (From the Nutrition Screening Initiative, a project of the American Academy of Family Physicians, the American Dietetic Association, and the National Council on the Aging, Inc, and funded in part by a grant from Ross Products Division, Abbott Laboratories, Inc.)

of the hip-to-waist ratio. This indicates that fat stored above the waist is associated with hypertension and cholesterol levels. Weight lower on the body (pear-shaped body) is benign. A man's waist should not exceed the hips at its largest diameter, and a woman's waist should not exceed 80% of her hip diameter (Crowley, 1988).

Anthropometric measurements. Anthropometric measurements are the third part of the nutritional assessment. These measurements obtain information about the status of the aged person's muscle mass and body fat in relation to height and weight. In some instances an individual is bedridden or confined to a chair, or the individual has a spinal curvature preventing accurate height measurement.

Muscle mass measurements are obtained by measuring the arm circumference of the nondominant upper arm. Body fat is assessed by measuring specific skinfolds with Lange or Harpenden calipers. The most accurate site is immediately below the tip of the scapula. This area provides uniformity of the fat layer.

Biochemical examination. The final step in a nutritional assessment is the biochemical examination. This includes an analysis of the pH; the presence or absence of protein, glucose, and acetone in the urine; the blood levels of hemoglobin, total protein, serum albumin, and cholesterol; and the hematocrit value. Data directly related to the present nutritional state can be gathered and evaluated.

Based on the nurse's assessment, it may be necessary to refer the aged person to a nutritionist for a more intensive evaluation. The nurse in many instances should be able to educate the aged about their nutritional needs and how to effectively meet them.

Interventions

Interventions are formulated around the identified nutritional problem or problems. Perhaps the most significant intervention for the community elder is nutrition education and problem solving with the elder as to how to best resolve the potential or actual nutritional deficit.

Education in the area of reading nutritional information on labels is needed. The Food and Drug Administration (FDA) has required makers of processed foods to list nutritional information based on daily values. Daily values represent the amount of nutrients and fiber that is desirable in daily diets of 2000 to 2500 calories. The nutrients were chosen based on evidence suggesting that eating too much or too little of these substances has the greatest impact on your health. The FDA defines a "good source" as a food that contains 10% to 19% of the daily value per serving. The daily totals for fat, cholesterol, and sodium need to be less than 100%. An emphasis on balance as the key to a healthful diet needs to be promoted (Daily Values, 1995). The addition of liquid supplements to the diet is valuable, if this is used as a supplement and not as a meal replacement. The most economical, least expensive supplement is Carnation Instant Breakfast, which provides both calories and nutrients (Peters, 1998).

Practical suggestions for increasing intake when an older person is experiencing a poor appetite were presented by Yen (1994). Suggestions include the following:
- Add nonfat dry milk powder to just about anything with liquid in it.
- Make nourishments part of routine care.
- Offer the most food when the patient is most hungry (usually morning).
- Emphasize taste and eye appeal.
- Offer finger foods.
- Add some fat—margarine—to vegetables, creamed foods and sauces, and cooked cereal.
- Use fortified milk.
- Conduct calorie counts, because they serve as a useful indicator that progress is being made and show foods that are tolerated.

It is important for those elders institutionalized in acute or long-term care facilities to receive appropriate supervision at mealtime so that they are able to eat their food, have their dentures in place and eyeglasses on, have their food cut for them, if necessary, and have any other requirements met that will enable them to meet their nutritional intake needs. It is also important to provide the elder with some degree of social interaction during mealtime. Table 10-2 provides age-related changes, outcomes, and interventions for the gastrointestinal system that directly or indirectly affect nutrition and elimination.

Improving the nutritional status of malnourished older adults in the community and institutional settings decreases dependence, recuperation time, and the burden on health care resources.

ETHICS OF NUTRITION

Feeding, intentional starvation, fads, and megavitamins are ethical issues to be addressed in nutrition of the older adult.

Feeding the Impaired Aged

It is not uncommon in long-term care facilities to hear over the public address system at mealtime, "Feeder trays are ready." This reference to the need to feed those unable to feed themselves is, in itself, degrading and erases any trace of dignity the aged person is trying to maintain in a controlled environment. It is not malicious intent by nurses or other caregivers but, rather, a habit of convenience. Feeding the aged who

Table 10-2

Age-Related Gastrointestinal Changes; Outcomes; and Health Prevention, Promotion, and Maintenance Approaches

Age-related changes	Outcomes	Health prevention, promotion, and maintenance
Decreased acuity of taste	Dry mouth	Take in adequate high fiber in diet
Decreased saliva production with increased alkalinity	Diminished taste	Adequate exercise
Brittle teeth/retracted gingiva	Pale gums	Bowel training
Less effective chewing	Vermilion border of mouth missing	No or little use of laxative
Decreased esophageal and intestinal motility	Atrophy of gums with loss of teeth or decay	Good oral care
Decrease in gastric secretions	Difficulty chewing	Suck on ice chips or hard candy
Loss of elasticity in intestinal wall	Decreased appetite	Hold cold water in mouth before swallowing
Decreased blood flow to intestines	Thirst	Use sodium-free flavorings
Reduced blood flow to liver	Coughing or choking	Consult dentist once or twice a year
Loss of or diminished anal sphincter control	Dysphagia	Use soft-bristled toothbrush and dental floss
Weaker neural impulses to lower bowel	Nausea/vomiting	For dentures, brush to clean between teeth
	Heartburn/indigestion	Cut food into small pieces; chew thoroughly
	Diarrhea	Have abdominal pain evaluated
	Constipation	Increase dietary fiber, fluids, and exercise
	Fecal impaction	Have a regular meal pattern
	Malnutrition	Respond promptly to the urge to defecate
	Drug toxicity	Report any change in bowel routine
		Manage diet within budget
		Utilize Meals on Wheels if needed
		Use dietary supplements
		Recognize signs of drug toxicity for drugs taken
Taste		
Fewer taste buds	Food tastes bland	Encourage social dining
	Overseasons food	Nutritional supplementation
		Use herbs for seasoning, lemon, spices (nonsalty)

do not respond intelligibly becomes mechanical and devoid of conversation and feeling. The feeding process becomes rapid, and if it bogs down and becomes too slow, the meal may be ended abruptly, depending on the time the caregiver has allotted for feeding the patient. Any pleasure that could be derived through socialization and eating is destroyed, as is any dignity that could be maintained by the elder while being dependent on others for food. Individuals who require feeding should be given food slowly and allowed to completely swallow the bite before more food is offered. The ability to swallow is more difficult and slower when food is rapidly placed in the mouth. Shoveling food into one's mouth is a precursor to a disaster such as choking or aspiration.

Food should be given with variety throughout the meal (i.e., serve a bite of one item, then another, and so forth). Not only does this eliminate the monotony of

eating all of one food before being given another, but it also changes the texture as one eats, enhancing eating enjoyment. Small, frequent servings of food should be offered when an elder needs encouragement to eat; smaller amounts of food may be better tolerated. Nutritional intake can be effectively increased in elders with severe cognitive dysfunction by means of touch, verbal cueing, and a combination of touch and verbal cueing (Lange-Alberts, Shott, 1994).

Adequate nutrition for the helpless aged depends on the conscientiousness of the individual doing the feeding. It is the nurse's responsibility to ensure that all patients unable to feed themselves not only receive a tray but also are actually fed the food that has been brought to them. Any time a patient has not eaten a meal or has refused as few as three consecutive meals, it is essential that a nutritional assessment be done to prevent malnutrition and its complications.

In the acute care hospital setting it is equally important to give consideration, care, and attention to the feeding of the dependent aged patient. Sufficient time should be provided to accommodate the aged person who has a slow eating pace or who has undiagnosed dysphagia.

Intentional Starvation

Refusal of food can be an acceptable means of suicide for the aged person. Some aged persons truly have given up and wish to die. Not eating is one last bastion of control over life and dignity. It is essential for the nurse to differentiate between the individual who is refusing food because it is unpalatable and the person who is depressed and really wishes to die.

Intentional starvation is easier and more successful when one is not institutionalized. The institutionalized person is often denied this right and is robbed of the option by forced feeding via a nasogastric tube. The American Nurses Association's position statement on forgoing artificial nutrition and hydration (1992) states: "The decision to withhold artificial nutrition and hydration should be made by the patient or surrogate with the health care team. The nurse continues to provide expert care to patients who are no longer receiving artificial nutrition and hydration."

Watching someone starve is difficult for the nurse, but if intentional starvation is the patient's desire, the nurse should continue to order the tray, take it to the person, and acknowledge that the individual has the right to eat or not eat. It is important to leave the tray so that the person can exercise the option to change his or her mind. If the person is unable to feed himself or herself, the nurse should check shortly after the first offering of food has been refused to see if the person does wish to eat. An empathetic and nonjudgmental approach by the nurse to the aged person who demonstrates starvation behavior will convey that the individual is still in control, and if for some reason the individual decides to exercise the option to eat again, that, too, is all right. Either way, the caregiver has provided support and respect for that individual. Professional team conferences are needed to deal with the client's mental status and ethical issues involved in refusal to eat and the right to die. Superficial judgments are not adequate to encompass these profound issues.

Food Fads

Aged individuals are not immune to food faddism and fall prey to advertisements that claim that specific foods maintain youth and vitality or rid one of chronic conditions. Fad foods are often more costly than a balanced diet and can sometimes be obtained only in health food stores or by mail order. Even if the food is easily obtained in a supermarket, such large quantities may be called for that some nutrients are obtained in excess whereas others are excluded.

Megavitamin therapy, or the ingestion of large amounts of a specific vitamin or many different vitamins, can also be considered a fad. Unless the individual is severely depleted of vitamins, which can usually be obtained in an adequate diet, megavitamin therapy is nonessential and dangerous. Risks exist in megavitamin therapy: bone meal, a source of calcium, may contain lead and thus cause lead poisoning; high doses of zinc cause zinc toxicity; and kelp, with its high iodine content, can cause goiter in those with preexisting thyroid enlargement. High intake of niacin is discouraged because of a high incidence of cardiac dysrhythmias, abnormal biochemical findings, and gastrointestinal problems. Intake of vitamin D has the potential for toxicity, and vitamins C and E have insufficient data to warrant recommendation now (Roe, 1992). The money spent on food fads and unneeded vitamins by the aged could buy more economical foods that benefit the individual's health. Megavitamin therapy has a role in maintaining nutrition when illness, malnutrition, or excessive demands are placed on body function.

Recently attention has been directed toward the lowering of cholesterol in the diet. A soy-containing diet, fatty fish (salmon, herring, mackerel, and anchovies) in the diet at least four times a week, and other low-fat diets have been found to decrease total cholesterol and LDL measurements (Anderson et al, 1995; Siscovick et al, 1995). Fat substitutes such as Olestra are currently appearing in the nation's food stores, but they are fraught with problems, among which are the depletion of fat-soluble vitamins, including A, D, E, and K, and a reduction of blood carotenoid levels (even though the substitutes may be fortified with the vitamins to make up for the depletion). Some individuals have noted diarrhea and/or abdominal cramping, as well as rectal leakage, after eating several ounces of food containing the fat substitute. The evidence for potentially adverse effects from the use of the fat substitutes is overwhelming, and the elderly need to be cautioned about their use of foods containing this substance. The FDA is requiring additional studies (Olestra: Just Say No, 1996).

Fast foods have become a stable part of the American diet. In a survey of older Americans who attend senior centers in two states, 6% in one state and 11% in the other state reported that they ate at a fast food restaurant once a week. They usually did not eat their main meal there. Elders also frequented fast food restaurants so that they would not have to cook. They visited fast food restaurants for discounts and low food costs because economics were important. Social reasons for frequenting fast food establishments were also cited (Morris et al, 1995).

Snack foods constitute a substantial component of the American diet. Cross et al (1995) evaluated snacking behavior among 335 noninstitutionalized older adults. They found that the majority of seniors snacked at least once daily, with only 2.1% reporting that they never snacked. Evening was the most common time for snacking, with the reported foods most often being salty/crunchy foods. When snacks were selected, taste outranked nutrition as a selection criterion.

BOWEL FUNCTION

Attention to bowel function occurs when there is a deviation from what is perceived as normal elimination. The aged are known for their concern with their bowel function and frequently complain to physicians and other health care personnel about problems, particularly constipation. Whatever the complaint, one needs to know exactly what the individual means when he or she says there is a problem.

Although bowel function of the aged normally is only slightly altered by physiologic changes of age, problems can develop that are severe enough to interfere with the ability to continue independent living and seriously threaten the body's capacity to function and survive. The major problem that the nurse will encounter among aged clients is constipation, which if not dealt with proactively, can lead to fecal impaction and fecal or bowel incontinence.

Constipation

The term *constipation* has different meanings to different people. Some individuals consider constipation to be infrequent bowel action; others perceive it as difficulty in passing feces; and others consider both of these problems to be indicative of constipation. To the health professional, constipation occurs when there are fewer than three bowel movements per week (Rousseau, 1990).

Evacuation of feces is accomplished by relaxation of the sphincters and contraction of the diaphragm and abdominal muscles, which raises intraabdominal pressure. When one strains at stool, pressure is elevated in the colon, which causes the formation of pouches, or diverticula, in the colon wall. Increased intraabdominal pressure pushes the stomach against and through the diaphragm, creating hiatal hernias. Downward pressure is transmitted to veins and can cause varicose veins and hemorrhoids.

Constipation appears to be a problem of the old because they use more laxatives than the young and because the advertisements are overwhelmingly directed toward the aged (Rousseau, 1990). It is perhaps more correct to consider the extensive use of laxatives by the aged as a cultural habit. During their formative years, weekly doses of rhubarb, cascara, castor oil, and other types of laxatives were consumed to promote health. This belief that cleaning out the colon is paramount to maintaining good health persists with many of the elderly.

Constipation is a symptom. It is a reflection of poor habits, postponed passage of stool, and a misunderstanding of the real definition of constipation. Most people believe that an individual must have a bowel movement daily, when in fact normal bowel function for 98% of the population varies from three movements daily to only three per week (Harari et al, 1993). There are numerous precipitating factors for constipation, which can be categorized as physiologic, functional, mechanical, psychologic, systemic, pharmacologic, and other. A list of these factors is provided in Table 10-3.

Diet has been shown to play a significant role in problems with intestinal motility and constipation. Some authorities believe that delayed passage of stool facilitates the action of carcinogenic chemical buildup caused by bacteria in the bowel, permitting higher concentrations of these chemicals to remain in contact with the colon wall for longer periods (Burkitt, 1982; Brocklehurst, 1986). However, it has been suggested that constipation in elders might be related to loss of colonic cells that determine water content of stool.

Assessment

The precipitating factors of constipation (see Table 10-3) need to be included in the assessment of the client to shed light on the possible cause or causes of altered bowel function. A review of these factors will also determine if a client is at risk for altered bowel function. It is recognized that the elderly at high risk for constipation and subsequent impaction are the aged who have hypotonic colon function, who are immobilized and debilitated, or who have central nervous system lesions. Specific questions for initial assessment of constipation with the rationale for obtaining the assessment data appear in Box 10-10. A review of food and fluid intake may be necessary to determine the amount of fiber and fluid ingested. It is also important to remember that confusion, increased agitation, incontinence, and elevated temperature and/or unexplainable falls may be the only presenting clinical symptoms of constipation in the elderly (Allison et al, 1994).

A physical examination is needed to assess conditions such as dry skin and poor skin turgor, decubitus ulcer, abdominal distention, masses, bowel sounds, flatus, and mobility. Light palpation of the abdomen can detect tenderness and muscular resistance associated with chronic constipation (Allison et al, 1994).

A rectal examination is important to reveal painful anal disorders, such as hemorrhoids or fissures, that will impede the evacuation of stool and to evaluate sphincter tone. Biochemical tests should include calcium and potassium levels, a complete blood count, and thyroid studies.

Interventions

Nonpharmacologic interventions. Nonpharmacologic interventions for constipation that have been implemented and evaluated can be grouped into four areas: (1) fluid/fiber, (2) exercise, (3) environmental manipulation, and (4) a combination of the first three areas.

ADEQUATE FIBER. Fiber is an important dietary component that facilitates regular bowel function. Some aged persons do not consume sufficient quantities of daily fiber to maintain normal bowel evacuation. Fiber, the undigestible material that gives plants their structure, is abundant in raw fruits and vegetables and in unrefined grains and cereals.

Fiber facilitates the absorption of water, increases bulk, and improves intestinal motility. It prevents constipation, hemorrhoids, and diverticulosis. Fiber also helps reduce caloric intake, aids in the control of obesity, and is thought to play a role in the prevention of "diseases of civilization" such as heart disease and colon cancer. Various types of fiber exist, but all possess the common characteristic of indigestibility. Individuals who can chew foods well could benefit from eating increased amounts of fresh fruits and vegetables daily or combining unsweetened bran with other types of food. Those who have difficulty chewing could sprinkle

---

Table 10-3

Precipitating Factors for Constipation

PHYSIOLOGIC	PSYCHOLOGIC
Dehydration	Avoidance of urge to defecate
Insufficient fiber intake	Confusion
Poor dietary habits	Depression
	Emotional stress

FUNCTIONAL	SYSTEMIC
Decreased physical activity	Diabetes mellitus
Inadequate toileting	Hypercalcemia
Irregular defecation habits	Hyperparathyroidism
Irritable bowel disease	Hypothyroidism
Weakness	Hypokalemia
	Pheochromocytoma
	Porphyria
	Uremia

MECHANICAL	PHARMACOLOGIC
Abscess or ulcer	Aluminum-containing antacids
Cerebrovascular disease	Anticholinergics
Defective electrolyte transfer	Anticonvulsants
Fissures	Antidepressants
Hemorrhoids	Bismuth salts
Hirschsprung's disease	Calcium carbonate
Neurological disease	Calcium channel blockers
Parkinson's disease	Diuretics
Postsurgical obstruction	Laxative overuse
Prostate enlargement	Iron salts
Rectal prolapse	Nonsteroidal antiinflammatories
Rectocele	Opiates
Spinal cord injury	Phenothiazines
Strictures	Sedatives
Tumors	Sympathomimetics

OTHER	
Lack of abdominal muscle tone	Obesity
Recent environmental changes	Poor dentition

From Allison OC, Porter ME, Briggs GG: Chronic constipation: assessment and management in the elderly, *J Am Acad Nurse Pract* 6(7):311, 1994.

Box 10-10   CONSTIPATION ASSESSMENT QUESTIONS AND RATIONALE

Question	Rationale
When did constipation begin?	Lifelong history of constipation is likely to be a functional disorder; sudden change may be an organic lesion, such as carcinoma.
Has anything in bowel function recently changed?	A sudden change even in constipation may signal an underlying disorder.
How often do bowel movements occur?	Frequency of defecation may actually be normal. The question may also unknowingly let clients describe their cathartic use.
Is the urge to defecate lacking or the stool difficult to expel?	Absent urge may indicate chronic suppression of normal function or neurologic disorder. Difficult passage of stool may be due to fiber or fluid deficit, medication use, or thyroid disorder.
Is pain associated with defecation?	Pain implies fecal impaction of rectum, anorectal fissures, or intestinal obstruction.
Is blood evident in bowel movement?	Witnessed, usually is hemorrhoid bleeding, tear, or fissure.
What medications are taken, including over-the-counter drugs?	Multiple drugs are capable of causing constipation.

Modified from Rousseau P: Aging and chronic constipation, *Geriatr Med Today* 9(3):35, 1990.

unsweetened bran on cereals or in soups, meat loaf, or casseroles. The quantity of bran used depends on the individual, but generally 1 to 2 tablespoons daily is sufficient to facilitate intestinal motility. Individuals who have not used bran should begin with 1 teaspoon and progressively increase the quantity until the fiber intake is enough to accomplish its purpose. Otherwise, bloating, gas, diarrhea, and other colon discomforts will initially occur and discourage further use of this important dietary ingredient.

Cooked dried beans are a good source of fiber. Pinto beans, split peas, red beans, and peanuts can be served in casseroles, soups, and dips. These are all relatively inexpensive and nutritious in addition to having high fiber content.

Wichita (1977) and Rodrigues-Fisher et al (1993) noted that prevention and correction of constipation could be obtained in nursing home residents if the residents ate two slices of whole-wheat bread daily and had 2 teaspoons of bran in their diet every day; the use of fiber and fluids resulted in bowel maintenance without the use of pharmacologic elimination aids in long-term care residents. Wheat and bran, and fiber and fluids are capable of increasing stool weight and transit time through the colon. Kovach (1992) promotes the use of bran fiber rather than fruit and vegetable fiber, since bran fiber will not degrade as readily in the intestinal tract. Bran fiber results in a functioning colon

with higher fecal bulking action and less constipation. Yet Kovach suggests that fruit and vegetable fiber are still important, because the products of their degradation could be essential for other physiologic and metabolic actions.

Gibson et al (1995) found that the use of the "standard recipe" of prune juice, applesauce, and bran was effective in decreasing the use of laxatives among elderly rehabilitation patients. The researchers caution that the mixture is not effective for everyone and that monitoring is essential. The recipe is used routinely in numerous long-term care facilities. Other dietary interventions have also been implemented. A mixture of dried fruit was found by Beverly and Travis (1992) to be a cost-effective alternative to laxative use, saving an estimated $4500 per year. It was well accepted by the elderly in a long-term care facility and was considered easy to administer. A "power pudding" similar to the standard recipe with the addition of whipped topping was reported to be effective and very acceptable in a group of homebound elderly (Neal, 1995). A selected list of recipes is presented in Box 10-11.

Besides the addition of bran to the diet, other dietary adjuncts have been found to be effective by individuals in promoting bowel elimination. These dietary adjuncts include prunes, rhubarb, apples, oranges, bananas, carrots, cabbage, greens, potatoes with the skin, oatmeal,

Box 10-11 NATURAL LAXATIVE RECIPES

Fruit Spread*

2 lbs raisins
2 lbs currants
2 lbs prunes
2 lbs figs
2 lbs dates
2 containers (28 oz each) undiluted prune concentrate

Put fruit through a grinder. Mix with prune concentrate in large mixer (mixture will be very thick). Store in large-mouthed plastic container. Refrigerate. Any dried fruit can be added.

Power Pudding†

$1/2$ cup prune juice
$1/2$ cup applesauce
$1/2$ cup wheat bran flakes
$1/2$ cup whipped topping
$1/2$ cup prunes (canned stewed)
(Diabetics may use "no added sugar" applesauce and "light" whipped topping.)

Blend ingredients, cover, and refrigerate, and keep as long as 1 week. Take $1/4$ cup portions of recipe with breakfast. Regulate dose as needed.

Standard Recipe

1 cup bran
1 cup applesauce
1 cup prune juice

Mix and store in refrigerator. Start with administration of 1 oz per day. Increase or decrease dosage as needed.

*Data from Beverley L, Travis I: Constipation: proposed natural laxative mixtures, *J Gerontol Nurs* 18(10):5, 1992.
†Data from Neal LJ: "Power pudding": natural laxative therapy for the elderly who are homebound, *Home Health Nurse* 13(3):66, 1995.

whole-grain cereals, and seeds (sunflower and sesame). Those with poor dentition can benefit from the same food if it is chopped, not pureed, and by soup with extra chopped vegetables added. Persons with swallowing difficulties need foods that are mashed, not pureed, and additional liquids. The acceptance, tolerance, and effectiveness of these dietary adjuncts need to be considered on an individual basis.

Increasing fiber intake has been found to be effective for prevention and management of bowel elimination problems. Yet the specific amount and type of fiber used in the intervention studies have varied.

One other dietary consideration besides fiber is senna tea. It is a good laxative that has a local action that increases colon peristalsis. Senna tea is slightly absorbed systemically and is effective in small doses. A cup taken in the morning and in the evening is sufficient. Taken in the evening with a bran muffin, raisin whole-wheat cookies, or a piece of whole-wheat toast, it will naturally facilitate regularity (Pearson and Kotthoff, 1979). Senna tea is nontoxic unless it is used in a manner that produces prolonged overdose.

EXERCISE. Exercise is important as an intervention to stimulate colon motility and bowel evacuation. Daily walking, pelvic tilt exercises, and range-of-motion (passive or active) exercises are beneficial for those who are less mobile. Exercise and abdominal massage were used as an intervention and shown by Resende et al (1993) to be effective for immobile patients to prevent and relieve constipation.

ENVIRONMENTAL MANIPULATION. Simple environmental manipulation can facilitate solving the problem of constipation. Sometimes placing the feet on a footstool puts the colon in the normal anatomic position for passing stool, a position closer to a squat. This may ease the evacuation if there is difficulty and straining. Clients should be encouraged to establish a regular bowel routine that includes attempting defecation after the morning meal. The gastrocolic reflex, the mass propulsion of material through the large intestines that occurs after a meal, is strongest after the morning meal. Adequate time and privacy need to be provided to promote a relaxing environment.

• • •

The combination of these approaches (dietary, exercise, and environmental modifications) has been found to be effective. Hall et al (1995) established a protocol intervention for constipation that included fiber, fluids, exercise (including abdominal exercises), and hygiene measures. The researchers evaluated the protocol over a 3-year period in a group of hospitalized immobile vascular surgery patients and found that the incidence of constipation was reduced from 59% to about 9% and the incidence of impaction was eliminated. A program to prevent, as well as treat, constipation that incorporates these approaches to promote a regular pattern of bowel elimination needs to be developed for each client. The interventions for clients in any setting are based on a thorough assessment.

Pharmacologic interventions. Pharmacologic measures can be instituted if nonpharmacologic measures have been tried and have failed. The least aggressive therapy needs to be used first. The bulk-forming agents are generally tried first because they are the most physiologic. An adequate intake of fluids is necessary with the use of bulk-forming agents. Stool softeners need to be used if the patient is having hard, pelletlike stools or if straining needs to be avoided. Saline or osmotic laxatives are recommended if the aforementioned agents are not effective. The stimulant or irritant agents are recommended for occasional use only. Long-term use of these agents can result in the risk of electrolyte disturbances and damage to the colon (Allison et al, 1994).

Fecal Impaction

Anyone can experience fecal impaction, but it is especially common in the incapacitated and institutionalized elderly. The causes are similar to constipation. Unrecognized, unattended, or neglected constipation eventually leads to fecal impaction and incontinence or paradoxic diarrhea, which results from a ball-valve effect that allows liquid stool to seep around the obstructing fecal mass during normal colon contractions. Removal of a fecal impaction is at times worse than the misery of the condition. Box 10-12 lists the causes and complications of fecal impaction.

Interventions

Management of fecal impactions requires the digital removal of the hard, compacted stool from the rectum after application of an anesthetic and lubrication with lidocaine jelly. Generally this is preceded by multiple enemas or an oil retention enema to soften the feces in preparation for manual removal. Use of suppositories is not effective, since their action is blocked by the amount and the size of the stool in the rectum compared with the capacity of the sphincter to dilate; nor do suppositories facilitate removal of stool in the sigmoid, which may continue to ooze once the rectum is emptied.

Several sessions or days may be required to totally cleanse the sigmoid colon and rectum of impacted feces. Once this is achieved, attention should be directed to planning a regimen that includes adequate fluid intake of at least 2 L or more per day, increased dietary fiber in the form of unsweetened bran, fresh fruits and vegetables with the skins, administration of stool softeners, and many of the suggestions presented for prevention of constipation. The provision of privacy and time to attend to defecation without feeling rushed will also facilitate easy and regular bowel function. Age-related changes of the gastrointestinal system create numerous problems. Table 10-3 should help the nurse identify the changes so that interventions can be planned for health promotion and maintenance, as well as illness prevention.

Box 10-12	COMMON CAUSES AND COMPLICATIONS OF FECAL IMPACTION

Causes
Medications
Diet
Lack of mobility
Illness
Habits

Complications
Fecal incontinence
Large bowel obstruction
Ischemic necrosis of colon wall (stercoral ulcer)

Modified from Wrenn K: Fecal impaction, *N Engl J Med* 321(10):658, 1989.

▶ KEY CONCEPTS

- Interruption of basic required nutrients may trigger subclinical or chronic disorders.
- Recommended dietary patterns for the aged are similar to those of younger persons, with some reduction in caloric intake based on decreased metabolic requirements.
- Adequate nutrition is affected by lifelong eating habits and patterns, accessibility of food, mood disorders, capacity for food preparation, and income.
- Medications may interfere with absorption, digestion, and elimination.
- Making mealtime pleasant and attractive for the aged who are unable to eat unassisted is a nursing challenge; mealtime *must* be made enjoyable.

NANDA and Wellness Diagnoses

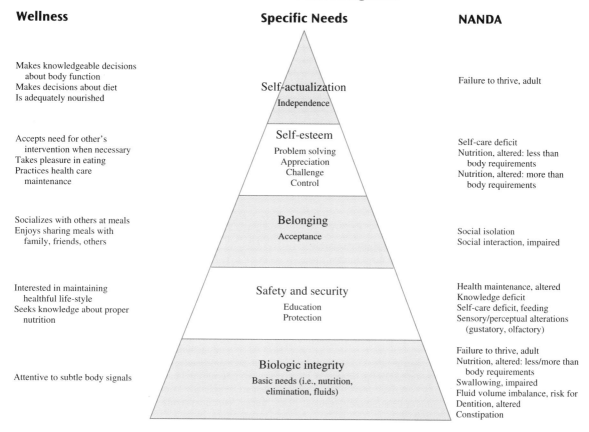

Wellness

Makes knowledgeable decisions
  about body function
Makes decisions about diet
Is adequately nourished

Accepts need for other's
  intervention when necessary
Takes pleasure in eating
Practices health care
  maintenance

Socializes with others at meals
Enjoys sharing meals with
  family, friends, others

Interested in maintaining
  healthful life-style
Seeks knowledge about proper
  nutrition

Attentive to subtle body signals

Specific Needs

Self-actualization
Independence

Self-esteem
Problem solving
Appreciation
Challenge
Control

Belonging
Acceptance

Safety and security
Education
Protection

Biologic integrity
Basic needs (i.e., nutrition,
elimination, fluids)

NANDA

Failure to thrive, adult

Self-care deficit
Nutrition, altered: less than
  body requirements
Nutrition, altered: more than
  body requirements

Social isolation
Social interaction, impaired

Health maintenance, altered
Knowledge deficit
Self-care deficit, feeding
Sensory/perceptual alterations
  (gustatory, olfactory)

Failure to thrive, adult
Nutrition, altered: less/more than
  body requirements
Swallowing, impaired
Fluid volume imbalance, risk for
Dentition, altered
Constipation

These are not all of the possible wellness or NANDA diagnoses that may be identified. The above are frequent examples of nursing diagnoses that should be considered when planning care for the older adult in whatever setting.

► Activities and Discussion Questions

1. What are the factors affecting the nutrition of the aged?
2. How can the nurse intervene to provide better nutrition for elders in the community, in acute care, and in long-term care settings?
3. What are the causes of malnutrition?
4. How would one assess malnutrition?
5. Define constipation.
6. List the causes and complications of constipation.
7. What proactive measures can the nurse take to prevent elders in the community, in acute care, and in long-term care settings from becoming constipated or developing a fecal impaction?
8. Develop a nursing care plan using wellness and NANDA diagnoses.

RESOURCES

National Dairy Council (Dairy and Nutrition Council)
  6300 N. River Road
  Rosemont, IL 60018-4233
      To Your Health . . . In Your Second Fifty Years
      For Mature Eaters Only: Guidelines for Good Nutrition
      Sticks and Stones Can Break Your Bones . . . and So Will
          Too Little Calcium
      The All American Guide to Calcium Rich Foods
American Association of Retired Persons (AARP)
  Health Advocacy Services (HAS)
  601 E Street NW
  Washington, DC 20049

REFERENCES

Allison OC, Porter ME, Briggs GC: Chronic constipation: assessment and management in the elderly, *J Am Acad Nurse Pract* 6(7):311, 1994.

American Nurses Association : *Position statement on forgoing artificial nutrition and hydration,* Washington, DC, 1992, The Association.

American Nurses Association: *Position statement on nutrition screening for the elderly,* Washington, DC, 1992, The Association.

Anderson JW, Johnstone BM, Cook-Newell ME: Meta-analysis of the effects of soy protein intake on serum lipids, *N Engl J Med* 333(5):276, 1995.

Beverly L, Travis I: Constipation: proposed natural laxative mixtures, *J Gerontol Nurs* 18(10):5, 1992.

Brocklehurst JC: Incontinence. In Ham RJ, editor: *Geriatric medical annals,* Ordell, NJ, 1986, Medical Economics Books.

Burkitt D: Dietary fiber: is it really helpful? *Geriatrics* 37:119, 1982.

Cape RDT: Obesity. In Abrams WB, Berkow R, editors: *The Merck manual of geriatrics,* Rahway, NJ, 1990, Merck Sharpe & Dohme Research Laboratories.

Cross AT, Babicz D, Cushman LF: Snacking habits of senior Americans, *J Nutr Elderly* 14(2/3):27, 1995.

Corwin J, Loury M, Gilbert AN: Workplace, age, and sex as mediators of olfactory function: data from National Geographic smell survey, *J Gerontol* 50B(4):P179, 1995.

Crowley S: Experts weigh heft vs health, *AARP Bull* 29:8, Sept 1988.

Daily Values, *Mayo Clin Health Lett* 13(4):6, 1995.

Feldman RS: Update on geriatric dentistry, *University of Pennsylvania Center for the Study of Aging Newsletter* 10:7, 1986.

Garofalo JA, Hynak-Hankinson MT: New Jersey's Nutrition Screening Initiative: activities and results, *J Am Diet Assoc* 95(12):1422-1424, 1995.

Gaspar PM: *Nutritional intake of nursing home residents and minimum data set variables.* Presentation at the ANA Council for Nursing Research Science Session, Washington, DC, 1996.

Gibson CJ et al: Effectiveness of bran supplement on the bowel management of elderly rehabilitation patients, *J Gerontol Nurs* 21(10):21, 1995.

Gupta K, Dworkin B, Gambert SR: Common nutritional disorders in the elderly: atypical manifestations, *Geriatr Nurs* 43:87, 1988.

Gurgoz Y, Vella B, Garry PJ: Mini-Nutritional Assessment: a practical assessment tool for grading the nutritional state of elderly patients, *Facts Res Gerontol* (suppl nutrition):15, 1994.

Hall GR et al: Managing constipation using a research-based protocol, *MedSurg Nurs* 4(1):11, 1995.

Harari D, Gurwitz J, Minaker K: Constipation in the elderly, *J Am Geriatr Soc* 41(10):130, 1993.

Kayser-Jones J et al: An instrument to assess the oral health status of nursing home residents, *Gerontologist* 35(6), 1995.

Kovach T: Managing geriatric chronic constipation, *Home Healthc Nurse* 10(5):57, 1992.

Krebs-Smith SM et al: Psychosocial factors associated with fruit and vegetable consumption, *Am J Health Promotion* 10(2):98, 1995.

Lange-Alberts ME, Shott S: Nutritional intake: use of touch and verbal cueing, *J Gerontol Nurs* 20(2):36, 1994.

Lipski PS et al: A study of nutritional deficits of long-stay geriatric patients, *Age Ageing* 220:244, 1993.

Morris B, Schnelders D, Macey S: A survey of older Americans to determine frequency and motivation for eating fast food, *J Nutr Elderly* 15(1):1, 1995.

Neal LJ: Power pudding: natural laxative therapy for the elderly who are homebound, *Home Healthc Nurse* 13(3):66, 1995.

Nutrition Screening Initiative, Project of American Academy of Family Physicians, American Dietetic Association, and National Council on Aging, Inc. Grant from Ross-Abbott Laboratories, Inc., 1991.

Olestra: just say no, *Wellness Letter* 12(5):1, 1996, University of California at Berkeley.

Payette H, Gray-Donald K: Risk of malnutrition in an elderly population receiving home care services, *Facts and Research in Gerontology (Supplement: Nutrition):* 71, 1994.

Pearson LJ, Kotthoff ME: *Geriatric clinical protocol,* Philadelphia, 1979, Lippincott.

Peters S: Helping older adults meet their unique nutrient needs, *Adv Nurse Pract* 6(8):66, 1998.

Pyle MA et al: A pilot study on improving oral care in long-term care settings, *J Gerontol Nurs* 24(10):35, 1998.

Resende TL, Brochlehurst JC, O'Neill PA: A pilot study on the effect of exercise and abdominal massage on bowel habit in continuing care patients, *Clin Rehabil* 7(3):204, 1993.

Rodrigues-Fisher L, Bourguigon C, Good BV: Dietary fiber nursing interventions: prevention of constipation in older adults, *Clin Nurs Res* 2(4): 464, 1993.

Roe D: *Geriatric nutrition,* Englewood Cliffs, NJ, 1992, Prentice-Hall.

Rounds MC, Papas AS: Preventive dentistry for the older adult. In Papas AS, Niessen LC, Chauncey HH, editors: *Geriatric dentistry: aging and oral health,* St Louis, 1991, Mosby.

Rousseau P: Aging and chronic constipation, *Geriatr Med Today* 9(3):35, 1990.

Shifflett PA: Future time perspective, past experience and negotiation of food use patterns among the elderly, *Gerontologist* 27:611, 1987.

Siscovick DS et al: Dietary intake and cell membrane level of long chain n-3 polyunsaturated fatty acids and the risk of primary cardiac arrest, *JAMA* 274(17):1363, 1995.

US Department of Health and Human Services, Public Health Service, Centers for Disease Control and Prevention: *Healthy people 2003: review 1994,* DHHS Pub No (PHS) 95-1256-1, Hyattsville, Md, 1995, US Government Printing Office.

van der Wielen RPJ et al: Dietary intake of energy and water-soluble vitamins in different categories of aging, *J Gertontol* 51A(1):B100, 1996.

Whitmyer CC et al: Clinical evaluation of the efficacy and safety of an ultrasonic toothbrush system in an elderly patient population, *Geriatr Nurse* 19(1):29, 1998.

Wichita C: Treating and preventing constipation in nursing home residents, *J Gerontol Nurs* 3:35, 1977.

Wilson WR: Nose and throat disorders. In Abrams WB, Beers MH, Berkow R, editors: *The Merck manual of geriatrics,* ed 2, Whitehouse Station, NJ, 1995, Merck Research Laboratories.

Wolanin MO: Nursing assessment. In Burnside IM, editor: *Nursing and the aged,* New York, 1976, McGraw-Hill.

Yen P: Boosting intake when appetite is poor, *Geriatr Nurse* 15:284, 1994.

Yen P: When food doesn't taste good anymore, *Geriatr Nurse* 17(1):44, 1996.

chapter 11
Fluids and Continence in the Aged

▶LEARNING OBJECTIVES

Upon completion of this chapter, the reader will be able to:

- Identify some manifestations of inadequate fluid intake.
- Discuss interventions to prevent or treat dehydration.
- Define *urinary* and *fecal incontinence.*
- List factors contributing to urinary and fecal incontinence.
- Explain the types of urinary incontinence and their cause.
- Discuss interventions for urinary and fecal incontinence.

▶GLOSSARY

Detrusor A body part that pushes down, such as the bladder muscle.

Iatrogenic An adverse condition resulting from treatment by a physician or nurse or other health care provider.

Incontinence The inability to control excretory function.

Micturition Urination.

▶THE LIVED EXPERIENCE

I know I must smell of urine and others don't want to be around me. It has gotten to the point where I don't want to go anywhere. I know Harry gets irritated with me when I need to stop so often to find a bathroom. But, even so, I can't always hold the urine no matter how I try. Beth told me about an incontinence clinic in the city. I guess I really need to find out if they can help me.

Maria, age 60, mother of eight children

It really is too bad so many women think nothing can be done about their problems with incontinence. Just today I met Maria, who has been unable to control her urination for such a long time. I think Kegel exercises may help, but she may need surgery. I'll need to get a consult for her.

Betty, director of an incontinence clinic

Water, an accessible and available commodity to all, is often overlooked as an essential part of nutritional requirements. Water's function to the body includes thermoregulation, dilution of water-soluble medications, facilitation of renal and bowel function, and creating and maintaining metabolic processes.

The percentage of total body water decreases from the time of infancy to old age. By older adulthood, body water composition has decreased to 50% or less of the elder's body weight. This is due to the loss of wa-

ter content and the increase of body fat, which contains less water. In addition to the age-related decreases in total body water, older adults take in less water and other fluids because of a diminished thirst sensation.

The mechanism responsible for decreased sensitivity to thirst in the elderly is unclear. Even when there is free access to water and their mouth is dry, elders do not respond by drinking fluids. If an elder drinks more frequently, he or she still does not imbibe adequate water to rehydrate to the previous levels (Phillips et al, 1984).

No accepted standard measure to calculate the total body water needs of elders is available at present (Gaspar, 1999). However, it has been recommended by a number of researchers that 1500 to 2000 ml of non-caffeinated fluids be consumed every 24 hours by the older adult to maintain adequate hydration. Despite this goal, the average intake continues to be a maximum of only 1500 to 1600 ml in 24 hours in the best of circumstances (Norton et al, 1962; Hart, Adametk, 1984; Adams, Marano, 1998; Gaspar, 1999).

HYDRATION/DEHYDRATION

According to Amella (cited in Peters, 1998), "Old people sit on the edge of dehydration." The aged are frequently vulnerable to fluid and accompanying electrolyte imbalance, acidosis and alkalosis, and confusion because of electrolyte imbalance (Rolls, 1989). Increased amounts of fluid not only prevent these problems but also are essential for individuals who, for example, are diagnosed with a bipolar disorder and are receiving the medication lithium. This medical regimen requires a fluid intake of as much as 3 L of fluid daily; the use of diuretics requires that fluid intake be maintained unless specifically ordered to the contrary; and coffee has a diuretic effect that requires fluid intake to compensate for fluid loss through diuresis. In hot weather increased perspiration and evaporation deplete the individual of needed body fluid. Fever and upper respiratory tract infections also cause dehydration in the aged. Under normal circumstances a healthy adult needs 1.5 L of oral fluids; an additional 700 ml comes from solid food, and 300 ml comes from oxidation of food during metabolism (Reedy, 1988).

Common manifestations of dehydration in elders are altered mental status, light-headedness, and syncope, all of which can also be symptoms of other disease entities. Standard indicators for dehydration among the aged are unreliable. Skin turgor assessment, if done improperly, is unreliable, and weight alone may not reveal the extent of dehydration in the community and nursing home setting. Dry mucous membranes may be misleading because many elderly persons are mouth breathers. Intake and output recordings are generally unreliable because they are not consistently maintained. Urine-specific gravity is poorly correlated with serum biochemical parameters of hydration status because the older kidney has difficulty concentrating urine (Peters, 1998). Laboratory parameters can be used, but other conditions that can occur in the elderly can alter these laboratory findings.

Weinberg et al (1995), in a review of the published literature regarding dehydration in older individuals, formulated a consensus statement. The statement recommends that the OBRA (Omnibus Budget Reconciliation Act of 1987 and 1990) Dehydration/Fluid Maintenance Triggers and Additional Risk Factors for Dehydration Among Residents of Long-Term Care Facilities be used for assessment of the elderly in nursing homes and in the home. The indicators are presented in Box 11-1.

Prevention of dehydration is essential. Nursing staff in a long-term care facility were able to identify dehydration based on poor oral intake (Pals et al, 1995). These authors conclude that observation by staff continues to be the first defense for fever and dehydration detection in residents. Staff education to increase awareness of atypical presentation of dehydration is encouraged. In the community setting it is particularly difficult to know the fluid intake of the older adult living alone.

Oral hydration is the first treatment approach when dehydration occurs and if the patient is able to ingest fluids. Sports drinks, although high in sugar, are often recommended over tap water because they can be easily absorbed by the stomach, are generally palatable to patients, and will more rapidly correct the situation. Other fluids such as Pedialyte or other commercial fluid-and-electrolyte solutions are also available. It is suggested that unless contraindicated by a medical condition such as heart failure, renal disease, or liver disease, 30 ml of fluid per kilogram of body weight be consumed to maintain an adequately hydrated state. The last-resort treatment approaches are hypodermoclysis and intravenous therapy (Weinberg et al, 1995).

In both rural and urban nursing home patients, water intake from food and fluid was found to be inadequate based on the standard of 1600 ml of water per square meter of body surface area (Gaspar, 1998, 1999). Variables that influence fluid intake of institutionalized elders were identified as decreased fluid intake occurring with age, speech problems, the ability to request fluids, visual impairment, opportunity to obtain water, the amount of time that fluid was in reach, functional ability, gender, and the length of stay in a long-term care facility (Gaspar, 1998, 1999). The findings suggest that those who are semidependent are at greater risk for inadequate fluid intake than those who are independent (able to obtain their own fluids) or dependent (care needs are anticipated). The longer the length of stay, the lower the water intake. Gaspar concluded that nursing care plans for those who are semidependent, female,

Box 11-1	OBRA 1987/1990 MINIMUM DATA SET: DEHYDRATION/FLUID MAINTENANCE TRIGGERS AND ADDITIONAL RISK FACTORS FOR DEHYDRATION AMONG RESIDENTS OF LONG-TERM CARE FACILITIES

Dehydration/Fluid Maintenance Triggers

Deterioration in cognitive status, skills, or abilities in last 90 days
Failure to eat or take medication(s)
Urinary tract infection in last 30 days
Current diagnosis of dehydration (*ICD*-9 code 276-5)
Diarrhea
Dizziness/vertigo
Fever
Internal bleeding
Vomiting
Weight loss ($\geq$5% in last 30 days; or 10% in last 180 days)
Insufficient fluid intake (dehydrated)
Did not consume all/almost all liquids provided during last 3 days

Leaves $\geq$25% food uneaten at most meals
Requirement for parenteral (intravenous) fluids

Additional Potential Risk Factors

Hand dexterity/body control problems
Use of diuretics
Abuse of laxatives
Uncontrolled diabetes mellitus
Swallowing problems
Purposeful restriction of fluids
Patients on enteral feedings (need free water in addition to feedings)
History of previous episodes of dehydration
Comprehension/communication problems

From Omnibus Budget Reconciliation Act of 1987 and 1990 (federal). *ICD*-9 indicates *International Classification of Diseases,* ed 9.

Box 11-2	MEASURES TO HELP PREVENT DEHYDRATION OF INSTITUTIONALIZED ELDERLY PERSONS

- Ensure a 24-hour intake of at least 1500 ml of oral fluid. (Food intake and metabolic oxidation should provide additional fluid for hydration.)
- Offer fluids hourly during the day. Include fluids with an evening snack.
- Ask the physician to order intravenous fluids if the elder is not able to take oral fluids.
- Accurately record intake and output on all elders. (The 24-hour urine volume should be 1000 ml to 1500 ml.)
- Note the urine color and specific gravity.
- Listen to bowel sounds. Note any change in activity. (Extra soft or loose stool means losing water, and hard stool means dehydration.)
- Be familiar with tests or examinations that the patient may have had. If they involved enemas or laxatives prior to the tests, there will be a fluid loss.
- Replace fluids when there has been nothing consumed orally or fluids have been lost from test preparation.
- Obtain a drug history.
- Provide cups, glasses, and pitchers that are not too big or heavy for the aged to handle. (Help those who can't help themselves to fluids.)
- Offer other fluids in addition to water. Find out the types of beverages liked and fluid temperature preferred.
- Remember that coffee acts as a diuretic. Fluid loss by coffee should be supplemented to compensate for the fluid loss.
- Note skin turgor and mucous membranes.
- Note increases in pulse and respirations and decrease in blood pressure (suggestive of dehydration).
- Check laboratory values for changes: sodium, blood urea nitrogen, hematocrit, hemoglobin, urine and serum osmolarity, and creatinine. Also check for signs of acidosis.
- Weigh the patient daily at the same time and on the same scale.

From Reedy DF: Fluid intake: how can you prevent dehydration? *Geriatr Nurs* 9:224, 1988.

and over the age of 85 should include nursing orders clearly stating the need to increase the number of times water and fluids are offered. Just placing pitchers or cups of water by the bedside or near a person is ineffective. If fluids are not consistently offered and drink-ing encouraged, the goal of adequate hydration cannot be met. Interventions to prevent dehydration appear in Box 11-2. The importance of hydration of elders cannot be overstated. Warren et al (1994) indicate that nearly one half of elders hospitalized for dehydration or dehydration associated with disease and who are on Medicare die within a year of admission, thus raising Medicare costs.

INCONTINENCE

Widespread advertising and availability of continence products aid in the "cover up of symptoms and abet the conspiracy of silence" (Maloney, Cafiero, 1999). This, along with the myths that urinary incontinence is a normal part of aging and that cognitively alert and mobile persons are not incontinent, causes older adults, their families, and nurses to brush off the possibility that successful interventions can be achieved. Most older adults, and society in general, don't know that treatment is possible.

Incontinence is a common chronic problem that is frequently misunderstood by the public and health professionals. It is estimated that 13 million Americans experience urinary incontinence; thousands more do not report their experience with urinary leakage because of embarrassment or misconceptions (Fantl et al, 1996). Incontinence is primarily a female condition, with twice as many women as men affected, but men are also incontinent. Brown et al (1996) and Nygaard and Lemke (1996) report that urinary incontinence in women is as high as 41%. More than 50% of nursing home residents are incontinent (Snyder et al, 1998), which translates into an annual cost for incontinence of $7 million in the community, $3.3 million in nursing homes (US Department of Health and Human Services, 1992), and $15 billion for care of incontinence of all persons, young and old (Fantl et al, 1996).

The public health costs associated with incontinence are approximately $11 billion (Hu et al, 1994). Medicare data indicate that failure to treat urinary incontinence results in extra hospital days at a cost of $3.8 billion, as well as $174 million for related skin conditions and $1.7 billion for additional nursing home admissions (Hu et al, 1994). A high correlation exists between urinary incontinence, pressure ulcers, infections, depression, increased social isolation, and self-esteem (Morishita, 1988; Colling et al, 1994).

Elders in rural settings and small towns are more likely than those in metropolitan areas to be institutionalized when afflicted with incontinence (Coward et al, 1995). Many community elders avoid physical activity to reduce episodes of incontinence and thus exacerbate physical debility and further reduce muscle tone and control. In one study it was shown that fewer than 23%

of primary care physicians routinely ask elderly patients about urinary incontinence, and 62% of those physicians believed that they were inadequately prepared to evaluate the condition (Branch et al, 1995). Therefore continence must be routinely addressed in the initial assessment of every aged person in the nurse's care within or outside a care facility. Initial and periodic assessments are necessary to maintain an individualized nursing care plan.

Bladder Function in Old Age

Nocturnal frequency is common in two thirds of women and men over age 65 who do not take medication and in over 80% of those elders with three chronic diseases (Wasson, Bruskewitz, 1990). Normal bladder function requires an intact brain and spinal cord, a competent bladder, and active sphincters that will sustain maximal urethral pressure against rising bladder pressure. A full bladder increases pressure and signals the desire to micturate to the spinal cord and the brainstem center. Social training then dictates whether micturition should be attended to or can be postponed until there is an appropriate opportunity to seek out toilet facilities. However, when the bladder contents reach 500 ml or more (in elders, less than 500 ml), the pressure is such that it becomes more difficult to control the urge to micturate. As volume increases, emptying the bladder becomes an uncontrollable act. The bladder of the aged retains its tone, but the volume that it can hold decreases. If cerebrovascular disease is present (dementia being the most severe form), the changes are exaggerated and bladder control becomes diminished.

Many healthy aged persons are bothered by frequency and some degree of urgency. The warning period between the desire to micturate and actual micturition is shortened or lost, resulting in many trips to the toilet to void small amounts of urine, or incontinence occurs because the signal and the act of voiding are too close together. Severe illness, difficulty in walking or handling a bedpan or urinal, problems manipulating clothing, and emotional disturbances (such as occur during a change in the living situation or resentment, anger, or bereavement) may be responsible for some incontinence. In some instances micturition is uncontrolled as a deliberate means to gain attention or demonstrate anger. Drugs that increase urinary output and sedatives, tranquilizers, and hypnotics, which produce drowsiness or confusion, promote incontinence by dulling the transmission of the desire to micturate.

Urinary Incontinence

Urinary incontinence is one of the most prevalent symptoms encountered in the care of the aged. Many families cannot cope with incontinent relatives. It is therefore not surprising that incontinence is judged to be the second leading precipitating cause of institutionalization of the aged (Ouslander, 1992; Fantl et al, 1996). Among the approximately 28 million elders in the community, 15% to 35% have urinary incontinence (Fantl et al, 1996). Incontinence is present in 50% or more of nursing home residents. This translates into 1.5 million elders.

The current definition of *urinary incontinence,* "involuntary loss of urine that is sufficient to be a problem" (Fantl et al, 1996, p. 1), varies little from the International Continence Society's definition that urinary incontinence is "a condition in which involuntary loss of urine is a social or hygienic problem and is objectively demonstrated" (National Institutes of Health Panel, 1989). Incontinence is not a result of advancing age, nor is it a disease. It is a symptom of existing environmental, psychologic, drug, or physical disturbances and can become a catastrophic event when it interferes with mobility, sociability, and the ability to remain in one's home. Box 11-3 enumerates risk factors associated with incontinence.

Incontinence ushers in dependence, shame, guilt, and fear. The aged who are aware of a problem of continence are mortified by their state. If it is assumed that all aged persons eventually become incontinent, a resolution of the problem will not be sought, and it will become a self-fulfilling prophecy. Goldstein et al (1992) point out that elders generally do nothing about incontinence because they consider it a normal part of aging, do not realize that treatment exists, do not think that treatment will help, worry about the cost, or are too embarrassed to discuss it. Staff who do not attend to the aged person's request for assistance often cause the aged to withdraw because no one seems to care.

Health care personnel must begin to change their thinking about incontinence and acknowledge that incontinence can be cured. If it cannot be cured, it can be treated to minimize its detrimental effects. The nurse who cares for the incontinent person either in the community or in other types of facilities needs sensitivity, insight, patience, and understanding. Reassurance rather than guilt should be promoted. The Agency for Health Care Policy and Research (AHCPR) increased awareness and knowledge about incontinence and has continued to disseminate factual information through the publication of the Clinical Practice Guideline, *Urinary Incontinence in Adults,* in 1992 and the updated version in 1996. This information attempts to improve reporting, diagnosis, and treatment of the ambulatory and nonambulatory individual and to educate health professionals and consumers about urinary incontinence (Fantl et al, 1996).

Types of Urinary Incontinence

The National Institutes of Health Panel of 1989 (US Department of Health and Human Services, 1992) identified the most common types of urinary incontinence in older adults as stress incontinence, urge incontinence, and overflow incontinence. Mobley et al (1991) added functional, iatrogenic, and mixed incontinence to the list. Transient urinary incontinence, the result of functional and iatrogenic causes, can be remembered by the mnemonic *DRIP* (Box 11-4). Table 11-1 lists the types of urinary incontinence with their signs and symptoms.

Stress incontinence occurs when intraabdominal pressure exceeds urethral resistance. A number of causes are rooted in anatomic damage to the urethral sphincter and weakened bladder neck supports. Urine loss may occur when an individual sneezes, coughs, bends over, or lifts a heavy object. The amount of urine leakage may vary in amount from small to large. Frequently, a postresidual urine is documented by catheter

Box 11-3	**RISK FACTORS FOR INCONTINENT OLDER ADULTS**

Immobility of chronic degenerative diseases
Diminished cognitive status, dementia
Delirium
Medications including diuretics
Smoking
Fecal impaction
Low fluid intake
Environmental barriers
High-impact physical exercise
Diabetes
Stroke
Estrogen difficiency
Pelvic muscle weakness

From Fantl JA et al: *Managing acute and chronic urinary incontinence,* Clinical Practice Guideline: Quick Reference Guide for Clinicians No 2, 1996 update, AHCPR Pub No 96-0686, Rockville, Md, 1996, US Department of Health and Human Services, Public Health Service, Agency for Health Care Policy and Research.

Box 11-4   CAUSES OF ACUTE OR TRANSIENT INCONTINENCE

D   Delirium, depression, dehydration, dementia
R   Restricted mobility, retention
I   Infection, inflammation, impaction (fecal)
P   Polyuria, pharmaceuticals

Modified from Kane RL, Ouslander JG, Abrass IB: *Essentials of clinical geriatrics,* ed 3, New York, 1994, McGraw-Hill.

or visualized by ultrasound to reveal the remaining volume of urine in the bladder.

Urge incontinence is caused by central nervous system lesions such as stroke, demyelinating diseases, and local irritating factors such as bladder tumors or urinary tract infections (UTIs). Individuals sense the urge to void but cannot inhibit urination long enough to reach a toilet. The volume of urine lost is moderate, and episodes occur every few hours. A postresidual urine is

Table 11-1

Common Classifications of Established Incontinence and Symptoms

Type	Symptoms
STRESS	
Related to a weakness of the pelvic floor muscles, position of the bladder or urethra, or loss of estrogen	Leakage of small amounts of urine with increased abdominal pressure or physical exertion (e.g., coughing, sneezing, laughing, exercise, transferring)
URGE	
Sometimes referred to as instability; related to an overactive or hypersensitive detrusor muscle; associated with disorders of the brain, bladder outlet obstruction, and irritative disorders	Frequent urination, feeling an urge but not getting to the bathroom in time
REFLEX	
Related to neurologic dysfunction (i.e., paraplegia); bladder instability without normal sensation	No sensory awareness of the need to void; constant dribbling
OVERFLOW	
Related to partial obstruction of the bladder neck, sphincter, or urethra	Difficulty starting stream, frequency, nocturia*
MIXED	
A combination of types, usually components of stress and urge incontinence	Related to each type of incontinence
FUNCTIONAL	
Results from barriers that prevent getting to the bathroom (e.g., mobility, dexterity, impaired cognition)	
IATROGENIC	
Related to other diseases or conditions involving extracellular fluids (e.g., congestive heart failure; chronic venous insufficiency; metabolic states such as glycosuria, calcemia); drugs	

Modified from Smith DB: A continence care approach for long-term care facilities, *Geriatr Nurs* 19(2):81, 1998; Resnick NM: Urinary incontinence. In Abrams WB, Beers MH, Berkow R, editors: *The Merck manual of geriatric,* ed 2, Whitehouse Station, NJ, Merck Research Laboratories; and Fantl JA et al: Managing acute and chronic urinary incontinence. In *Clinical practice guidelines: quick reference guide for clinicians,* No 2, 1996 update, AHCPR, Pub No 96-0686, Rockville, Md, 1996, US Department of Health and Human Services, Public Health Service, Agency for Health Care Policy and Research.
*Complete obstruction of urine flow is a medical emergency.

useful in establishing the amount of remaining urine in the bladder.

Overflow incontinence is a result of neurologic abnormalities of the spinal cord that affect the contractility of the detrusor muscle of the bladder. Any factor disrupting detrusor stability, such as drugs, tumors, strictures, and prostatic hypertrophy, will cause the bladder to become overdistended, leading to frequent or constant loss of urine.

In *functional incontinence* the lower urinary tract is intact but the individual is limited by musculoskeletal disability or severe cognitive impairment. Urine is lost because the individual is unaware of the need to void or is unable to reach a toilet because of, for example, arthritis or Parkinson disease or, in the case of hospitalized patients, their condition or raised bed rails. Environmental conditions and prescribed drug use are additional examples of factors that can create functional incontinence.

Iatrogenic incontinence is associated with medication side effects. This can be managed by decreasing the dosage of medication to maintain the primary drug effect but eliminate the secondary effects. It may be necessary to change a drug to another class of medication that is not associated with incontinence. Other iatrogenic causes of incontinence include expanded extracellular fluid compartmentalization with the development of nocturia and polyuria, as occurs in heart failure, in chronic venous insufficiency, and in metabolic states such as polyuria with increased glycosuria or increased calcemia.

In *mixed incontinence,* more than one urinary incontinence problem exists in the same individual. These conditions can be caused by anatomic, physiologic, or pathologic factors (internal factors) or by outside factors such as mobility, dexterity, motivation, and environment.

Assessment

Nurses are often the ones to identify urinary incontinence, but neither nurses nor physicians have been particularly aggressive in its treatment. Assessment is multidimensional. It includes a health history, physical examination, and urinalysis. More extensive examinations are considered after the initial findings are assessed. A thorough health history should focus on the medical, neurologic, and genitourinary history; medication review of both prescribed and over-the-counter drugs; a detailed exploration of the symptoms of the urinary incontinence; and associated symptoms and other factors. Nurses, in general, should be able to gather data that will help the physician or the advanced

practice nurse in accurate diagnosis and treatment. Box 11-5 includes the type of data nurses should obtain in assessing urinary incontinence. One of the best ways to validate and describe incontinence problems is with a voiding diary. This is applicable to both community-dwelling and institutionalized elders. Pfister (1999) indicates that maintaining a detailed bladder diary for 3 days involving a weekend (either Friday, Saturday, and Sunday, or Saturday, Sunday, and Monday) was as good as maintaining a diary for a full week. Bladder diaries should include the type and amount of fluid ingested, the occurrence and timing of voluntary voiding, involuntary urine leakage episodes, and activity that occurred at the time of leakage. It also requires that once a day the individual measure the amount of urine voluntarily eliminated during any one voiding (Fig. 11-1). Older adults in the community can usually do this without much difficulty. Bladder diaries for those in long-term care are usually maintained by the staff. Following the Minimum Data Set (MDS) requires only a summary of incontinence using the following five categories:

0—Complete control
1—Usually continent (incontinent once a week or less)
2—Occasionally incontinent (two or more times a week but not daily)
3—Frequently incontinent (tends to be incontinent daily but has some control)
4—Incontinent (has inadequate control of bladder and multiple daily episodes)

Unfortunately, the MDS does not provide data that are addressed in the bladder diaries; thus its use is limited in any ability to develop a nursing care plan that is beneficial to the patient or that considers the cause of the urinary incontinence.

The value of the bladder diaries enables not only identification of problems but also a means of evaluating the effectiveness of nursing interventions and treatment.

Whether a bladder diary is maintained by a community elder or by nursing staff, accurate notations should also be made of significant burning, itching, or pressure; the character of the urine (odor, color, sedimentary, or clear); and difficulty starting and stopping the urinary stream. Activities of daily living such as ability to reach a toilet and use it and finger dexterity for clothing manipulation should be documented.

Use of medications such as sedatives, hypnotics, anticholinergics, and antidepressants should be assessed (Box 11-6). Furosemide (Lasix), diazepam (Valium), amitriptyline (Elavil), and phenothiazines are among the common drugs prescribed. In addition, the nurse should not forget to ask about vaginal discharge and/or constipation

Box 11-5   ELEMENTS OF AN INCONTINENCE ASSESSMENT

History

Duration and characteristics of urinary incontinence
Most bothersome symptom(s) for the aged person
Frequency, timing, and amount of continent and incontinent episodes
Other urinary tract symptoms
Daily fluid intake
Bowel habits
Alteration in sexual function because of urinary incontinence
Amount and type of perineal pads or protective devices used
Previous treatment and effect on urinary incontinence
Expectations of treatment

Mental Evaluation

Cognition
Motivation to self-toilet

Functional Assessment

Manual dexterity
Mobility:
    Observe toileting
        Unaided
        Chemical or physical restraints being used

Environmental

Access and distance to toilet or toilet substitute
Chair/bed allows ease of getting up

Social Factors

Relationship of urinary incontinence to activities
Living arrangements
Identified caregiver and degree of caregiver involvement
Lives alone

Bladder Records

Frequency, timing, and amount of voids
Number of incontinence episodes
Activity associated with urinary incontinence
Fluid intake

Physical Examination
General

Edema
Neurologic abnormalities

Abdomen

Diastasis rectii
Organomegaly
Masses
Peritoneal irritation
Fluid collection

Rectal examination

Perineal sensation
Resting and active sphincter tone
Fecal impaction
Masses
Consistency and contour of prostate (males)

Genital examination

Male:
    Skin condition
    Abnormalities of foreskin, penis, perineum
Female:
    Pelvic examination
    Skin
    Genital atrophy
    Pelvic organ prolapse
    Pelvic masses
    Perivaginal musculature

Direct observation of urine loss

With a full bladder under cough stress test
Estimate of postvoid residual volume

Urinalysis

From Fantl JA et al: *Managing acute and chronic urinary incontinence,* Clinical Practice Guideline: Quick Reference Guide for Clinicians No 2, 1996 update, AHCPR Pub No 96-0686, Rockville, Md, 1996, US Department of Health and Human Services, Public Health Service, Agency for Health Care Policy and Research.

or fecal impaction. The nurse may also do all or part of the physical examination, which includes evaluation of mental status; mobility; dexterity; and a neurologic, abdominal, rectal, and pelvic examination (see Box 11-5).

In summary, assessment of urinary incontinence can identify incontinence as either acute/transient—the result of temporary conditions that are amenable to medication, surgery, or psychologic intervention—or established—the result of neurologic involvement or damage to the urinary system. Transient incontinence is curable; established incontinence is treatable or controllable but not generally curable.

Sample Voiding or Bladder Diary

Name_____   Date_____

Time	Type of intake	Amount of intake	Urge to void	Voided	Leak	Activity

Measured Urine:

Time: Amount:

Fig. 11-1   Sample voiding or bladder diary.

Box 11-6	MEDICATIONS THAT MAY AFFECT BLADDER CONTROL

Anticholinergics
Inhibit bladder contractility and may cause retention

Antispasmodics
Relax muscles and sphincter

Antihistamines
May cause retention

Calcium Channel Blockers
Reduce detrusor contractions

Diuretics
Increase frequency and volume

Sedatives, Hypnotics, Alcohol
Decrease sensation

††From Smith DB: A continence care approach for long-term care facilities, *Geriatr Nurs* 19(2):81, 1998.

Interventions

When there is sufficient understanding of the problem, various therapeutic modalities and concomitant nursing interventions can be initiated. Selection of a modality and interventions will depend on the type of incontinence and its underlying cause and whether the outcome is to cure or to minimize the extent of the incontinence. Box 11-7 lists the numerous modalities available in the treatment of incontinence. Nursing in-terventions focus primarily on the therapeutic modality of supportive measures. However, the nurse is involved and must remain aware of the prescriptions, implications, and outcomes associated with the other therapeutic modalities.

Attitude. An appropriate attitude is most important when providing nursing care to an incontinent individual. Caregivers are often unaware of the many causes of incontinence and passively accept a client's urinary incontinence and believe that it is an inevitable part of aging, which only adds to the elder's feelings of low self-worth, dependence, and social isolation (Long, 1985; Wyman et al, 1990). Caregivers who regard incontinence as an unpleasant and demanding hygienic problem emphasize only keeping the patient clean and dry, with little consideration of what causes the problem. Ouslander et al (1987) studied an incontinent nursing home population and found that the incontinence was not associated with most clinical conditions or medications, except for bacteriuria. The fact that incontinence is curable and that the nurse and other health care providers will work with the elder to resolve the incontinence is an important idea to foster in the elder who is not cognitively impaired. The role of the nurse in the community is to give the older adult information and tools that will allow the individual to maintain body control.

Toilet accessibility. Accessibility to the toilet is an intervention that is often not considered in providing assistance for the incontinent patient. Environmental circumstances can contribute to incontinence. If the distance the aged person must either walk or travel by wheelchair to reach the toilet is longer than the time be-

Box 11-7   THERAPEUTIC MODALITIES IN THE TREATMENT OF INCONTINENCE

Support Measures
Appropriate attitude
Accessible toilet substitutes (bedpan, urinal, commode)
Avoidance of iatrogenic complications (urinary tract infection, excessive sedation, inaccessible toilets, and drugs adversely affecting bladder or urethral function)
Protective undergarments
Absorbent bed pads
Behavioral techniques (bladder training, toilet scheduling, prompted toileting, Kegel exercises, biofeedback, urge suppression techniques, fluid/dietary management, environmental review)
Good skin care

Drugs
Urge incontinence
Pseudoephedrine (Sudafed)
Phenylpropanolamine (Entex LA)

Stress incontinence
Tolterodine (Detrol)
Oxybutynin (Ditropan and Ditropan X-L)
Propantheline (Pro-Banthine)
Imipramine (Tofranil)
Estrogen, oral or local

Diet (removal of potential bladder irritants)
Tea/coffee
Cola
Alcohol
Citrus fruits/juices
Spicy foods
Artificial sweeteners
Chocolate
Tomatoes

Nonsurgical Devices (mechanical and electric)
Urethral cap
Urethral insert
Pessary
Electrical stimulation
Biofeedback

Surgery
Suspension of bladder neck
Urethral sling
Bladder augmentation
Prosthetic sphincter implant
Transurethral resection of prostate

Catheters
External (condom or "Texas" catheter)
Intermittent
Suprapubic
Indwelling

Modified from Ebersole B, Hess P: *Toward healthy aging: human needs and nursing response,* ed 5, St Louis, 1998, Mosby; and Maloney C, Cafiero MR: Urinary incontinence: noninvasive treatment options, *Adv Nurse Pract* 7(6):37, 1999.

tween the onset of the desire to micturate and actual micturition, incontinence is certain to occur. Using this formula, the nurse can predict some episodes of incontinence.

$$\frac{D}{T_2} > T_1 = \text{Incontinence}$$

where

T_1 = Time between onset and desire of micturition and uncontrolled micturition

T_2 = Rate at which individual can walk

$\frac{D}{T_2}$ = Distance individual must walk to reach toilet

An absolute last resort in dealing with incontinence is the use of urinary appliances.

Toilet substitutes. Toilet substitutes for the infirm and ill have been around for hundreds of years. Four types are used: commodes for the bedside; over-toilet chairs for transport; bedpans for beds or commodes; and urinals for both men and women that can be used in bed, in a chair, or in a standing position. The criterion for use of a commode is that the toilet is too far for the elder's mobility or it requires too much energy for the elderly person to get to the toilet. A commode can also substitute for an inadequate number of available toilets (Wells, Brink, 1980). Over-toilet-chair criteria are similar to those for a commode. However, it cannot be used as a substitute for available toilets. Urinals are generally used by men; however, bottle-shaped urinals have been designed for women and are used on occasion. They can be obtained from a surgical supply store or various mail-order catalogues.

Protective undergarments. A variety of protective undergarments or adult briefs are available for the incontinent older adult. A list of factors to be considered when selecting protective garments appears in Box

Box 11-8	FACTORS TO CONSIDER FOR USE OF ABSORBENT PRODUCTS

Functional disability of person
Type and severity of incontinence
Gender
Availability of caregivers
Failure with previous treatment program
Client preference
Co-morbidity

11-8. Disposable types come in several sizes determined by hip and waist measurements, or one size may fit all. The lining of these disposable pants may contain fiberfill or an absorbent polymer or gel substance. Polymer and gel substances are more absorbent and tend to keep a protective layer between the skin and wet material. Washable garments with inserts also do a reasonable job of containing urine. However, they tend to be made of plastic or rubber and therefore are hot and cause skin discomfort. If pants are going to leak, they will do so at the groin. It is important to fit them firmly but comfortably around the leg.

Protective padding. A variation of the standard drawsheet is a protective washable pad used along with a plastic sheet. The Australian Kylie pad is a sophisticated version of the drawsheet that is successful in keeping both the bed and the incontinent person dry. It is composed of two layers, with a water-repellent layer next to the individual. Urine is absorbed by the liner. Disposable protective pads are available in the United States, but it is important to know the amount and type of fill in the pads. A polymer gel is more economical. It is unwise to purchase pads because they are inexpensive if it means using several more per day than if more expensive and more absorbent pads were bought.

Behavioral techniques. Behavioral techniques such as scheduled toileting, habit training, bladder training, biofeedback, and conditioning focus on improving the person's awareness of his or her lower urinary tract (see Box 11-7). These techniques are usually effective in urge and stress incontinence. In some instances the goal is not to regain a normal voiding pattern but to decrease the number of wetting episodes, to decrease laundry costs and use of absorbent protection, and to improve the person's quality of life and social activity. The methods are free of side effects and do not limit future options. However, they do require time, effort, practice,

and an individual who is cognitively intact and highly motivated.

Scheduled toileting consists of a fixed toileting schedule, such as every 2 hours, with techniques to trigger voiding and emptying the bladder completely (National Institutes of Health Panel, 1989; Newman, 1992; Palmer, 1996).

Habit training uses frequent checks (every 1 to 2 hours) for dryness. The client is reminded to void and is praised frequently when successful. The objective of habit training is to allow the person to regain a normal voiding pattern and continence. It involves cognitive function, mobility, dexterity, and motivation (Newman, 1992; Rousseau, Fuentevilla-Clifton, 1992; Palmer, 1996).

Bladder retraining uses an interplay of methods. It teaches the individual to void at regular intervals and attempts to lengthen intervals between voidings. Bladder training has been effective in reducing the frequency of urge and stress incontinence (National Institutes of Health Panel, 1989; Newman, 1992; Palmer, 1996). Box 11-9 provides suggestions for caregivers who are toileting residents with dementia.

Conditioning or pelvic muscle exercises employ use of Kegel exercises. Conditioning also involves improving mobility. Pelvic floor exercises strengthen the periurethral and pelvic floor muscles. The contractions exert a closing force on the urethra. Kegal exercises are one approach to the problem of stress incontinence. They can be either slow or rapid. The muscle contraction is held for 3 seconds and then relaxed. This is repeated 10 times, working up to 20 times. The exercise is repeated five times a day. Quick Kegel exercises begin with tightening and relaxing the pubococcygeal muscle without pausing. These are done as fast as possible, beginning with a count of 15 seconds and working up to 2 minutes. Initially it is difficult to identify, tighten, and relax this muscle, but with repeated practice it becomes easier (National Institutes of Health Panel, 1989; Jette et al, 1990; US Department of Health and Human Services, 1992; Palmer, 1996). Mandelstam and Robinson (1977) describe the following exercise routine to improve perineal and sphincter muscle control: Standing, sitting, or lying, tighten the anal sphincter (as if to control the passage of flatus or feces) and then the urethral/vaginal muscles (as if to stop the flow of urine). This should be done at least four times each hour and can be done in any position or any place.

Biofeedback uses both visual or auditory instruments to give the individual immediate feedback on how well he or she is controlling the sphincter, the detrusor muscle, and/or abdominal muscles. Those who

Box 11-9	HINTS FOR CAREGIVERS TOILETING RESIDENTS WITH DEMENTIA

Have the word "bathroom" or "toilet" on the door.
Have a picture of a bathroom on the door.
Decrease clutter in and around the toilet.
Increase environmental safety (i.e., use good lighting, hand rails, elevated toilet).
Use simple verbal or behavioral cues.
Hold out your hand and say pleasantly, "Come with me."
Sing with the resident or use another pleasant distraction.
Avoid complicated commands or questions (i.e., "Mr. Jones, is it time for you to go to the bathroom?").
Avoid grabbing the resident's wrist and pulling.
Stay with a routine.
Use a familiar caregiver.
Have residents wear elastic waistbands or other easy-to-remove clothing.
Stay pleasant and avoid confrontation or hurrying.
Use timing with fluids and toileting.
Avoid bladder irritants.
Provide skin care cleanser, moisturizer, and protection.
Keep containment gaments simple and similar to regular underpants.

From Smith DB: A continence care approach for long-term care facilities, *Geriatr Nurs* 19(2):81, 1998.

are successful learn to contract the sphincter and/or relax the detrusor and abdominal muscles automatically. Complete continence can occur in 20% to 25% of individuals, and improvement in an additional 30%. Biofeedback requires sophisticated equipment (Newman, 1992; US Department of Health and Human Services, 1992). Table 11-2 provides a summary of behavioral modalities, the type of incontinence, outcomes, and appropriate populations for these approaches.

Skin care. Skin care maintains the first line of defense against infection. Skin that is in contact with urine should be washed with mild soap and warm water, then dried thoroughly. Application of a skin lubricant or an ointment such as A & D or skin barrier cream provides a thin protective layer to skin repeatedly exposed to urine. It is tempting to neglect an individual who wears protective pants, but it is important that the person be checked every few hours for wetness in order to maintain skin intactness. To minimize the episodes of incontinence, it is prudent to establish the incontinence pattern and place the individual on a toilet or commode before voiding.

Drugs. Drugs to eliminate or improve incontinence include bladder relaxants and bladder stimulants. Bladder relaxants include anticholinergic agents that delay, decrease, or inhibit detrusor muscle contractions, especially the involuntary contractions, and may increase bladder capacity. The most commonly used drug is propantheline (Pro-Banthine). Undesirable side effects such as dry mouth, dry eyes, constipation, confusion, or the precipitation of glaucoma may occur with high doses of this drug. Smooth muscle relaxants such as flavoxate (Urispas), oxybutynin (Ditropan), and dicyclomine (Bentyl) work directly on the bladder detrusor muscle. These drugs exert mild anticholinergic side effects. Calcium channel blockers, also used for cardiovascular problems, have a depressant effect on the bladder. More study is needed to determine if there is a significant benefit for their use in urge incontinence. Imipramine (Tofranil), a tricyclic antidepressant, exerts both anticholinergic and direct relaxant effects on the detrusor muscle, as well as a contractile effect on the bladder outlet, thus enhancing continence. Two important side effects to be aware of in the elderly are hypotension and sedation. Bladder outlet stimulants include alpha-adrenergic agonist agents and estrogen replacement preparations. Alpha-adrenergic agonists—pseudoephedrine and ephedrine—cause contractions of smooth muscle at the bladder outlet and improve stress incontinence. Estrogen replacement therapy, although not definitively used for stress incontinence, has been effective in improving postmenopausal urgency, frequency, and urge incontinence. Box 11-7 presents drugs used in the management of stress and urge incontinence.

Surgery. Surgical intervention is appropriate for some conditions of incontinence. Surgical suspension of the bladder neck in women has proved effective in 80% to 95% of persons electing to have this surgical corrective procedure. Outflow obstruction incontinence secondary to prostatic hypertrophy is generally corrected by prostatectomy. Sphincter dysfunction resulting from nerve damage following surgical trauma or radical perineal procedures is 70% to 90% repairable through sphincter implantation. Complications for this type of surgery are greater than 20% and may require an additional surgery. A urethral sling of fascia increases urethral elevation and compression. Continence is restored in approximately 80% of clients who have this surgery. Currently periurethral bulking has been added to the number of surgical procedures that address urinary incontinence. Collagen or polytetrafluoroethylene (PTFE) is injected into the periurethral area to increase pressure on the urethra. This adds bulk to the in-

Table 11-2

Behavioral Intervention Options for Incontinence

Type of incontinence	Intended population	Behavioral intervention	Purpose of intervention	Expected outcome
Urge, stress, mixed	Cognitively intact; able to discern urge sensation; able to understand or learn how to inhibit urge; able to toilet themselves with or without assistance	Bladder training	Restore normal pattern of voiding and normal bladder function Inhibit involuntary detrusor contractions	↓Number of wet episodes ↓Amount of urine lost ↓Number of voidings ↑Bladder capacity ↑Quality of life
Urge, functional	Cognitively impaired; functionally disabled; incomplete bladder emptying; caregiver dependent	Scheduled toileting	Timed with individual's voiding habits Decrease wet episodes; no attempt to regain normal voiding pattern	↓Number of wet episodes ↓Laundry costs and/or use of absorbent devices ↑Life quality ↑Social activity
Functional, urge, mixed	Same as above	Habit training	Develop a pattern for voiding	↓Frequency of incontinent episodes ↑Comfort ↑Quality of life
Urge, functional	Functionally able to use toilet or toileting device; able to feel urge sensation; able to request toileting assistance; caregiver is available	Prompted voiding	Heighten individual awareness of need to void	↑Interaction between caregiver and individual ↓Wet episodes
Stress, urge, mixed	Able to identify and contract pelvic muscles; able and willing to follow instructions and committed to actively participate	Pelvic floor training	Strengthen pubococcygeus muscle for efficient urethral closure during sudden increases in intravesical pressure	↑Strength and size of pubococcygeus ↑Duration of muscle contraction with increased urethral pressure ↓Urine loss ↑Ability to stop urine flow once initiated Self-report of ↓urine loss ↑Self-esteem; enhance quality of life ↓Reliance on pads, pantyliners, or absorbent products

Data from Fantl JA et al: Managing acute and chronic urinary incontinence. In *Clinical practice guideline: quick reference guide for clinicians,* No 2, 1996 update, Rockville, Md, US Department of Health and Human Services, Agency for Health Care Policy and Research, AHCPR, Pub No 96-0686, 1996; Staab AS, Hodges LC: *Essentials of gerontological nursing,* Philadelphia, 1996, Lippincott; Palmer MH: *Urinary incontinence,* Gaithersburg, Md, 1996, Aspen; Anderson MA, Braun JV: *Caring for the elderly client,* Philadelphia, 1995, Davis.

Continued

Table 11-2—cont'd

Behavioral Intervention Options for Incontinence

Type of incontinence	Intended population	Behavioral intervention	Purpose of intervention	Expected outcome
Stress, urge, mixed	Cognitively intact Compliant with instructions Able to stand Sufficient muscle strength to contract muscle and retain the lightest weight No pelvic organ prolapse	Vaginal weight training	Same as above	Same as above
Stress, mixed	Ability to understand analog or digital signals using auditory or visual display Motivated, able to learn voluntary control through observation of biofeedback A health care provider who can appropriately assess the incontinence problem and provide behavior interventions	Biofeedback	Same as above	Same as above
Stress, urge, mixed	Ability to discern stimulation	Electrical stimulation	Reeducation of pelvic muscle; inhibit bladder instability and improve striated sphincter and levator ani contractility and efficiency	↑Resistance of the pelvic floor; block unhibited bladder contractions

ternal sphincter and closes the gap that allowed leakage to occur (Mayo Foundation for Medical Education and Research, 1994; Palmer, 1996). Bladder augmentation is more specific and limited to neurologic disorders such as a contracted bladder. A segment of the bowel is used to increase bladder capacity and to facilitate release of excess pressure (Rosenberg, 1992).

Nonsurgical devices. The Food and Drug Administration (FDA) has approved two devices, available through prescription, to manage stress incontinence.

The Miniguard is about the size of a postage stamp and fits over the urethral opening. It is contoured with an adhesive foam backing. The other device, the Reliance Urinary Control Insert, is designed for moderate to severe incontinence in women. The device is a balloon-tipped plug, about one-fifth the diameter of a tampon, which is inserted by an applicator. The force of the insertion inflates the balloon, so that the neck of the bladder is then obstructed. The device must be removed by pulling a string before urination or intercourse. Trials of both of these devices have been on a limited number of women at present. Women using the devices gained complete or limited continence but also experienced UTIs, particularly with the Reliance Control Insert. However, it was thought that as the women gained skill in use of the device, the frequency of UTIs would diminish (More Ways to Stay Dry, 1998). A third option, the pessary, has been around for many years and has primarily been used to prevent uterine prolapse. The pessary is a device that is fitted into the vagina and that exerts pressure to elevate the urethrovesical junction or the pelvic floor. The patient is taught to insert and remove the pessary much like the insertion and removal of a diaphram used for contraception. The pessary is removed weekly or monthly for cleaning with soap and water and then reinserted (see Box 11-7).

Catheters. As a last resort, appliances may need to be used. Too frequently, abuse of appliances occurs because they are convenient for the caregivers. Foley and condom catheters, diapers, and rubber pants carry with them inherent hazards of iatrogenic infection and skin irritation and breakdown. Psychologically the aged person feels and is treated differently—no longer as an adult but, rather, as a dependent and, perhaps, childlike individual. The aged person who has an indwelling catheter soon loses awareness of the sensations of bladder pressure and the habit of toileting. Persons with catheters often lose the micturition function completely. Women have fewer appliance options than men. In addition to the Foley catheter, men can use condom and sheath catheters, which are soft and pliable.

Catheter care is important regardless of the type of catheter used. The condom catheter should be removed

daily to allow the penis to be scrupulously cleansed, dried, and aired to prevent irritation, maceration, and the development of pressure areas and skin breakdown. Foley catheter care should be performed at least twice a day. Cleansing of the external urethral meatus with a gentle cleanser, maintaining a closed system with unobstructed flow, maintaining an acid urine (see Box 11-7), and meticulous care of equipment are essential in acute care or long-term care facilities, as well as at home if a Foley catheter is used. Regular Foley catheter care ensures cleansing and removal of secretions and fecal matter, which can become the media for bacterial growth in the perineal area.

Constant use of condom catheters is not a safe practice with elders. Skin under the catheter is prone to the development of fungal skin infections, irritation, edema, fissures, contact burns from urea, UTIs, and septicemia (Wells, Brink, 1980). Long-term use of indwelling catheters should be discouraged because of the complications that can occur. These include fever, bacteremia, acute and chronic pylonephritis, urethral abscesses, bladder or renal stones, renal failure, and possibly death (Greengold, Ouslander, 1986).

Evaluation. The success of interventions in urinary incontinence is measured against phased accomplishment such as the following:
1. The individual voids when placed on the toilet.
2. The individual drinks at least 2000 ml of fluid daily.
3. The individual remains continent 25% of the time.
4. The individual has fewer accidents in each successive phase.
5. The individual is continent all the time.

Table 11-3 provides a standard protocol for urinary incontinence.

Table 11-3

Nursing Standard-of-Practice Protocol: Urinary Incontinence in Older Adults Admitted to Acute Care

I. Background
   A. UI is the involuntary loss of urine sufficient to be a problem.
   B. UI affects approximately 13 million Americans and is prevalent in hospitalized elders.
   C. Risk factors associated with UI include immobility, impaired cognition, medications, fecal impaction, low fluid intake, environmental barriers, diabetes mellitus, and stroke.
   D. Nurses play a key role in assessing and managing UI.

II. Assessment Parameters
   A. Document the presence or absence of UI for all patients on admission.
   B. Document the presence or absence of an indwelling urinary catheter.
   C. For patients who are incontinent:
      1. Determine whether the problem is transient, established, or both.

From Bradway C et al: Urinary continence in older adults admitted to acute care, *Geriatr Nurs* 19(2):100, 1998.
UI, Urinary incontinence; *AHCPR,* Agency for Health Care Policy and Research.

Continued

Table 11-3—cont'd

Nursing Standard-of-Practice Protocol: Urinary Incontinence in Older Adults Admitted to Acute Care

    2. Identify and document the possible etiologies of the UI.

    3. Elicit assistance with assessment and management from multidisciplinary team members.

III. Care Strategies

  A. General principles that apply to prevention and management of all forms of UI:

    1. Identify and treat causes of transient UI.

    2. Identify and continue successful prehospital management strategies for established UI.

    3. Develop an individualized plan of care using data obtained from the history and physical examination and in collaboration with other team members.

    4. Avoid medications that may contribute to UI.

    5. Avoid indwelling urinary catheters whenever possible.

    6. Monitor fluid intake and maintain an appropriate hydration schedule.

    7. Modify the environment to facilitate continence.

    8. Provide patients with usual undergarments in expectation of continence.

    9. Prevent skin breakdown by providing immediate cleansing after an incontinent episode.

   10. Use absorbent products judiciously.

  B. Strategies for specific problems:

    1. Stress UI:

      a. Teach pelvic muscle exercises (PME).

      b. Provide toileting assistance and bladder training prn.

      c. Consider referral to other team members if pharmacologic or surgical therapies are warranted.

    2. Urge UI:

      a. Implement bladder training or habit training.

      b. Teach PME to be used in conjunction with *a*.

      c. Consider referral to other team members if pharmacologic therapy is warranted.

      d. Initiate referrals for patients who do not respond to the above.

    3. Overflow UI:

      a. Allow sufficient time for voiding.

      b. Instruct patients in double voiding and Credé maneuver.

      c. Consider use of external collection devices for men.

      d. Provide sterile intermittent or indwelling catheterization prn.

      e. Initiate referrals to other team members for patients requiring pharmacologic or surgical intervention.

    4. Functional UI:

      a. Provide scheduled toileting or habit training.

      b. Provide adequate fluid intake.

      c. Collaborate with other team members to eliminate any medications adversely affecting continence.

      d. Refer for physical and occupational therapy PRN.

IV. Evaluation of Expected Outcomes

  A. Patients will have fewer or no episodes of UI or complications associated with UI.

  B. Health care providers:

    1. Will document continence status at admission and throughout hospital stay

    2. Will use multidisciplinary expertise and interventions to assess and manage UI during hospitalization

    3. Will include UI in discharge planning needs and refer PRN

  C. Institution:

    1. Will see a decrease in incidence and prevalence of acute UI

    2. Will implement policies that require assessing and documenting continence status

    3. Will provide access to AHCPR guidelines for managing acute and chronic UI

    4. Will give staff administrative support and ongoing education regarding assessment and management of UI

V. Follow-up to Monitor the Condition

  A. Provide the patient and caregiver discharge teaching regarding outpatient referral and management.

  B. Incorporate continuous quality improvement criteria into existing program.

  C. Identify areas for improvement and enlist multidisciplinary assistance in devising strategies for improvement.

Fecal or Bowel Incontinence

Fecal incontinence is defined as the inability to control the passage of stool or gas via the anus (Basch, Jenson, 1992) or involuntary loss of stool from the rectum at inappropriate times (Staab, Hodges, 1996). The prevalence of fecal incontinence is approximately 3% to 4% of community-dwelling elders, and approximately 16% to 60% of the institutionalized aged have some fecal incontinence (Richter, 1995). Often fecal incontinence is associated with urinary incontinence. Fecal incontinence is a relatively benign condition, but like urinary incontinence it has devastating social ramifications for the individuals and families who experience it. Many factors are similar to urinary incontinence. The factors affecting fecal incontinence include intestinal transit time, rectal factors (sensory), pelvic floor and sphincter tone, pelvic musculature, medications, muscular flaccidity, and the inability to get to the toilet when the urge to eliminate is present. This translates into such causes as sphincter dysfunction, anatomic disarrangement, neurologic impairments, and musculoneural dysfunction (Hanauer, Sable, 1991; Basch, Jenson, 1992; Wald, 1995). Other factors distinct to bowel evacuation problems are long-term dependence on laxatives, lack of sufficient bulk in the diet, insufficient fluid intake, lack of exercise, hemorrhoids, and depression. Many instances of fecal incontinence result from fecal impaction, or there may be a neurologic origin. Serious illness accompanied by delirium and excessive doses of iron, antibiotic, and digitalis preparations may precipitate incontinence. Sedatives, too, can account for incontinence through depression of cerebral awareness and control over sphincter response.

Assessment

Assessment should include a complete client history in urinary incontinence (described earlier in this chapter) and a bowel record. The following questions should be included in a bowel incontinence assessment:

- What is the availability of the toilet or commode, and what is the time required to get to it?
- What medications, if any, is the aged person taking that influence peristaltic action, lucidity, or fluid balance?
- How much bulk is provided in the food? (Pureed food does not help.)
- What is the manual dexterity required to remove clothing once the aged person is in the bathroom?
- Is there any neurologic or circulatory impairment of the cerebral cortex?

Interventions

The nurse's attitude in assisting the person who is incontinent of feces should be the same as for the individual with urinary incontinence. Fecal incontinence is a symptom. It requires that the patient be accepted as a person, that the incontinence problem not be advertised or ridiculed, and that the person not be made to feel ashamed or guilty. A great deterrent to successful intervention in incontinence is inconsistency in implementing the planned strategy and unrealistic expectations of rapid, full recovery. Time and patience are essential ingredients of success. Nursing interventions should include several days' surveillance of the patient's bowel function. A chart similar to that used to monitor urinary incontinence can be constructed.

Nursing intervention should work to manage and/or restore bowel continence. Therapies similar to those used in treating urinary incontinence are effective with fecal incontinence, such as environmental manipulation, diet alterations, bowel training, sensory reeducation, sphincter training exercises, biofeedback, electrical stimulation, medication, and/or surgery to correct underlying defects (Wald, 1995). Instituting a diet adequate in dietary fiber (6 to 10 g daily) (Ellickson, 1987) will add bulk, weight, and form to the stool and improve colon evacuation of the sigmoid and rectum rather than producing a continuous or intermittent oozing of fecal material. This may assist in the attainment of more controlled and complete bowel movements.

When the incontinence has a cerebral or neurologic cause, it is often necessary to identify triggers that initiate incontinence. For example, eating a meal stimulates defecation 30 minutes following the completion of the meal, or defecation occurs following the morning cup of coffee. If the fecal incontinence is only once or twice a day, it can be controlled by being prepared. Placing the individual on the toilet, commode, or bedpan at a given time following the trigger event facilitates defecation in the appropriate place at the appropriate time.

When fecal incontinence is continual, as often happens in nursing homes and hospitals, it may be necessary to develop a plan that controls the specific time of day when the individual has a bowel movement or movements. Generally, this is accomplished by establishing constipation for several days and evacuating the bowel (e.g., every fourth day) by enema or suppository. Diet plays a role in this also. Creating the proper diet will affect intestinal motility and help evacuation.

Box 11-10 BOWEL TRAINING PROGRAM

1. Obtain bowel history and establish a schedule for the bowel training program that is normal and comfortable for the patient and conforms to his or her life-style.
2. Ensure adequate fiber and fluid intake (normalize stool consistency).
   Fiber
      Add high-fiber foods to diet (dried fruit, dried beans, vegetables, and wheat products).
      Suggest adding 1 to 3 tbsp bran or Metamucil to diet one or two times a day. (Titrate dosage based on response.)
   Fluid
      Two to 3 liters daily (unless contraindicated)
      Four ounces of prune, fig, or pear juice (or a warm fluid) may be given daily as a stimulus (for example, 30 minutes to 1 hour before the established time for defecation).
3. Encourage exercise program.
   Pelvic tilt, modified sit-ups for abdominal strength
   Walking for general muscle tone and cardiovascular system
   More vigorous program if appropriate
4. Establish a regular time for the bowel movement.
   Established time depends on patient's schedule.
   Best times are 20 to 40 minutes after regularly scheduled meals, when gastrocolic reflex is active.
   Attempts at evacuation should be made daily within 15 minutes of the established time and whenever the patient senses rectal distention.
   Instruct patient in normal posture for defecation. (The patient normally sits on the toilet or bedside commode; for the patient who is unable to get out of bed, the left side lying position is best.)
   Instruct the patient to contract the abdominal muscles and "bear down."
   Have patient lean forward to increase the intraabdominal pressure by use of compression against the thighs.
   Stimulate anorectal reflex and rectal emptying if necessary.
      Insert a rectal suppository or mini-enema into the rectum 15 to 30 minutes before the scheduled bowel movement, placing the suppository against the bowel wall, or
      Insert a gloved, lubricated finger into the anal canal and gently dilate the anal sphincter.

From Basch A, Jensen L: Management of fecal incontinence. In Doughty DB: *Urinary and fecal incontinence: nursing management,* St Louis, 1991, Mosby.

Bowel training of this type allows for predictability of colon evacuation and more freedom and less embarrassment for the aged person (Box 11-10). If protective garments are necessary, they will allow the patient more opportunity to participate actively in events and to be more mobile in the institutional community.

The effectiveness of interventions in fecal incontinence will be self-evident but will take time. As in treatment of urinary incontinence, goals must be realistic. It cannot be stated too often or too strongly that the nurse must always provide immaculate skin care to the incontinent aged because self-esteem and skin integrity depend on it.

▶ KEY CONCEPTS

- Older adults do not experience thirst and therefore do not drink sufficient fluids to maintain adequate hydration. Certain medications and fluids such as coffee tend to abet dehydration.
- Urinary incontinence is not a part of normal aging. It is a symptom, not a disease, caused by drugs or by environmental, psychologic, or physiologic disturbances.
- Urinary incontinence can be minimized or cured.
- Nurses who perform thorough assessments are generally the ones who identify the presence of incontinence.
- A number of interventions for urinary incontinence are applicable to the management of bowel incontinence.

NANDA and Wellness Diagnoses

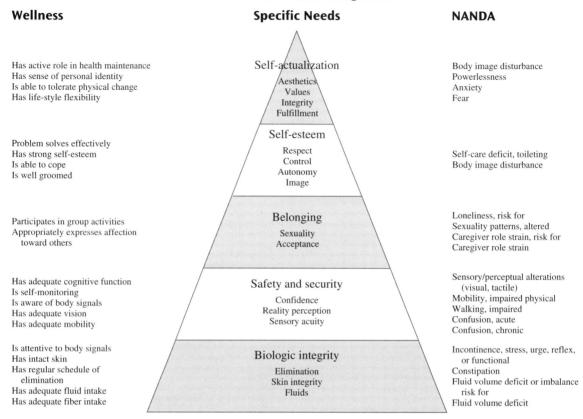

Wellness	Specific Needs	NANDA

Self-actualization
Aesthetics
Values
Integrity
Fulfillment

Has active role in health maintenance
Has sense of personal identity
Is able to tolerate physical change
Has life-style flexibility

Body image disturbance
Powerlessness
Anxiety
Fear

Self-esteem
Respect
Control
Autonomy
Image

Problem solves effectively
Has strong self-esteem
Is able to cope
Is well groomed

Self-care deficit, toileting
Body image disturbance

Belonging
Sexuality
Acceptance

Participates in group activities
Appropriately expresses affection
   toward others

Loneliness, risk for
Sexuality patterns, altered
Caregiver role strain, risk for
Caregiver role strain

Safety and security
Confidence
Reality perception
Sensory acuity

Has adequate cognitive function
Is self-monitoring
Is aware of body signals
Has adequate vision
Has adequate mobility

Sensory/perceptual alterations
   (visual, tactile)
Mobility, impaired physical
Walking, impaired
Confusion, acute
Confusion, chronic

Biologic integrity
Elimination
Skin integrity
Fluids

Is attentive to body signals
Has intact skin
Has regular schedule of
   elimination
Has adequate fluid intake
Has adequate fiber intake

Incontinence, stress, urge, reflex,
   or functional
Constipation
Fluid volume deficit or imbalance
   risk for
Fluid volume deficit

These are not all of the possible wellness or NANDA diagnoses that may be identified. The above are frequent examples of nursing diagnoses that should be considered when planning care for the older adult in whatever setting.

▶ Activities and Discussion Questions

1. Explain the problems associated with dehydration in the older adult.
2. Identify the signs and symptoms of dehydration in the elderly.
3. Discuss interventions to prevent and treat dehydration.
4. Explain the implications of urinary incontinence for the older adult.
5. What measures can be taken to cure or decrease urinary incontinence?
6. What interventions can be instituted for managing fecal incontinence?
7. Devise a nursing care plan for an elder with urinary incontinence or fecal incontinence.

RESOURCES

Managing Incontinence: A Guide for Living With Loss of Bladder Control. Available from the Simon Foundation, Box 835, Wilmette, IL 60091; (800) 23SIMON ($12.95).

Resource Guide of Continence Aids and Services. Available from Help for Incontinent People (HIP), PO Box 544, Union, SC 29379 ($4.00).

American Foundation for Urologic Disease
PO Box 8306
Spartanburg, SC 29305-8306
(800) 579-7900

Society of Urologic Nurses and Associates
E. Holly Avenue, PO Box 56
Pittman, NJ 08071-0056
(609) 256-2335

REFERENCES

Adams PF, Marano MA: Current estimates from the national health interview survey, 1994, National Center for Health Statistics, *Vital Health Stat* 10(193):1995, 1998.

Basch A, Jenson L: Management of fecal incontinence. In Doughty DB, editor: *Urinary and fecal incontinence,* St Louis, 1992, Mosby.

Branch L, Resnick N, Dubeau C: Knowledge, attitudes and practices of physicians regarding urinary incontinence in persons aged >65 years—Massachusetts and Oklahoma, 1993, *MMWR Morb Mortal Wkly Rep* 44(40):747, 1995.

Brown JS et al: Urinary incontinence in older women: who is at risk? *Obstet Gynecol* 87(5, pt 1):715, 1996.

Colling JC, Owns TR, McCreedy MR: Urine volumes and voiding patterns among incontinent nursing home residents, *Geriatr Nurs* 15(3):188, 1994.

Coward R, Horne C, Peek D: Predicting nursing home admissions among incontinent older adults: a comparison of residential differences across six years, *Gerontologist* 35(6):732, 1995.

Ellickson EB: Bowel management plan for the homebound elderly, *J Gerontol Nurs* 14(1):16, 1987.

Fantl JA et al: *Managing acute and chronic urinary incontinence,* Clinical Practice Guideline: Quick Reference Guide for Clinicians No 2, 1996 update, AHCPR Pub No 96-0686, Rockville, Md, 1996, US Department of Health and Human Services, Public Health Service, Agency for Health Care Policy and Research.

Gaspar PM: Fluid intake: what determines how much patients drink? *Geriatr Nurs* 9:221, 1998.

Gaspar PM: Water intake of nursing home residents, *J Gerontol Nurs* 25(4):23, 1999.

Goldstein M et al: Urinary incontinence: why people do not seek help, *J Gerontol Nurs* 18(4):15, 1992.

Greengold BA, Ouslander JG: Bladder retraining, *J Gerontol Nurs* 12:31, 1986.

Hanauer SB, Sable KS: Pathology of fecal incontinence. In Doughty DB, editor: *Urinary and fecal incontinence,* St Louis, 1991, Mosby.

Hart M, Adametk C: Do increased fluids decrease urinary stone formation? *Geriatr Nurs* 5:245, 1984.

Hu T et al: Clinical guidelines and cost implications in the case of urinary incontinence, *Geriatr Nephrol Urol* 4:85, 1994.

Jette AM, Branch LG, Berlin J: Musculoskeletal impairments and physical disablement among the aged, *J Gerontol* 45(6):M203, 1990.

Long ML: Incontinence, *J Gerontol Nurs* 11:30, 1985.

Maloney C, Cafiero MR: Urinary incontinence: noninvasive treatment options, *Adv Nurse Pract* 7(6):37, 1999.

Mandelstam D, Robinson W: Support for the incontinent patient, *Nurs Mirror* 144(15):xix, 1977.

Mayo Foundation for Medical Education and Research: Incontinence: collagen injections offer a new solution to bladder control problems, *Mayo Clin Health Lett* 12(1):1, 1994.

Mobley D, Goldberg K, Wilson S: Management of urinary incontinence, *Geriatr Med Today* 10(9):18, 1991.

More Ways to Stay Dry, *Harvard Women's Healthwatch* 5(7):2, 1998.

Morishita L: Nursing evaluation and treatment of geriatric outpatients with urinary incontinence: geriatric day hospital model: a case study, *Nurs Clin North Am* 23:189, 1988.

National Institutes of Health Panel: Teaching a consensus in incontinence, *Geriatr Nurs* 10:78, 1989.

Newman D: *Continence control: vision for the future: biofeedback and other techniques for bowel and bladder control,* Senior Focus, Mills-Peninsula Hospitals Conference, San Francisco, Oct 26-27, 1994.

Norton D, McLaren R, Exton-Smith AN: *An investigation of geriatric nursing problems in the hospital,* London, 1962, National Corporation for the Care of Older People.

Nygaard IE, Lemke JH: Urinary incontinence in rural older women: prevalence, incidence and remission, *J Am Geriatr Soc* 44(9):1049, 1996.

Ouslander JG: *Continence control: vision for the future: medical ramifications of incontinence,* Senior Focus, Mills-Peninsula Hospitals Conference, San Francisco, Oct 26-27, 1992.

Ouslander JG et al: Clinical, functional, and psychological characteristics of an incontinent nursing home population, *J Gerontol* 46:631, 1987.

Palmer MH: *Urinary continence assessment and promotion,* Gaithersburg, Md, 1996, Aspen.

Pals JK et al: Clinical triggers for detection of fever and dehydration: implications for long-term care nursing, *J Gerontol Nurs* 21(4):13, 1995.

Peters S: Helping older adults meet their unique nutrient needs, *Adv Nurse Pract* 6(8):66, 1998.

Pfister SM: Bladder diaries and voiding patterns in older adults, *J Gerontol Nurs* 25(3):36, 1999.

Phillips PA et al: Reduced thirst after water deprivation in healthy elderly men, *N Engl J Med* 311:753, 1984.

Reedy DF: Fluid intake: how can you prevent dehydration? *Geriatr Nurs* 9(6):224, 1988.

Richter JE: Functional disorders of the gastrointestinal tract. In Abrams WB, Beers MH, Berkow R, editors: *Merck manual of geriatrics,* ed 2, Whitehouse Station, NJ, 1995, Merck Research Laboratories.

Rolls BJ: Regulation of food and fluid intake in the elderly, *Ann NY Acad Sci* 561:217-225, 1989.

Rosenberg A: *Continence control: vision for the future,* Senior Focus, Mills-Peninsula Hospitals Conference, San Francisco, Oct 26-27, 1992.

Rousseau P, Fuentevilla-Clifton A: Urinary incontinence in the aged, Parts 1 and 2, *Geriatrics* 47(6):22, 1992.

Snyder M et al: Barriers to progress in urinary incontinence: achieving quality assessments, *Geriatr Nurs* 19(2):77, 1998.

Staab A, Hodges LC: *Essentials of gerontological nursing,* Philadelphia, 1996, Lippincott.

US Department of Health and Human Services: *Urinary incontinence in adults,* Clinical Practice Guideline, AHCPR Pub No 92-0038, Rockville, Md, 1992, US Department of Health and Human Services, Public Health Service, Agency for Health Care Policy and Research.

Wald A: Lower gastrointestinal tract disorders. In Abrams WB, Beers MH, Berkow R, editors: *The Merck manual of geriatrics,* ed 2, Whitehouse Station, NJ, 1995, Merck Research Laboratories.

Warren JL et al: The burden and outcome of dehydration among U.S. elderly, *Am J Public Health* 84:1265, 1994.

Wasson JH, Bruskewitz RC: Disorders of the lower genitourinary tract: bladder, prostate, testes. In Abrams WB, Beers MH, Berkow R, editors: *The Merck manual of geriatrics,* Rahway, NJ, 1990, Merck Sharpe & Dohme Research Laboratories.

Weinberg AD, Minaker KL, and the Council on Scientific Affairs, American Medical Association: Dehydration: evaluation and management in older adults, *JAMA* 274(19):1552, 1995.

Wells T, Brink C: Helpful equipment, *Geriatr Nurs* 1:264, 1980.

Wyman JF, Hawkins SW, Fantl JA: Psychosocial impact of urinary incontinence in the community dwelling population, *J Am Geriatr Soc* 38:282, 1990.

12

Rest, Sleep, and Activity in the Aged

▶LEARNING OBJECTIVES

Upon completion of this chapter, the reader will be able to:

- Identify age-related changes that affect rest, sleep, and activity.
- List the types of outcomes that occur because of age-related changes in rest, sleep, and activity.
- Describe nursing assessment relevant to rest, sleep, and activity.
- Explain nursing interventions useful in the promotion of rest, sleep, and activity.

▶GLOSSARY

Circadian rhythm The regular recurrence of certain phenomena in cycles of approximately 24 hours.
Dyssomnia Bad or difficult sleep.
Hypersomnia Excessive sleep or drowsiness.
Insomnia Inability to fall asleep easily or to remain asleep throughout the night.
Isometrics Active exercise performed against stable resistance without change in length of the muscle.
Isotonics Active exercise without appreciable change in force of muscular contraction, with shortening of the muscle.

Myoclonus Shocklike contractions of a part of a muscle, an entire muscle, or a group of muscles.
Non–rapid eye movement (NREM) sleep The first four stages of sleep.
Parasomnia Interruption of sleep as a result of disruptive physiologic conditions (e.g., restless leg syndrome).
Rapid eye movement (REM) sleep A wakeful and active form of sleep during which dreaming or tension is discharged.
Sleep apnea Temporary cessation of breathing during sleep.
Sundowning Describes behavior of one who habitually becomes confused or disoriented in the evening.

▶THE LIVED EXPERIENCE

You know, I never get a decent night's sleep. I wake up at least four times every night, and I just know I won't get back to sleep. I really don't want to keep taking pills for sleep, but when I lie there awake, I just think of all the difficult times and situations I can't manage. After a while, I'm really in a stew about everything.

Richard, a 67-year-old recent retiree

This is really beginning to tire me out. Richard keeps waking me at night because he can't sleep. I try to tell him to get up and read or something. I really need my sleep if I'm going to get to work on time. I wonder if Richard needs to see a doctor. Maybe he is depressed about being retired and alone while I'm at work. I'll talk to him about it.

Clara, Richard's wife

*R*est, sleep, and activity are dependent on each other. Inadequacy of rest and sleep affects activity, whether it is strenuous or performing activities of daily living. Activity is necessary to maintain physical and physiologic integrity, such as cardiopulmonary endurance and function, musculoskeletal strength, agility, and structure, and it helps a person obtain adequate sleep. Rest, sleep, and activity greatly contribute to overall physical and mental well-being.

REST AND SLEEP

The human organism needs rest and sleep to conserve energy, prevent fatigue, provide organ respite, and relieve tension. Sleep is an extension of rest, and both are physiologic and mental necessities for survival. Rest depends on the degree of physical and mental relaxation. It is often assumed that lying in bed constitutes rest, but worries and other related stressors cause muscles throughout the body to continue to contract with tension even though physical activity has ceased. Attainment of rest depends on the interrelationship of psyche and soma. Body functions possess refractory times and rest periods in the continuous cycle of activity (biorhythms). Drastically or continually altered sleep and rest cycles disrupt homeostatic balance and create physical or mental aberration.

Rest "par excellence" (Henderson, Nite, 1978) is sleep that occurs for sustained, unbroken periods. Sleep is restorative and recuperative and is necessary for the preservation of life. Contrary to popular belief, sleep does not significantly decrease with age. A healthy adult sleeps 4 to 10 hours in a 24-hour period, with the average elder sleeping approximately 6.5 hours in a 24-hour period (Moiser et al, 1998). Because of changes in the circadian rhythm, older adults may experience a decrease in sleep hours with age.

Biorhythm and Sleep

Our lives are a series of rhythms that influence and regulate physiologic function, chemical concentrations, performance, behavioral responses, moods, and the ability to adapt. The most obvious rhythm is the day-night cycle known as *diurnal* or *circadian rhythm.*

The most important and obvious biorhythm is the circadian sleep-wake rhythm. Abnormalities of this endogenous cycle may be responsible for some of the difficulties of old age. Gerontologists are beginning to seriously study the relevance of age-related changes in circadian rhythms to health and the process of aging. It is clear that body temperature, pulse, blood pressure, neurotransmitter excretion, and hormonal levels change significantly and predictably in a circadian rhythm. In old age there is a reduction in the amplitude of all of these circadian endogenous responses.

Cycles also exist that are less than 24 hours (infradian) or longer than 24 hours (ultradian). Rhythms can be disrupted by time zone changes, varying work schedules, and physical conditions. Alterations in the usual sleep-wake cycle—sleeping during the day and wakefulness at night—can signal serious illnesses.

Institutions that provide care for the aged adhere to specific time schedules, which may not correspond to the biorhythm of the aged person and which may place the individual out of synchronization with his or her body functions. Attention to biorhythms can help establish the normal sleep-wake pattern of the aged person and identify the best times to introduce activities, periods of rest, and therapeutic measures.

Normal Sleep Pattern

The mystery of sleep has been researched for more than 30 years. The body progresses through the five stages of the normal sleep pattern consisting of rapid eye movement (REM) sleep and non–rapid eye movement (NREM) sleep (Kleitman, 1960; Jouvet, 1967). One third of life is spent in sleep; REM sleep consumes 20% to 25% of sleep time; stage I sleep, 5%; stage II, 50% to 55%; stage III, 10%; and stage IV, 10% (Henderson, Nite, 1978). Webb (1982) estimates the amount of wake time for the aged after sleep onset to be about $2^{1}/_{2}$ times greater after age 60 for stage I sleep, with little change in REM and stage II sleep time. Lerner (1982) indicates that stage IV sleep time is reduced 50% by age 50. The number of awakenings increases from one or two to six per night (Webb, 1982; Bixler, Vela-Bueno, 1987).

Two phases of sleep, REM and stage IV, have received the most attention and study. Sleep begins with a nodding or dropping off to sleep (stage I, NREM), which is characterized by easy arousal by noise, touch, or other varied stimuli. If awakened, the individual does not realize that dozing has occurred and would describe the state as being similar to daydreaming. At times, as stage I is entered, the individual is awakened by muscle jerks or by the sensation of falling, which is a phenomenon attributed to initial muscle relaxation. If the individual is undisturbed, stage II is quickly entered, followed by stage III, a period of medium-deep sleep; stage IV, deep sleep from which arousal is extremely difficult, soon follows. From the stage of deepest sleep, the individual ascends to the level of REM sleep, which resembles the sleep pattern of stage I. REM sleep occurs four or five times each night but is most prominent in the early-morning hours; it is a more wakeful and active form of sleep, in which mounting excitement and tension are discharged.

REM (dreaming) sleep facilitates the release of emotional tension and working through mental issues and serves to nourish and aid metabolism of the central nervous system, a necessity for well-being. Deprivation of REM sleep has been shown to produce irritability, anxiousness, and, on occasion, truly disturbed behavior such as hallucinations and psychosis. Stage IV NREM sleep is a nightly occurrence that is essential for restoring the well-being of the body's physiologic processes. This sleep period is characterized by the depth of sleep and the difficulty of arousal. Individuals deprived of stage IV sleep report feelings of depression, general body malaise, apathy, and general lethargy. Stage IV, considered the restorative stage of sleep, is markedly reduced in the aged.

NREM sleep is predominantly a quiet period when body secretions in the nose, mouth, throat, eyes, stomach, and bile tract are minimal; small intestine motility is reduced; the heart rate slows and systolic pressure is diminished; the basal metabolic rate is low; there is generalized muscle relaxation; body temperature falls; breathing is slower and more shallow; and there is no definite eye position, just notable constriction of the pupils. A list of the characteristics of each stage of sleep appears in Box 12-1.

Sleep in the aged is generally characterized by numerous awakenings, periods of subdued respiration, marked temperature drops, less resilience in response to jet-lag conditions or other biorhythmic disturbances, and less stage III and stage IV (slow-wave) sleep. A small but significant number of women continue to display sustained periods of stage IV sleep, but men over 60 years of age show very little. The work of Bliwise et al (1989) suggests that slow-wave sleep decline may be a close correlate of the aging process in the central nervous system across the adult life span. This would explain significant differences observed in the sleep of old persons. Ordinarily the amount of REM sleep remains appreciably the same throughout adulthood until extreme old age, but it has been found that REM sleep declines follow the trend of reduced intellectual function and are implicated in the presence of dementia and reduced cerebral function (see Sundowner's Syndrome, p. 211). When REM sleep is decreased, the physiologic concomitants of REM sleep, such as muscle twitching and increased respirations, heart rate, and blood flow, are also suppressed. It appears that the integrity of sleep

---

Box 12-1   CHARACTERISTICS OF SLEEP STAGES

Stage I (Light Sleep)
Drops off to sleep
Relaxed
Fleeting thoughts
Easily awakened
Remembers being drowsy but not asleep

Stage II (Medium-Deep Sleep)
Enters within minutes of stage I
More relaxed
Vague, dreamlike thoughts (fragmentary dreams)
Can observe the eyes moving slowly under the eyelids
Unmistakably asleep but easily aroused

Stage III (Medium-Deep Sleep)
About 20 minutes after stage I
Muscles relaxed
Slower pulse
Decreased body temperature
Undisturbed by moderate random stimuli (doors closing, etc.)

Stage IV (Deep Sleep)
Restorative sleep
Very relaxed
Rarely moves
Awakens only with vigorous stimuli
Period during which most sleepwalking, screaming, nightmares, and bedwetting occur
Lasts 10 to 20 minutes

REM Sleep (Active Sleep)
Relieves tensions
Drifts up from stage IV every 90 to 100 minutes (REM sleep resembles stage I by electroencephalogram monitoring)
Rapid eye movement
Head and neck lose tonus, body feels flaccid
Increased and fluctuating pulse, blood pressure, and respirations
Most dreaming and sleep talking occur
When medical crisis occurs (e.g., angina, dyspnea), most often because of anxiety or fear induced by dreams

REM, Rapid eye movement.

---

patterns not only is indicative of central nervous system status but also may conversely be significant in the maintenance of central nervous system integrity. Persons with pulmonary and cardiac disorders may be severely compromised during REM sleep.

Quality of Sleep

"Good" or "poor" sleep is a subjective judgment based on body position, movement, and personal opinion. One may appear to sleep "well," as nurses' notes frequently record, based on closed eyes and no movement in the bed, but other factors are significant in determining sleep quality.

Good sleepers have been described as registering a normal body temperature on awakening and less of a temperature drop in stage IV sleep than do poor sleepers. Those who sleep poorly have body temperatures that do not rapidly return to normal by the time they awaken. The question arises whether those who are poor sleepers have a different time sequence or rhythm that is longer than the established circadian rhythm. Those with a physiologic rhythm that is not synchronous with the local time clock may sleep longer and arise later than is socially convenient. This is true in institutional settings that have specific schedules; thus an individual's body time may lag behind clock time. Ancoli-Israel et al (1986, 1989) found that nursing home patients' sleep was more fragmented and averaged an hour longer than that of independently living elders. Sleep patterns can be disturbed when REM sleep is altered or stopped through the administration of sedatives and hypnotics or by repeated awakening, such as for monitoring of vital signs and administration of nighttime procedures and medications.

The quality of sleep deteriorates with age. Most older people do not have a problem falling asleep but experience difficulty in staying asleep. Often when asked about the quality of sleep, the aged respond with remarks or complaints that they hardly slept the night. Sleep of the aged is more fragmented than that of the young. Frequent and long periods of wakefulness occur during the night. These interruptions may be a result of nocturnal micturition; leg cramps (usually in men); nightmares (characteristic of women); mental stimulation through worry, bereavement, or extraneous noises in the environment; medical conditions (e.g., cardiac and musculoskeletal); or use of over-the-counter and/or prescription drugs (Moiser et al, 1998). Women tend to go to bed earlier than men, but both rise later than younger adults in the morning. Monk et al (1991) noted that elders had an earlier habitual time of awakening and a circadian orientation associated with longer sleep in the morning. Older people spend more total time in bed to achieve the same amount of restorative sleep that they had in their younger years. Ancoli-Israel et al (1989) found that the institutionalized elderly spent substantially more time in bed to obtain the same amount of sleep as independent elders. There is

scarcely an hour that goes by without the elder awakening, with the subsequent loss of deep, restorative sleep (Lerner, 1982).

Sleep complaints of the elderly are numerous. Data on the majority of sleep problems of the elderly were obtained through questionnaires (Frisoni et al, 1993). Using a qualitative approach to study sleep complaints of the elderly, Floyd (1993) identified four themes concerning factors contributing to sleep problems: (1) physical pain or bodily discomfort; (2) external environmental factors—noises, poor-quality air, or uncomfortable room temperature; (3) emotional discomforts; and (4) changes in the sleep pattern—longer time to fall asleep, awakening after falling asleep, difficulty in returning to sleep, or awakening in the morning earlier than desired. Floyd found that the qualitative findings were similar to the quantitative results of the study.

It was thought at one time that the aged needed more sleep, but this is not necessarily true. The aged seem to sleep less. If an elder sleeps more, it is usually because of boredom, sedation, or symptoms of disease conditions such as uremia or cardiac or renal failure (Prinz et al, 1990). Long periods of sedation can reverse sleep patterns, causing the aged to sleep during the day and be awake at night. Discontinuation of sedation can reestablish the aged person's sleep pattern. Often the aged are lonely, cold, and bored and go to bed about 6:00 or 7:00 in the evening. When they awaken in the early-morning hours, they do not understand why sleep does not return. To them, this constitutes insomnia. The changes that occur with aging are summarized in Box 12-2.

Box 12-2   AGE-RELATED SLEEP CHANGES

Total sleep time decreases until age 80, then increases slightly.

Time in bed increases after age 65.

Onset to sleep is lengthened (>30 minutes in about 32% of women and 15% of men).

Awakenings are frequent, increasing after age 50 (>30 minutes of wakefulness after sleep onset in over 50% of older subjects).

Naps are more common, although only about 10% of elders report daily napping.

Sleep is subjectively and objectively lighter (more stage I, less stage IV, more disruptions).

Frequency of abnormal breathing events is increased.

Frequency of leg movements during sleep is increased.

Dyssomnias

Insomnia

Of the 13 million persons over age 65, more than half of those residing at home and two thirds of those in long-term care facilities complain of insomnia (National Institutes of Health, 1996). Spiegel et al (1990) cite that one in three persons age 65 or older complains of insomnia. Old people with minimal environmental stimulation or who doze for extended periods of time during the day are prone to insomnia. The prevalence of insomnia is difficult to document because *insomnia* has a number of definitions, depending on who is defining it. Generally, insomnia is considered to be the inability to sleep despite the desire to do so (Prinz et al, 1990; Vitiello et al, 1992).

The elderly are particularly susceptible to insomnia because of changing sleep patterns, particularly in stage IV, or deep, sleep. Complaints concerning insomnia include inability to fall asleep, frequent awakenings, inability to return to sleep, and early-morning arousal.

Insomnia is a symptom. Successful resolution depends on understanding and addressing the individual's special mix of contributing factors, including biologic, medical, and emotional factors, as well as bad habits. Insomnia may be short term, transient, or chronic. Short-term insomnia results from environmental changes, stress, anxiety, or depression. Resolution occurs without medical intervention when the individual adapts to the changes or removes them. Transient insomnia is similar to short-term insomnia but generally lasts 1 to 3 weeks. Chronic insomnia comprises sleep problems lasting more than 3 weeks or recurring throughout one's life. Chronic insomnia occurs most frequently in persons with psychiatric disorders, chronic drug and alcohol dependency, dementia, or serious physical illnesses or conditions. This form of insomnia requires concentrated medical and/or psychiatric attention. These disorders are described in the manual of the International Classification of Sleep Disorders Diagnosis and Coding (ISCD) under the classification of dyssomnias, parasomnias, or medical-psychiatric sleep disorders (Beck-Little, Weinrich, 1998).

Hypersomnia

Persons who have hypersomnia routinely sleep more than 8 to 9 hours in a 24-hour period and complain that they sleep excessively. The individual may state, or the family or nurse may observe, that the person exhibits persistent daytime drowsiness, appears in a drugged state, has sleep "attacks," or seems to be in a comatose state or experiences postencephalitic drowsiness (Dement et al, 1982). The client complains of weakness, fatigue, and learning and memory difficulties.

Sleep Apnea

Sleep apnea syndrome is a disorder characterized by repetitive cessation of respiration during sleep. Sleep apnea is considered widespread among those over age 60. According to Kotagal and Dement (1985), approximately 35% of adults over age 60 experience sleep apnea. Of nursing home residents, 42% had 5 or more episodes of apnea per hour of sleep; 4% of 427 elders at home had 20 or more episodes of apnea per hour (Ancoli-Israel et al, 1989).

Recognition of this disorder is usually through the symptoms of snoring, interrupted breathing of at least 10 seconds, and unusual daytime sleepiness. Medical illness such as congestive heart failure raises the incidence of patients with 10 or more episodes of apnea per hour to 21% of hospitalized elders over age 65. Sleep apnea has been linked with high relative risk of nonhemorrhagic cerebral infarction, angina pectoris, congestive heart failure, pulmonary hypertension, and hypertension. It is recognized as a significant factor for mortality among the elderly. McGinty et al (1988) studied events associated with sleep apnea that may alter nocturnal circulatory function among the elderly. Hypotensive episodes were found to occur among subjects and were associated with hemoglobin desaturation below 80% (secondary to sleep-related breathing disorders) and elevated supine nasopharyngeal airway resistance. These researchers suggest that sympathetic reflexes may be impaired, permitting hypotension and risk of circulatory failure in some elderly persons.

Sleep apnea may occur in individuals who may not have any respiratory problem while awake. During sleep, breathing may be interrupted as many as 300 times and apneic episodes may last from 10 to 90 seconds (Oesting, Manza, 1988). It is thought that sleep apnea occurs for two reasons:

1. Central nervous system mechanisms in which thoracic breathing movements cease cause a complete absence of ventilatory effort and a constant intrathoracic pressure. Respiration resumes when a person is aroused. Central apnea is associated with brainstem disorders and bulbar damage or is idiopathic.

2. Oropharyngeal membranes collapse or are obstructed by excess tissue. Individuals make increasingly greater attempts to breathe against the obstruction until air is forced through the upper airway with a loud snorting sound. Obstructive apnea is associated with hypertrophy of adenotonsillar or buccal tissue or may be idiopathic (Fernandes, Strollo, 1998).

Persons most likely to have sleep apnea are adult men with a long history of loud, intermittent snoring. Hypertension and cardiac dysrhythmias are common, and persons who have had a stroke may be at increased risk. Commonly these individuals have upper body obesity and short, thick necks of ≥17 inches (Oesting, Manza, 1988; Fernandes, Strollo, 1998).

Another group of patients at risk for sleep apnea are individuals diagnosed with Alzheimer's disease. These patients have been found to have a significantly higher proportion of sleep apnea than healthy elderly persons (Hoch et al, 1987). Those patients with Alzheimer's disease who had sleep apnea had significantly more awake time during the course of the night than patients with Alzheimer's disease who did not experience apnea. Hoch et al (1987) also found that the higher the level of dementia, the greater the severity of apnea experienced by patients with Alzheimer's disease. One wonders if the long-range effects of cerebral anorexia during apneic attacks contribute to the dementia.

Symptoms of sleep apnea include loud and periodic snoring; broken sleep with frequent nocturnal waking; and unusual nighttime activity, such as sitting upright, sleepwalking, or falling out of bed. It seems that additional symptoms such as memory changes, depression, excessive daytime sleepiness, morning headaches, nocturia, and orthopnea result from sleep apnea.

Assessment. Information from the sleeping partner, as well as observation of signs and symptoms, should be noted. Assessment of patients during sleep is important. Emphasis should be placed on describing the respiratory rate, the number of apneic episodes, the length of apneic periods, and the effect of central nervous system depressants (e.g., sleeping pills). Sleep assessment is detailed later in the chapter.

Interventions. Specific treatment of sleep apnea may involve weight loss, surgery to remove redundant tissue, or medical management. The most effective treatment, but one that is followed by only 50% of the individuals for whom it is prescribed, is a continuous positive airway pressure (CPAP) mask worn at night over the nose and attached to a compressor. Room air under high pressure is delivered by mask to maintain an open airway. Persons are counseled to avoid drugs with analeptic effects, particularly alcohol. Anything that interferes with the arousal response is exceedingly dangerous. Use of extra pillows or sleeping in a chair is sometimes helpful. Ordinarily the individual has quite spontaneously made compensatory adjustments during sleeping hours.

Parasomnias

Nocturnal Myoclonus

Nocturnal myoclonus is the syndrome of periodic leg jerks or movements in sleep. It is diagnosed when the number of periodic leg jerks or movements is equal to or greater than five per hour of sleep (Ancoli-Israel, Kripke, 1986; Herrera, 1990). As many as 40% of persons over age 65 experience this disorder. The stereotypic movements consist of flexion of the hip, knee, and ankle with extension of the toes, which occurs sometimes as often as every 20 to 40 seconds during sleep or occurs in clusters (Johnston, 1994; Beck-Little, Weinrich, 1998). The incidence of this syndrome increases with age and is estimated to affect 44% of those over age 65 (Montplaisier et al, 1994). Because of the repeated awakenings from this condition, complaints of insomnia and excessive daytime sleepiness occur. It is thought that nocturnal myoclonus is associated with sleep apnea. It is, however, more common in association with chronic renal failure and tricyclic antidepressants (Kales et al, 1990). Johnston (1994) indicates that individuals with signs and symptoms of this condition should be referred to a sleep disorder clinic for specific diagnosis and treatment.

Restless Leg Syndrome

The major difference between this syndrome and nocturnal myoclonus is when the leg movement occurs. Restless leg syndrome is characterized by a nonpainful dysesthesia of the lower leg, described as a pulling, creeping, or crawling sensation that is often associated only with rest. The discomfort interferes with sleep onset. Relief is obtained by movement of the legs. Exercise during the day may relieve the movements (Johnston, 1994). The individual should be referred to a sleep disorder clinic for specific diagnosis and treatment (Beck-Little, Weinrich, 1998).

Sleep Disorders Associated With Medical Problems

Many medical problems cause sleep disturbance in the older adult (Table 12-1). These include cardiovascular diseases, diabetes, gastrointestinal reflux, and arthritis, to mention a few. Cardiovascular disease can manifest with nocturnal cardiac ischemia and may result in alteration in respiration or transient angina, thus causing frequent awakenings. Diabetes may contribute to nightmares or early-morning awakening as a result of the fluctuation in blood glucose levels. Gastric reflux (gastroesophageal reflux disease [GERD]) attributable to the slow acid move-

Table 12-1

Causes, Reasons/Symptoms, Assessment, and Interventions for Sleep Alterations in the Aged

Causes	Reasons/symptoms	Assessment	Potential/actual interventions
Alcoholism	Abnormal EEG pattern results as effects wear off; sleeper may awaken with withdrawal symptoms and a hangover; early-morning awakening	Sleep log and interview with bed partner or caregiver	No alcoholic beverages; explain that reformed alcoholics may experience insomnia a year or so after withdrawal of alcohol; may require temporary medication to relieve symptoms that interfere with sleep
Alzheimer's disease (AD)	AD patients' sleep shows reduction in stage III and stage IV sleep early in disease; late in AD, these stages disappear; daytime sleepiness increases as disease progresses; nighttime wandering; sundowning	Sleep history from family or caregivers	Assist family and/or staff with wandering behavior and sundowning syndrome; major tranquilizers may be needed; be sure person has comfortable chair in which to rest; strict schedule of nighttime bed hours, daytime naps, and activity periods and attendance to needs; for wanderers and behavior problems, stop all drug treatment to see if normal sleep rhythm returns
Anxiety	A feeling of dread, doom, or uneasiness; pacing, irritable, fidgety; stomach or nerve trouble	Psychosocial history; 24-hour sleep diary; Hamilton scale	Supportive care; explain new routines and treatments; encourage decision making; support previous life-style
Arthritis	Early-morning awakening secondary to pain of muscle/joint stiffness; wearing off of pain medication	Medical history; sleep history	Sustained-release analgesic 30 minutes before sleep; provide comfortable pillows to support joints; careful use of electric blankets for warmth
Cardiovascular	Frequent awakenings, nocturia	Medical history; sleep history	Sustained-release nitroglycerin; nitroglycerin at bedside; take diuretic in morning; restrict fluids close to bedtime; prop up on pillows
Cognitive deficit	Agitation at bedtime; nighttime wandering	Folstein Mini-Mental State Examination; psychologic history; at times, physical examination	Antipsychotic medications; structure environment
Chronic obstructive pulmonary disease (COPD)	Abnormal increase in alveolar tension; decrease in oxygen saturation; prone position causes dyspnea and stasis of mucus	Medical history; sleep history	Patient education regarding self-care; pulmonary toilet before bedtime; use of bronchial dilators; need to prevent fatigue; rest during day; no diuretics in late afternoon; need to avoid cola, coffee, tea, chocolate; need to use caution with sedatives and OTC medication

Modified from Ebersole P, Hess, P: *Toward healthy aging: human needs and nursing response,* ed 5, St Louis, 1998, Mosby, and Beck-Little R, Weinrich SP: Assessment and management of sleep disorders in the elderly, *J Gerontol Nurs* 24(4):21, 1998.
SSRI, Selective serotonin reuptake inhibitors; *EEG,* electroencephalogram; *OTC,* over the counter; *REM,* rapid eye movement; *NREM,* non–rapid eye movement.

Continued

Table 12-1—cont'd

Causes, Reasons/Symptoms, Assessment, and Interventions for Sleep Alterations in the Aged

Causes	Reasons/symptoms	Assessment	Potential/actual interventions
Depression	Difficulty falling asleep, sustaining sleep, or early-morning awakening; feelings of helplessness, hopelessness, or sadness; decreased energy, low self-esteem; withdrawal; confusion or disorientation; history of recent loss	Psychosocial history; medical history and history of current medication use (prescribed and OTC; Beck Depression Inventory	Counseling; SSRIs or tricyclic antidepressants if depression confirmed; socialization, reminiscence
Diabetes mellitus	Early-morning awakening secondary to hypoglycemia; unpleasant dreams or nightmares; nocturia	Medical history; sleep history; eating schedule; fasting blood glucose levels	Carbohydrate bedtime snack; reevaluate medication regimen (oral hypoglycemic agent or insulin)
Disturbed sensory perception	Early-morning awakening; poor environmental lighting; visual difficulties; nocturnal hallucinations; alteration in REM-NREM cycle	Medical history, check hearing and vision; sleep history	Modify environment; check hearing aid; put glasses nearby; reduce noise in home or hospital; frequent reassurance
Gastrointestinal reflux (GERD)	Difficulty falling asleep or early-morning awakening secondary to abdominal or chest discomfort due to gastric secretions	Medical history; sleep history	Restrict intake after evening meal; antacid medication 2 hours before bedtime; elevate head and shoulders for sleeping; ensure that medication for reflux is taken appropriately (e.g., H_2 inhibitors, acid pump inhibitors, promotility agents)
Obstructive sleep apnea (OSA)	Frequent awakenings with nocturia; snoring; morning headache; unusual daytime drowsiness or sleepiness; frequent daytime naps	24-hour sleep diary; interview bed partner; clinical sleep studies (polysomnography)	Continuous positive airway pressure via mask; weight loss; surgery
Parkinson disease	Difficulty with sleep in general; total wake time increases; decreased REM sleep	Medical history; 24-hour sleep diary	Levodopa (L-Dopa) at bedtime may help decrease rigidity that occurs during night
Peptic ulcers	Periodic awakenings when in REM sleep (gastric juices increase during REM sleep, causing epigastric pain)	Medical history	Take appropriate prescribed medication
Periodic limb movement disorder	Frequent awakenings; nocturnal restlessness; muscle soreness; daytime fatigue	Interview bed partner; medication history; clinical sleep studies (polysomnography)	Administration of prescribed medications such as benzodiazepines

Continued

Table 12-1—cont'd

Causes, Reasons/Symptoms, Assessment, and Interventions for Sleep Alterations in the Aged

Causes	Reasons/symptoms	Assessment	Potential/actual interventions
Restless leg syndrome	Difficulty falling asleep; crawling, pulling sensation in legs, especially at night when sitting or lying down	Sleep history; medication history	Vitamin E; quinine tablets or capsules or quinine water (tonic water); low-dose narcotic analgesics
Situational insomnia	Difficulty falling asleep and staying asleep on admission to institution; after visiting a relative; after moving to a new residence; after recent loss or death; change in nighttime routine	Usually transient but helpful to get a brief sleep history	Establish a one-to-one relationship; if necessary, use hypnotics for short term only (e.g., 1 week)
Surgical procedures	Premature arousal related to blood drawn in early morning; anxiety, worry about outcome and pain		Analyze rituals and routines in place; can they be changed? Keep pain free; monitor vital signs frequently and promote rest

ment resulting from depressed swallowing and salivation during sleep may cause chest or abdominal pain. Musculoskeletal pain of arthritis, which usually occurs early in the morning, may result in early-morning awakening. Musculoskeletal pain tends to be the most common complaint related to sleep (Floyd, 1993). In a large study of community-dwelling elders, poor self-rated health and the presence of chronic conditions were associated with complaints of poor sleeping (Blazer et al, 1995).

Sleep Disorders Related to Psychiatric Problems

Anxiety, depression, and cognitive deficits are responsible for inability to fall asleep, awaking and not being able to return to sleep, or early-morning awakening (see Table 12-1). Life events of the elderly, such as loss of a spouse, situational disruptions, retirement, and change in living arrangements, often result in anxiety and depression. Cognitive deficits are often accompanied by altered sleep patterns. Alzheimer's disease frequently results in impaired sleep continuity (Bliwise et al, 1995). Daytime sleep hours seem to increase as nighttime sleep decreases in elders with cognitive impairment, decreased physical activity, and neurologic lesions (Meguro et al, 1995).

Sundowner's Syndrome

The term *sundowner's syndrome* describes behavior; the syndrome is not a disease. Sundowning is recurring confusion and exacerbation of disruptive behavior and agitation in the late afternoon or early evening. It has also been called *nocturnal delirium* (Duckett, Scotto, 1992). Sundowning is a temporary condition but is disruptive and dangerous when it occurs. Elderly persons may wander out of a home or a facility, or the caregiver may become sleep deprived trying to cope with the night behavior. This presents a major problem to nursing staff in acute care and long-term care facilities. As the name implies, sundowner's syndrome is generally associated with an occurrence in the late afternoon and early evening. Limited research has documented the time of occurrence. In a pilot study conducted by Beel-Bates and Rogers (1990) the activity of patients with dementia and those without dementia was quite different between 4:00 and 6:30 PM. Subjects with dementia increased their activity, whereas those without dementia decreased their activity.

The causes of sundowning, based on the limited research in this area, have been grouped by Duckett (1993) as psychologic, environmental, and physiologic. A combination of variables in these three groups is supported. Karl et al (cited in Duckett, Scotto, 1992) argue that psychosocial stressors in conjunction with impaired cognitive function may account for sundowning. Evans (1985) presents the idea that sundowning is a result of brain hypoxia caused by biologic or biochemical factors, such as the effects of drugs, cardiovascular disorders, or dehydration; sensory overload or deprivation; circadian rhythm disruption; psychologic stress; isolation; fear; influence of the lunar cycle; and the weather.

Satlin et al (1992) found that pulsating bright light ameliorated the sundowning behavior of some patients with Alzheimer's disease. The study speculated that the pulsating bright light changed the sleep-wake cycle disturbance. The effect may be attributed to mediation in the chronobiologic mechanism.

Assessment and interventions. Assessment of an individual for risk factors includes age and history of delirium or sundowning, cardiovascular disease or dementia, polypharmacy, and electrolyte imbalance. Nursing measures might include providing environment-orienting cues, minimizing the relocation of a person within a nursing facility, frequent nighttime monitoring, turning on the lights before dark, and offering soft music or social stimulation in the late afternoon. Wallace (1994) studied the outcome of providing specialized training of nurse aides that incorporated a background understanding of the syndrome and approaches to deal with it. The total number of sundowning behaviors decreased after the educational program. Although the study was limited by sample size, the findings do support the need for interventions.

Duckett (1993) presents a decision-making flow chart for intervening with the sundowning patient based on the research to date. The first questions to be answered are related to the existence of dementia and reversible medical condition(s). Staff-patient conflict is evaluated next. Then the physical environment, social environment, and psychologic status of the patient are assessed and interventions planned.

Vitiello et al (1992) suggest restriction of daytime sleep, which may lead to better night sleep, and exposure to bright light. If all else fails, the use of neuroleptics (such as haloperidol) or thioridazine is recommended. However, long-term use of these drugs has major sequelae, and monitoring of the individual's responses is needed.

Naps

Napping is a sequence of sleeping and waking from less deep sleep. It is a normal pattern that seems to increase with age and is indicative of a different distribution of sleep; one should not worry about napping.

There tends to be a correlation between age and the length of napping: the older the person, the longer the nap (Hayter, 1985). An increased frequency of daytime napping in elders may indicate a change in circadian rhythm (Buysse et al, 1992). Naps tend to peak in late afternoon. In a pilot study of geriatric patients in a rehabilitation hospital, Creighton (1995) found that afternoon drowsiness was decreased by a nap, making therapy more effective.

Napping is not an attempt to compensate for sleep lost at night. Sleep and napping are independent of each other (Hayter, 1985). Naps augment sleep and increase the total amount slept. Afternoon naps provide deep sleep, a necessity for physical rest. It is speculated that the individual may need napping to restore energy. Napping may be based more on physical health, psychologic health, and volitional factors, which may mediate daytime sleepiness (Buysse et al, 1992).

The average nap lasts from 15 to 60 minutes; this usually occurs several times a day. In a study of 14 healthy elderly subjects, Evans and Rogers (1994) found that all took one or more naps during the daytime. Yet napping time composed only a small fraction of their total sleep time—an average of 60 minutes. These subjects took frequent, yet short naps of less than 10 minutes.

Sleep and Drugs

Institutions and the aged themselves disrupt sleep quality and patterns and attempt to counteract this by administering sleeping medications. People age 60 and older consume the majority of sleep medications. Often nurses think they are helping the aged person who is awake most of the night to get a "good night's rest" by giving medication. However, few hypnotic drugs are compatible with the normal sleep cycle. Instead, these drugs depress the REM sleep necessary for the relief of mental stress, such as tension and anxiety. When medication is discontinued, there may be a rebound period of insomnia before normal sleep patterns return. Dreaming and nightmares are also increased until natural sleep cycles are reestablished. Some researchers believe that this compensates for dreams that have been depressed or obliterated by REM sleep suppression.

Drug tolerance, physical dependence, daytime delirium, drowsiness, and depression of mental alertness occur with chronic use of bedtime hypnotic agents. Some major tranquilizers (used at bedtime for their sedating side effects) and sedatives are responsible for loss of equilibrium. Hypnotic drugs often induce night terrors, hallucinations, and such paradoxical responses as agitation instead of relaxation; hangover; depression; and changes in memory, balance, and gait. If hypnotic drugs are necessary, those that are the least disruptive to the sleep cycle should be used. A number of prescribed and over-the-counter agents have effects on sleep even if the agent is being taken for an unrelated condition. Table 12-2 presents commonly used medications and their sleep-related effects on the aged.

Patients should be treated nonpharmacologically before any medication is prescribed. Jenkins's classic study (1976) reported that elderly patients in her fa-

cility were not given routinely prescribed sleeping medication; rather, nursing actions were substituted. Since that time, many facilities have also done so quite successfully. Few patients needed sleep medication if attention was given to specific bedtime needs and rituals. Tablaski et al (1998) describe a procedure for the withdrawal of sleep medication in women who were long-term users of sedatives and hypnotics. The women's medication was reduced by half for a week or two and then eliminated altogether. The change in bedtime ritual can precipitate or aggravate insomnia, so an inert replacement capsule or tablet was substituted to maintain the nightly routine of taking some-

Table 12-2

Sleep-Related Effects of Commonly Used Medications by the Aged

Therapeutic category	Sample drugs	Common sleep-related effect(s)
Antiparkinson agents	Amantadine HCl (Symmetrel) Pergolide mesylate (Permax)	Somnolence, insomnia, dizziness, anxiety, confusion, orthostatic hypotension
Agents for Alzheimer's disease	Donepezil HCl (Aricept)	Insomnia, fatigue, muscle cramps
Asthma preparations	Theophylline (Marax) Albuterol (Ventolin)	Hypertension, insomnia, headache, dizziness
Cardiovascular agents	Acebutolol (Sectral) Diltiazem HCl Guanfacine HCl (Tenex) Nifedipine (Procardia) Captopril (Capoten) Digoxin (Lanoxin)	Somnolence, insomnia, hallucinations, fatigue, headache, hypotension, dizziness
Combined diuretics	Hydrocholorothiazide-triamterene (Dyazide, Maxide)	Dizziness, somnolence, insomnia, fatigue, headache
Conjugated estrogens	Conjugated estrogen (Premarin)	Headache, migraine, depression
H₂ blockers	Ranitidine (Zantac)	Headache, malaise, insomnia
Mood disorders	Amitriptyline (Elavil)	Drowsiness, CNS overstimulation, confusion, dry mouth, blurred vision
Muscle relaxants	Cyclobenzaprine (Flexeril)	Drowsiness, dizziness, blurred vision, ataxia, vertigo, hypotension, headache
NSAIDs	Indomethacin (Indocin) Ketoprofen (Orudis) Naproxen (Naprosyn, Aleve)	Dizziness, drowsiness, headache, heartburn, dyspepsia, GI bleeding, peptic ulcers, CNS disturbance
Psychotropics	Alprazolam (Xanax) Clozapine (Clozaril) Fluoxetine HCl (Prozac)	CNS depression, drowsiness, paradoxical excitation, hypotension, headache, ataxia, somnolence, insomnia, sedation

HCl, Hydrochloride; *CNS,* central nervous system; *NSAIDs,* nonsteroidal antiinflammatory drugs; *GI,* gastrointestinal.

thing. The outcome indicated no significant complaints of sleep problems. This suggests the potential for combining a planned withdrawal that includes the following:

- Carefully assess the long-term user for readiness to stop the medication.
- Examine the nighttime ritual of pill taking as a necessary link to sleep.
- Substitute a non-sleep-inducing medication, such as a vitamin pill or inert medication.
- Substitute another ritual for pill taking, such as calming music or relaxation exercises.
- Offer emotional supports during the withdrawal process.
- Provide careful clinical monitoring for withdrawal effects and increased complaints about the quality of sleep.

Melatonin, which is classified as a dietary supplement, has been the topic of talk shows and numerous popular magazines over the past several years. It has been cited not only as a sleep aid but also as an age-reversing, disease-fighting, and sex-enhancing hormone. Research supporting the use of melatonin, a hormone secreted by the pineal gland, has been conducted. Haimov et al (1994) noted that all patients with insomnia had a significantly lower sleep efficiency and a higher activity level during sleep. The elderly subjects had a 49% lower peak excretion than that in young subjects. The study suggested a relation between deficiency of melatonin or disruption of its rhythms and an increased prevalence of sleep disorders with advancing age. The researchers suggested that lack of exposure to bright light in institutions may lead to diminution of melatonin excretion in old age.

Although no side effects have been found from the use of melatonin, the long-term use and its effect on cycles, especially seasonal and lifetime events, have not been studied (Murray, 1995). If melatonin is used, 1 to 5 mg of melatonin at bedtime is recommended, with effective doses varying among individuals. Advise the client to begin with 1 mg at bedtime. If unable to fall asleep within 30 minutes, the client may take another 1 mg and continue to take 1 mg every 20 to 30 minutes up to 5 mg. If unable to go back to sleep, the client may take 1 to 3 mg to fall back asleep. It is important to remember that as a dietary supplement the manufacture of melatonin is unregulated and there are no standards for quality, purity, or dosage. The quality of the inactive fillers to form tablets or capsules and the amount of melatonin actually used in the pills may vary widely.

Assessment

Nurses are in an excellent position to assess sleep, to improve the quality of the aged person's sleep, and to study sleep or assist in sleep research by being available at customary sleep times. Sleep history interviews are important and should be obtained from all elderly clients. The nurse should learn how well the person sleeps at home, how many times the aged person is awakened at night, what time the person retires, and what rituals occur at bedtime. Rituals include bedtime snacks, watching television, listening to music, or reading—activities that unless carried out, interfere with the individual's ability to fall asleep. Other assessment data should include the amount and type of daily exercise; favorite position when in bed; room environment, including temperature, ventilation, and illumination; activities engaged in several hours before bedtime; and sleep medications, as well as other medications taken routinely. Some medications taken regularly produce side effects that interfere with the ability to sleep. Information about the individual's involvement in hobbies, life satisfaction, and perception of health status is also important in assessing for possible depression. The history should be cross-checked with the caregiver and/or family members.

A nursing standard-of-practice protocol for sleep disturbances in elderly patients was developed as part of the Nurses Improving Care of the Hospitalized Elderly (NICHE) Project, supported by a grant from the Hartford Foundation. Assessment standards are presented in Table 12-3. The assessment is focused to elicit information relative to indicators or defining characteristics of sleep disturbance.

The sleep diary or log is noted as an important part of assessment. This information will provide an accurate account of the person's sleep problem and identify the sleep disturbance. Usually a family member or the caregiver, if the aged person is institutionalized, records specific behaviors on a flow sheet. A period of 2 to 4 weeks is required to obtain a clear picture of the sleep problem. Important items to record are the following:

1. The number of times a call for assistance to the bathroom or for pain medication, or subjective symptoms of inability to sleep (such as anxiety) occur
2. If the person is out of bed
3. Whether the person appears to be asleep or awake when the nurse is on rounds
4. Episodes of confusion or disorientation
5. If sleep medication was given and if repeated
6. The time the person awakens in the morning (approximation)

Table 12-3

Nursing Standard-of-Practice Protocol: Sleep Disturbance in Elderly Patients

Assessment	Health promotion and maintenance intervention	Evaluation
SLEEP-WAKE PATTERNS	**MAINTAIN NORMAL SLEEP PATTERN**	**OBJECTIVE EVIDENCE**
Inquire about usual times for retiring and rising, time for falling asleep, frequency and duration of nighttime awakenings; frequency and duration of daytime naps; daytime physical and social activity	Maintain usual bedtime/wake time	Time required to fall asleep; should fall asleep within 30-45 minutes
	Avoid staying in bed beyond waking hours	Time for awakening, at usual reported time
	Encourage to get up at regular time even if did not sleep well	Behavior, alertness, attention, ability to concentrate, reaction time
	Schedule nighttime activities to provide uninterrupted periods of sleep of at least 2-3 hours	Observe duration of sleep: patient should remain asleep for at least 4-hour intervals
Have person provide a subjective evaluation of the quality of sleep	Balance daytime activity and rest	
Have person complete sleep log for 2 weeks	Encourage keeping daytime naps to a minimum	**SUBJECTIVE EVIDENCE**
	Promote social interaction	Verbalizations about the quality and quantity of sleep (e.g., statements of difficulty falling asleep, of frequent awakenings, of having slept well, of feeling well rested/refreshed, of an increased sense of well-being)
	Encourage exercise before evening	
BEDTIME ROUTINES/RITUALS	**SUPPORT BEDTIME ROUTINES/RITUALS**	
Inquire about activities performed by the individual before bedtime (e.g., personal hygiene, prayer, reading, watching TV, listening to music, snacks)	Offer a bedtime snack or beverage	
	Enable bedtime reading or listening to music	
	Assist with aspects of personal hygiene at bedtime (e.g., bath)	
	Encourage prayer or meditation	
	Assist in establishing a relaxing bedtime routine	
MEDICATIONS	**AVOID/MINIMIZE DRUGS THAT NEGATIVELY INFLUENCE SLEEP**	
Obtain information relative to all prescribed and self-selected over-the-counter medications used by person, especially sleep aids, diuretics, laxatives	Pharmacologic treatment of sleep disturbances is treatment of last resort	
	Discontinue or adjust the dose or dosing schedule of any/all offending medications	
Determine types of medications and length of time used by person	Consider drug-drug potentiation	
	Administer medications to promote sleep (e.g., give diuretics at least 4 hours before bedtime)	
DIET EFFECTS	**MINIMIZE/AVOID FOODS THAT NEGATIVELY INFLUENCE SLEEP**	
Obtain information about consumption of caffeinated and alcoholic beverages	Discourage use of beverages containing stimulants (e.g., coffee, tea, sodas) in afternoon and evening	
	Encourage use of food naturally containing L-tryptophan	
	Provide snacks according to patient preference	
	Generally, discourage use of alcoholic beverages	
	Decrease fluid intake 2-4 hours before bedtime	
	Encourage to have lighter meal in evening	

Modified from Forman MD, Wykle M: Nursing standard-of-practice protocol: sleep disturbances in elderly patients, *Geriatr Nurs* 16(5):238, 1995.

Continued

Table 12-3—cont'd

Nursing Standard-of-Practice Protocol: Sleep Disturbance in Elderly Patients

Assessment	Health promotion and maintenance intervention	Evaluation
ENVIRONMENTAL FACTORS	**CREATE OPTIMAL ENVIRONMENT FOR SLEEP**	
Evaluate noise, light, temperature, ventilation, bedding Inquire about distance of bathroom from bedroom Inquire about use of night-lights	Keep noise to an absolute minimum Set room temperature according to preference Provide blankets as requested Use night-light as desired Provide soft music or white noise to mask noise Encourage bed and bedroom for sleep and not other activities Use light exposure during day and evening to maintain wakefulness	
PHYSIOLOGIC FACTORS	**PROMOTE PHYSIOLOGIC STABILITY**	
Evaluate breathing pattern with sleep, with attention to pauses Observe for periodic movement or jerking during sleep Inquire about sleeping position Note diagnoses of sleep disorder Note diagnoses of specific health problems that adversely affect sleep (e.g., CHF, COPD)	Elevate head of bed as required Provide extra pillows per preference Administer bronchodilators, if prescribed, before bedtime Use medical therapeutics (e.g., continuous positive airway pressure machine) as prescribed	
ILLNESS FACTORS	**PROMOTE COMFORT**	
Inquire about pain, affective disturbances (e.g., depression, anxiety, worry, fatigue, and discomfort)	Provide analgesia as needed 30 minutes before bedtime (Note that some over-the-counter analgesics may have caffeine.) Massage back or foot to help relax Warm and cool compresses to painful areas as indicated Use relaxation methods—deep breathing, progressive relaxation, mental imagery Encourage to urinate before going to bed Keep path to bathroom clear/provide bedside commode	

CHF, Congestive heart failure; *COPD,* chronic obstructive pulmonary disease.

Interventions

Interventions begin after a thorough sleep history has been recorded and, if possible, a sleep log obtained. Interventions for sleep disturbances among the elderly have been the focus of several research studies in the past 5 years. Mornhinweg and Voignier (1995) tested the effect of music (classical music and New Age) on sleep promotion. The majority of subjects believed that the music helped them fall asleep, return to sleep quicker if awakened during the night, or sleep longer in the morning. Music allowed them to "turn off" their mind so that they could relax enough to fall asleep.

Campbell et al (1993) evaluated the efficacy of exposure to bright light in the treatment of sleep maintenance insomnia in elderly persons who had experienced a sleep disturbance for at least a year. Exposure to bright light resulted in substantial changes in sleep quality. Waking time within sleep was reduced by an hour, and sleep efficiency improved from 77.5% to 90% without altering time spent in bed. Exposure to 2 hours daily of sunlight among elderly institutionalized patients with dementia was investigated by Castor et al (1991). Overall beneficial effects from exposure to sunlight were shown by increased mean sleep hours, increased uninterrupted nighttime sleep hours, decreased nighttime wake hours, and decreased daytime sleep hours. Disrupted sleep patterns resumed in the first 24 hours after sunlight deprivation in week 3 of the study.

Bedtime routine was found by Johnson (1991) to be a factor related to sleep patterns of the elderly. Fewer sleep complaints were recorded among the elderly who maintained a bedtime routine. It is important to remember that the bedtime routine is that which is established by the individual, not by the institution.

Noise was found by Alessi et al (1995) to be at a very high level at night in the nursing home. A University of California, Los Angeles (UCLA) study was designed to promote sound slumber through a nighttime-incontinence management program coupled with noise abatement (UCLA Study, 1995). Incontinence care was provided primarily during time periods when the residents were awake. Nurse aides checked incontinent residents hourly during nighttime hours. Residents who happened to be awake were either helped to the toilet, if they desired, or were checked and changed, if necessary. Residents found sleeping after several consecutive checks were awakened to prevent incontinence as a precaution against pressure sore development. There was also an in-service training session for the staff to heighten their sensitivity to sleep and noise. Feedback on noise levels twice per nighttime shift was provided to the staff. The noise levels of telephones, buzzers, and intercom systems were reduced after 9 PM each night. Preliminary results after 2 years of testing suggested that these interventions increased the residents' average length of sleep time at night.

Progressive whole-body relaxation using controlled breathing and alternation contractions was not effective in older adults, possibly because they have more difficulty using this technique.

Intervention standards are a part of the nursing standard-of-practice protocol (see Table 12-3 for sleep disturbances [NICHE Project]). The interventions are based on the principle that to be effective, first, the intervention must be individualized, considering the specific characteristics of the patient and the nature of the sleep disturbance; and second, pharmacologic treatment should be considered an intervention of last resort. Additions were incorporated into the protocol based on a review of the literature.

Drugs should be a last resort and are not intended for long-term treatment. Rebound insomnia, as well as episodes of confusion and nightmares, is common when sleep medications are withdrawn. The key to selection of a hypnotic is to consider the half-life and the adverse effects of the agent. For example, flurazepam (Dalmane) has active metabolites, some of which have a half-life of 50 to 100 hours. Because of this half-life and the adverse effects of confusion, dizziness, and ataxia, it is not a good choice. Triazolam (Halcion), which has an intermediate onset and rapid elimination, is frequently recommended. Yet there is controversy surrounding this drug because of the adverse effects observed in the elderly. A newer drug of the imidazopyridine class is zolpidem. It has been found to be as effective as triazolam, yet with less confusion resulting. A high risk of hangover has been reported. Table 12-4 presents the characteristics of selected medications used as hypnotics in treatment of elderly patients.

Evaluation

The nursing standard-of-practice protocol presented in Table 12-3 includes an evaluation component. Observation of the person when awake and asleep is necessary. Physiologic changes observable for each stage of sleep reviewed previously can be evaluated to give clues to the phases of the sleep cycle experienced. It is essential to obtain the subjective evidence of the quality and quantity of sleep.

ACTIVITY

Activity is a direct use of energy in voluntary and involuntary physical and mental ways that alter the microenvironment and macroenvironment of the individual. The National Institutes of Health (NIH)–sponsored Consensus Development Conference on Physical Activity and Cardiovascular Health (1996) defined *physical activity*

Table 12-4

Hypnotics and Sedatives Often Prescribed for Older Adults

Medications	Class	Hypnotic efficacy	Risk of hangover	Risk of tolerance/ dependence	Other complications
Quazepam (Doral)	Benzodiazepine	Very high	Very high	High	Falls, GI distress, anticholinergic effect, paradoxical excitement
Flurazepam (Dalmane)	Benzodiazepine	Very high	Very high	High	Falls, worsens obstructive sleep apnea
Estazolam (ProSom)	Benzodiazepine	Very high	High	High	Confusion
Temazepam (Restoril)	Benzodiazepine	Very high	High	High	Falls, worsens obstructive sleep apnea
Lorazepam (Ativan)	Benzodiazepine	Very high	High	High	Confusion, potential falls, anxiety
Oxazepam (Serax)	Benzodiazepine	Very high	High	High	Worsens sleep apnea
Triazolam (Halcion)*	Benzodiazepine	Very high	Low	High	Memory disturbance
Zolpidem tartrate* (Ambien)	Nonbenzodiazepine	Very high	Low	High	Confusion
Amitriptyline (Elavil)	Tricyclic	Unpredictable	High	Low	Anticholinergic effects
Trazodone (Desyrel)	Triazolopyridine	High	High	Low	Priapism

*Have the shortest half-life of 2-4 hours; all others range from 2-4 days to 10-20 hours. Always give the older adult the lowest possible dose.

as "bodily movement produced by skeletal muscles that requires energy expenditure and produces progressive healthy benefits." *Exercise,* a type of physical activity, was defined as "a planned, structured, and repetitive bodily movement done to improve or maintain one or more components of physical fitness." Activities of daily living are another type of physical activity.

Physical activity is often the barometer by which an individual's health and wellness are judged. The inability to exercise, do physical work, or perform activities of daily living is among the first indicators of decline. Research in gerontologic exercise physiology is relatively young, but in general, results indicate that maintenance of a physically active life-style arrests or significantly delays age changes associated with cardiovascular, respiratory, and musculoskeletal function.

Public perceptions of the aged and how they spend their time continue to reflect the belief that retirement ushers in the pursuit of sedentary, private, isolated ac-

tivity and the assumption of a passive role in society. The prevalence estimates for leisure activity among those age 65 years or older in the United States are low. Thirty percent exercise regularly, and fewer than 10% exercise vigorously (Barry, Eathorne, 1994). The 1990 Behavioral Risk Factor Surveillance System found that leisure-time activity of those 65 years or older was less than that of younger age-groups. Regular walking (20 minutes three times a week) was higher for the older age-groups, with 31% of those 65 to 74 years of age and 24.3% of those 75 years or older reporting regular walking (Siegel et al, 1995). A similar finding was reported by Uriri and Thatcher-Winger (1995). Among a group of 68 volunteers who were enrolled in a community seniors' health service and who took the Healthier People Health Risk Appraisal, 38% exercised 20 minutes three times a week on a regular basis before the initiation of the project. The aged underestimate their own capacity to engage in activity, using the justification that vigorous activity is a great risk and emphasizing that light and sporadic exercise is physiologically better, or that they garden, shop, and do household chores, which is adequate activity.

Physical inactivity is a risk factor for many conditions experienced by the elderly, including obesity; diabetes; and cardiovascular, respiratory, and musculoskeletal diseases. These conditions and other changes generally attributed to aging may in fact be due to inactivity. Functional changes that are associated with inactivity include the following: (1) reduced aerobic fitness, (2) loss of postural reflexes, (3) altered lipid metabolism, (4) negative nitrogen balance, (5) loss of muscle mass, and (6) calcium extraction (Barry, Eathorne, 1994). Rather than attributing much of the functional decline seen among the elderly to the aging process, Barry and Eathorne (1994) propose a model that depicts a cycle of aging and reduced physical activity. Deconditioning, weakness, and fatigue result from the reduced physical activity. With the addition of disease, disability, and injury, there is an even greater tendency toward inactivity and further physical decline. A deterioration in the sense of wellness, resulting in poor self-esteem, anxiety, and depression, occurs. Poor motivation and a further reduction in physical activity result. This model reveals the complexity of physical activity and aging.

The benefits of exercise are well known and for the aged include maintenance of a level of functional capacity and strength to enhance self-sufficiency and independence; improvement of general life-style; maintenance of mental functional integrity; self-confidence; decreased depression; and decreased risk of medical problems. Physical benefits include improved cardiac muscle tone, decreased blood pressure, decreasing percentage of body fat, improved ability to breath deeply and effectively, reduced tension, favorable bowel control, and appetite control. Exercise is also credited as a factor in the retardation of the progress of degenerative conditions and some diseases. Donahue et al (1988) found that in persons 64 years or older, the rate of definite coronary heart disease in active men was less than half the rate experienced by those who led more sedentary lives. This early study upholds continuing observations that physical activity is beneficial to middle-age and elderly persons.

A nurse-led exercise group of 215 overweight older women reported various types of improvements as a result of the exercise (Gillett et al, 1993). The improvements reported were in range of motion, mobility, strength, sleep, bowel function, ability to manage stress, and posture. The women also reported decreased lower back and joint pain and marked increases in energy and endurance. The perception of improvements in physiologic and psychosocial areas has been substantiated in research through objective measurements.

The San Diego Adult Fitness Program, one of the few longitudinal studies on exercise and aging to date, found that maintenance of conditioning over time results in the maintenance of fitness. Also, conditioning will increase the health of sedentary individuals with low fitness to the level of moderately active persons.

Psychosocial benefits of exercise were demonstrated as early as 1975 when deVries found that the elderly who walked and maintained a heart rate of 100 beats/min had a better degree of anxiety control than a group of aged given meprobamate to control their anxiety.

Movement therapy is defined as the use of body motion and language to meet therapeutic goals such as body awareness, improved breathing patterns, increased attentiveness, increased periods of relaxation and stimulation, increased physical mobility and flexibility, increased sense of individuality, increased socialization, increased morale, and increased self-esteem of older persons (Goldberg, Fitzpatrick, 1980). Emery and Blumenthal (1990) demonstrated that adults ages 60 to 83 perceived positive changes in their lives, as well as improved physiologic outcomes, following a 4-month aerobic training program.

Range of motion was found to improve among the elderly who participated in an exercise program. The Sit and Get Fit program for sedentary older adults in a long-term care facility showed a significant improvement in shoulder, hip, and elbow range of motion among the exercisers (Kinion et al, 1993). Community-living elderly persons increased range of motion of select joints after involvement in exercise (Misner et al, 1992; Mills, 1994). Misner et al (1992) reported that the increase in range of motion was long term (5 years) with regular exercise.

Improved quadriceps strength and reduced body sway among the elderly subjects resulted from a 20-week exercise session that included a walking component and a gentle exercise component (Lord, Castell, 1994), and from a 9-week water exercise program (Lord et al, 1993). Koroknay et al (1995) reported an improvement in ambulatory status and a decrease in falls after nursing home residents participated in a walking program. Yet no significant difference in balance was found after exercise programs between exercise and nonexercise groups in studies conducted by

Mills (1994) and Topp et al (1993) among community-dwelling elderly persons.

Physical and psychosocial aspects of aquatic exercise among community-living elderly persons included significantly better bone mineral densities of the hips and spine in those who regularly exercised. Those who exercised regularly expressed more positive attitudes toward their bodies and had higher morale than the nonexercisers. Interestingly, depression levels were not significantly different, even though happiness and well-being were significantly improved (Benedict, Freeman, 1993; Moore, Bracegirdle, 1994).

Dawes and Moore-Orr (1995) looked at the effect of a single session of mild exercise on tests of cognitive performance (set test) in a group of 20 cognitively unimpaired institutionalized elderly patients. Results indicated that nonstrenuous exercise of low intensity (range-of-motion type) does improve the ability to recall immediately following exercise and for at least a half an hour.

In a group of 30 nursing home residents with moderate to severe cognitive impairment caused by Alzheimer's disease, Friedman and Tappen (1991) studied the effect of walking and talking on the communication abilities of the subjects. Residents were randomly assigned to either a group that walked 30 minutes three times a week while talking with an investigator or to a group that spent the same amount of time in conversation. The investigators postulated that because the neurons that control the physical activities of communication and walking are located in the motor cortex, walking would "prime" the motor circuitry involved in communication, and communication would improve. After 10 weeks the walking-and-talking group improved on two tests of communication, whereas the talking-only group did not.

Benefits in both physical and psychosocial aspects of function have been found for community-living and institutionalized elderly persons. The frail and the healthy, independent elderly have both benefited from various forms of exercise programs.

Assessment

An assessment should be initiated before allowing an older adult to participate in an exercise program. The assessment needs to include a medical history; knowledge of the individual's physical activity level and/or physical limitations; current medication regimen; and emotional, psychologic, and social needs.

In addition to the medical history, a physical examination with emphasis on cardiovascular, pulmonary, musculoskeletal, and neurologic systems should be done. The examination should focus on those aspects that may have an impact on functional status and that may give clues to potential risk. Attention should be focused on joint range of motion, flexibility, and strength. Previous injuries and the presence of active inflammation need to be assessed.

Laboratory analysis should include a hematocrit ratio and a hemoglobin level. A low hematocrit ratio and hemoglobin level will increase the workload on the heart to maintain an adequate oxygen supply. In addition, analysis of electrolyte and fluid balance is necessary to evaluate conductivity and contractility of the cardiac muscle and its ability to function adequately.

The American College of Sports Medicine recommends exercise tolerance testing (ETT) for the elderly before they begin a moderately intense or vigorous exercise program. This test provides information regarding metabolic equivalents and the target heart rate of the older person. Yet ETT is not recommended for the frail elderly. A frail elder's functional impairments may hinder the ability to perform an adequate test. The strength required for ETT may exceed the aerobic capacity of a frail elder. ETT is not essential for the elderly who desire to start a simple walking program or perform a level of exercise aimed at improving mobility and performance of activities of daily living. The patient's exercise goals and functional capacity need to be considered in the decision to use ETT (Barry, Eathorne, 1994).

The American Heart Association suggests that the quickest way to monitor one's activity tolerance is through the pulse rate. An accurate resting pulse is the baseline for activity and should increase to approximately 60% to 80% of the cardiopulmonary capacity (Kligman, Pepin, 1992). Those individuals 65 years old and over who are certified as medically healthy can safely attain a pulse rate as high as 165 beats/min during sustained activity for a training effect (Hagberg, 1987). The sustained pulse rate of 99 to 132 beats/min is the expected (Tobis, 1979). For individuals with a resting pulse of 100 beats/min and who after light activity and a rest period maintain a pulse of 120 beats/min, activity should be carefully chosen. A pulse rate over 130 beats/min indicates excessive stress to the cardiac system. In severe cardiac conditions the heart should not be stressed more than 20 beats above the baseline pulse and should return to normal in 5 minutes.

The nurse can establish the safe activity pulse of the healthy by two methods or formulas:

Safe cardiac function = 200 − Age +
        60% (Lower heart rate) + 80% (Upper heart rate)
                    or
Safe cardiac function = Resting pulse + 160% + 180%

If a resting pulse is 72, multiply by 60% and add the result (43) to the resting pulse for the lower limit (115). Then multiply 72 by 80% and again add the result (57) to the resting pulse for the upper limit (129) of safe cardiac function. In this instance the activity should be sustained with the heart rate between 115 and 129 beats/min. Above this limit, excessive demands on the cardiopulmonary function of the person could be deleterious.

A rule of thumb is the ability to talk while doing exercise. The nurse should consider the increase in pulse from the baseline before, during, and at 3-, 5-, and 10-minute intervals after activity. Baseline values can be obtained anytime during a resting state except in REM sleep, when physiologic activity is erratic. It is important to remember that there is variation in maximal heart rate and that variability increases with age. Therefore the standard of 60% and 80% of cardiopulmonary capacity may be too high for the older person. Gillett et al (1993) recommend 40% to 70%.

The respiratory system indicates intolerance to activity when dyspnea is evident or when a decrease in respiratory rate occurs during the activity. The cheeks, lips, and nail beds become red (flushed), pallid, or cyanotic with intolerance. Fatigue, tiredness, dizziness, and requests to sit down are additional signs of inability to tolerate the activity. Obviously, tightness and heaviness in the chest and tightness in the legs are indicative of diminished capacity for activity. If nothing occurs within the expected tolerance level but the nurse notices that the aged person is slowing down, shows signs of decreased dexterity or coordination, and needs frequent rests, then that aged person is not able to tolerate that level of activity.

A rating of perceived exertion can be used to assess tolerance to exercise. The Borg scale has been used successfully to measure perceived exertion among elderly individuals. The scale ranges from 6 to 20 points, with a rating of 6, 7, or 8 for very, very light intensity; 13 or 14 for somewhat hard intensity; and up to 19 or 20 for very, very hard intensity. Gillett et al (1993) recommend that a rating of perceived exertion be used rather than a pulse rate for monitoring exertion during exercise.

Intervention and Evaluation

The Centers for Disease Control and Prevention and the President's Council on Physical Fitness and Sports, in collaboration with the American Council of Sports Medicine, proposed that "every American adult should accumulate 30 minutes or more of moderate intensity physical activity over the course of most days of the week." Yet exercise is not commonly recommended or incorporated into health prevention care of most elderly persons (Kligman, Pepin, 1992). The benefits of activity on the health of elderly persons support the need for incorporation of activity into the plan of care. The nurse's role has implications for knowledge about fitness and approval of exercise programs in which the aged may participate. Attention should be paid to the simplicity, effectiveness, and adaptability of a program for the aged in whatever setting they may live. Acceptable exercise programs for the aged should have realistic objectives and provide for improvement and maintenance of endurance, strength, flexibility, balance, and coordination while minimizing the risk of injury.

Exercise Programs

Participation in exercise programs is influenced by a number of factors. Fitzgerald et al (1994) found that participation of African-American and white females is influenced by their perception of obstacles, especially the amount of time required for exercise and the time they have available. Among a group of mall walkers, those told to exercise by their physician perceived significantly greater susceptibility to and severity of health problems if they did not walk than those not told by their physician to walk. The mall walkers had more cues and fewer barriers to walking (Sommers et al, 1995).

Motivating elders to change behavior is not always easy. A successful exercise program needs to address perceived barriers to exercise (dispel misconceptions about exercise as dangerous, uncomfortable, exhausting, or embarrassing and address poor weather and lack of facilities and transportation); tailor the exercise to the current fitness status and abilities of each individual; provide various forms of social support (leader, class members, family, friends, and assigned partners); use a decision balance sheet that has participants contrast potential benefits with barriers to exercise; cue exercise participants to focus on how they feel during exercise; and agree on appropriate exercises. The use of goals has been stressed as an important point in planning an exercise program (Schuster et al, 1995).

The following are critical characteristics of exercise programs that improve long-term compliance:
1. Low probability of musculoskeletal injury (low to moderate intensity, duration, and frequency)
2. Group participation
3. Emphasis on variety and pleasure (use of games as exercise)

4. Setting of personal goals; contracts
5. Assessment of response to training
6. Recruitment of friends, family, or spouse for support
7. Monitoring of progress (use of charts to display changes visually)
8. Use of music
9. Provision of positive feedback
10. Provision of enthusiastic leadership and role models

Gillett et al (1993) incorporated these characteristics into an exercise program and had 88% of the 244 women who entered the program complete it.

Kinion et al (1993) evaluated the effects of the Sit and Get Fit program for sedentary older adults in a long-term care facility. The program was designed so that it could be implemented by paraprofessional caregivers with minimal supervision. The uniqueness and positive regard for each participant were incorporated into the protocol. They concluded that the importance lies not only in the development of an effective exercise program, but also in the creation of an atmosphere that stimulates engagement and breaks down the barriers erected by the apathetic outlook of many elderly persons. Enjoyment and individualization of the program to meet individual goals and needs are key factors in improving long-term participation. Another consideration for many older adults is the expense associated with the exercise program. Many elderly persons have limited financial reserves for recreational purposes; however, many of today's health, fitness, and recreation centers have low fee rates specifically for those over age 55.

It is also important that individuals who conduct aerobic exercise programs and classes consider differences between the abilities of the young and the old. Classes are generally taught by young and fit persons who become so involved in what they are doing that they are unaware that adults over age 60 may not be able to do the number of repetitions at the intensity they consider necessary for toning muscles, increasing flexibility, or gaining cardiorespiratory benefit. These programs can damage the muscles, tendons, ligaments, and joints of the older adult, as well as discourage their participation. Gillett et al (1993) trained nonathletic female nurses between the ages of 50 and 60 years as group leaders for exercise classes for the elderly. Bonding with the leaders was apparent within the first 2 weeks of the programs. The participants repeatedly mentioned the effectiveness of the leaders.

A variety of exercise programs exist for the elderly. The existing programs need to be evaluated on an individual basis to determine if they are appropriate.

Three programs have been developed by the Administration on Aging. Each program is accompanied by pretest exercises to establish the correct starting level. Instructions are carefully stated for starting positions, sequence of exercises, and precautions when doing the exercises. These exercises include jog-walking, walking, bending, head rotation, leg raising, walking a straight line, knee push-ups, and the "stork stand." Some require incremental participation to ensure individual safety.

Senior Games

Senior centers throughout the United States have instituted physical fitness programs, which include Ping-Pong, boccie, golf, horseshoes, and many other activities enjoyed by the aged. These activities incorporate rhythmic action and stretching and provide improvement in or maintenance of cardiopulmonary function, muscle tone, and mental stimulation.

Nearly all of the states of the United States promote "senior games" in collaboration with public service and private corporations. These are Olympic-style competitions for men and women 55 years of age and older (Neville, 1988). Some companies have established par courses or 1-mile exercise fitness trails for the older adult.

A sustained brisk walk is one of the most popular and accessible forms of activity for the aged. Those who have done little walking are encouraged to start slowly by first walking to the corner of the block and eventually work up to distance walking of several miles. Those limited to institutional facilities should also be encouraged to increase the amount of walking. The walk may be only from the bed to the bathroom at first; then it may be down the hall, and eventually it may be around the total facility. If the person can go outside, walking around the block might be a long-term goal. Siegel et al (1995) found that the elderly had more regular walking habits than younger adults.

Dancing

For those accustomed to it, ballroom, folk, or square dancing should be encouraged. This form of activity done properly can have as much aerobic benefit as workouts to music videotapes. Dancing is kind to the joints and can burn as many calories as swimming, biking, or walking. However, it should not be done as the only form of activity, since it does not develop upper body strength. To enhance cardiovascular and respiratory fitness, one would have to engage in 20 to 30 minutes of sustained dancing (Social Dancing, 1990).

Dancing provides another means of obtaining pleasant, sociable, vigorous exercise that tones the body and benefits cardiopulmonary and mental health.

Swimming

Swimming—one of America's most popular sports—or water exercise improves muscle tone, circulation, muscle strength, endurance, flexibility, and weight control, and in addition it can be relaxing and a mood elevator. The benefits of aquatic activity or exercise therapy are that arm and leg movements against water are less painful and do not seem to require as much effort because of the buoyancy of the water. Some aged persons maintain a swimming program begun earlier in life; others enjoy this as a relaxing new way to get activity and socialize. Those who are nonswimmers or who do not swim well might benefit from water exercise classes held in the shallow end of the pool. The YMCA, YWCA, American Red Cross, and various health and fitness and recreation centers offer classes in these types of activities. Some areas of the country have "senior splash" aerobic swim classes or arthritic aquatic programs, which conform to guidelines set by the Arthritis Foundation. Swimming, however, may be hazardous to those with ischemic heart disease because horizontal water immersion can increase central blood volume, thus stressing the limited cardiac reserve of the individual. Those with ischemic heart disease who want to swim should be under a physician's care.

Isotonic and Isometric Exercises

Yoga is another form of exercise that can be practiced regardless of one's condition. It can foster mental alacrity, independence, and good health in the aged through simple exercise, relaxation, meditation, and emphasis on nutrition. Tai Chi, originally developed as a martial arts form, has for years been used as abdominal exercise for elders in China. Wolf et al (1993) examined the effects of Tai Chi on frailty and balance among 200 community elders after 15 weekly sessions of Tai Chi. Schaller (1996) studied the effects of Tai Chi Chih on balance, flexibility, mood, health status, and blood pressure in a group of community elders. These studies found Tai Chi to be effective in improving muscle strength, flexibility, and balance and providing a feeling of physical and mental well-being.

Isotonic exercises train the cardiovascular and skeletal muscles. Isometrics primarily work with the cardiovascular system. Persons who are confined to a bed or chair, as well as those who are ambulatory, can do these rhythmic tasks or calisthenics. Exercise should be aerobic in nature, easily attained, and not produce an oxygen debt. Numerous programs have been developed in which simplicity and flexibility of the program make it easily adaptable to a variety of settings.

Guidelines for developing an exercise program and/or modifying an existing program for the elderly have been developed by Marsiglio and Holms (1988) and Gillett et al (1993) and appear in Box 12-3.

Special Needs of the Elderly

It is also important to address special needs of the elderly when initiating an exercise program. The elderly are less able to adapt to the environment during exercise. They should dress in layers to adjust to different environmental temperatures. Well-fitting footwear and socks are essential to prevent injury because of impaired foot sensation. Blisters and friction injuries may occur without the elderly person knowing it. Maintaining hydration is essential. Total body water is decreased in the elderly. Consumption of fluid before exercising and regularly while exercising is recommended. Environments with poor air quality, including areas near roadways when exercising outside, should be avoided.

Often when one is beginning a physical exercise program, muscles will be sore. Warm, not hot, baths or soaks are excellent. Another way to minimize muscle soreness is to maintain a 5- to 10-minute cool-down period of slow walking or stretching to keep the primary muscle groups active, to decrease venous pooling and increase venous return to the heart, and to prevent vagal responses.

When planning activities for the elderly, the age-related changes of the musculoskeletal system need to be considered. Table 12-5 addresses age-related changes of the musculoskeletal system with outcomes and management approaches. Musculoskeletal function is essential to activity.

Nurses should capitalize, more than they do, on activities of daily living, such as providing the aged with bath brushes to wash their own backs in the shower or bathtub and encouraging the aged to dry body parts or rub the back dry with a towel. Reaching for objects while cleaning house can be included in an activity program, as can washing dishes in warm water to provide finger exercises. Warm water aids in the relief of stiffness and enables the fingers to move more easily without discomfort. Various exercises to maintain flexibility are presented in Fig. 12-1. Strengthening exercises have been shown to improve balance and prevent falls in the older adult, regardless of age (Ciaccia, 1995).

Box 12-3   GUIDELINES FOR DEVELOPING OR MODIFYING AN EXERCISE PROGRAM

1. Base program on individual assessment data (underlying conditions, medications, present activity level).
2. Establish mutual goals.
3. Teach to use correct body mechanics, wear appropriate clothing (layer so can change to environment), wear exercise-specific (supportive) shoes, and maintain sufficient hydration (drink water before, during, and after).
4. Begin at a very low level (40% to 50% of predicted maximal heart rate), and follow very gentle exercise progression.
5. Teach to avoid sudden twisting movements, rapid movements, and rapid transitions from one movement to the next.
6. Avoid exercises that tax vision and balance.
7. Avoid sustained isometric contractions of greater than 10 seconds.
8. Assess ability to tolerate low-level activity without signs and symptoms of muscle fatigue, shortness of breath, angina, dysrhythmias, abnormal blood pressure, or intermittent claudication.
9. Stop exercising if cardiac dysrhythmias, angina, or excessive breathlessness occurs.
10. Instruct to avoid exercise during acute viral infections.
11. Increase activity slowly in relation to intensity (workload), duration (time), and frequency (time interval or length of time).
12. Monitor exercise intensity by perceived exertion and exercise heart rate.
13. Perform a gradual, extended exercise warm-up (i.e., 15 minutes) to maximize flexibility and decrease muscle injury.
14. Perform cool-down until heart rate returns to resting level to decrease postural hypotension and cardiac dysrhythmias.
15. Modify exercise program based on individual's responses.

Table 12-5

Age-Related Musculoskeletal Changes; Outcomes; and Health Prevention, Promotion, and Maintenance Approaches

Age-related changes	Outcomes	Health prevention, promotion, and maintenance
Bones become more porous (osteoporosis)	Dowager's hump (kyphosis)	Have good lighting, dry floors, nonskid rugs
Demineralization of vertebral trabecular bone	Risk of hip fracture	Diet high in calcium
Intervertebral disks dehydrate and narrow	Tremors	Calcium supplements as necessary
Reduced height	Back pain	Do moderate exercise: walking or swimming
Erosion of cartilage through exposure and wearing	Joint swelling	Use assistive devices: cane, walker, if needed
Subchondral bone becomes hyperemic and fibrotic	Ankylosis	Do range-of-motion activity
Synovial membranes become fibrotic	Crepitation	Seek medical evaluation of back pain
Synovial fluid thickens	Decreased range of motion	Wear shoes with low heels, nonskid soles, and support
Muscle wasting of hand dorsum	Stiffness	Use leg muscles rather than back muscles when lifting
Diminished protein synthesis in muscle cells	Muscle wasting	Rest joints when pain occurs
Glucose mobilizes slowly in response to exercise	Reduced muscle strength	Lose weight when necessary
Diminished muscle mass decreases glucose stores	Night leg cramps	Develop an appropriate exercise program
Bone and muscle weakness changes the center of gravity	Gait problems	Pace activities
	Smaller steps	Allow for rest periods
	Wider stance base	Break big jobs into small parts
	Poor posture	Adjust activities to periods of day when energy is high
		Remove scatter rugs
		Use nonskid rubber mats in tub and shower
		Take stretch breaks
		Eat more potassium- and calcium-rich foods
		Coordinate and balance exercise

LYING DOWN

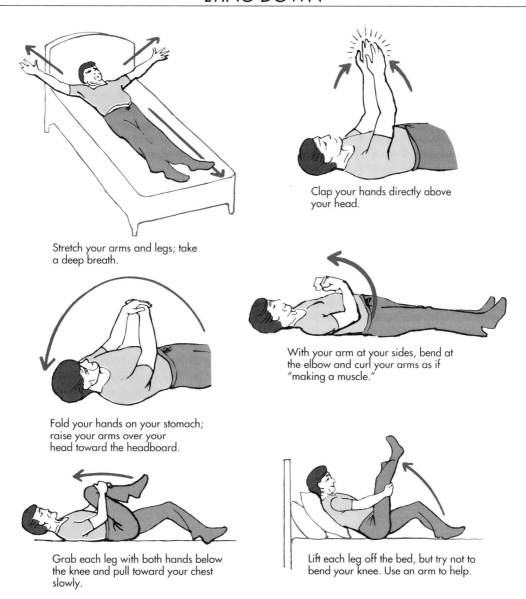

Stretch your arms and legs; take a deep breath.

Clap your hands directly above your head.

Fold your hands on your stomach; raise your arms over your head toward the headboard.

With your arm at your sides, bend at the elbow and curl your arms as if "making a muscle."

Grab each leg with both hands below the knee and pull toward your chest slowly.

Lift each leg off the bed, but try not to bend your knee. Use an arm to help.

Fig. 12-1   Exercises: lying down, sitting, standing up, and walking places. (From Johnson-Pawlson JE, Koshes R: Exercise is for everyone, *Geriatr Nurs* 6[6]:322-325, 1985.)   *Continued*

Housekeeping activities can be utilized for strength and flexibility. Community-dwelling elders can be taught simple approaches in utilizing household chores for activity. The elderly in long-term care who respond to the work ethic can be encouraged to push wheelchairs, clean tables, and run errands.

Other activities that can be done while watching television or whenever there are a few spare minutes during the day are rolling a pencil between the hand and a hard surface, exaggerating the chewing motion of the jaw, holding the stomach in, tightening the buttocks, flexing the fingers, and rotating the head and

SITTING

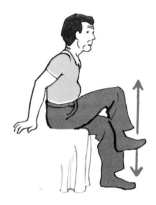

Touch your elbows together in front of you.

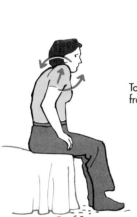

Shrug your shoulders forward, then move them in a circle, raising them high enough to reach your ears.

While still sitting, move each of your knees up and down as if you are walking; each time your right foot hits the ground, count it as one. Lift your knee high.

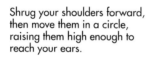

Twist your whole upper body from side to side with your hands on your hips.

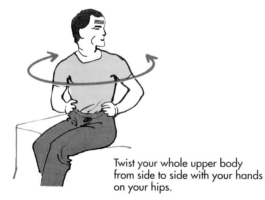

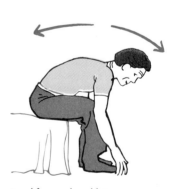

Bend forward and let your arms dangle; try to touch the floor with your hands.

Fig. 12-1, cont'd See legend on p. 225.

STANDING UP

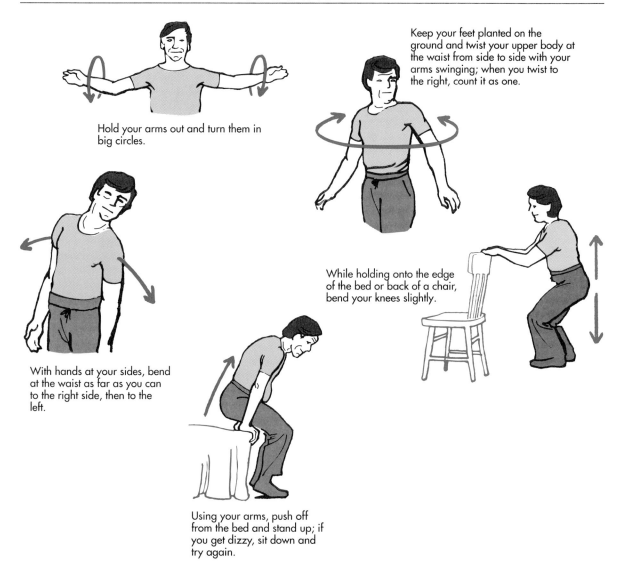

Hold your arms out and turn them in big circles.

Keep your feet planted on the ground and twist your upper body at the waist from side to side with your arms swinging; when you twist to the right, count it as one.

With hands at your sides, bend at the waist as far as you can to the right side, then to the left.

While holding onto the edge of the bed or back of a chair, bend your knees slightly.

Using your arms, push off from the bed and stand up; if you get dizzy, sit down and try again.

Fig. 12-1, cont'd   See legend on p. 225.   *Continued*

the ankles. Benison and Hogstel (1986) elaborate on specific total-body exercises for the older immobile patient.

Activity, in general, should be paced and occur regularly every day. Activities that will help eliminate stiff-ness should be done in the morning, when stiffness is most prevalent. Relaxation exercises should be per-formed before bedtime to help induce sleep. With any activity in which the aged are involved, sufficient inter-mittent rest periods should be provided.

WALKING PLACES

Walking is good exercise. It helps tone muscles, helps maintaining flexibility of joints, and also is good exercise for the heart and circulatory system. Walking briskly for 20 minutes a day, 3 times a week can be as effective a heart conditioner as jogging, but it does take a longer time to achieve the same effect as jogging. For those who cannot walk rapidly for long periods, walking to the point of muscular fatigue also helps maintain good muscle tone.

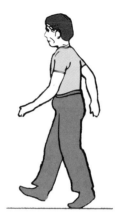

There are signs your body may give you to indicate you are overdoing exercise. Stop, rest, and if necessary call your physician if you experience any of these symptoms:

- SEVERE SHORTNESS OF BREATH
- CHEST PAIN
- SEVERE JOINT PAIN
- DIZZINESS OR FAINT FEELING
- HEART FLUTTERS

In all walking exercises, go only as fast as you are able to walk and still carry on a conversation. If you cannot, slow down.

INSIDE

It is important to maintain walking ability. Determine how far you can walk and each day walk to $3/4$ of that distance, building endurance. Wear supportive shoes and use whatever aids are necessary.

OUTSIDE

Wear soft-soled shoes with good support, i.e., jogging shoes. When walking, push off *from* your toes and land on your heels. Swing arms loosely at your sides. Begin with 10-minute walks and build to 20 to 30 minutes.

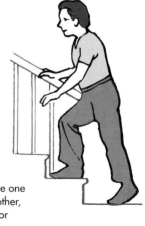

Walking upstairs requires effort. Place one foot flat on a step, push off with the other, and shift your weight. Use a railing for balance if necessary.

Fig. 12-1, cont'd   See legend on p. 225.

Table 12-6

Benefits of Exercise on Chronic Conditions

Condition	Types of exercise	Benefits
Chronic lung disease	Aerobic	Improve diaphragmatic breathing Reduce reliance on accessory muscles
Cognitive dysfunction	Aerobic	Improve cerebral function Increase cerebral perfusion Increase beta-endorphin secretion
Coronary heart disease	Aerobic Endurance type	Reduce blood pressure Increase HDLs and reduce body fat Increase maximal oxygen consumption
Diabetes mellitus	Aerobic Endurance type	Fat loss Increase insulin sensitivity Decrease glucose intolerance risk
Hypertension	Aerobic Endurance type Leisure-time activity	Decrease systolic blood pressure Decrease total peripheral resistance
Osteoarthritis	Resistance stretching Endurance type	Maintain range of motion; muscle mass Increase muscle strength
Osteoporosis	Resistance Weight-bearing	Strengthen postural muscles Stimulate bone growth Decrease rate of bone loss

Data compiled from Kligman EW, Pepin E: Prescribing physical activity for elder patients, *Geriatrics* 47(8):33, 1992; Edward K, Larson EB: Benefits of exercise for older adults, *Clin Geriatr Med* 8(1):35, 1992; and Barry HC, Eathorne SW: Exercise and aging: issues for the practitioner, *Med Clin North Am* 78(2):357, 1994.
HDLs, High-density lipoproteins.

Safety and Other Considerations

Those who are frail should not engage in strenuous activity, nor should their joints be forced past the point of resistance or discomfort. If frail individuals have regularly participated in activity that the nurse deems too stressful to their skeletal systems, it is important to keep in mind that an activity done for many years is not as difficult as it would be if it were just introduced. When the activity is new, serious consideration should be given to the levels of stress produced.

Many aged persons are fearful of falling because of altered balance or the inability to reach or bend. Some fear that if they get down on the floor, they will not be able to get up again. Sometimes all that is necessary to alleviate this fear is to ensure that the aged person has his or her glasses or other appliances that provide security, stability, and mobility.

Mental activity should be planned as carefully as physical activity. These activities should be consistent with the individual's interests. New hobbies may develop; involvement in raising or keeping pets may foster caring and affection for others and a rebirth of socialization.

Activity should not be thought of as something to keep the aged busy but should be purposeful to enhance their physical and mental well-being. The benefits of exercise for those with chronic conditions appear in Table 12-6.

• • •

In summary, this chapter has looked at the need for rest and sleep and the need for activity individually. It is apparent that each area influences the function of the other. The quality and the overall perception of life can be augmented when the nurse monitors these specific functions and provides support or assistance according to identified problems.

▶ **KEY CONCEPTS**

- Many chronic conditions often interfere with the quality and quantity of sleep. Rest and sleep are restorative, recuperative, and necessary for the preservation of life. Drastic reductions or continually altered or interrupted sleep disrupts homeostatic balance and creates physical and mental aberrations.
- Medication is not always the solution to problems with sleep disturbance.
- Napping may be based more on physical and psychologic health. It does not compensate for a good night's sleep but restores energy by providing the body with needed physical rest.
- Activity is an indication of an individual's health and wellness; inability to exercise, do physical

NANDA and Wellness Diagnoses

Wellness	Specific Needs	NANDA
Has appropriate thought process Has energy to engage in interests	**Self-actualization** Fulfillment Self-expression	Sensory/perceptual alterations Thought processes, altered
Is able to cope Problem solves Makes rational decisions Functions at own pace Is well groomed	Self-esteem Appreciation Autonomy Image Challenge	Coping, ineffective Self-esteem disturbance Sensory/perceptual alterations Social interaction, impaired
Has energy to participate in social activities Has patience to accept others	**Belonging** Acceptance	Family processes, altered Anxiety Coping ineffective, individual Self-esteem disturbance
Is alert to surroundings Makes decisions Is rested	Safety and security Protection Sensory acuity Reality perception Problem solving	Injury, risk for Altered thought processes Sleep deprivation Sleep pattern disturbance Sensory/perceptual alterations
Has restful sleep Is able to perform activities without difficulty	**Biologic integrity** Rest Sleep Activity	Sleep deprivation Sleep pattern disturbance Activity intolerance Activity intolerance, risk for Fatigue

These are not all of the possible wellness or NANDA diagnoses that may be identified. The above are frequent examples of nursing diagnoses that should be considered when planning care for the older adult in whatever setting.

work, or perform activities of daily living is one of the first indicators of decline.

- Lack of physical activity increases the risk for many medical conditions experienced by elders. Exercise can be done by elders who are ambulatory, chair bound, or bedridden and should include an aspect of aerobics, flexibility, and balance (if the elder is ambulatory).
- The benefits of exercise are that it provides maintenance of functional capacity, enhances self-confidence and self-sufficiency, decreases depression, improves one's general life-style, maintains mental functional capacity, and decreases the risk of medical problems.

▶ **Activities and Discussion Questions**

1. What age-related changes affect rest, sleep, and activity in the aged?
2. How would you assess an elder for adequacy or inadequacy of rest, sleep, and activity?
3. Discuss the nursing interventions to promote rest, sleep, and activity.
4. Develop a nursing care plan using wellness and NANDA diagnoses.

RESOURCES

Sleep

A to Zzzz Guide to Better Sleep. Available from the Better Sleep Council, PO Box 13, Washington, DC 20044.

Sleep Disorders. Available from the Association of Professional Sleep Society, 604 2nd Street SW, Rochester, MN 55902.

National Sleep Foundation
  1367 Connecticut Avenue NW, Suite 200
  Washington, DC 20036

Activity

Armchair Fitness Video Programs. Available from CC-M Productions, 7755 16th Street NW, Washington, DC 20012; (301) 588-4095.

National Senior Sports Organization
  14323 S. Outer Forty Road, Suite N300
  Chesterfield, MO 63017

Local YMCA/YWCA activity programs

REFERENCES

Alessi CA et al: Psychotropic medications in incontinent nursing home residents: association with sleep and bed mobility, *J Am Geriatr Soc* 43(7):788, 1995.

Ancoli-Israel S, Kripke D: Sleep and aging. In Calkins E, Davis PJ, Ford AB, editors: *The practice of geriatrics,* Philadelphia, 1986, Saunders.

Ancoli-Israel S et al: Sleep fragmentation in patients from a nursing home, *J Gerontol* 44(1):M18, 1989.

Barry HC, Eathorne SW: Exercise and aging: issues for the practitioner, *Med Clin North Am* 78(2):357, 1994.

Beck-Little R, Weinrich SP: Assessment and management of sleep disorders in the elderly, *J Gerontol Nurs* 24(4):21, 1998.

Beel-Bates CA, Rogers AE: An exploratory study of sundown syndrome, *J Neurosci Nurs* 22(1):51, 1990.

Benedict A, Freeman R: The effect of aquatic exercise on aged persons' bone density, body image, and morale, *AAAA* 17(3):67, 1993.

Benison B, Hogstel MO: Aging and movement therapy: essential interventions for the immobile elderly, *J Gerontol Nurs* 12:8, 1986.

Bixler EO, Vela-Bueno A: Normal sleep: physiological behavior and clinical correlates, *Psych Ann* 17:437, 1987.

Blazer D, Hays J, Foley D: Sleep complaints in older adults: a racial comparison, *J Gerontol Med Sci* 50A(3):M280, 1995.

Bliwise DL et al: Sleep apnea and mortality in an aged cohort, *Am J Public Health* 78(5):544, 1989.

Bliwise DL et al: Observed sleep/wakefulness and severity of dementia in an Alzheimer's disease special care unit, *J Gerontol Med Sci* 50A(6): M303, 1995.

Buysse DJ et al: Napping and 24-hour sleep/wake patterns in healthy elderly and young adults, *J Gerontol* 40(8):779, 1992.

Campbell SS, Dawson D, Anderson MW: Alleviation of sleep maintenance insomnia with timed exposure to light, *J Am Geriatr Soc* 41(8):829, 1993.

Castor D et al: Effect of sunlight on sleep patterns of the elderly, *J Am Acad PA* 4(4):321, 1991.

Ciaccia J: Moderate exercise reduces the risk of falls, *Senior Wellness Letter* 1(1)1-5, 1995.

Creighton C: Effects of afternoon rest on the performance of geriatric patients in a rehabilitation hospital: a pilot study, *Am J Occup Ther* 49(8):775, 1995.

Dawes D, Moore-Orr R: Low-intensity, range-of-motion exercise: invaluable nursing care for elderly patients, *J Adv Nurs* 21(4):675, 1995.

Dement WC, Miles LE, Carskadon MA: White paper on sleep and aging, *J Gerontol* 30:25, 1982.

deVries HA: Physiology of exercise and aging. In Woodruff DS, Birren JE, editors: *Aging, scientific perspectives, and social issues,* New York, 1975, Van Nostrand Reinhold.

Donahue R et al: Physical activity and coronary heart disease in middle-aged and elderly men: the Honolulu program, *Am J Public Health* 78:683, 1988.

Duckett S: Managing the sundowning patient, *J Rehabil* 59(1):24, 1993.

Duckett S, Scotto M: An unusual case of sundown syndrome subsequent to a traumatic head injury, *Brain Inj* 6(2):189, 1992.

Emery CF, Blumenthal JA: Perceived change among participants in an exercise program for older adults, *Gerontologist* 30(4):516, 1990.

Evans BD, Rogers AE: 24-Hour sleep/wake patterns in healthy elderly persons, *Appl Nurs Res* 7(2):75, 1994.

Evans LK: Sundown syndrome in the elderly: a phenomenon in search of exploration, *University of Pennsylvania Center for the Study of Aging Newsletter* 7:7, 1985.

Fernandes K, Strollo PJ: Sleep apnea: a common problem, *Clin Advisor* 1(11/12):63, 1998.

Fitzgerald JT et al: Activity levels, fitness status, exercise knowledge, and exercise beliefs among healthy, older African American and white women, *J Aging Health* 6(3):296, 1994.

Floyd JA: The use of across-method triangulation in the study of sleep concerns in healthy older adults, *Adv Nurs Sci* 16(2):L70, 1993.

Friedman R, Tappen RM: The effects of planned walking on communication in Alzheimer's disease, *J Am Geriatr Soc* 39:650, 1991.

Frisoni GB et al: Night sleep symptoms in an elderly population and their relation with age, gender, and education, *Clin Gerontol* 13(1):51, 1993.

Gillett PA et al: The nurse as exercise leader, *Geriatr Nurs* 14(3)133, 1993.

Goldberg WG, Fitzpatrick JL: Movement therapy with the aged, *Nurs Res* 29:339, 1980.

Hagberg JM: Effects of training on the decline of VO-2 max with aging, *Fed Proc* 46:16, 1987.

Haimov I et al: Sleep disorders and melatonin rhythm in elderly people, *BMJ* 309(6948):167, 1994.

Hayter J: To nap or not to nap, *Geriatr Nurs* 6:104, 1985.

Henderson V, Nite G: *Principles and practices of nursing,* ed 6, New York, 1978, Macmillan.

Herrera CO: Sleep disorders. In Abrams WB, Berkow R, editors: *The Merck manual of geriatrics,* Rahway, NJ, 1990, Merck, Sharpe, & Dohme Research Laboratories.

Hoch CC, Reynolds CF, Houck PR: Sleep apnea in Alzheimer's patients and the healthy elderly, *Sch Inq Nurs Pract* 1(3):221, 1987.

Jenkins BL: a case against sleepers, *J Gerontol Nurs* 2:10, 1976.

Johnson JE: Effect of benzodiazepines on older women, *J Community Health Nurs* 5(2):119, 1988.

Johnson JE: A comparative study of bedtime routines and sleep of older adults, *J Community Health Nurs* 8(3):129, 1991.

Johnston JE: Sleep problems in the elderly, *J Am Acad Nurs Pract* 6(4):161, 1994.

Jouvet M: The state of sleep, *Sci Am* 216:62, 1967.

Kales JD, Cavell M, Kales A: Sleep disorders and their management. In Cassel CK et al, editors: *Geriatric medicine,* ed 2, New York, 1990, Springer-Verlag.

Kinion ES, Christie N, Willella AM: Promoting activity in the elderly through interdisciplinary linkages, *Nurs Connections* 6(3):19, 1993.

Kleitman N: The nature of dreaming. In Walslenhome GEW, O'-Conner M, editors: *CIBA Foundation symposium on the nature of sleep,* Boston, 1960, Little, Brown.

Kligman EW, Pepin E: Prescribing physical activity for older patients, *Geriatrics* 47(8):33, 1992.

Koroknay VJ et al: Maintaining ambulation in the frail nursing home resident: a nursing administered walking program, *J Gerontol Nurs* 21(11):18, 1995.

Kotagal S, Dement W: Overview of sleep apnea and its prevalence in the elderly, *Consultant* 25:86, 1985.

Lerner R: Sleep loss in the aged: implications for nursing research, *J Gerontol Nurs* 8:323, 1982.

Lord S, Castell S: Effect of exercise on balance, strength and reaction time in older people, *Aust J Physiother* 40(2):83, 1994.

Lord S, Mitchell D, Williams P: Effect of water exercise on balance and related factors in older people, *Aust J Physiother* 39(3):217, 1993.

Marsiglio A, Holms K: Physical conditioning in the aging adult, *Nurse Pract* 13:33, 1988.

McGinty D et al: Nocturnal hypotension in older men with sleep-related breathing disorders, *Chest* 4(2):305, 1988.

Meguro K et al: Sleep disturbance in elderly patients with cognitive impairment, decreased daily activity and periventricular white matter lesions, *Sleep* 18(2):109, 1995.

Mills EM: The effect of low-intensity aerobic exercise on muscle strength, flexibility, and balance among sedentary elderly persons, *Nurs Res* 43(4):207, 1994.

Misner JE et al: Long-term effects of exercise on the range of motion of aging women, *J Orthop Sports Phys Ther* 16(1):37, 1992.

Moiser WA, Nelson AS, Walgren KD: Wanted: a good night's sleep, *Adv Nurs Pract* 6(5):31, 1998.

Monk TH et al: Circadian characteristics of healthy 80-year-olds and their relationship to objectively recorded sleep, *J Gerontol* 46(5):M171, 1991.

Moore C, Bracegirdle H: The effects of a short-term, low-intensity exercise program on the psychological well-being of community dwelling elderly women, *Br J Occup Ther* 57(6):213, 1994.

Montplaisier J et al: Restless leg syndrome and periodic limb movement during sleep. In Kryger MH, Roth T, Dement WC, editors: *Principles and practice of sleep medicine,* Philadelphia, 1994, Saunders.

Mornhinweg GC, Voignier RR: Music for sleep disturbance in the elderly, *J Holistic Nurs* 13(3):248, 1995.

Murray F: Awakening to a better life with melatonin, *Better Nutrition for Today's Living* 57(12):50, 1995.

National Institutes of Health, Consensus Development Conference on Physical Activity and Cardiovascular Health: *Development conference statement draft,* Kensington, Md, 1996, NIH Consensus Program, Information Service.

Neville K: Promoting health for seniors, *Geriatr Nurs* 9:42, Jan/Feb 1988.

Oesting H, Manza R: Sleep apnea, *Geriatr Nurs* 9:232, July/Aug, 1988.

Prinz PN et al: Geriatrics: sleep disorders in aging, *N Engl J Med* 323:520, 1990.

Satlin A et al: Bright light treatment of behavior and sleep disturbance in patients with Alzheimer's disease, *Am J Psychiatry* 149(8):1028, 1992.

Schaller KJ: Tai Chi Chih: an exercise option for older adults, *J Gerontol Nurs* 22(10):12, 1996.

Schuster C, Petosa R, Petosa S: Using social cognitive theory to predict intentional exercise in post-retirement adults, *J Health Educ* 26(1):14, 1995.

Siegel PZ, Brackbill RM, Heath GW: The epidemiology of walking for exercise: implications for promoting activity among sedentary groups, *Am J Public Health* 85(5):706, 1995.

Social dancing, *Mayo Clin Nutr Lett* 3(11):5, 1990.

Sommers JM, Andres FF, Price JH: Perceptions of exercise of mall walkers utilizing the Health Belief Model, *J Health Educ* 26(3):158, 1995.

Spiegel R, Azcoma A, Morgan K: Sleep disorders. In Pathy MS, editor: *Principles and practices of geriatric medicine,* ed 2, New York, 1990, Wiley.

Tabloski PA, Cooke KM, Thoman EB: A procedure for withdrawal of sleep medication in elderly women who have been long-term users, *J Gerontol Nurs* 24 (9):20, 1998.

Tobis JS: Rehabilitation of the geriatric patient. In Rossman I, editor: *Clinical geriatrics,* ed 2, Philadelphia, 1979, Lippincott.

Topp R et al: The effect of a 12-week dynamic resistance strength training program on gait velocity and balance in older adults, *Gerontologist* 33(4):501, 1993.

UCLA study aims to improve sleep in nursing homes, *UCLA News,* pp 1-3, April 10, 1995.

Uriri JT, Thatcher-Winger R: Health risk appraisal and the older adult, *J Gerontol Nurs* 21(5):25, 1995.

Vitiello MV, Bliwise DL, Prinz PN: Sleep in Alzheimer's disease and the sundown syndrome, *Neurology* 42(7, suppl 6):83, 1992.

Wallace M: The sundown syndrome: will the specialized training of nurse's aides help elders with sundown syndrome? *Geriatr Nurs* 15(3):164, 1994.

Webb WB: Sleep in older persons: sleep structures of 50- to 60-year-old men and women, *J Gerontol* 37:581, 1982.

Wolf SL et al: The Atlanta FICSIT Study: two exercise interventions to reduce frailty in elders, *J Am Geriatr Soc* 41(3):329, 1993.

chapter 13

Integument and Feet of the Aged

▶ LEARNING OBJECTIVES

Upon completion of this chapter, the reader will be able to:

- Identify normal age-related changes of the integument and feet.
- Identify common skin and foot problems.
- Use standard assessment tools to assess the skin and feet.
- Identify preventive, maintenance, and restorative measures for skin and foot health.

▶ GLOSSARY

Emollient An agent that softens and smooths the skin.

Hyperemia Increased amount of blood in a part of the body caused by increased blood flow, which causes redness, as in the inflammatory process.

Induration Hardening of tissue as a result of edema or inflammation.

Podiatric Pertaining to the feet.

Pruritus A symptom of itching; an uncomfortable sensation leading to the urge to scratch.

Rhinophyma A form of rosacea in which there is sebaceous hyperplasia, redness, prominent vascularity, swelling, and distortion of the skin of the nose.

Rosacea A chronic form of acne seen in adults of all ages, causing the nose, forehead, and cheeks to look inflamed.

Telangiectasis A spot usually on the skin produced by dilation of a capillary or terminal artery.

Tissue tolerance The amount of pressure a tissue (skin) can endure before it breaks down, as in a pressure sore.

Xerosis Another term for dry skin.

▶ THE LIVED EXPERIENCE

I can hardly reach my feet anymore. I suppose if I lost weight and did some sort of stretching exercises, I might be able to. I have forgotten how long it has been since I could comfortably clip my toenails. I do know that if my feet aren't taken care of, I may have difficulty walking, so I guess I'll call my doctor and see about getting a recommendation for a podiatrist. I really hadn't given it much thought until he said I was developing diabetes and foot care would be extremely important.

Joe, age 72 and portly

I just can't believe Joe let his toenails grow so far they had turned under. I did see him 6 months ago, but I don't remember any such problem. I don't know how the poor man can walk comfortably. Maybe that is why he has gained weight—no exercise. I'll have to really keep on top of this situation.

Joe's physician

INTEGUMENT

The skin is looked on as having aesthetic and cosmetic appeal. Artists have portrayed its delicate, flawless qualities, and poets have extolled its virtues through descriptive phrases. Today, art, poetry, and conversation still include similar depictions. Changes in the skin are part of the normal aging process. Changes occur as a result of genetic (intrinsic) factors and environmental (extrinsic) factors such as the sun and harsh weather. Whether these changes are genetic or environmental, all older persons will have some degree of dryness, thinning of the skin, decreased elasticity, and prominence of small blood vessels. Changes thought to be part of the initial process of aging are products of extrinsic causes such as cigarette smoking, which causes coarse wrinkles, and the sun, which is responsible for photodamage, including rough, leathery texture, itching, and mottled pigmentation of the skin (Talarico, 1998).

The integument does more than keep the skeleton from falling apart. As the largest, most visible organ of the body (Gilchrest, 1986), its various layers mold and model the individual to give much of his or her identity; glands and hair provide recognizable characteristics and sexual orientation. The skin is important both in health and in illness. It provides clues to hereditary, racial, dietary, physical, and emotional conditions. It is also an important means of communication. The integument provides at least seven physiologic functions. It protects underlying structures, serves as a heat-regulating mechanism, serves as a sense organ, is involved in the metabolism of salt and water, and stores fat. The skin facilitates two-way gaseous exchange and converts sunshine into vitamin D (Saxon, Etten, 1994). When the integument malfunctions or is overwhelmed by outside trauma, discomfort, disfigurement, or death may ensue. Despite exposure to heat, cold, water trauma, friction, and pressure, it maintains a homeostatic environment. The skin is durable, pliable, and strong enough to protect the body by absorbing, reflecting, cushioning, and restricting various substances and forces that might enter and alter its function. Yet it is sensitive enough to relay messages to the brain.

The rate at which the skin ages is proportional to the degree of exposure to environmental elements such as wind and the irradiation of the sun. The face and hands are the most constantly exposed areas of the body; thus aging is considerably faster in these areas than in those that are rarely exposed. Visible changes of the skin—

quality of color, firmness, elasticity, and texture—affirm that one is aging. Skin coloration varies with blood flow. Paleness is apparent with diminished blood blow; conversely, flushing occurs when blood flow increases. Decreased hemoglobin in capillary blood flow that has lost most of its oxygen produces cyanosis. Circulatory disorders affect skin coloration; skin loses its color, and blood vessels become more fragile. Although the aged may appear less attractive physically, like most people, they take pride in their appearance and should not be slighted because of wrinkles and saggy tissue.

The epidermis, dermis, and subcutaneous layers of the skin have specific functions that will affect nursing assessment and intervention.

Epidermis

The aged epidermis produces varying cell shapes and sizes. The loss of conelike projections, called *rete ridges,* changes the previously textured skin to thinner, fragile, shiny, and flatter tissue. The skin serves as an impermeable barrier, preventing the loss of fluids and intrusion of substances from the environment. Melanocytes are in the basal layer of the epidermis. Melanin gives the skin its color. Areas of the skin exposed to the sun have two to three times the melanocytes as unexposed skin. Hormonal activity causes changes in skin pigmentation. Melanin is affected by the melanocyte-stimulating hormone (MSH), which is similar to adrenocorticotropic hormone (ACTH). Moles, nevi, and freckles are all products of melanin distribution. Melanocytes increase in size but decrease in number over time; it is the degree of this activity that creates the uneven pigmentation. In darker-pigmented races the melanocytes work harder than in light-skinned races. If pigmentation is lacking or insufficient, it is thought that epinephrine, a known MSH antagonist, may have blocked melanin synthesis.

Pigmented moles and nevi are thought to be benign neoplasms, or melanocytes. Freckles are a result of the inability of the melanocytes to produce even pigmentation of the skin. Lentigines, called *age spots* or *liver spots,* are similar to freckles. These can occur at any age; however, from the sixth decade on, they are thought to be sun related (Lombardo, 1979). The development of lentigines is also thought to be from uneven melanin production. Lentigines are dramatically seen on the back of the hands and wrists of light-skinned persons (Porth, Kapke, 1983).

Dermis

The dermis, lying beneath the epidermis, is a supportive layer of connective tissue composed of a matrix of yellow elastic fibers that provide stretch and recoil, white fibrous collagen fibers that provide tensile strength, and an absorbent gel between the two types of fibers. In addition, the dermis also supports hair follicles, sweat and sebaceous glands, nerve fibers, muscle cells, and blood vessels (which provide nourishment to the epidermis, which does not contain blood vessels). With age, the dermis elasticity and suppleness are lost as a result of cross-link changes of the elastin and collagen components (Box 13-1). Studies suggest that estrogen replacement therapy (ERT) slows skin aging in the first few years of menopause (Wallis, 1995; Wasaha, Angelopoulos, 1996; Dunn et al, 1997). Dermal cells also are replaced more slowly, and tactile sensory receptors do not transmit sensations as rapidly.

Subcutaneous Layer

The subcutis is the inner layer of fat tissue that protects underlying tissue from trauma. It is responsible for insulation and the regulation of heat loss. With age, some areas of subcutaneous tissue atrophy. This is particularly true of the hands, face, and lower legs, which are frequently exposed to the sun. Other areas of subcutaneous fat (such as around the thighs of women and the waist, which is more prominent in women than in men) hypertrophy.

Glands

Eccrine, apocrine, and sebaceous gland activity is influenced by the hormonal and nervous systems; thus if the effectiveness of hormonal and nervous stimulation decreases, glandular activity diminishes significantly.

Eccrine glands, or sweat glands, are located all over the body and respond to thermostimulation and neurostimulation. The usual body response to heat is to produce moisture or sweat from these glands and thus cool the skin by evaporation. Since sweating is diminished in the aged, overheating and heat intolerance become important problems. The aged should avoid spending long periods in the heat, both indoors and outdoors. The summer, in particular, poses a major threat in areas in which there are persistent high humidity and heat. In these areas the death rate among the aged from heat is high. The aged should be encouraged to wear a hat when in the sun; to wear light, cool clothing; and to drink sufficient amounts of fluid.

Box 13-1   STRUCTURAL AND FUNCTIONAL CHANGES OF THE AGING SKIN AND THEIR IMPLICATIONS

Altered Cell Proliferation

Wound-healing capability ↓
  Blister formation ↑

Altered Immune Response

Cell-mediated immune response ↓
  Barrier function ↓
  Clearance of foreign substances ↓
  Incidence of infection ↑
  Incidence of cancer ↑

Altered Pigmentation

Melanocytes ↓
  Graying of hair ↑
  Tanning ↓

Altered Subcutaneous Tissue and Gland Function

Thermoregulation ↓
Sweat and oil production ↓

Altered Elastic Fibers, Tissue Density, and Vascularity

Elasticity ↓
  Fragility ↑
Thickness ↓
Roughness ↑
Dryness ↑

Altered Nail Changes

Thickness ↑
Fragility ↑
Sensory deprivation ↑

Apocrine glands are associated with hair follicles and are located in the axillary, genital, and perianal areas and in the external ear canal. These glands are larger than the eccrine glands, depend on hormones, and are responsive to emotions. They become active at puberty, but this activity diminishes slightly with advanced age. They are also responsible for characteristic body odors that occur under stress or excitement (Marks, 1987; Ferrell and Osterweil, 1989). The secretions are odorless until bacteria begin to act on the moisture to produce odors. Deodorants and antiperspirants are often used to suppress odors from the apocrine glands. Dusting powder with baking soda is a natural, inexpensive substance that can keep the axillae dry and free from odor.

Sebaceous glands secrete sebum and depend on hormonal stimulation. Because of a decrease in androgen levels and in the blood supply to sebaceous glands, sebum production decreases with age. Sebum protects the skin by preventing the evaporation of water from the keratin, or horny, layer of the epidermis; it possesses bactericidal properties and contains a precursor of vitamin D. When the skin is exposed to sunlight, vitamin D is produced and absorbed into the skin. Box 13-1 notes implications to an elder's health as a result of aging skin.

Hair

Hair, as part of the integument, has a biologic, psychologic, and cosmetic value for both men and women. Hair is composed of tightly fused horny cells that arise from the dermal layer and obtain coloration from melanocytes. Hair coloration usually correlates with skin coloration; however, there are exceptions. The hormone testosterone influences hair distribution in both men and women. Axillary and pubic hair tends to diminish with age in women and in some instances disappears. Hair on the head becomes thinner and depleted of melanin, giving it the characteristic gray color. Older women develop chin and facial hair because of decreased estrogen production. Men become bald or develop a receding hairline. Hair growth is also affected by diet, radiation, physical conditions, and drugs.

The various races have definite hair characteristics, which should be kept in mind when caring for or assessing the aged. Almost all Asians have sparse facial and body hair that is dark, straight, and silky. Blacks have slightly more head and body hair than Asians; however, the hair texture varies widely. It can be fragile, and it ranges from long and straight to short, spiraled, and thick. Whites have the most head and body hair, with an intermediate texture and form ranging from straight to curly, fine to thick, and coarse (Jarvis, 1996; Giger, Davidhizar, 1999; Seidel et al, 1999).

Nails

The aged nail becomes harder and thicker, more brittle, dull, and opaque. It changes shape, becoming at times flat or concave instead of convex. Vertical ridges appear because of decreasing water, calcium, and lipid content. The blood supply, as well as the rate of nail growth, de-

creases. The half moon (lunule) of the fingernail may entirely disappear, and the color of the nails may vary from yellow to gray (Staab, Lyles, 1990; Timaris, 1994; Gilchrest, 1995).

Photoaging

Solar elastosis, or photoaging, is a result of environmental damage to the skin from ultraviolet sun rays. Many of the changes associated with photoaging are preventable. Ideally, preventive measures should begin in childhood, but clinical evidence has shown that some improvement can be achieved through avoidance of sun exposure and the regular use of sunscreens, even after actinic damage has occurred. Sunscreens offer protection from harmful ultraviolet A and B rays.

Sun-induced damage varies with skin type. Individuals who always burn, never tan, or minimally tan, or who burn moderately and tan to a light brown, should be considered to have sensitive to very sensitive skin, which requires a sun protection factor (SPF) of 15 or more.* Individuals who minimally burn and always tan to a moderate brown should use a sunscreen with an SPF of 6 to 10. Those individuals who rarely burn and tan to a dark brown require a sunscreen with an SPF of only 4 to 6. The use of sunscreens should not be limited to summer use or sunny days. Damaging ultraviolet rays penetrate clouds and overcast skies.

It must be remembered that the normal skin changes, such as fragility and diminished melanocyte activity, that occur in older adults may not correlate with the level of SPF protection that was adequate when they were younger. The aged individual may require a sunscreen with a higher SPF.

Topical tretinoin (all-*trans*-retinoic acid) has been found to reverse some structural damage caused by excessive sun exposure. New capillary formation, collagen synthesis, and regulation of epidermal melanin distribution, as well as the disappearance of premalignant actinic keratoses, have been noted with the use of tretinoin over a period of 6 to 9 months. However, individuals who apply this topical medication may initially experience erythema and peeling of the treated area. There tends to be more improvement in individuals

---

*The effectiveness of sunscreens is measured in terms of the SPF. The equation of minimal erythema dose (MED), the amount of time it takes to cause the skin to become red, times the SPF provides the length of time, in minutes, that an individual can be in the sun without burning.

with slight to moderate sun damage than in those with severe photoaging (Phillips, Gilchrest, 1990).

Common Skin Problems

Common skin problems of the aged include dry skin, pruritus, dermatitis, seborrheic and actinic keratoses, skin cancer, vascular lesions, and pressure sores (Phillips, Gilchrest, 1990; Talarico, 1998).

Dry Skin

Dry skin (xerosis) is perhaps the most common problem of the aged and is poorly understood. The thinner epidermis allows more moisture to escape from the skin. Inadequate fluid intake has the systemic effect of pulling moisture from the skin to assist in overall hydration of the body. Diminished amounts of sebum, secreted by the sebaceous glands, lessen the availability of the protective lipid film that normally retards the evaporation of water from the stratum corneum (horny layer). Exposure to environmental elements, decreased humidity, use of harsh soaps, frequent hot baths, nutritional deficiencies, smoking, stress, and excessive perspiration contribute to skin dryness and dehydration of the stratum corneum. Hospital care promotes dry skin through routine bathing, use of soap, prolonged bed rest, and the action of bed linen on the patient's skin. Repeated wetting and drying of the skin layer cause subsequent swelling and tissue drying. Chapping, drying, and major skin changes occur more slowly and later in those individuals who routinely use emollient skin care products that afford good skin protection. These skin care items are apt to contain moisturizers and sunscreening agents. Based on the number of commercial skin preparations on the market today, it is obvious that dry skin and protection from ultraviolet rays are recognized problems.

Treatment of dry skin in the aged is focused on the relief of symptoms; the underlying problem cannot be cured. The nurse should be alert to signs of rough, scaly, flaking skin on the face, neck, hands, forearms, sides of the lower trunk, and exterior and lateral aspects of the thighs. Itching frequently accompanies dryness and may be evident as skin irritation or scratch marks in these areas. Dry skin may be just dry skin, but it may also be a symptom of more serious systemic disease (e.g., diabetes mellitus, hypothyroidism, or renal disease).

The treatment of dry, itchy skin is to rehydrate the epidermis, especially the keratin, or horny, layer. The skin's only moisturizer is water. Substances may be used to enhance water's ability to stay in the skin. These include binders (bind water to the skin) and humectants (attract moisture from the air to the skin). Other products such as oils, petroleum jelly, and zinc oxide serve to keep moisture that is already in the skin from evaporating. Oils and ointments also are designed to coat the skin and replace the skin's natural oil barrier (sebum) (Motta, 1992). The use of superfatted soaps without hexachlorophene is effective in helping to restore the protective lipid film to the skin surface. Basis, Dove, Tone, and Caress are the most common of the superfatted soaps used (Hardy, 1996).

Incorporation of bath oils and other hydrophobic preparations into the bathing routine temporarily helps hold moisture and retards its escape from the skin. However, bath oil poured into the bathtub creates the potential for falls. It is safer and more effective to have the aged person bathe or shower, lightly towel dry, and apply the oil directly onto the moist skin; mild, water-laden emulsions are best. Light mineral oil as a bath aid is equally as effective and more economical than commercial brands.

Application of lotion or emollients to the body several times each day is another way to keep the epidermal layer lubricated and hydrated; vegetable oil is an inexpensive emollient but may smell or stain clothing. Emollients applied to nonhydrated skin act by trapping the water, which constantly enters the subcutaneous layer from below. "Heavy" (very greasy) emollients have an additional ability to coat the skin, providing a smooth-surface film. This seems to be a better barrier against evaporation than cosmetic preparations. Lubricants are most effective when applied to the skin immediately after bathing. Most skin products in the pH range of 6.0 to 7.0 are effective, even though the skin pH ranges from 4.5 to 6.0. Cleansing agents with a pH of 7.0 are mild and will cleanse the skin better than cleansers with a lower pH. A moisturizing lotion with a pH of 6.0 to 7.0 will have a softening effect on the skin. The skin absorbs beneficial ingredients more easily when a product pH is neutral (Renaissance Medical Inc, 1992).

Maintaining the environmental humidity at 60%, alleviating mechanical irritation caused by clothing, encouraging baths and showers with water temperatures at 90° to 105° F (32.2° to 40.5° C) without limiting bathing, and applying mineral oil after bathing are measures that help to control dry skin (Hardy, 1996). Eczema may occur as a result of dry skin in the extreme and in response to pruritus. The skin may fissure, appear shiny, and crack, with subsequent inflammatory changes. Treatment of skin dryness and resolution of itching help to eliminate this condition.

Pruritus

Pruritus (itching) is the most common complaint of the elderly (Elewski, 1990; Talarico, 1998). It is described as an "unpleasant cutaneous sensation" (Montagu, 1992). Pruritus is a symptom, not a diagnosis or a dis-ease, and is a threat to skin intactness. It is aggravated by heat, sudden temperature changes, sweating, contact with articles of clothing, fatigue, and emotional upheavals and may accompany such systemic disorders as chronic renal failure, biliary or hepatic disease, and iron deficiency anemia. Box 13-2 lists the various causes of pruritus in the elderly.

Scratching is an ineffective response to the urge to remove the irritant itch from the skin. When one scratches, a counterstimulus is introduced, which is stronger than the original itch stimulus. The nerve messages become confused or eliminate the itching sensation by the intensity of the counterstimulation scratch stimulus. Itching is akin to pain. The nerve endings that produce cutaneous pain also produce itching. When rehydration of the stratum corneum is not sufficient to control itching, cool compresses of saline solution or oatmeal or Epsom salt baths may be indicated. Using a lotion such as Lubriderm, Nutraderm, or Eucerine is helpful. Vigorous towel drying intensifies pruritus by overstimulating the skin and by removing the needed water from the stratum corneum. Guidelines for the treatment of pruritus appear in Box 13-3.

Candidiasis *(Candida albicans)*

Candida albicans is present in healthy persons but proliferates in those with malnutrition or diabetes and in persons receiving antibiotic or steroid therapy. Intertriginous *C. albicans* occurs when there are opposing skinfolds that become moist and create friction, as in the case of obesity and pendulous breasts. It can also occur with incontinence, poor hygiene, immune deficiencies, and angular cheilitis (fissures in the corners of the mouth that develop as a result of an edentulous state, ill-fitting dentures, vitamin deficiency, or drool-

---

Box 13-2   CAUSES OF PRURITUS IN THE ELDERLY

Dermatitis
Eczema
Contact
Seborrhea
Lichen simplex chronicus (neurodermatitis)
Xerosis (dry skin)
Microvascular (stasis dermatitis, erythema)

Papular Scaling Disorders
Psoriasis, lichen planus

Drug Reactions
Drug withdrawal (delerium tremens)
Erythema multiforme
  Antidepressants, opiates
  Acetylsalicylic acid, idiosyncratic responses

Metabolic Responses
Liver and biliary disorders
Renal failure (uremia)
Diabetes mellitus
Hypothyroidism

Neoplastic Disorders
Benign (seborrheic keratosis)
Malignant (central nervous system tumors)

Hematopoietic Responses
Iron deficiency anemia
Leukemia, lymphoma

Psychogenic Etiologies
Involutional psychoses
Hallucinatory aberrations (dementias)

Infections and Infestations
Bacterial (impetigo, chlamydia)
Viral (herpes zoster)
Yeast infections (candidiasis, monilial intertrigo)
Parasitic (scabies, pediculosis)

Box 13-3   GUIDELINES FOR DEALING WITH PRURITUS

1. Take tepid baths using bath oil so as not to further dehydrate skin.
2. Apply soothing creams or emollients several times daily, especially on hands, feet, and face.
3. Wear soft, absorbent clothing, such as cotton.
4. **Be careful of and use with caution:**
   • Topical steroid creams (unpredictable absorption)
   • Low-dose systemic steroids (likely to result in complications)
   • *Do not use* antihistamines with persons over age 75 (experience sudden, severe side effects).

ing) when there is an overlap of tissue where saliva can pool (Reichel, 1995). White satellite pustules surrounded by a glazed, bright red (erythema) maceration; at times ulceration or erosion; itching; and burning are characteristic of *C. albicans* dermatitis. In the mouth it may look a little like cottage cheese, with the surrounding mucosa bright red and ulcerated, making it painful to swallow or eat.

The best approach is prevention through directing attention to situations where potential causes of candidal infection can manifest as intertrigo at skinfolds or as thrush in the mouth, through preventing residual moisture from incontinence, and through correcting malnutrition. For pendulous breasts or extensive skinfolds, light absorbent pads such as panty liners can be used. The sticky sides should be placed together and placed between the opposing skin surfaces. These should be changed whenever they are wet. Wearing loose-fitting cotton clothing and cotton underwear (and changing it when damp), as well as limiting activity that promotes sweating, is helpful.

The goal of treatment is to reduce the moisture, eliminate maceration, decrease friction, and aerate between skinfolds. Treatment for candidiasis includes maintaining dry, clean skin. A mild soap or cleansing agent such as Cetaphil should be used, followed by drying the skin well and applying an antifungal preparation in either powder, cream, or lotion form for 7 to 14 days. These antifungal medications include miconazole (Micatin), clotrimazole (Lotrimin), nystatin (Mycostatin), and econazole (Spectazole). Cornstarch should never be used because it promotes the growth of *Candida* organisms. A skin barrier cream such as SBR-Lipocream may be of value in patients who are incontinent.

Anyone who is diaphoretic or who sweats profusely should be considered for prevention of candidiasis. Treatment of angular cheilitis and oral *C. albicans* infection includes mouth swishing with Mycostatin suspension, sucking on antifungal troches, and applying an antifungal ointment to the corners of the mouth for cheilitis. If the *C. albicans* cannot be eliminated in the usual course of therapy, it may be necessary to use ketoconazole or fluconazole tablets systemically for a prescribed period of time. Conditions such as psoriasis, seborrhetic dematitis, and contact dermatitis may aggravate *C. albicans* dermatitis and may contribute to secondary infections (Riechel, 1995; Talarico, 1998; Miller, 1999).

Keratoses

Seborrheic keratosis is a benign growth that appears mainly on the trunk, face, and scalp as single or multi-ple lesions. Multiple keratotic lesions are commonly distributed on the body (Elewski, 1990; Talarico, 1998). A keratotic lesion is a superficial, circumscribed, raised area that thickens and darkens in color over time. The greasy, dry to rough appearance resembles a "blob of wax." Because the growth gets its coloration from melanin, some individuals fear that it will become malignant. When there is concern about this type of lesion, a biopsy may be necessary to definitively establish that it is benign, not a melanoma. Generally, if it is cosmetically distressing or in an area of chronic irritation, this neoplasm can be removed by a dermatologist.

Actinic or solar keratosis, unlike the benign seborrheic keratosis, is a precancerous lesion. It is a result of years of overexposure to the sun and is found on sun-exposed areas such as bald heads, hands, faces, ears, noses, and upper chests. Numerous lesions may occur at the same time and appear as a reddish or brownish, localized, scaly patch or patches on superficial areas, eventually thickening and becoming crusty. Early recognition, treatment, and removal of this lesion are important to prevent serious problems later.

Skin Cancers

Squamous cell carcinoma. Squamous cell carcinoma is the second most common skin cancer; it is more prevalent in fair-skinned, elderly men who live in sunny climates. It is a direct result of extensive sun exposure by an elder. Less common causes include chronic stasis ulcers, scars from injury, chemical carcinogens such as topical hydrocarbons, exposure to arsenic, and radiation exposure. It begins as a firm, irregular, fleshy, pink-colored nodule that becomes reddened and scaly, much like actinic keratosis, but it may increase in size rapidly. It may be hard and wartlike with a gray top and horny texture, or it may be ulcerated and indurated with raised, defined borders. Individuals in their mid-60s who are fair skinned and have been or are chronically exposed to the sun are prime candidates for this type of skin cancer. Squamous cell carcinoma is an aggressive carcinoma; it has a higher incidence of metastasis and cannot be ignored.

Basal cell carcinoma. Basal cell carcinoma is the most common malignant lesion of epidermal tissue and frequently appears around the fifth decade. It is a slower-growing neoplasm than squamous cell carcinoma. A basal cell lesion is precipitated by extensive sun exposure, chronic irritation, and chronic ulceration of the skin. It is more prevalent in light-skinned races. This neoplasm begins as a pearly papule with prominent telangiectasis (blood vessels) or as a scarlike area where no history of trauma has occurred. Basal cell carcinoma is also known to ulcerate. Even though metastasis is rare, early detection and treatment are advisable because it can be quite disfiguring.

Melanoma. Melanoma is a neoplasm of melanocytes that can spread throughout the body through the lymph and blood. It is becoming more prevalent, but it is still less common than squamous cell or basal cell carcinomas. Melanoma has a high mortality rate and also can be a result of sun exposure. Blistering sunburns before the age of 18 are thought to damage the Langerhans cells, which affect the immune response of the skin. The legs and backs of women and backs of men are the most common sites for this neoplasm. Two thirds of melanomas develop from preexisting moles; only one third arise from new moles. In addition, nonexposed areas of the body are not exempt from the appearance of melanoma (Elewski, 1990; Mayfield, 1992). Additional criteria for identifying the *ABCD*'s (asymmetry, border irregularity, color, diameter) of melanomas are suggested by Flory (1992) and McGrann (1994): *E* for elevation and the *S* factor, or shadow around the lesion. The shadow is a slight erythematous haze extending beyond the normal margins of the mole or suspected lesion.

Vascular Lesions

Capillary friability or abnormalities are more common with age. These include red and blue spider veins (telangiectasis), which are found mainly on the legs and face but can be anywhere and are due in part to sun exposure, hormone imbalance, liver disease, drug reaction, or radiation treatment. Tight-fitting clothing and alcohol use may also contribute to the formation of these benign but rather unsightly lesions. Cherry angiomas, which are smooth, dome-shaped, bright red lesions, are found mainly on the trunk and extremities.

Rosacea

Rosacea can occur in middle and late life. Eruptions are localized to the same areas as acne in young adults, but unlike acne, rosacea does not create plugs. The eruptions are associated with vascular dilation, papules, and pustules. The vascular component is aggravated by extensive sun exposure in fair-skinned persons. Those individuals with sensitive or ruddy skin and those who flush easily are most at risk for this condition. Vasodilating drugs and use of strong topical corticosteroids may also produce flushing.

Initially in rosacea a vascular erythema, telangiectasia, and flushing are distributed symmetrically on the nose, cheeks, forehead, and chin. In its later stages it may progress to rhinophyma and conjunctivitis. It is sug-

gested, since there is no definitive treatment, that extrinsic causes of the vasodilation be eliminated to decrease the occurrence of the signs and symptoms of this condition and help prevent additional episodes. It is highly recommended that an individual who has rosacea avoid spicy foods, alcoholic and hot beverages, extremes of heat, sun exposure, and stressful situations. Today, complete clearing of facial redness and discrete vessels can be achieved with laser therapy.

Vascular Insufficiency

Vascular insufficiency includes both arterial and venous systems and involves the disruption of skin integrity by stasis dematitis, ulceration, and/or gangrene, depending on the source of vascular involvement. Table 13-1 compares arterial and venous insufficiency.

Arterial insufficiency. Arterial insufficiency of the lower extremities often requires surgical intervention if the circulation cannot be improved adequately with vasodilating medication. Not infrequently, arterial insufficiency leads to gangrene and amputation of all or a portion of the extremity.

Venous insufficiency. Venous insufficiency affects approximately 500,000 Americans, most of whom are older than 60 years of age (Leg Ulcers, 1995). Fortunately, venous insufficiency and stasis ulcers respond to conservative treatment, although it takes many weeks and months to resolve, depending on the extent of tissue involvement.

The microvascular changes that occur with age often leave the vein walls weakened and unable to respond to increased venous pressure. This pressure is due to poor venous flow, vasculitis (inflammation), or thrombophlebitis (venous blood clot), all of which add to the weakening of the vein walls. Heredity and obesity are additional factors that contribute to the altered venous integrity of the lower extremities. Weakened vein walls are also responsible for varicose veins. The backflow that occurs from venous pressure occurs in the small veins in the feet and ankle area, causing leakage of fluid into the tissues with subsequent foot and ankle edema. If the congestion is sufficient, the lower leg also becomes involved. Skin tissue becomes vulnerable to insignificant trauma such as an insect bite or snug elastic-topped ankle socks. Either of these or other events could precipitate the beginning of venous ulcer formation. In individuals with dark-pigmented skin, the skin discoloration is darker than the surrounding tissue.

Usually symptoms begin with pruritus, edema, and stasis dermatitis (also called *varicose* or *gravitational eczema*) or with ulceration from a minor trauma (Gilchrest, 1995; Friedman, 1995). An ulceration will

Table 13-1

Comparison of Arterial and Venous Insufficiency of the Lower Extremities

Characteristics	Arterial	Venous
Pain	Sudden onset with acute; gradual onset with chronic Exceedingly painful Claudication relieved by rest Rest pain relieved by dependency (with total occlusion, no position will give complete relief)	Deep muscle pain with acute deep vein thrombosis Relieved by elevation
Pulses	Absent or weak	Normal (unless there is also arterial disease)
Associated changes in leg and foot	Thin, shiny, dry skin Thickened toenails Absence of hair growth Temperature variations (cooler if there is no cellulitis) Elevational pallor Dependent rubor Atrophy or no change in limb size	Firm ("brawny") edema Reddish brown discoloration with post-phlebitic syndrome Evidence of healed ulcers Dilated and tortuous superficial veins Swollen limb Increased warmth and erythema with acute deep vein thrombosis
Ulcer location	Between toes or at tips of toes Over phalangeal heads On heels Over lateral malleolus or pretibial area (for diabetic patients), over metatarsal heads, on side or sole of foot	"Garter area" around ankles (rich in perforator veins), especially the medial malleolus
Ulcer characteristics	Well-defined edges Black or necrotic tissue Deep, pale base Nonbleeding	Uneven edges Ruddy granulation tissue Superficial Bleeding

generally appear on the medial aspect of the tibia above the malleolus. Evidence of previously healed ulcers can be identified by brown or tannish discoloration over the skin.

A conservative treatment approach is usually taken, and the elder is generally treated at home with the intent of maintaining his or her activities (in some instances increasing the activity). Box 13-4 details information and treatment strategies for venous ulcers. Treatment usually consists of one or a combination of therapies such as leg elevation whenever the person is sitting, topical antibiotics when an ulceration is present, use of wet to moist compresses and soaks, débridement with medications that contain fibrinolysin and deoxyribonuclease enzymes, or, if necessary, surgical débridement. For those who are active, an Unna boot may be the most effective and practical treatment.

Elastic support stockings are frequently prescribed to enhance the efficiency of venous circulation. For the aged individual, it can be energy depleting to bend over and pull and tug on the elastic hose. It is sometimes helpful for both men and women with this problem to put on knee-high nylon stockings (not pantyhose) under the elastic hose. This method achieves minimal energy expenditure and might permit the aged person who needs assistance with that part of dressing to become independent. A few minor annoyances do exist: the legs tend to get hot in warm weather, women find themselves wearing two (or three) pairs of hose, and men may be reluctant to wear women's stockings. In winter, however, it does have the benefit of keeping the legs warm, particularly for those aged persons who live in cold climates.

Treatment and resolution of venous stasis ulcers are not the only role for the nurse. Education of the aged person is essential as a means of preventing further episodes or minimizing the severity should ulceration recur.

Box 13-4	TREATMENTS FOR VENOUS STASIS ULCERS	

Conservative Treatment

Dressings	
Wet	To absorb weeping fluid
	Prevent tissue drying out
Change daily initially	Decreases risk of infection
(If not infected, an adhesive film or absorbent gel or foam is possible.)	Keeps clean and protected from bacteria
Application of fibrinolytic agents	
Cleaning	Mild soap and water
	Mechanically removes loose tissue without additional trauma
	Removes creams/lotions/medications applied
Compression wrap	Increases venous flow
	Should continue to wear even after lesion is healed
Elevation of legs	Decreases swelling
	Improves venous return
Ambulation	Improves venous return

Treatment for Severe Ulcers

Mechanical pump compression	Provides intermittent compression for several hours daily
Elastic stockings or wrap	
Surgery	
Skin graft	For large ulcers
Vein stripping	

Treatment for Chronic Recurring Stasis Ulcers

Growth factor from human blood platelets applied to ulcer in combination with other treatment	Stimulates new skin formation over ulcer, enhances healing
Cultured skin grown in laboratory (under Food and Drug Administration [FDA] review)	To cover ulcer and enhance healing

Pressure Ulcers (Pressure Sores)

Pressure ulcers, or pressure sores, are significant problems affecting 32% of patients (Pieper, 1998) and tend to be a chronic disorder of debilitated elders who are largely bed bound or chair bound. The primary cause is pressure on bony prominences. Just how much pressure can be endured by tissue (tissue tolerance) between the force and the bony prominence determines where an ulcer will form. Tissue tolerance is affected by moisture, pressure, friction, shearing, nutrition, age, and low arterial pressure. Pressure ulcers can develop anywhere on the body but are most frequently seen from the waist down. The prevalence is as high as 23% in long-term care settings (Bergstrom et al, 1994) and 30% in acute care settings (Anderson, Braun, 1995). It is often extremely difficult to predict, even with the use of the highly reliable Braden scale, which individuals will develop pressure ulcers, and

it is even more difficult to restore skin integrity once they have developed (Vandenbosch et al, 1996).

Pressure sores are a consequence of ischemia and anoxia to tissue. Tissues are compressed, blood is diverted, and blood vessels are forcibly constricted by persistent pressure on the skin and underlying structures; thus cellular respiration is impaired, and cells die. The sequence of events in pressure sore formation begins with erythema, which is followed by edema, blister formation, and, finally, ulceration if the blister sloughs.

Intervention at any point in the developing process can stop the advancement of the pressure sore. Fig. 13-1 illustrates the development of pressure sores. Anyone can develop pressure sores, but the aged have more friable tissue and more of the predisposing factors that lead to the development of pressure sores: poor nutritional status, such as anemia, hypoproteinemia, and vit-

Stage I

Erythema not resolving within thirty (30) minutes of pressure relief. Epidermis remains intact. REVERSIBLE WITH INTERVENTION.

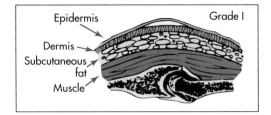

Stage II

Partial-thickness loss of skin layers involving epidermis and possibly penetrating into but not through dermis. May present as blistering with erythema and/or induration; wound base moist and pink; painful; free of necrotic tissue.

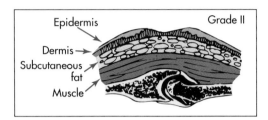

Stage III

Full-thickness tissue loss extending through dermis to involve subcutaneous tissue. Presents as shallow crater unless covered by eschar. May include necrotic tissue, undermining, sinus tract formation, exudate, and/or infection. Wound base is usually not painful.

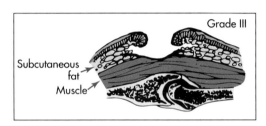

Stage IV

Deep tissue destruction extending through subcutaneous tissue to fascia and may involve muscle layers, joint, and/or bone. Presents as a deep crater. May include necrotic tissue, undermining, sinus tract formation, exudate, and/or infection. Wound base is usually not painful.

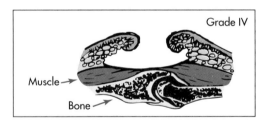

Fig. 13-1   Pressure sore development.

amin deficiencies; impaired sensory feedback systems; lack of fat padding over bony prominences; corticosteroid therapy; and immobilization by restraint or sedation. All of these contribute to tissue breakdown. Tissue breakdown is aggravated by heat, moisture, and decomposing and irritating substances on the skin. Those 70 years of age and older are particularly vulnerable (Pajk, 1995) to these conditions and situations. The particularly high risk groups include those hospitalized for femoral fractures, critical care patients, quadriplegic individuals, and those in skilled nursing facilities.

Pressure sores are not limited to those confined to bed. Individuals in wheelchairs or who sit in one place for a long time are equally vulnerable. In the recumbent position, the shoulders, lower back, and heels are susceptible to pressure breakdown. If one is lying on the abdomen, the knees, shins, and pelvis sustain undue pressure. The hips or trochanters receive undue pressure when one is in the side-lying position, and the buttocks receive undue pressure when one is in a sitting position. On occasion the outer rim of the ear can break down if it is pressed firmly against the side of the head for prolonged periods. It is particularly important to consider the underside of the scrotum and inspect it for pressure and excoriation. This area is subject to the friction and shearing force of the sheets without the benefit of a pull sheet. The warm, moist tissue is particularly susceptible to bacterial action from sustained moisture and soil.

Two tools, the Braden scale, developed in 1987, (Bergstrom et al, 1994) (see Appendix 13-B) and the Norton scale (Norton et al, 1962), are being used more frequently in the clinical setting in predicting individuals at risk for pressure sores. Since development of pressure sores is a dynamic process, it requires constant vigilance and repeated assessment (Kresevic, Naylor, 1995). Not clearly understood by nurses, physicians, and other caregivers is that it may take as long as 2 weeks of non–weight bearing or total pressure relief to heal a pressure area completely (Pires, Muller, 1991). The use of either the Braden or Norton assessment tools provides the means for a systematic evaluation and periodic reevaluation of a person's risk for pressure sores. Six subscales of the Braden scale are sensory perception, skin moisture, activity, mobility, friction and shearing, and nutritional status. Each category is rated as 1 (least favorable) to 4 (most favorable). The maximum score possible is 24 points; thus the lower the score, the more at risk a patient is for pressure sores and the greater the need for preventive interventions.

A more recent tool (developed in 1992), the Pressure Sore Status Tool (PSST) (Bates-Jensen, 1996), provides a framework for assessment of the actual pressure sore once it has developed. The revised Clinical Practice Guideline, *Treatment of Pressure Ulcers* (Bergstrom et al, 1994), suggests that this tool "with further research may prove useful for monitoring and reassessment" (p. 26). The PSST focuses on 13 macroscopic parameters, which allows the tracking over time of the status of the pressure sore. This is a dynamic method that is research based and reliable (Bates-Jensen, 1996). The 13 indexes include the 1-to-4 staging of the pressure ulcer (see Fig. 13-1). The complete PSST (Bates-Jensen) is found in Appendix 13-A; the Braden scale is found in Appendix 13-B.

The advantages of the PSST include validity, reliability, sensitivity to wound status, objectivity, quantifiability and subjective impression of the wound status, wound-healing parameters, and potential help in prescribing therapy. The disadvantages of the PSST revolve around the fact that people are not familiar with it. There is a learning curve that occurs with first use, and the tool is valid only with pressure sores, not other wounds (Bates-Jensen, 1996).

It has become apparent that a combination tool to address pressure sores is needed. Use of both the Braden scale for risk factor assessment and the PSST (actual pressure sore assessment) could provide a comprehensive and reliable approach to pressure sore risk and monitoring (Fig. 13-2).

Nurses play a vital role in the prevention of pressure sores. They must be able to identify early signs and initiate appropriate interventions to prevent further skin breakdown and to promote healing. Failure to do this jeopardizes the health and life of the elderly person. Pressure sores are costly to treat and may require extended separation from friends and loved ones. For many, it can prolong recovery and extend rehabilitation. The acquisition of iatrogenic complications such as pressure ulcers and complications from them, such as the need for grafting or amputation, sepsis, or even death, may lead to legal action by the individual or his or her representative against the caregiver. Box 13-5 lists the associated complications of pressure sores.

Clinical Practice Guidelines were developed by a multidisciplinary panel of experts under the auspices of the Agency for Health Care Policy and Research (AHCPR) of the U.S. Department of Health and Human Services to help professional and nonprofessional caregivers become knowledgeable about pressure sores and establish a baseline of care (US Department of Health and Human Services, 1994; Bergstrom et al, 1994). No particular approach is suggested, but a suggested protocol or guideline is offered.

Assessment. Visual and tactile inspection is essential to establish a normal skin characteristic baseline for a particular patient or client. Inspection is best achieved when performed in nonglare daylight or, if that is not possible, under the illumination of a 60-watt lightbulb (Jarvis, 1996; Seidel et al, 1999; Giger, Davidhizar, 1999). We also highly recommend Polaroid photographic recording. With the present sophisticated equipment available, accurate documentation is absolute (Morey, 1996; Pieper, 1999). Photographic documentation and inspection should include actual and potential areas for breakdown, with special attention directed to specific areas when an individual uses orthotic devices such as corsets, braces, prostheses, postural supports, splints, slings, or casts. Visual inspection should look for hyperemia, and if present, the area should be rechecked in an hour. Even though it is more difficult to see hyperemia in dark-skinned people, a red tone can be detected no matter how dark the skin may be (Giger, Davidhizar, 1999).

Blisters or pimples with or without hyperemia and scabs over weight-bearing areas in the absence of trauma should be considered suspicious. The location, color, and size of the area or areas should be noted. Tactile inspection should test hyperemic areas for blanch-

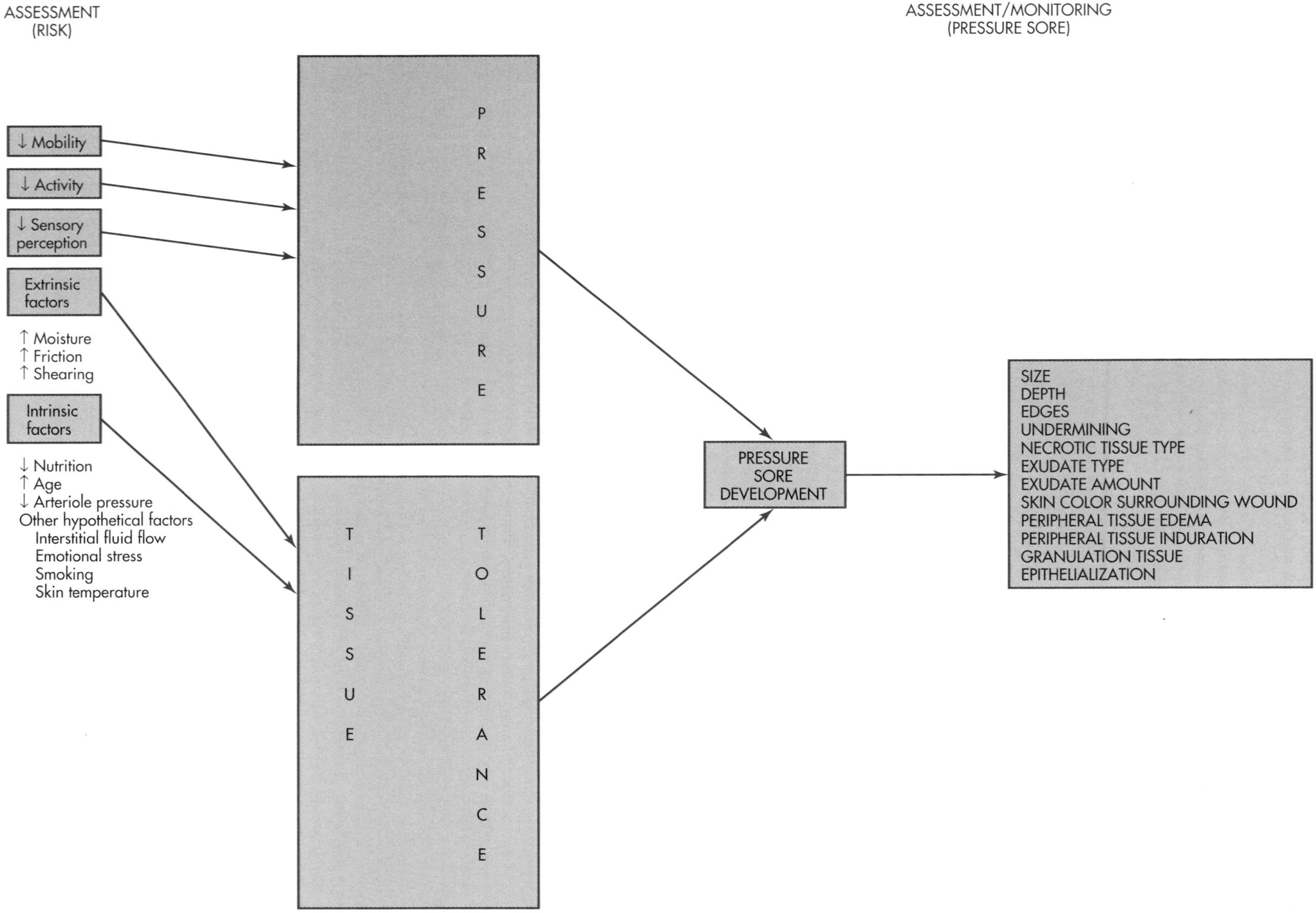

ASSESSMENT/MONITORING
(PRESSURE SORE)

| | | | | | | | | | | | | | |
| SIZE |
| DEPTH |
| EDGES |
| UNDERMINING |
| NECROTIC TISSUE TYPE |
| EXUDATE TYPE |
| EXUDATE AMOUNT |
| SKIN COLOR SURROUNDING WOUND |
| PERIPHERAL TISSUE EDEMA |
| PERIPHERAL TISSUE INDURATION |
| GRANULATION TISSUE |
| EPITHELIALIZATION |

PRESSURE
SORE
DEVELOPMENT

P R E S S U R E

T O L E R A N C E

T I S S U E

ASSESSMENT
(RISK)

↓ Mobility

↓ Activity

↓ Sensory
perception

Extrinsic
factors

↑ Moisture
↑ Friction
↑ Shearing

Intrinsic
factors

↓ Nutrition
↑ Age
↓ Arteriole pressure
Other hypothetical factors
Interstitial fluid flow
Emotional stress
Smoking
Skin temperature

Fig. 13-2   Comprehensive risk assessment and pressure sore monitoring.

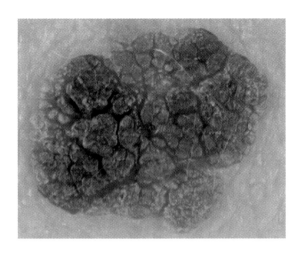

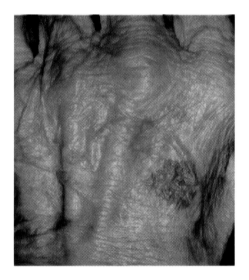

Fig. 1 Seborrheic keratosis in older adult. (From Habif TP: *Clinical dermatology: a color guide to diagnosis and therapy*, ed 3, St Louis, 1996, Mosby.)

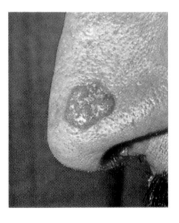

Fig. 2 Lentigo, a brown macule that appears in chronically sun-exposed areas. (From Habif TP: *Clinical dermatology: a color guide to diagnosis and therapy,* ed 3, St Louis, 1996, Mosby.)

Fig. 3 Basal cell carcinoma, the most commonly occurring skin cancer. (Courtesy Gary Monheit, MD, University of Alabama at Birmingham School of Medicine. In Seidel HM et al: *Mosby's guide to physical examination,* ed 4, St Louis, 1999, Mosby.)

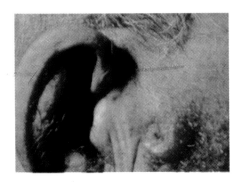

Fig. 4 Squamous cell carcinoma. (Courtesy Gary Monheit, MD, University of Alabama at Birmingham School of Medicine. In Seidel HM et al: *Mosby's guide to physical examination,* ed 4, St Louis, 1999, Mosby.)

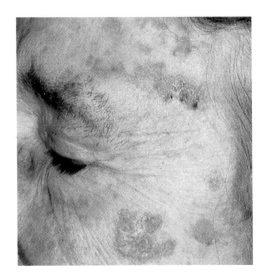

Fig. 5 Actinic keratosis in older adult in area of sun exposure. (From Habif TP: *Clinical dermatology: a color guide to diagnosis and therapy,* ed 3, St Louis, 1996, Mosby.)

Box 13-5	COMPLICATIONS OF PRESSURE SORES

Amyloidosis
Endocarditis
Heterotopic bone formation
Maggot infestation
Meningitis
Perineal-urethral fistula
Pseudoaneurysm
Septic arthritis
Sinus tract or abscess
Squamous cell carcinoma in the ulcer
Iodine toxicity or uncover subclinical hyperthyroidism (from use of iodine-based cleansing)
Hearing loss from use of topical aminoglycosides
Osteomyelitis
Bacteremia
Advanced cellulitis

From Bergstrom N et al: *Treatment of pressure ulcers,* Clinical Practice Guidelines No 15, AHCPR Pub No 95-0652, Rockville, Md, 1994, US Department of Health and Human Services, Public Health Service, Agency for Health Care Policy and Research.

Box 13-6	GENERAL SKIN ASSESSMENT GUIDELINES

General Inspection
Exposed body parts
  Color: generalized with regard to light- and dark-skinned individuals; variations
Unexposed parts (if individual is inactive, confined to bed or chair)

General Palpation
Texture, temperature, moisture, turgor, edema
Inspection and palpation of lesions
  Size, location, mobility, consistency, pattern, type (primary/secondary)
Hair: Inspection and palpation
  Color, amount, distribution, texture, parasites
Scalp: Inspection and palpation
  Texture, lesions
Nails: Inspection and palpation
  Color, shape, texture, condition of nail bed

ing and palpate for induration, noting hardness and temperature and comparing these characteristics with those of surrounding skin. The use of a risk assessment tool should be an integral part of any skin assessment. An assessment of nutritional status should be obtained, and if possible, a serum albumin value obtained. It has been demonstrated that a serum albumin value below 3.5 g/dl has a positive correlation with the severity of the pressure sore (Hanan, Scheele, 1991). Malnutrition ranks second only to excessive pressure in the etiology, pathogenesis, and nonhealing of pressure sores. Refer to Box 13-6 for general skin assessment guidelines.

The goal of nurses is to help maintain skin integrity against the various environmental, mechanical, and chemical assaults that are potential causes of skin breakdown. The nurse should assess the frequency of position change, adding pillows so that skin surfaces do not touch, and establish a turning schedule. Sitting and activity, skin care, incontinence care, and the use of heel protectors or the use of pillows to keep the heels off the bed, with or without so-called protective booties or blocks, should be assessed. In addition, a nutrition assessment with a body mass index (BMI) should be documented. Heels are a problematic site because they are particularly prone to pressure and are small surfaces that receive a high degree of pressure.

Elevating the heels off the bed with pillows or commercial products is helpful and especially important for individuals with diabetes mellitus and peripheral neuropathy.

Interventions. A wound in a person over 60 years of age takes approximately 100 days to heal. The estimated cost of treating a pressure sore is more than $20,000, not considering the emotional and physical discomfort that results. Miller and Delozier (1994) estimate that the cost to the health care system exceeds $1.3 billion. Nursing interventions should focus on prevention: actions that eliminate friction and irritation to the skin by lifting, turning, placing, and rolling (using two or more persons) the patient; reduction of moisture so that tissues can breathe and do not macerate; and displacement of body weight from prominent areas to facilitate circulation to the skin. The nurse should be familiar with the types of supportive surfaces so that the most effective surface can be used. Nutritional intake should be monitored, as well as the serum albumin level, hematocrit, and hemoglobin. Diets high in protein, carbohydrates, and vitamins are necessary to maintain and promote tissue growth. If appetite is lacking, appetite stimulants may be prescribed. Supplements of vitamin B help in the metabolism of carbohydrates, and pyridoxine and vitamin C assist in protein use.

Box 13-7   INTERVENTIONS BY RISK FACTOR

Bed or Chair Confinement

Inspect skin at least once daily.
Bathe when needed for comfort or cleanliness.
Prevent dry skin.

Bed confinement

Change position at least every 2 hours.
Use a special mattress that contains foam, air, gel, or water.
Raise head of bed as little and for as short a time as possible.

Chair confinement

Change position every hour.
Use foam, gel, air, or cushion to relieve pressure.
Reduce friction by:
    Lifting rather than dragging when repositioning
    Using cornstarch on skin
Avoid use of donut-shaped cushions.
Participate in a rehabilitation program.

Inability to Move
Bed confinement

Place pillow under legs from midcalf to ankles to keep heels off bed.

Chair confinement

Reposition every hour *if unable* to do by self.
Shift weight and position at least every 15 minutes *if able* to do by self.
Use pillows or wedges to keep knees or ankles from touching each other.

Loss of Bowel and Bladder Control

Clean skin as soon as soiled.
Assess and treat urine leaks.
If moisture cannot be controlled:
    Use absorbent pads and/or briefs with a quick-drying surface.
    Protect skin with a cream or ointment.

Poor Nutrition

Eat a balanced diet.
If a normal diet is not possible, talk to health care provider about nutritional supplements.

Lowered Mental Awareness

Choose preventive action that applies to person with lowered mental awareness. For example: if person chair bound, refer to specific prevention action as outlined in the above risk factors.

From *Preventing pressure ulcers: a patient's guide,* Clinical Practice Guideline, Rockville, Md, 1992, US Department of Health and Human Services, Public Health Service, Agency for Health Care Policy and Research.

Once ulcers have developed, treatments include débridement of necrotic tissue and debris, wound cleansing, appropriate dressings, and cultivation of the growth of granulation tissue (US Department of Health and Human Services, 1994). The number of treatments that exist for pressure sores indicates that no one approach has been entirely successful. However, through the collaborative efforts of the consultants who developed the AHCPR guidelines (Clinical Practice Guideline No. 3:

Pressure Ulcers in Adults: Prediction and Prevention and Clinical Practice Guideline No. 15: *Treatment of Pressure Ulcers*) significant progress has been made that may lead to a uniform manner of addressing the care of pressure sores. Within these guidelines the individuality of the patient is maintained, as are the possible choices of equipment and treatment modalities.

Interventions for prevention and early skin care treatment are presented in Box 13-7. It is important to note that solutions such as alcohol, certain soaps, and hydrogen peroxide are damaging to newly formed fragile skin. Povidone iodine placed on an open sore can be absorbed by tissues and is also a drying agent. Wounds heal best in their own natural environment (clean, moist, normal pH). Never occlude an infected wound. Various types of dressings are used depending on the condition of the pressure ulcer. These include transparent or film dressings, hydrocolloid, foam, hydrogels or alginate dressings, and collagen dressings. A wound care specialist is the best person to decide the most appropriate type of dressing to be used.

Realistically, it is not always possible to prevent pressure sores from occurring because of the physiologic or psychologic condition of the patient. Tissue injury is proportional to the amount and duration of the pressure exerted on the area. Obese people exert more pressure per square inch on tissue than do those who are thin. The deeper the sore penetration, the longer it will take to heal.

It is important not to use reverse staging of pressure ulcers as a description of ulcer healing. Staging is only appropriate as an indication of the depth of tissue involvement. As they heal, pressure ulcers fill with granulation tissue composed of endothelial cells, fibroblasts, collagen, and an extracellular matrix. Muscle, subcutaneous fat, or dermis is not replaced. *A pressure sore retains its initial stage rating.* For example, a stage IV pressure sore that is healing does not become a stage III and then a stage II as it heals. It remains defined as a stage IV; said another way, a patient has/would be recovered from a stage IV pressure ulcer. The change in its status provides objective data as to the healing process.

Pain caused by pressure ulcers has not been taken seriously until recently. Krasner (1995) indicates that 59% of persons with pressure ulcers do report pain. It was also noted that these individuals do not receive pain-relieving analgesics. Patients who cannot respond should not be considered pain free. Stage IV pressure ulcers are associated with more pain than other sources of pain. This is thought to be due to chemicals from the damaged tissue, erosion of tissue with destruction of nerve terminals, subsequent regeneration of nociceptive nerve terminals, infection, and/or dressing changes and débridement. Appropriate medication should be given to decrease or alleviate pain. In addition, occupational or physical therapy may decrease spasms caused by the wound; positioning and adaptive equipment may also help diminish pain.

Evaluation of pressure ulcers should be objective. The surface area, exudate quality, and tissue appearance should be noted. Pressure ulcer stages should not be used as a guide for determining ulcer resolution; rather, the percent of reduction in size after 2 weeks of treatment should be used. Pressure ulcers should be reassessed after each dressing change.

FEET

The feet undergo a great deal of use, trauma, misuse, and neglect as part of everyday living. Most aged persons accept foot problems as an inescapable accompaniment of aging. Nurses and people in general have a fairly strong negative reaction to having contact with the feet. The foot is aesthetically unpleasant (Pelican et al, 1990). Yet, adequate care of the feet can alleviate disability, pain, and the tendency for falling. It is for these reasons that the importance of feet to the well-being of the aged is emphasized more extensively in this chapter than in most texts.

The feet influence the physical, psychologic, and social well-being of the individual. The feet carry one's body weight, hold the body erect in an upright and stationary position, coordinate and maintain balance in walking, and must be rigid yet loose and adaptable enough to conform to the surfaces underfoot (all the while holding the legs and body in an upright position). Little attention is given to these valuable appendages until the feet interfere with ambulation and the ability to maintain independence.

The feet often reflect systemic disease conditions or give clues to physical ailments before their actual appearance (Echevarria et al, 1988; Burning Feet, 1992). Sudden or gradual changes in nail or skin conditions of the feet and/or the appearance of recurring infections may be a precursor of more serious health problems. The feet have a significant effect on one's productivity, amiability, and mobility. The effect is comparable to the influence that the automobile has had in our society. Like the automobile, if there is something wrong, it is difficult to get around, and the routine of the day is upset. The feet, like the automobile, are taken for granted and accorded little attention as long as they work. Unlike the automobile, though, the feet do not have easily replaceable parts. Neglect of the feet throughout one's active years results in painful conditions later (Collet, 1995).

Uncomfortable and painful feet may force the elderly person to become sedentary and deprived of social contacts. Foot discomfort can cause irritability, fatigue, and chronic complaints. Socrates is thought to have said, "To him whose feet hurt, everything hurts" (An Assessment, 1977, p. 102). This sums up the essence of foot problems.

The aged person's feet are subjected to functional and physical neglect and traumatic stresses over the years. The residual effects from these varied stresses, compounded by a decreased ability of the aged to clearly see their feet (because of visual impairment) and to bend to give their feet routine care often result in conditions that need not exist or at least could be controlled.

Mobility for the aged may mean the difference between an independent, active community life, self-respect, motivation, and responsibility for one's health versus institutionalization. Even in an institution, foot problems may mean the difference between confinement to bed or wheelchair and the ability to ambulate in the protective setting.

Foot Problems in Old Age

The foot begins to change shape in females soon after birth, but in males changes in shape begin in about the fourth decade. There is a gradual loss of fat padding of the adult foot, resulting in greater stress on feet and the potential for the development of musculoskeletal disorders (Echevarria et al, 1988; Helfand, 1989).

Fifty percent of the general population have foot problems. The number and severity of the problems increase with age. Almost 80% of persons over the age of 50 will have at least one significant foot problem. Three of every four persons 65 years and over complain of foot pain. Individuals over 55 years of age (88% of women and 83% of men) demonstrate arthritic changes in the foot on x-ray examination. Of these older adults, 25% have symptoms of foot problems (Gudas, 1986; Common Foot Problems, 1993).

Major abnormalities occur gradually with discomfort, not with pain. Without proper care and treatment these conditions become disabling and a threat to the person's independence.

Diseases also endanger the foot. Osteoarthritis can cause pain in the feet. Rheumatoid arthritis may lead to hammer toes and dislocated toes. Peripheral vascular disease can lead to infections of the feet, pain resulting from decreased circulation, and amputation. Gout creates difficulty in walking as a result of the pain of uric acid crystal accumulation and swelling of toe joints, particularly the joint of the great toe. Diabetes, with the development of peripheral neuropathy, predisposes the foot to injury, infection, and in some instances amputation.

Corns

Corns, the cone-shaped layers of compacted skin, usually on toes, occur as a result of friction and pressure on the skin rubbing against bony, protuberant areas of the toes when shoes are worn. Once the small, hard, white corn is established, continued pressure elicits pain. Unless the cause of the corn is removed, it will continue to enlarge and cause increasing pain. Soft corns form in the same manner but occur between opposing surfaces of the toes. Corns interfere with the ability to walk comfortably and wear shoes. This condition is symptomatic of underlying problems of feet that are subjected to prolonged or recurrent friction and pressure.

Most individuals have attempted do-it-yourself remedies for corns. The aged usually follow what they have done for years to correct their foot discomfort. Over-the-counter preparations for corns, in particular, damage normal tissue in addition to removing the corn. Chemical burns and ulcerations can result in the loss of toes or a leg for the aged person with diabetes, neurologic impairment, or poor circulatory function to the lower extremities. Some elderly persons use razor blades and scissors to remove corns. In light of the aforementioned problems with vision and flexibility, this is a dangerous solution.

Oval corn pads, which seem to aid in the relief of corns, actually create greater pressure on the toes and can decrease circulation to the tissue within the oval pad. Oval corn pads can be adapted for effective use. Instead of using the oval pad as it is, the upper or lower section of the corn pad can be cut out so that the pad resembles the letter U. This can be placed around three aspects of the corn, protecting it from pressure without restricting circulation to healthy tissue. Newer gel-type pads are also useful to protect against friction and pressure. Irritation from soft corns between the toes can be eased by loosely wrapping small amounts of lamb's wool around the involved toe.

Calluses

Calluses are also layers of compacted skin that usually occur on the soles and heels of the feet because of chronic irritation and friction from shoes. Calluses can be eased with moleskin applied to those areas that receive undue friction. Moleskin adheres for several days or longer but should be removed when it becomes wet or excessively soiled. Removing moleskin from the feet of the elderly should be done slowly to prevent tearing of skin.

The nurse should be very careful when using adhesive tape on the aged foot. Older foot skin is thinner and more delicate and does not tolerate adhesive tape well (Jahss, 1979).

Decreased sebaceous activity, dehydration of the horny layer, and environmental influences are responsible for the majority of dry and scaly foot problems that the elderly exhibit. Metabolic or nutritional alterations and dysfunctions of keratin formation are considered other possible causes of problems with dry feet. Dryness leads to fissures in the soles of the feet, particularly the heels. Feet itch and are scratched to relieve the discomfort. It is necessary to lubricate the feet with lotion at least twice each day to retain tissue hydration. Lotion helps keep water in the tissue rather than letting it evaporate and cause dryness. Vegetable and mineral oils are inexpensive and effective substitutes for the standard over-the-counter lotions. Lotion or oil should be applied and massaged into the foot tissue and the excess removed, particularly between the toes.

Bunions

Bunions (hallux valgus) are bony prominences that occur over the medial aspect of the first metatarsal head (the joint of the great toe) and, at times, at the lateral aspect of the fifth metatarsal head (the joint of the little toe), which is often called a *tailor bunion* or a *bunionette.* Bunions are long-standing residual effects from occupational activity and the influence of shoe styles. Women's shoes, which draw the toes together and cause improper weight transmission, and restrictive hose contribute to the problem. Bunions may also be hereditary in nature (Common Foot Problems, 1993).

The nurse should focus on obtaining shoes that properly support, protect, and provide comfort for the foot and encourage the client to wear them. Shoes should provide enough forefoot space laterally and dorsally with a wide toe box and comfortable fit, such as found in ultralight walking shoes and running shoes. Fabric shoes (not recommended for diabetic persons) are perhaps the most comfortable for the aged person with a bunion because fabric stretches more than leather and synthetic materials. Cloth shoes should have a good-quality walking surface. Protective pads are also available to cushion bunion joints.

Shoe stores have devices that will stretch the shoe at the pressure area, but the customer must purchase the shoe before this easement is made. Shoe repair shops have shoe-stretching devices and charge a reasonable fee for stretching a shoe. At home, leather shoes can be eased while they are being worn by wetting the shoe with alcohol. This allows the leather to stretch to the shape of the foot and will not leave a permanent water-

mark because the alcohol evaporates. Custom-made shoes, although expensive, are available to the aged person with bunions.

Hammer Toe

A hammer toe is a permanently flexed and rotated toe (or toes) that has a clawlike appearance; the condition is a result of muscle imbalance and is aggravated by poor-fitting shoes. Over time, the toe, usually the second toe, is pushed by the bunioned great toe slanting toward and under the toe. The toe then contracts, leaving a bulge on top of the joint. Balance and comfort are affected. Treatment includes professional orthotics; properly fitting, nonconstricting shoes; and/or surgical intervention to rectify this problem (Common Foot Problems, 1993).

Metatarsalgia

Metatarsalgia is pain in the ball of the foot caused by a narrow, high-arched foot, which focuses stress on the ball of the foot; legs that are unequal in length, thus adding stress to the metatarsal joints of the shorter leg; rheumatoid arthritis; stress fractures; fluid accumulation; muscle fatigue; flat feet; or overloaded feet, as in the case of obesity. Bunions or tender calluses under the metatarsophalangeal joint or a Morton neuroma may also be responsible for this foot problem. Relief is often obtained with foot freedom (i.e., when the foot is not restricted by shoes, or shoe length and width are adequate). Orthotics and the use of nonsteroidal antiinflammatory medications are also helpful. Orthotics can be a reasonably priced alternative (rather than custom-made shoes) for the elder with foot problems (Metatarsalgia, 1991).

Burning Feet

Burning feet, although usually temporary, are a common problem with the aged. This annoyance occurs as a result of irritating fabrics, poorly fitting shoes, fungal infections, or contact with toxic substances such as poison ivy or poison oak. Generally, burning feet are not serious but can be symptomatic of such underlying diseases as diabetes mellitus, alcoholism, poor nutritional state (folic acid, B_{12} deficiency), chronic kidney failure, or liver disease. In addition, medications and exposure to such poisons as arsenic and lead may cause burning feet.

Self-help measures that can help alleviate burning feet include wearing cotton or cotton-blend socks. Shoes made of natural materials that breathe, provide a good fit, and have fitted insoles can help greatly to reduce the burning sensation. Cold tap water foot baths 15 minutes twice a day to cool the feet, in conjunction with rest and avoidance of activities that aggravate the problem, can reduce burning. The use of prescribed and over-the-counter preparations also can bring relief.

Fungal and Bacterial Infections

Fungal and bacterial infections are common in the aged foot. These conditions usually develop because the foot is encased in a warm, dark, and moisture-holding shoe. Nail fungus is characterized by dirty yellow streaks or total nail discoloration. The nail becomes opaque, scaly, and hypertrophied. A fine powdery substance forms under the center of the nail and pushes it up, causing the sides of the nail to dig into the flesh like an ingrown toenail. Culturing is the only definitive way to identify onychomycosis (Tosti, 1995). Hands should be washed each time the feet of a patient with a fungal infection are handled. Feet, especially between the toes, should be dry and exposed to sun and air. If the feet are prone to fungal and bacterial conditions, a daily dusting with antifungal powder or spray is appropriate. This condition requires a podiatrist to control and eliminate it. Itraconazole (Sporanox) was approved by the U.S. Food and Drug Administration (FDA) to treat and cure most nail fungal infections. It causes fewer side effects than previous oral drugs and provides for a shorter treatment time (New Drugs, 1996).

Care of the Feet

Foot care is a prime factor in determining mobility and the quality of existence in retaining independence. Elders with painful foot problems and resultant activity limitations are usually forced to remain within the boundaries of their homes.

Nursing care of the aged foot should be directed toward maintaining comfort and function, removing possible mechanical irritants, decreasing the likelihood of infection, and helping to enhance and preserve maximal function. These goals are consistent with podiatric goals.

The nurse has the important function of assessing the feet of the aged person for clues to well-being and functional ability, not just bathing and applying lotion to the feet. Nurses can identify potential and actual problems and refer or seek podiatric assistance for the foot problems of the patient.

Assessment

Nursing care of the feet should include a thorough assessment (Pelican et al, 1990). King (1978, 1980) de-

veloped an assessment tool for the lower extremities of the aged that any caregiver can learn to use. As shown in Fig. 13-3, the tool provides illustrations of some of the important aspects to look for and evaluate and simple explanations of specific items to ensure uniform evaluation regardless of who performs the assessment. Until the nurse is familiar with this tool, it will take about 20 minutes or more to complete, but with increased proficiency, the time required can be reduced. The assessment itself includes the essentials of foot care: inspection of the feet for irritation, abrasions, and other lesions; determination of functional and other acquired deviations; checks for hazards to the maintenance of adequate circulation to the lower extremities and the existing circulatory status; and observation of the individual's mobility.

Other tools for foot assessment have been developed. The Kelechi and Lukas (Kelechi, 1991) assessment tool is a form for regular and follow-up assessment and care. It is divided into five sections, each with a list of data to obtain either by questioning or through direct observation. An intervention list is included that provides a list of what action was taken and the results. The final section of the tool is completed with the follow-up plan and appointment, which is then signed by the person who provided the care. Pelican et al (1990) used a shorter form for assessing the feet. They listed those observations that should be part of a plan of care. The types of interventions that might have been done are listed, and a follow-up section is provided. The variety of tools available speaks to the need for individualization to the client population with whom one is working and to the expertise of the individual who is doing the assessment and giving the care.

Assessment is the key to maintenance of the aged person's highest level of function and mobility. Elderly persons with diabetes mellitus; cardiac, hyperthyroid, or kidney conditions; or pernicious anemia are naturally prone to foot problems. Those individuals with residual foot and leg impairment from strokes may develop foot ulcers from pressure exerted by their shoes or braces and from pressure and persistent friction and irritation caused by altered walking patterns. Box 13-8, p. 255, gives essential assessment items for obtaining a thorough foot assessment.

Interventions

Care of the toenails. The inability of the aged to care for their toenails is influenced by poor vision, hand tremors, the inability to bend, obesity, or increased nail thickness. Nails that are neglected or that do not receive

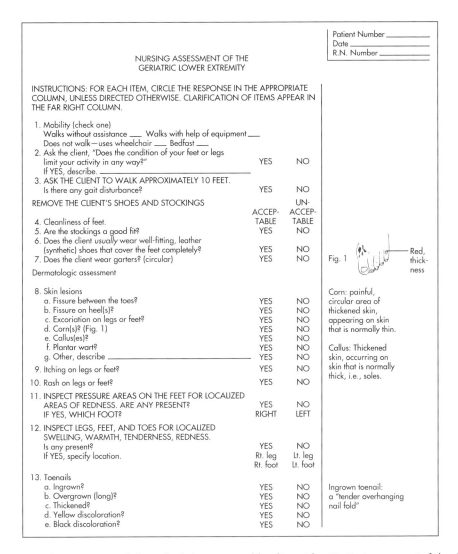

Fig. 13-3   Nursing assessment of the geriatric lower extremities. (From King PA: Foot assessment of the elderly, *J Gerontol Nurs* 4:47, Nov/Dec 1978.)

Continued

treatment may become unusually long and curved. This type of nail is known as *ram's horn* because of its appearance. Hard, thickened nails indicate inadequate nutrition to the nail matrix from trauma or poor circulation. Once the nail becomes thickened, it will remain so. These conditions should be brought to the attention of the podiatrist. Any attempt by the nurse or other caregiver to cut these nails may result in further damage to the matrix or precipitate an infection.

Normal nails that become too long or begin to interfere with stockings, hose, or shoes should be cut straight across and even with the top of the toe (Turner, 1996). Nails that are hard can easily split, causing trauma to the matrix, pain, and possibly infection. Feet should be soaked in warm water to soften the nails before they are clipped. Ideally, toenails should be trimmed after the bath or shower, but if this is not appropriate, soaking the feet for 20 to 30 minutes will facilitate the procedure. However, foot soaks are not recommended for diabetic persons, nor is it recommended that nurses cut the nails of an elder with diabetes mellitus. A podiatrist should do this.

Circulatory status (Questions 14-18 relate to FEET ONLY)

14. Do the feet have any red, reddish blue, or bluish discoloration?	YES	NO
15. Is there any brownish discoloration around the ankles?	YES	NO
16. Is the dorsalis pedis present? (Fig. 2) If NO, which foot?	YES RIGHT	NO LEFT
17. Is the posterior tibial pulse present? (Fig. 3) If NO, which foot?	YES RIGHT	NO LEFT
18. Is the skin dry?	YES	NO

The following relate to BOTH FEET AND LEGS

19. Is edema present?	YES	NO

CHECK THE TEMPERATURE OF THE LEGS AND THE FEET WITH THE BACKS OF YOUR FINGERS, COMPARING ONE EXTREMITY WITH THE OTHER.

20. Are the feet the same temperature?	YES	NO
21. Are the legs the same temperature?	YES	NO
22. Does the client have any pain in the legs or feet? If YES, DESCRIBE	YES	NO

INSPECT THE LEGS, SIDES OF ANKLES, SOLES, TOES FOR ULCERATION.

23. Is any ulceration present? If YES, specify location.	YES Rt. leg Rt. foot	NO Lt. leg Lt. foot

Structural deformities

24. Hallux valgus (bunion)? (Fig. 4)	YES	NO
25. Hammer toes? (Fig. 5)	YES	NO
26. Overlapping digits?	YES	NO

ASK THE CLIENT TO STAND

27. Are the legs the same relative size?	YES	NO
28. Are the legs the same relative length?	YES	NO
29. Are varicosities present?	YES	NO

Use three fingers on the dorsum of the foot usually just lateral to the extensor tendon of the great toe.

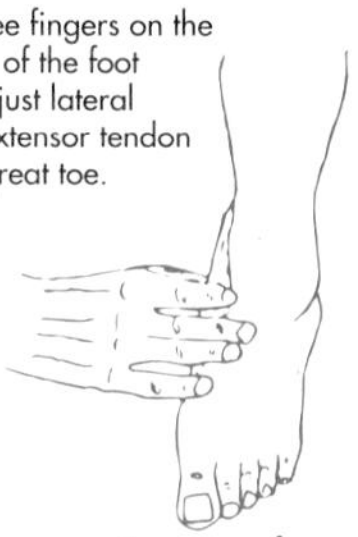

Fig. 2

Curve your fingers behind and slightly below the medial malleolus of the ankle.

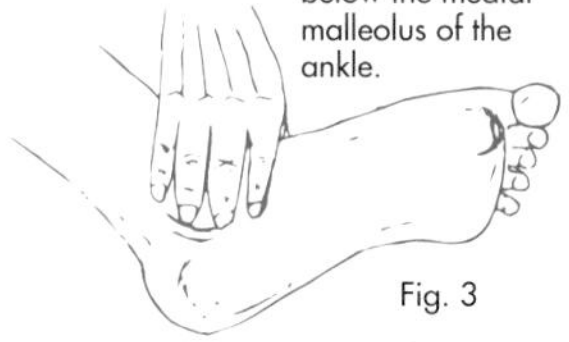

Fig. 3

Figs. 2 and 3. Questions 16 & 17. (The instructions and illustrations for palpating the pulses are from *A Guide to Physical Examination*, 1974, by Barbara Bates, M.D., used by permission of J.B. Lippincott Co., publisher).

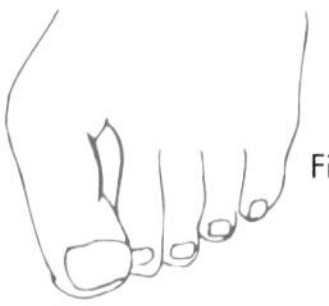

Fig. 4

Hallux valgus (Outward deviation of great toe)

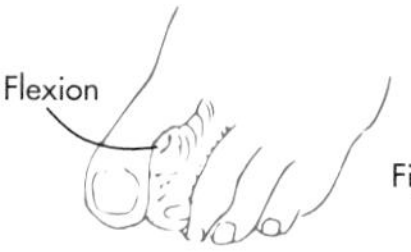

Flexion

Fig. 5

Hammer Toe (Flexion contracture)

Fig. 13-3, cont'd   See legend on p. 253.

An ingrown toenail is a fragment of nail that pierces the skin of the nail lip. Often this problem is a consequence of improper cutting of the nail. An additional cause is pressure exerted on the toes by short or supportive hose. This problem, too, should be seen by the podiatrist, but as a temporary measure it is simple enough for the nurse to insert a wisp of cotton under the section of the nail that is growing into the nail lip, which will lift it and reduce the pressure and pain.

Shoes. Shoes should be worn that cover, protect, and provide stability for the foot, maximize toe space, and minimize the chance of falls. In essence, shoes should be considered as clothing and be functional. Slip-on shoes are helpful for those aged persons who are unable to bend or lace shoes. Velcro closures are also useful to those who have limited finger dexterity. Low-heeled shoes with a wide toe box and a ridged sole minimize falls, place less stress on the legs and back, and are ideal for comfort. The proverbial "thumb's width" is the correct space between the big toe and the toe tip of the shoe. One should also be able to pinch the leather or fabric across the widest part of the upper shoe.

Box 13-8   ESSENTIAL DATA OF FOOT ASSESSMENT

Observation of Mobility

Gait
Ambulation
Foot hygiene
Footwear

Past Medical History

Systemic diseases
Musculoskeletal problems
Vascular/ulcerations/peripheral vascular disease
Vision problems
Falls
Trauma
Smoking history
Pain

Bilateral Assessment

Color
Circulation
Pulses
Structures (hammer toe, bunion, overlapping digits)
Temperature
Dermatologic aspects
  Skin lesions (fissures, corns, calluses, warts, excoriation)
  Edema
  Itching
  Rash
Toenails
  Long, thick
  Discoloration

Reduction of dependent edema. Circulatory efficiency in the lower extremities, especially the feet, is sluggish. Edema of the ankles and feet is evident after periods of prolonged sitting and standing. It is helpful if the aged do not wear constricting circular garters, socks with snug bands, or support hose, which constrict the feet. Sitting with the feet elevated on a footstool or hassock is helpful in reducing edema and facilitating better venous circulation. Foot exercises, too, are a means of reducing edema by encouraging more efficient venous return. Exercises can be done anytime. It would be good to develop the habit of doing foot exercises on rising and going to bed. Other times could be during television commercials.

The exercises are simple, and in addition to helping reduce edema, they facilitate foot flexibility. Toe bends, or curling and relaxing the toes, should be done at least five times on each foot. These can be done one foot at a time or both feet together, followed by rotating the feet at the ankles clockwise and then counterclockwise 5 to 10 times, and, finally, bringing the knees to the chest 5 to 10 times. These exercises can be done consecutively or with short rest periods in between, depending on the stamina of the individual.

Two areas of the foot in older persons may appear to be edematous. The upper outer aspect near the ankle is actually muscle. This can usually be identified by wiggling the toes; it will move. The other area is below and in front of the ankle bone. This occurs in some, but not all, women and is a fat pad. Its size remains constant.

Singly or together these may look like edema, but they are not. Awareness of these anatomic phenomena will help in assessing edema correctly.

Foot massage. Foot massage is another useful means of reducing edema, stimulating circulation, and improving pedal flexibility. Not only does massage aid in accomplishing these things, but also it relaxes the feet and stimulates relaxation of the rest of the body. However, not all elderly persons are candidates for foot massage. Individuals with foot lesions or vascular problems of the lower extremities should be seen by the physician for a definitive decision before massage is considered.

▶ **KEY CONCEPTS**

- The skin is the largest and most visible organ of the body; it is the direct mediator with the environment.
- Showering is best for elders and then only two to three times a week, followed by the use of moisturizing lotion.
- The elderly should avoid prolonged direct sun exposure.
- Mobility is fundamental to independence; therefore care of the feet and toenails is important and should not be neglected.
- The feet often reflect systemic disease and give clues to physical ailments before the actual appearance of these ailments.

- Individuals with foot lesions or vascular problems of the extremities should have a qualified podiatrist routinely care for their feet.
- Foot massage with a good lubricating lotion reduces edema, stimulates circulation, improves pedal flexibility, and tends to relax the entire body. Massage should be done only with medical approval if there are foot lesions or vascular problems.

 Activities and Discussion Questions

1. Describe the normal age-related changes of the skin.
2. What are the common skin problems of the older adult?
3. Explain what assessment tools are useful to the nurse for skin and foot assessments.
4. List several interventions that apply to skin care; to foot care.
5. Develop a nursing care plan using wellness and NANDA diagnoses.

NANDA and Wellness Diagnoses

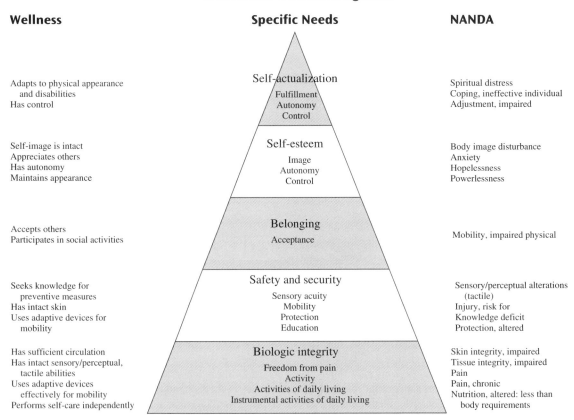

Wellness	Specific Needs	NANDA
Adapts to physical appearance and disabilities Has control	**Self-actualization** Fulfillment Autonomy Control	Spiritual distress Coping, ineffective individual Adjustment, impaired
Self-image is intact Appreciates others Has autonomy Maintains appearance	**Self-esteem** Image Autonomy Control	Body image disturbance Anxiety Hopelessness Powerlessness
Accepts others Participates in social activities	**Belonging** Acceptance	Mobility, impaired physical
Seeks knowledge for preventive measures Has intact skin Uses adaptive devices for mobility	**Safety and security** Sensory acuity Mobility Protection Education	Sensory/perceptual alterations (tactile) Injury, risk for Knowledge deficit Protection, altered
Has sufficient circulation Has intact sensory/perceptual, tactile abilities Uses adaptive devices effectively for mobility Performs self-care independently	**Biologic integrity** Freedom from pain Activity Activities of daily living Instrumental activities of daily living	Skin integrity, impaired Tissue integrity, impaired Pain Pain, chronic Nutrition, altered: less than body requirements

These are not all of the possible wellness or NANDA diagnoses that may be identified. The above are frequent examples of nursing diagnoses that should be considered when planning care for the older adult in whatever setting.

RESOURCES

Pressure Ulcers in Adults: Prediction and Prevention, Clinical Practice Guideline No. 3. Available from AHCPR Publications Clearing House, PO Box 8547, Silver Spring, MD 20907.

American Cancer Society publications:

The Diagnosis and Management of Common Skin Cancer, No. 2558

Facts on Skin Cancer, No. 825

Fry Now, Pay Later, No. 901

Melanoma/Skin Cancer—Can You Recognize the Signs? No. 904

Krames Communications

312 90th Street

Daly City, CA 94015-1898

Brochure briefly explains how to examine your skin, conditions to look for, prevention of problems, and risk factors.

Local podiatric society

Local and regional podiatric referral service

Local podiatric college/clinic

REFERENCES

Anderson MA, Braun JV: *Caring for the elderly,* Philadelphia, 1995, Davis.

An assessment of foot health problems and related health utilization and requirements, *J Am Podiatr Assoc* 69:102, 1977 (abstract).

Bates-Jensen BM: *Why and how to assess pressure ulcers,* Presented at the Ninth Annual Symposium on Advanced Wound Care, Atlanta, April 20, 1996.

Bergstrom N et al: *Treatment of pressure ulcers,* Clinical Practice Guideline No 15, AHCPR Pub No 95-0652, Rockville, Md, 1994, US Department of Health and Human Services, Public Health Service, Agency for Health Care Policy and Research.

Burning feet, *Mayo Clin Health Lett* 10(1):1, 1992.

Collet BS: Foot problems. In Abrams WB, Beers MH, Berkow R, editors: *The Merck manual of geriatrics,* ed 2, Whitehouse Station, NJ, 1995, Merck Research Laboratories.

Common foot problems: prevention and treatment, *Perspect Health Promot Aging* 8(2):1, 1993.

Dunn LB et al: Does estrogen prevent skin aging? *Arch Dermatol* 133:339, 1997.

Echevarria KH et al: A team approach to foot care, *Geriatr Nurs* 9(6):338, 1988.

Elewski BE: Dermatologic disorders of aging. In Bosker G et al, editors: *Geriatric emergency medicine,* St Louis, 1990, Mosby.

Ferrell BA, Osterweil D, issue editors: Aging skin, *Focus Geriatr Care Rehabil* 2(9):1, 1989.

Flory C: Skin assessment: perfecting the art, *RN* 55(60):22, 1992.

Friedman SA: Peripheral vascular diseases; aneurysms. In Abrams WB, Beers MH, Berkow R, editors: *The Merck manual of geriatrics,* ed 2, Whitehouse Station, NJ, 1995, Merck Research Laboratories.

Giger JN, Davidhizar RE: *Transcultural nursing: assessment and intervention,* ed 3, St Louis, 1999, Mosby.

Gilchrest BA: Dermatologic disorders in the elderly. In Rossman I, editor: *Clinical geriatrics,* ed 3, Philadelphia, 1986, Lippincott.

Gilchrest BA: Skin changes and disorders. In Abrams WB, Beers MH, Berkow R, editors: *The Merck manual of geriatrics,* ed 2, Whitehouse Station, NJ, 1995, Merck Research Laboratories.

Gudas CJ: Common foot disorders. In Calkins E, Davis PJ, Ford AB, editors: *The practice of geriatrics,* Philadelphia, 1986, WB Saunders.

Hanan K, Scheele L: Albumin vs weight as a predictor of nutritional status and pressure ulcer development, *Ostomy Wound Manage* 33:22, 1991.

Hardy MA: What can you do about your patient's dry skin? *J Gerontol Nurs* 22(5), 1996.

Helfand AE, issue editor: The aging foot, *Focus Geriatr Care Rehabil* 2(10):1, 1989.

Jahss MH: Geriatric aspects of the foot and ankle. In Rossman I, editor: *Clinical geriatrics,* ed 2, Philadelphia, 1979, Lippincott.

Jarvis C: *Physical examination and health assessment,* ed 2, Philadelphia, 1996, Saunders.

Kelechi T: Clinical outlook: nursing foot care for the aged, *J Gerontol Nurs* 17(9):40, 1991.

King PA: Foot assessment of the elderly, *J Gerontol Nurs* 4:47, 1978.

King PA: Foot problems and assessment, *Geriatr Nurs* 1:182, 1980.

Krasner D: Using a gentler approach: reflections on patients with pressure ulcers who experience pain, *Ostomy Wound Manage* 41:20, 1995.

Kresevic DM, Naylor M: Preventing pressure ulcers through use of protocols in a mentored nursing model, *Geriatr Nurs* 16(5):225, 1995.

Leg ulcers, *Mayo Clin Health Lett* 13:1, 1995.

Lombardo PC: Dermatological disorders in the elderly. In Rossman I, editor: *Clinical geriatrics,* ed 2, Philadelphia, 1979, Lippincott.

Marks R: *Skin disease in old age,* Philadelphia, 1987, Lippincott.

Mayfield P: Skin. In Hogstel MO, editor: *Clinical manual of gerontological nursing,* St Louis, 1992, Mosby.

McGrann GE: Diagnosis and management and preventing skin cancer, *Adv Nurse Pract* 2(7):36, 1994.

Metatarsalgia, *Mayo Clin Health Lett* 9(2):1991.

Miller CA: *Nursing care of older adults,* ed 3, Philadelphia, 1999, Lippincott.

Miller H, Delozier J: *Cost implications of the pressure ulcer treatment guideline,* Contract No 282-91-0070, Columbia, Md, 1994, Center for Health Policy Studies.

Montagu A: *Touching,* ed 2, New York, 1992, Harper & Row.

Morey SE: The Health Cam 2 in use: photos supplement written documentation, *Dev Photo Documentation* 1(1):1, 1996.

Motta G: *Care of mature skin,* Unpublished manuscript, 1992.

New drugs cure most nail infections, *UCSF to Our Neighbors* 21(1):1, 1996.

Norton D, McLaren R, Exton-Smith AN: *An investigation of geriatric nursing problems in the hospital,* London, 1962, National Corporation for the Care of Old People.

Pajk M: Pressure sores. In Abrams WB, Beers MH, Berkow R, editors: *The Merck manual of geriatrics,* ed.2, Whitehouse Station, NJ, 1995, Merck, Sharpe & Dohme Research Laboratories.

Pelican P, Barbieri E, Blair S: Toe the line: a nurse-run well foot care clinic, *J Gerontol Nurs* 16(12):6, 1990.

Phillips TJ, Gilchrest BA: Skin changes and disorders. In Abrams WB, Beers MH, Berkow R, editors: *The Merck manual of geriatrics,* Rahway, NJ, 1990, Merck Sharpe & Dohme Research Laboratories.

Pieper B: Pressure ulcer management, *Adv Nurs Pract* 6(10):55, 1998.

Pires M, Muller A: Detection and management of early tissue pressure indicators: a pictorial essay, *Progressions* 3(3):3, 1991.

Porth C, Kapke K: Aging and the skin, *Geriatr Nurs* 4:158, 1983.

Reichel W: *Care of the elderly,* ed 3, Baltimore, 1995, Williams & Wilkins.

Renaissance Medical, Inc, Dana Point, Calif, 1992.

Saxon SV, Etten MJ: *Physical changes and aging,* ed 3, New York, 1994, Tirasias.

Seidel HM et al: *Mosby's guide to physical examination,* ed 4, St Louis, 1999, Mosby.

Staab A, Lyles M: *Manual of geriatric nursing,* Glenview, Ill, 1990, Scott Foresman/Little, Brown Higher Education.

Talarico LD: Aging skin: best approaches to common problems, *Patient Care Nurse Pract* 1(5):28, 1998.

Timaris PS, editor: *Physiological basis of aging and geriatrics,* ed 2, Boca Raton, Fla, 1994, CRC Press.

Tosti A: Onychomycosis is often misdiagnosed on clinical exam: culture is the key, *Mod Med* 63(12):3, 1995.

Turner C: Nurses' knowledge, assessment skills, experience and confidence in toenail management of elderly people, *Geriatr Nurs* 17(6):273, 1996.

US Department of Health and Human Services: *Treatment of pressure ulcers,* Clinical Practice Guideline No 15, AHCPR Pub No 95-0652, Rockville, Md, 1994, US Department of Health and Human Services, Public Health Service, Agency for Health Care Policy and Research.

Vandenbosch T et al: Predictive validity of the Braden scale and nurse perception in identifying pressure ulcer risk, *Appl Nurs Res* 9(2):80, 1996.

Wallis C: The estrogen dilemma, *Time* 145:46, June 26, 1995.

Wasaha S, Angelopoulos T: What every woman should know about menopause, *Am J Nurs* 96(1):25, 1996.

appendix 13-a *Pressure Sore Status Tool*

INSTRUCTIONS FOR USE

General Guidelines

Fill out the attached rating sheet to assess a pressure sore's status after reading the definitions and methods of assessment described below. Evaluate once a week and whenever a change occurs in the wound. Rate according to each item by picking the response that best describes the wound and entering that score in the item score column for the appropriate date. When you have rated the pressure sore on all items, determine the total score by adding together the 13-item scores. The HIGHER the total score, the more severe the pressure score status. Plot total score on the Pressure Sore Status Continuum to determine progression of the wound.

Specific Instructions

1. Size: Use ruler to measure the longest and widest aspect of the wound surface in centimeters; multiply length × width.
2. Depth: Pick the depth, thickness, most appropriate to the wound using these additional descriptions:
   1 = tissues damaged but no break in skin surface.
   2 = superficial, abrasion, blister, or shallow crater. Even with, and/or elevated above skin surface (e.g., hyperplasia).
   3 = deep crater with or without undermining of adjacent tissue.
   4 = visualization of tissue layers not possible due to necrosis.
   5 = supporting structures include tendon, joint capsule.
3. Edges: Use this guide:

Indistinct, diffuse	= unable to clearly distinguish wound outline.
Attached	= even or flush with wound base, *no* sides or walls present; flat.
Not attached	= sides or walls *are* present; floor or base of wound is deeper than edge.
Rolled under, thickened	= soft to firm and flexible to touch.

Hyperkeratosis	= callous-like tissue formation around wound and at edges.
Fibrotic, scarred	= hard, rigid to touch.

4. Undermining: Assess by inserting a cotton-tipped applicator under the wound edge; advance it as far as it will go without using undue force; raise the tip of the applicator so it may be seen or felt on the surface of the skin; mark the surface with a pen; measure the distance from the mark on the skin to edge of the wound. Continue process around the wound. Then use a transparent metric measuring guide with concentric circles divided into four (25%) pie-shaped quadrants to help determine percent of wound involved.
5. Necrotic Tissue Type: Pick the type of necrotic tissue that is *predominant* in the wound according to color, consistency, and adherence using this guide:

White/gray non-viable tissue	= may appear prior to wound opening; skin surface is white or gray.
Nonadherent, yellow slough	= thin, mucinous substance; scattered throughout wound bed; easily separated from wound tissue.
Loosely adherent, yellow slough	= thick, stringy clumps of debris; attached to wound tissue.
Adherent, soft, black eschar	= soggy tissue; strongly attached to tissue in center of base of wound.
Firmly adherent, hard, black eschar	= firm, crusty tissue; strongly attached to wound base and edges (like a hard scab).

6. Necrotic Tissue Amount: Use a transparent metric measuring guide with concentric circles divided into four (25%) pie-shaped quadrants to help determine percent of wound involved.
7. Exudate Type: Some dressings interact with wound drainage to produce a gel or trap liquid. Before assessing exudate type, gently cleanse wound with normal saline or water. Pick the exudate type that is predominant in the wound according to color and consistency, using this guide:

Bloody	= thin, bright red

©1990 Barbara Bates-Jensen

Note: This tool may be copied and used without specific permission of the author. However, it may not be published without specific permission of the author.

Serosanguineous = thin, watery pale red or pink
Serous   = thin, watery, clear
Purulent   = thin or thick, opaque tan to yellow
Foul purulent   = thick, opaque yellow to green with offensive odor

8. Exudate Amount: Use a transparent metric measuring guide with concentric circles divided into four (25%) pie-shaped quadrants to determine percent of dressing involved with exudate. Use this guide:

None   = wound tissues dry.
Scant   = wound tissues moist; no measurable exudate.
Small   = wound tissues wet; moisture evenly distributed in wound; drainage involves <25% dressing.
Moderate = wound tissues saturated; drainage may or may not be evenly distributed in wound; drainage involved >25% to <75% dressing.
Large   = wound tissues bathed in fluid; drainage freely expressed; may or may not be evenly distributed in wound; drainage involves >75% of dressing.

9. Skin Color Surrounding Wound: Assess tissues with 4 cm of wound edge. Dark-skinned persons show the colors "bright red" and "dark red" as a deepening of normal ethnic skin color or a purple hue. As healing occurs in dark-skinned persons, the new skin is pink and may never darken.

10. Peripheral Tissue Edema: Assess tissues within 4 cm of wound edge. Non-pitting edema appears as skin that is shiny and taut. Identify pitting edema by firmly pressing a finger down into the tissues and waiting for 5 seconds; on release of pressure, tissues fail to resume previous position and an indentation appears. Crepitus is accumulation of air or gas in tissues. Use a transparent metric measuring guide to determine how far edema extends beyond wound.

11. Peripheral Tissue Induration: Assess tissues within 4 cm of wound edge. Induration is abnormal firmness of tissues with margins. Assess by gently pinching the tissues. Induration results in an inability to pinch the tissues. Use a transparent metric measuring guide with concentratic circles divided into four (25%) pie-shaped quadrants to determine percent of wound and area involved.

12. Granulation Tissue: Granulation tissue is the growth of small blood vessels and connective tissue to fill in full-thickness wounds. Tissue is healthy when bright, beefy red, shiny, and granular with a velvety appearance. Poor vascular supply appears as pale pink or blanched to dull, dusky red color.

13. Epithelialization: Epithelialization is the process of epidermal resurfacing and appears as pink or red skin. In partial-thickness wounds it can occur throughout the wound bed as well as from the wound edges. In full-thickness wounds it occurs from the edges only. Use a transparent metric measuring guide with concentric circles divided into four (25%) pie-shaped quadrants to help determine percent of wound involved and to measure the distance the epithelial tissue extends into the wound.

PRESSURE SORE STATUS TOOL   NAME _____

Complete the rating sheet to assess pressure sore status. Evaluate each item by picking the response that best describes the wound and entering the score in the item score column for the appropriate date.

Location: Anatomic site. Circle, identify right (**R**) or left (**L**), and use "X" to mark site on body diagrams:

_____ Sacrum and coccyx   _____ Lateral ankle   _____ Trochanter
_____ Medial ankle   _____ Ischial tuberosity   _____ Heel   _____ Other Site

Shape: Overall wound pattern; assess by observing perimeter and depth. Circle and *date* appropriate description:

_____ Irregular   _____ Linear or elongated   _____ Round/oval
_____ Bow/boat   _____ Square/rectangle   _____ Butterfly   _____ Other Site

Item	Assessment	Date Score	Date Score	Date Score
1. Size	1 = Length × width <4 sq cm 2 = Length × width 4-16 sq cm 3 = Length × width 6.1-36 sq cm 4 = Length × width 36.1-80 sq cm 5 = Length × width >80 sq cm			
2. Depth	1 = Non-blanchable erythema on intact skin 2 = Partial-thickness skin loss involving epidermis and/or dermis 3 = Full-thickness skin loss involving damage or necrosis of subcutaneous tissue; may extend down to but not through underlying fascia; and/or mixed partial and full thickness and or tissue layers obscured by granulation tissue 4 = Obscured by necrosis 5 = Full-thickness skin loss with extensive destruction, tissue necrosis or damage to muscle, bone, or supporting structures			
3. Edges	1 = Indistinct, diffuse, none clearly visible 2 = Distinct, outline clearly visible, attached, even with wound base 3 = Well-defined, not attached to wound base 4 = Well-defined, not attached to base, rolled under, thickened 5 = Well-defined, fibrotic, scarred or hyperkeratotic			
4. Undermining	1 = Undermining <2 cm in any area 2 = Undermining 2-4 cm involving <50% wound margins 3 = Undermining 2-4 cm involving >50% wound margins 4 = Undermining >4 cm in any area 5 = Tunneling and/or sinus tract formation			
5. Necrotic Tissue Type	1 = None visible 2 = White/gray non-viable tissue and/or non-adherent yellow slough 3 = Loosely adherent yellow slough 4 = Adherent, soft, black eschar 5 = Firmly adherent, hard, black eschar			
6. Necrotic Tissue Amount	1 = None visible 2 = <25% of wound bed covered 3 = 25% or 50% of wound covered 4 = >50% and <75% of wound covered 5 = 75% to 100% of wound covered			
7. Exudate Type	1 = None or bloody 2 = Serosanguineous: thin, watery, pale red/pink 3 = Serous: thin, water, clear 4 = Purulent: thin or thick, opaque, tan/yellow 5 = Foul purulent; thick, opaque, yellow/green with odor			
8. Exudate Amount	1 = None 2 = Scant 3 = Small 4 = Moderate 5 = Large			
9. Skin Color Surrounding Wound	1 = Pink or normal for ethnic group 2 = Bright red and/or blanches to touch 3 = White or grey pallor or hypopigmented 4 = Dark red or purple and/or non-blanchable 5 = Black or hyperpigmented			
10. Peripheral Tissue Edema	1 = Minimal swelling around wound 2 = Non-pitting edema extends <4 cm around wound 3 = Non-pitting edema extends ≥4 cm around wound 4 = Pitting edema extends <4 cm around wound 5 = Crepitus and/or pitting edema extends ≥4 cm			
11. Peripheral Tissue Induration	1 = Minimal firmness around wound 2 = Induration <2 cm around wound 3 = Induration 2-4 cm extending <50% around wound 4 = Induration 2-4 cm extending ≥50% around wound 5 = Induration >4 cm in any area			
12. Granulation Tissue	1 = Skin intact or partial-thickness wound 2 = Bright, beefy red; 75% to 100% of wound filled and or tissue overgrowth 3 = Bright, beefy red; <75% and >25% of wound filled 4 = Pink and/or dull, dusky red and/or fills ≤25% of wound 5 = No granulation tissue present			
13. Epithelialization	1 = 100% wound covered, surface intact 2 = 75% to <100% wound covered and/or epithelial tissue extends >0.5 cm into wound bed 3 = 50% to <75% wound covered and/or epithelial tissue extends to <0.5 cm into wound bed 4 = 25% to <wound covered 5 = <25% wound covered			

TOTAL SCORE

SIGNATURE

PRESSURE SCORE STATUS CONTINUUM

0   10   13   15   20   25   30   35   40   45   50   56   60   65

Tissue   Wound   Wound
Health   Regeneration   Degeneration

Plot the total score on the Pressure Sore Status continuum by putting an "X" on the line and the date beneath the line. Plot multiple scores with their dates to see-at-glance regeneration or degeneration of the wound. © 1990 Barbara Bates-Jensen

appendix 13-b   *Braden Scale for Predicting Pressure Sore Risk*

Patient's Name		Evaluator's Name
SENSORY PERCEPTION Ability to respond meaningfully to pressure-related discomfort	**1. COMPLETELY LIMITED:** Unresponsive (does not moan, flinch, or grasp) to painful stimuli, due to diminished level of consciousness or sedation, OR limited ability to feel pain over most of body surface.	**2. VERY LIMITED:** Responds only to painful stimuli. Cannot communicate discomfort except by moaning or restlessness, OR has a sensory impairment which limits the ability to feel pain or discomfort over one half of body.
MOISTURE Degree to which skin is exposed to moisture	**1. CONSTANTLY MOIST:** Skin is kept moist almost constantly by perspiration, urine, etc. Dampness is detected every time patient is moved or turned.	**2. MOIST:** Skin is often but not always moist. Linen must be changed at least once a shift.
ACTIVITY Degree of physical activity	**1. BEDFAST:** Confined to bed.	**2. CHAIRFAST:** Ability to walk severely limited or nonexistent. Cannot bear own weight and/or must be assisted into chair or wheelchair.
MOBILITY Ability to change and control body position	**1. COMPLETELY IMMOBILE:** Does not make even slight changes in body or extremity position without assistance.	**2. VERY LIMITED:** Makes occasional slight changes in body or extremity position but unable to make frequent or significant changes independently.
NUTRITION Usual food intake pattern	**1. VERY POOR:** Never eats a complete meal. Rarely eats more than a third of any food offered. Eats 2 servings or less of protein (meat or dairy products) per day. Takes fluids poorly. Does not take a liquid dietary supplement, OR is NPO and/or maintained on clear liquids or IV for more than 5 days.	**2. PROBABLY INADEQUATE:** Rarely eats a complete meal and generally eats only about half of any food offered. Protein intake includes only 3 servings of meat or dairy products per day. Occasionally will take a dietary supplement, OR receives less than optimum amount of liquid diet or tube feeding.
FRICTION AND SHEAR	**1. PROBLEM:** Requires moderate to maximum assistance in moving. Complete lifting without sliding against sheets is impossible. Frequently slides down in bed or chair, requiring frequent repositioning with maximum assistance. Spasticity, contractures, or agitation leads to almost constant friction.	**2. POTENTIAL PROBLEM:** Moves feebly or requires minimum assistance. During a move skin probably slides to some extent against sheets, chair, restraints, or other devices. Maintains relatively good position in chair or bed most of the time but occasionally slides down.

Copyright © 1988 Barbara Braden and Nancy Bergstrom.
NPO, Nothing by mouth; *IV,* intravenously; *TPN,* total parenteral nutrition.

	Date of Assessment				

3. SLIGHTLY LIMITED:

Responds to verbal commands but cannot always communicate discomfort or need to be turned,
OR
has some sensory impairment which limits ability to feel pain or discomfort in one or two extremities.

4. NO IMPAIRMENT:

Responds to verbal commands. Has no sensory deficit which would limit ability to feel or voice pain or discomfort.

3. OCCASIONALLY MOIST:

Skin is occasionally moist, requiring an extra linen change approximately once a day.

4. RARELY MOIST:

Skin is usually dry; linen requires changing only at routine intervals.

3. WALKS OCCASIONALLY:

Walks occasionally during day but for very short distances, with or without assistance. Spends majority of each shift in bed or chair.

4. WALKS FREQUENTLY:

Walks outside the room at least twice a day and inside room at least once every 2 hours during waking hours.

3. SLIGHTLY LIMITED:

Makes frequent though slight changes in body or extremity position independently.

4. NO LIMITATIONS:

Makes major and frequent changes in position without assistance.

3. ADEQUATE:

Eats over half of most meals. Eats a total of 4 servings of protein (meat, dairy products) each day. Occasionally will refuse a meal, but will usually take a supplement if offered,
OR
is on a tube feeding or TPN regimen, which probably meets most of nutritional needs.

4. EXCELLENT:

Eats most of every meal. Never refuses a meal. Usually eats a total of 4 or more servings of meat and dairy products. Occasionally eats between meals. Does not require supplementation.

3. NO APPARENT PROBLEM:

Moves in bed and in chair independently and has sufficient muscle strength to lift up completely during move. Maintains good position in bed or chair at all times.

Total Score

14

Physical, Cognitive, Psychosocial, and Environmental Assessment Tools

Upon completion of this chapter, the reader will be able to:

• State the purposes of primary, secondary, and tertiary health care.
• Ask questions that elicit significant data from an elder regarding his or her health status.
• State the importance of basic activities of daily living (BADLs), instrumental activities of daily living (IADLs), and advanced activities of daily living (AADLs).
• Identify the various health assessment tools and the information that they can provide.

AADLs Advanced activities of daily living.
BADLs Basic activities of daily living.
Confusion Disturbed orientation in regard to time, place, or person.

IADLs Instrumental activities of daily living.
Dementia Severe impairment or loss of intellectual capacity and personal integration.
Depression Morbid sadness, dejection.

HEALTH ASSESSMENT

Health assessment has been referred to as *health appraisal, physical examination,* and *health screening.* Regardless of the nomenclature, it is a process of collecting and analyzing data. This approach is the initial step in the nursing process. Assessment provides information critical to the development of a plan of action that can enhance personal health status, decrease the potential for or the severity of chronic conditions, and assist the individual to gain control over health through self-care.

A comprehensive geriatric assessment requires not only physical data but also an integration of the biologic, psychosocial, and functional aspects of the aged person. Inquiries into physiologic and anatomic function, growth and development, family relationships, group involvement, and religious and occupational pursuits are essential in a health assessment interview. Questions regarding genetic background, although important, have less significance for the aged because genetic consequences usually appear in earlier phases of life. One cannot entirely eliminate concern for genetic inheritance, since latent changes do occur and affect physical and mental well-being.

Health assessment data enable development and implementation of primary, secondary, and tertiary care regimens. Primary care is aimed at prevention of disease and promotion and maintenance of health. Care is directed toward limiting health risks and avoidance of sequelae from common health problems, uncomplicated illness, chronic illness, or mental states induced by a stressful environment, and the individual is usually able to receive the benefits of such care either at home or on an outpatient basis. Secondary care involves specific illness or pathologic conditions and focuses its efforts on the retardation or termination of physical, mental, social, or environmental situations that have induced the condition or situation. Care is provided in a health care setting by professionals who have specific knowledge and skill in the area of concern. Tertiary care deals with restorative measures that will enable the aged individual to achieve an optimal level of function, whatever that might be. Appropriate care requires professionals with specialized knowledge and skill in either an institutional health care setting or in the home or outpatient environment.

Aged persons do not usually seek assistance from health professionals until there is obvious physical or emotional difficulty. Some aged individuals have had adverse experiences with the health care system; others assume that their problems are age related and do not realize that relief and assistance are possible.

The initiation of the health history marks the beginning of the nurse-client relationship, ushers the aged person into the health care system, and initiates the assessment process. The interview that follows requires skill in establishing client trust and confidence and in avoiding offending the individual. A considerable amount of time is required to complete a health assessment of the aged client, often because of the lack of schooling, the use of English as a second language, or impaired communication skills resulting from previous illness. It is difficult for the interviewer to proceed slowly, one question at a time, and to wait for the slow response as a result of perceptive and receptive changes that occur in the nervous system of the aged. The client may find giving certain types of health information stressful and may even decline to discuss changes or problems that might confirm fears of illness, limitations, or old age. Any illness is seen as a threat to independence and is viewed as leading to eventual institutionalization. In this era of managed care, the time allotted to see patients or to address their multiple conditions is very limited. It is valuable for the client to complete an initial health questionnaire (if vision and intellectual ability are not problems) before coming to the practitioner's office or while waiting to see the practitioner; otherwise a family member or caregiver should fill in the questionnaire as completely as possible. The client often feels freer to respond to the printed question; doing so reduces time needed with the practitioner; and the completed questionnaire provides a background from which the interview can develop. In addition, if the aged client can complete the questionnaire at home, doing so often provides time for the client to remember or find the information about his or her health that is requested. The health caregiver can clarify questionnaire answers, and the client can elaborate with details.

Many of our present assessment tools do not provide for the attainment of accurate data with the rapidly changing ethnic mix of elders. Assessment must find ways to elicit health care beliefs from the ethnogeriatric groups. Cultural/ethnic sensitivity on the part of the care provider is important in order to disentangle cultural normative behavior from behavior that mimics a pathologic condition. The tools that can facilitate this type of assessment data are very limited. Pfeifferling (1981) and Kleinman (1980)

have both developed tools to assist caregivers in gleaning pertinent assessment information to provide appropriate health promotion, prevention, maintenance, and interventions. The tool is not limited to any one population and is useful for all groups in eliciting the individual's thinking about his or her illness and the suspected cause and allowing the patient an opportunity to discuss and provide the nurse with insight about his or her health beliefs. The nurse then has information that can be analyzed according to the symptom or symptoms. Box 14-1 provides an approach to the cultural history.

Assessment of the aged requires special abilities of the nurse: the ability to listen patiently, to allow for pauses, to ask questions that are not often asked, to observe minute details, to obtain data from all available sources, and to recognize normalities of late life that would be abnormal in one who is younger (see Chapter 7). The quality and speed of the assessment are an art born of experience. Novice nurses should neither be expected nor expect themselves to do this proficiently. According to Benner (1984), it is a task for the expert. Preferably, all initial assessments when an aged individual enters the health care system through any of the doors should be conducted by the most knowledgeable and experienced person available. When this is not possible, it would be useful to have a checklist format that would alert even the novice to pressing concerns.

Any health history form or interview should include a patient profile and social history, a history of current problems, a review of symptoms and systems, a medication history (prescribed and over-the-counter), assessment of caregiver stress, a family history, assessment of the patient's ability to perform activities of daily living (ADLs), and community services currently provided. Additional data should consider psychologic parameters such as cognitive and emotional well-being; the individual's self-perception; and social parameters such as the individual's economic resources and concerns, pattern of health and health care, education, family structure, plans for retirement, and living environment. Areas or problems not frequently addressed by the care provider or mentioned by the aged are sexual dysfunction, depression, incontinence, musculoskeletal stiffness, alcoholism, hearing loss, and dementia (Ham, 1996). Much of this information is obtained orally, but it can also be evaluated by observation of personal grooming, facial expression, responsiveness to the interview, and physical examination. Information about involvement with the surrounding community and group participation should reveal additional informa-

Box 14-1   CULTURAL ASSESSMENT RELATED TO CLIENT'S HEALTH PROBLEM

The clinician may need to identify others who can facilitate the discussion of the client's problem(s).

1. How would you describe the problem that has brought you here? (What do you call your problem; does it have a name?)
   a. Who in the community and your family helps you with your problem?
2. How long have you had this problem?
   a. When do you think it started?
   b. What do you think started it?
   c. Do you know anyone else with it?
   d. Tell me what happened to them when dealing with this problem.
3. What do you think is wrong with you?
   a. What does your sickness do to you?
   b. How severe is it?
   c. What might other people think is wrong with you?
   d. Tell me about people who don't get this problem.
4. Why do you think this happened to you?
   a. Why has it happened to the involved part?
   b. Why do you get sick and not someone else?
   c. Will it have a long or short course?
   d. What do you fear most about your sickness?
5. What are the chief problems your sickness has caused you?
6. What do you think will help clear up this problem? (What treatment should you receive; what are the most important results you hope to receive?)
   a. If specific tests, medications are listed, ask what they are and do.
7. Apart from me, who else do you think can make you feel better?
   a. Are there therapies that make you feel better that I don't know? (May be in another discipline.)

Modified from Kleinman A: *Patient and healers in the context of culture: an exploration of the borderland between anthropology, medicine, and psychiatry,* Berkeley, 1980, University of California Press; and Pfeifferling JH: A cultural prescription for mediocentrism. In Eisenberg L, Kleinman A, editors: *The relevance of social science for medicine,* Boston, 1981, Reidel.

Box 14-2   QUESTIONS TO ELICIT INFORMATION SIGNIFICANT TO HEALTH STATUS*

1. What is the first health problem you can remember? What happened, and how was it taken care of? (traumatic expectations)
2. When you were young, what did you think about old people? What did you expect to be like when you were old? (ageist attitudes)
3. How old do you feel now? (health status, grief, depression)
4. What was your most gratifying experience? (expression, elaboration, imagination exhibited in description)
5. How did your mother describe you as a child? How did your father describe you as a child? (incorporation, self-evaluation, self-fulfilling prophecies)
6. How would you describe yourself as a child? (identity, self-concept)
7. What is the most important thing that you have done? (values)
8. What is the most difficult thing that you have done? (strength, integrity, endurance, courage)
9. How did you manage to do that? (coping style and patterns)
10. What would you change if you could? (life satisfaction, integrity, acceptance)

*These are only a few thoughts that can be modified or expanded on in any particular situation.

tion about the emotional state and feelings of self-worth of the aged client. The essentials of a comprehensive geriatric assessment must include functional, physical, social, and mental assessment of the aged and of the caregiver (if used) and assessment of the environment to plan care and prevent problems (Box 14-2).

Home visit assessment complements or provides information that is difficult to gauge in a clinic, physi-cian's office, or other formal settings. Especially difficult to ascertain are such areas as nutrition, alcoholism, actual level of function on a daily basis, and suitability and safety of the environment. Even when the individual is relatively independent, an appreciation for the difficulty encountered in food preparation, use of the bathroom, showering, and heating and cooling the house can be acquired (Box 14-3).

Box 14-3	HOME VISIT INFORMATION AND INDICATIONS

Necessary Home Visit Information

Suitability and safety of home for client's functional level

Attitude and presence of other persons at home

Proximity and helpfulness of neighbors and relatives

Emergency assistance arrangements

Nutrition and alcohol habits

Actual and required daily living skills

Hygiene habits

Safety and convenience modification needed

Problems in getting to local community store and services

Indications for Home Visit

Lives alone (especially if recently bereaved)

Mental impairment

Major mobility problems

Several risk factors for dependency

History of falls or accidents

Recent hospital discharge (especially if recovery is incomplete)

Imminent institutionalization

From Ham RJ: *Geriatrics. I. AAFP home study of self-assessment monograph 89,* Kansas City, Mo, 1986, American Academy of Family Physicians.

The nurse must be cognizant of inherent obstacles and benefits of the health assessment, particularly the potential for developing a stereotyped view of the aged and perceiving the elderly as objects rather than persons. This is especially true when assessment is viewed in terms of potentially meeting the nurse's need for data instead of meeting the needs of the aged person, and as a task rather than as the basis of care.

ASSESSMENT TOOLS

An abundance of assessment tools exist that can broadly categorize motor capacity, manual ability, self-care ability, more complex or instrumental abilities, and cognitive and social function. Some community agencies and nursing care facilities routinely use health assessment tools designed to obtain specific information needed. Other institutions have developed or modified available tools because the available assessment tools are too complex and too time consuming to be of prac-

tical value. Regardless of the method used (established or self-developed), most health forms contain variants of the same basic information. It is important to remember that most of the assessment tools are screening in nature and do not provide for a definite diagnosis. Their use should provide signals or clues that a problem or potential problem exists and needs referral for more thorough investigation by the physician or nurse practitioner. To use assessment tools most effectively, the following guidelines should be followed:

- Ask the question on the tool.
- Spend time to develop rapport with the client.
- Avoid bias or leading the client.
- Probe appropriately.
- Do not avoid difficult situations.

Knowledge of the tool is important for accuracy; approaching a question and not avoiding it because you think it would be embarrassing to the client or because you, the nurse, are uncomfortable asking it alters the accuracy of the assessment. Approach difficult issues in a matter-of-fact manner. Older adults who feel comfortable with an assessor will tend to speak more openly, the information will be obtained more quickly, and the conversation will be more informative and mutually enjoyable. Talk about the assessment before beginning; engage in some small talk. Reassure the older adult that the assessment is important and worthwhile. Listen to the elder and make mental notes about his or her communication style. Always begin professionally, but do not be afraid to enjoy the process as well. If you relax, the elder will tend to relax also.

An area in which most professionals err is with bias. "A bias is any influence that changes an answer or opinion from what it might have been without that influence" (King, 1997). Be aware of your own bias and how it will affect the assessment. Keep your opinions to yourself, and do not suggest answers. Do not rush the elder or use leading questions. Some of these bias errors overlap into the area of probing. It is necessary to probe, but probing should be for correctness, clarity, and completeness. A correct probe is a prompt that encourages further conversation without biasing the response.

The assessor should not shy away from difficult situations. If a person is crying, acknowledge the situation; stop what you are doing; and be direct, polite, and sensitive. Say, "This must be very difficult for you" or "I'm sorry." Do not pity the elder; the individual wants respect and sensitivity. If at all possible, continue with the assessment. Be tolerant of pauses. Not finishing the assessment may cause the elder to have feelings of failure or unfinished business. A comment such as "I hope I didn't upset you" is often helpful.

Ideally, assessment tools should be used to gather baseline data before the older adult has a health crisis. Periodically, the older adult should be reassessed using the same tools. An individual who has confusion precipitated by an illness or drug therapy should be reassessed to see if the confusion is better or worse. Consider the results of assessment a yardstick of an individual's status at any given time. Just as children are periodically measured for their weight and height, so, too, should elders be assessed periodically for their physical, functional, social, and cognitive status in health and illness. When a baseline exists, this allows for a comparison from which care can be planned and resources utilized.

Physical Assessment

The physical examination process is not presented here. Many books provide the essential discussion of examination tools, techniques, and methods. The focus here is on FANCAPES, an assessment tool that uses a survival-needs framework with an emphasis on function. The acronym *FANCAPES* represents *F*luids, *A*eration, *N*utrition, *C*ommunication, *A*ctivity, *P*ain, *E*limination, and *S*ocialization and social skills. The information provided is helpful in the appraisal of the aged person's ability to meet his or her needs and the extent to which assistance is necessary. FANCAPES is applicable to all types of care environments in which the aged are found, may be used in part or total (depending on the need), and is easily adaptable to the functional pattern grouping if nursing diagnoses are used in planning care. Assessment data obtained from this method are based on the following considerations in each area.

Fluids

Evaluation of fluids requires the functional assessment of the client's state of hydration and those physiologic, situational, and mental factors that contribute to the maintenance of adequate hydration. Attention is directed to the ability of the client to obtain adequate fluids on his or her own, to express feelings of thirst, to effectively swallow, and to evaluate medications that affect intake and output (see Chapter 11).

Aeration

In considering aeration, one looks at the adequacy of oxygen exchange. Observations include respiratory rate

and depth at rest and during activity; talking, walking, and situations requiring added exertion; and the presence or absence of edema in the extremities or abdomen. Breath sounds should be auscultated and medication reviewed to evaluate the effects on aeration.

Nutrition

Nutrition involves mechanical and psychologic factors in addition to the type and amount of food consumed. It is necessary to ascertain the client's ability to bite, chew, and swallow. Edentulous clients may have dentures that fit improperly and are not worn. Alteration in diet because of culture, medical restrictions, available economic resources, and living conditions should be considered. Visual and neurologic impairment, which might interfere with the client's ability to prepare a meal or feed himself or herself, should be noted (see Chapter 10).

Communication

The sending and receiving of verbal and nonverbal information in the external world and signals in the internal environment of the body require mechanical function of body parts and psychosocial responses from others in the environment. Assessment includes sight and sound acuity; voice quality; and adequate function of the tongue, teeth, pharynx, and larynx. Appraisal of the client's ability to read, write, and understand the spoken language should be ascertained. This is an important issue, since an undetected disability in these skills can lead to erroneous conclusions (see Chapters 3 and 9).

Activity

Activity includes aspects other than exercise. ADLs provide an estimate of the individual's ability to maintain self-care and independent living. The nurse looks at the ability to feed, toilet, dress, and groom oneself; to prepare meals; to dial the telephone; and to move around with or without assistive devices. Coordination and balance, finger dexterity, grip strength, and other actions necessary to daily life should also be assessed. Ambulation should be considered a major component in activity. The timed "get up and go," which has the person rise from a chair, walk 8 feet, return to the chair, and sit down, correlates with functional dysfunction (Podsiadlo, Richardson, 1991).

Pain

Pain, both physical and mental, is important to consider. The presence or absence of pressure and discomfort are also aspects of pain assessment. Information about recent losses or visible symptoms of anxiety may help determine manifestations of pain. The manner by which a client customarily attains relief from pain or discomfort will provide further sources of information (see Chapter 17).

Elimination

Bladder and bowel elimination should be investigated for mechanical factors such as evidence of dribbling or incontinence, for use of assistive devices or altered body structures resulting from surgical intervention, and for medications that affect voiding and intestinal peristalsis.

Bowel function can be helped or hindered by what the client uses to purge himself or herself, by how concerned the client seems to be about bowel function, and by the amount of privacy needed for excretory functions. Colloquialisms used by the client must be recognized and used to accommodate obtaining assessment data (see Chapter 11).

Socialization and Social Skills

Socialization and social skills assess the individual's ability to negotiate in society, to give and receive love and friendship, and to feel self-worth. Responses to such influences as hearing and visual losses and approved gestures of friendship are considered under this category. Attention should focus on the individual's ability to deal with loss and to interact with other people in give-and-take situations. Behavioral responses not previously observed may become evident through discussion of the client's feelings of self-worth.

Functional Assessment

As part of the health assessment, it is important to include an appraisal of basic activities of daily living (BADLs) and instrumental activities of daily living (IADLs)—referred to as *functional assessment*—and advanced activities of daily living (AADLs), which include occupational, recreational, and leisure-time activities. These latter activities are based on choice, not necessity, as are those of the BADLs and IADLs. A functional assessment consists of the fundamental tasks and demands of daily life. BADLs are those abilities that are fundamental to self-care, such as bathing, dressing, toileting, transferring from bed or chair, feeding, and continence. The IADLs include more complex daily activities, such as using the telephone, preparing meals, and managing money, which

are necessary activities for living independently in the community

The goal of *Healthy People 2000* (1991) is to increase the life span of all Americans. Rather than delay mortality, focus has been directed at the preservation of function and extending active life expectancy. Functional assessment speaks to the "quality of life" in ways that medical diagnoses do not (Gallo et al, 1995).

Functional assessment can be defined as the evaluation of a person's ability to carry out basic tasks for self-care and tasks needed to support independent living. It is based on physical and psychosocial evaluation, with the assumption that any clinical condition can be diagnosed and properly treated (Williams, 1995). Additional reasons why functional assessment is so important are that the objective data obtained in a functional assessment accomplish the following:

- Define the elder's concerns
- May indicate a manifestation of disease
- Assist in determining a need for service(s)
- Assist in determining the type of placement
- Assist in determining cost/benefit of treatment/intervention
- Assist in realistic goal setting for those with chronic conditions
- Decrease fragmentation of care by reviewing goals according to functional status
- Assist in ethical/quality-of-life issues
- Help track untreated conditions (i.e., effects of arthritis)

Functional assessment tools that assess the individual's ability to perform BADLs and IADLs should provide numerically qualified data regarding an individual's capacity to be or remain independent.

The BADLs (eating, toileting, ambulation, bathing, dressing, and grooming) are tasks needed for self-care and are international as well as cross-cultural in nature. Three of these tasks (grooming, dressing, and bathing) require cognitive function. When the BADLs are vertically listed, it is not unusual for the individual who performs an activity to be able to do the activities above it but not below it. Change in or loss of ability occurs in the reverse order of acquisition.

The IADLs are tasks needed for independent living. The progression of loss of IADLs begins with cognitive functions, especially finances and shopping. Cooking is least important to community-dwelling elders, even when adjusted for gender differences (Williams, 1995).

Numerous tools are available that describe, screen, assess, monitor, and predict functional ability. Generally, the assessment does not break down a task into its component parts, such as picking up a spoon or cup or swallowing water when assessment of eating is done; instead, eating is seen as a total task. Functional assessment also shows the result, not the cause, of an altered task. This is particularly true with persons who have varying degrees of dementia (Tappan, 1994). The Katz index (Katz et al, 1963) provides a basic framework to evaluate a person's self-care ability to live independently and serves as a focal point to provide remedies. There are several versions of the Katz index; one is based on a 3-point scale and allows one to score client performance abilities as independent, assistive, or dependent. Another version of the tool assigns 1 point to each BADL if the activity as described for independent function is accomplished and zero (0) if supervision, direction, personal assistance, or total care is required. Scores will range from a maximum of 6 (totally inde-

pendent) to 0 (totally dependent). A score of 4 indicates moderate impairment, whereas 2 or less indicates severe impairment (Table 14-1).

The value of the Katz index is that it can be administered by anyone, with minimal training, and it can provide data that identify the functional abilities of an aged person and the kinds of services that might be needed. Historically, the Katz tool was intended for acute care patients as a measure to determine their readiness for discharge; that was 30 years ago. Despite its continuous use, tests and retests of reliability have not been reported in the literature (Wallace, Fulmer, 1998; Bennett, 1999). The tool is sensitive to changes in declining health status; it cannot measure small incremental changes, which are seen in rehabilitation of older adults. Scoring variations can also occur based on what one interprets as the cutoff for establishing what

Table 14-1

Katz Index of Independence in Activities of Daily Living

Activities (points [1 or 0])	Independence (1 point)	Dependence (0 points)
	NO supervision, direction, or personal assistance	WITH supervision, direction, personal assistance, or total care
BATHING	(1 point) Bathes self completely or needs help in bathing only a single part of the body such as the back, genital area, or disabled extremity.	(0 points) Needs help with bathing more than one part of the body, getting in or out of the tub or shower. Requires total bathing.
Points: _____		
DRESSING	(1 point) Gets clothes from closets and drawers and puts on clothes and outer garments complete with fasteners. May have help tying shoes.	(0 points) Needs help with dressing self or needs to be completely dressed.
Points: _____		
TOILETING	(1 point) Goes to toilet, gets on and off, arranges clothes, cleans genital area without help.	(0 points) Needs help transferring to the toilet, cleaning self or uses bedpan or commode.
Points: _____		
TRANSFERRING	(1 point) Moves in and out of bed or chair unassisted. Mechanical transferring aids are acceptable.	(0 points) Needs help in moving from bed to chair or requires a complete transfer.
Points: _____		
CONTINENCE	(1 point) Exercises complete self-control over urination and defecation.	(0 points) Is partially or totally incontinent of bowel or bladder.
Points: _____		
FEEDING	(1 point) Gets food from plate into mouth without help. Preparation of food may be done by another person.	(0 points) Needs partial or total help with feeding or requires parenteral feeding.
Points: _____		
TOTAL POINTS = _____	6 = High (patient independent)	0 = Low (patient very dependent)

From Katz S et al: Progress in the development of the index of ADL, *Gerontologist* 10:20-30, 1970.

is considered dependent, and even if that is established, there is no differentiation among the severe levels of disability. Also, by using one simple score, the Katz tool places equal importance on all tasks (Bennett, 1999). Despite these limitations, the tool is useful because it creates a common language about patient function for all caregivers involved in planning overall care and discharge.

Another tool used to assess self-care of the elderly is the Barthel index (1981) (Table 14-2). This instrument was devised to evaluate the amount of physical assistance required when a person can no longer carry out BADLs. Because it is so detailed, a modified Barthel index was developed that has proved useful in any setting. It is particularly useful in the home care setting. The index is divided into two categories: independent and dependent. Under each of these headings activities are rated as independent (intact and limited ability) or dependent (requiring a helper or unable to do an activity or activities at all).

The Barthel index provides data to determine the type of support that is needed in ADLs and can serve in rehabilitation settings as a method of documenting improvement of a patient's ability. The IADLs, considered to be more complex activities than the BADLs, include such abilities as traveling, shopping, preparing meals,

doing housework, dialing a telephone, and handling money. Although these tasks may seem more specific to women, the activities are required of most individuals in modern society today. Box 14-4 gives an example of a self-rated IADL instrument.

A current question being asked is whether the BADLs and IADLs are "old fashioned" or still useful as a means of assessing an older adult's functional abilities. Bennett (1999) suggests that performance tests that address balance, gait, strength, and endurance be added to the existing ADLs and that more studies be completed using improved scales. The three performance tests suggested are simple and quick: the ability to stand with feet together in a side-by-side manner and in a tandem and semitandem position; a timed walk of 8 feet; and a timed rise from a chair and return to a seated position five times (Box 14-5).

Mental Assessment

An evaluation of mental ability is essential. Frequently a combination of scores on mental status questions incorporates BADL and IADL items and can sometimes improve the detection of dementia. One such tool is the *Functional Dementia Scale* (Moore et al, 1983), a brief tool that can be administered in a written or oral form.

Table 14-2

Modified Barthel Index

	Independent		Dependent	
	Intact	Limited	Helper	Null
Feed from dish	10	5	3	0
Dress upper body	5	5	3	0
Dress lower body	5	5	2	0
Don brace or prosthesis	0	0	−2	0
Grooming	5	5	0	0
Wash or bathe	4	4	0	0
Bladder incontinence	10	10	5	0
Bowel incontinence	10	10	5	0
Care of perineum/clothing at toilet	4	4	2	0
Transfer, chair	15	15	7	0
Transfer, toilet	6	5	3	0
Transfer, tub or shower	1	1	0	0
Walk on level 50 yards or more	15	15	10	0
Up and down stairs for one flight or more	10	10	5	0
Wheelchair 50 yards (only if not walking)	15	5	0	0

Modified from Granger C, Gresham O: *Functional assessment in rehabilitation medicine,* Baltimore, 1984, Williams & Wilkins, p. 74.

It provides a way to quantify the severity of dementia, as well as a review of symptoms. Whether this tool provides data, over time, of diminished capacity is not evident (Gallo et al, 1995). The *Blessed Dementia Score* is based on a 22-item tool that can be scored from 0 to 27. The higher the score, the greater the degree of dementia. This tool incorporates aspects of the BADLs (issues with eating, dressing, and sphincter control) and IADLs (such as the inability to perform household tasks, cope with small sums of money, remember a short list of items, recall events, and find one's way outdoors). Several items (eating, dressing, sphincter control) are subdivided into three components, each with specific point values above 1 point. The remainder of the items receive 1 point each.

The *Clock Drawing Task,* which has been used since 1992 (Mendez et al, 1992), is a screening tool that differentiates normal elders from those with cognitive impairment. It is particularly sensitive for constructional apraxia, but it also can reflect general deficits in conception of time (Mendez et al, 1992; Tuokko et al, 1992; Nolan, Mohs, 1994). Less threatening to elders than the Folstein Mini-Mental State Examination (MMSE), it can be administered as sort of a game. There are several ways of scoring the completed drawing. A simple 0 to 4 score is brief, sensitive, and easy to apply (Pfizer, Inc.). This tool does not establish criteria for dementia, but if performance on the clock drawing is impaired, it suggests the need for further investigation and analysis (Box 14-6). A complete diagnostic evaluation for dementia is warranted, and the MMSE should be considered (Nolan, Mohs, 1994). This latter test can be done by the nurse following the clock results, if appropriate.

To complete the Clock Drawing Task, the individual needs to be able to adequately hold a pen or pencil, since it does require some manual dexterity. Individuals with severe arthritis, parkinsonism, or stroke that affects their dominant hand would be, in many cases, at a disadvantage if this tool were used. It does, however, have a good correlation with the MMSE.

The *Folstein Mini-Mental State Examination (MMSE)* is a short, convenient mental function test composed of two parts: one component requires verbal response and assesses orientation, memory, and attention, and the other component requires the ability to write a sentence, draw a complex design, respond to written and oral commands, and name objects. It can be administered in 10 minutes; however, additional time may be necessary if the person being tested has pronounced impairments. As with other assessment tools,

---

Box 14-4   INSTRUMENTAL ACTIVITIES OF DAILY LIVING

1. Telephone:
   I: Able to look up numbers, dial, receive and make calls without help
   A: Able to answer phone or dial operator in an emergency but needs special phone or help in getting number or dialing
   D: Unable to use telephone
2. Traveling:
   I: Able to drive own car or travel alone on bus or taxi
   A: Able to travel but not alone
   D: Unable to travel
3. Shopping:
   I: Able to take care of all shopping with transportation provided
   A: Able to shop but not alone
   D: Unable to shop
4. Preparing meals:
   I: Able to plan and cook full meals
   A: Able to prepare light foods but unable to cook full meals alone
   D: Unable to prepare any meals
5. Housework:
   I: Able to do heavy housework (like scrub floors)
   A: Able to do light housework but needs help with heavy tasks
   D: Unable to do any housework
6. Medication:
   I: Able to take medications in the right dose at the right time
   A: Able to take medications but needs reminding or someone to prepare it
   D: Unable to take medications
7. Money:
   I: Able to manage buying needs, write checks, pay bills
   A: Able to manage daily buying needs, but needs help managing checkbook, paying bills
   D: Unable to manage money

From *Multidimensional Functional Assessment Questionnaire,* ed 2, by Duke University Center for the Study of Aging and Human Development with permission of Duke University, 1978.
I, Independent; *A,* assistance; *D,* dependent.

---

there is a rating scale to quantify ability or disability (Table 14-3). Although this test is sensitive to and tests short-term memory, it lacks a degree of accuracy or sensitivity when used with minority or non-English-speaking people (Zarit, 1997). A score of 23 points or

Box 14-5 **FUNCTIONAL PERFORMANCE TESTS**

Standing Balance
Instructions: semi-tandem stand.* The nurse:
a. First demonstrates the task.
   (The heel of one foot is placed to the side of the first toe of the other foot.)
b. Supports one arm of the older adult while he or she positions the feet as demonstrated above. The elder can choose which foot to place forward.
c. Asks if the person is ready, then releases the support and begins timing.
d. Stop timing when the older adult moves the feet or grasps the nurse for support, or when 10 seconds have elapsed.

*Start with the semi-tandem stand. If it cannot be done for 10 seconds, then the **side-by-side** test should be done. If the semi-tandem can be accomplished for the requisite 10 seconds, follow the same instructions as above, except the **full tandem** requires placing the heel of one foot directly in front of the toes of the other foot.

Scoring	Full tandem	Semi-tandem	Side-by-side
0	_____	<10 seconds or unable	<10 seconds or unable
1	_____	<10 seconds or unable	10 seconds
2	<3 seconds or unable	10 seconds	_____
3	3 to 9 seconds	10 seconds	_____
4	10 seconds	10 seconds	_____

Standing Balance score: _____

Walking Speed
Instructions: The nurse:
a. Sets up an 8-foot walking course with an additional 2 feet at both ends free of any obstacles.
b. Places an 8-foot rigid carpenter's ruler to the side of the course.
c. Instructs the older adults to "walk to the other end of the course at your normal speed, just like walking down the street to go to the store." Assistive devices should be used if needed.
d. Times two walks. **The fastest of the two is used as the score.**

Scoring:
0	Unable
1	>5.6 seconds
2	4.1 to 5.6 seconds
3	3.2 to 4 seconds
4	<3.2 seconds

Walking Speed score: _____

Chair Stands
Instructions: The nurse:
a. Places a straight-backed chair next to a well.
b. Asks the older adult to fold the arms across the chest and stand up from the chair one time. If successful,
c. Asks the older adult to stand and sit five times as quickly as possible.
d. Times from the initial sitting position to the final standing position at the end of the fifth stand.
Scores are for the five rise-and-sits only. If the older adult performs less than five repetitions, the score is 0.

Scoring
0	Unable
1	>16.6 seconds
2	13.7 to 16.5 seconds
3	11.2 to 13.6 seconds
4	<11.2 seconds

Chair Stands score: _____   **Total of all performance tests (0-12)** _____

Modified from Guralnik et al: A short physical performance battery assessment of lower extremity function: association with self-reported disability and prediction of mortality and nursing home admission, *J Gerontol Med Sci* 49(2):M85-M94, 1994; and Bennett JA: Activities of daily living: old-fashioned or still useful? *J Gerontol Nurs* 25(5):22-28, 1999.

Box 14-6   CLOCK DRAWING TASK

Instructions

On a blank piece of paper:
  Ask the elder to draw a circle.
  Place the numbers inside the circle.
  Place the hands at 3:45.

Scoring

Draws closed circle	Score 1 point
Places numbers in correct position	Score 1 point
Includes all 12 correct numbers	Score 1 point
Places hands in correct position	Score 1 point

Interpretations

Errors such as grossly distorted contour or extraneous markings are rarely produced by cognitively intact persons.

Clinical judgment must be applied, but a low score indicates the need for further evaluation.

Data from Tuokko H et al: The clock test: a sensitive measure to differentiate normal elderly from those with Alzheimer disease, *J Am Geriatr Soc* 40:579-584, 1992; Mendez MF, Ala T, Underwood KL: Development of scoring criteria for the Clock Drawing Task in Alzheimer's disease, *J Am Geriatr Soc* 40:1095-1099, 1992; Morris JC: Differential diagnosis of Alzheimer's disease, *Clin Geriatr Med* 19:257-276, 1994; Nolan KA, Mohs RC: Screening for dementia in family practice. In Richter RW, Blass JP, editors: *Alzheimer's disease: a guide to practical management,* part II, St Louis, 1994, Mosby; Data on file, Pfizer, Inc., New York: American Psychiatric Association: *Diagnostic and statistical manual of mental disorders (DSM-IV),* ed 4, Washington DC, 1994, American Psychiatric Association; and Folstein MF, Folstein SE, McHugh PR: Mini-mental state: a practical method for grading the cognitive state of patients for the clinician, *Psychiatr Res* 12:189-198, 1975.

less (out of 30) for an individual with more than 8 years of formal education is indicative of cognitive impairment. Scores increase with educational level, and lower scores must take into account the extent of formal schooling (Crum et al, 1993).

A frequently used mental status examination is the *Short Portable Mental Status Questionnaire (SPMSQ)* (Pfeiffer, 1979). Its effectiveness as a method for clarifying cognitive function is still undetermined. The questionnaire asks 10 questions that assess the person's orientation, remote memory, and calculation ability; however, there is no task to evaluate short-term memory. The SPMSQ should be used with individuals who have a short attention span and cannot sit long enough for the MMSE to be administered. Its value as an as-

sessment tool is its ease of administration and the fact that it requires no equipment (Gallo et al, 1995). This tool has several significant flaws. Patients in nursing homes who view their life the same from day to day may be unaware of the day or date (Hays, Borger, 1985). It is also difficult to accurately use the normal cutoff points (3 wrong answers) with patients with delirium because of its variable presentation. Depression is often difficult to differentiate from dementia because many of the initial presenting symptoms are similar between the two. Depression is seen in the elderly at home but is often missed by the home care nurse. It is recommended by Covinsky (1996) that all hospitalized elders be screened for depression because the risk of increased dependency in ADLs is directly related to depressive symptomatology.

The *Zung Self-Rating Depression Scale* (Zung, 1965) has been used more extensively with older adults than any other depression instrument (Box 14-7, p. 277). The tool, however, did not construct norms based on an aged population. It also may interpret inaccurately the normal physiologic slowing of aging or subclinical or clinical disease such as depression.

The *Geriatric Depression Scale (GDS),* developed by Yesavage et al (1983), is a 30-item tool designed for geriatric patients and based almost entirely on psychologic discriminators. A short version is also available (Box 14-8, p. 278). The GDS has been extremely successful in determining depression because it deemphasizes physical complaints, libido, and appetite. It is viewed as a more accurate measure of depression in the elderly than other tools.

The *General Health Questionnaire (GHS)* is an integrated instrument that detects the presence of psychiatric distress. Four general categories (seven questions each)—somatic symptoms, anxiety and insomnia, social dysfunction, and depression—compose this tool (Box 14-9, p. 279), which was developed for the acute care setting. Respondents rate the presence of anxious or depressive symptoms "over the past few weeks" into four categories, which are coded as follows: "not at all" (coded 1), "not more than usual" (coded 2), "more than usual" (coded 3), or "much more" (coded 4). A score of 1 is assigned to either of the two answers consistent with depression, and a score of 0 is assigned to the other two.

The *Social Dysfunction Rating Scale* is another integrated tool that looks at major areas related to social factors associated with depression: self-esteem, interpersonal system; performance system (Box 14-10, p. 279).

Table 14-3

MiniMental LLC

NAME OF SUBJECT _____ Age _____

NAME OF EXAMINER _____ Years of School Completed ____

Approach the patient with respect and encouragement   Date of Examination _____

Ask: Do you have any trouble with your memory?   ☐Yes ☐No

May I ask you some questions about your memory?   ☐Yes ☐No

SCORE   ITEM

5 ( )   TIME ORIENTATION
Ask:
What is the year _____ (1), season _____ (1),
month of the year _____ (1), date _____ (1),
day of the week _____ (1)?

5 ( )   PLACE ORIENTATION
Ask:
Where are we now? What is the state _____ (1), city _____ (1),
part of the city _____ (1), building _____ (1),
floor of the building _____ (1)?

3 ( )   REGISTRATION OF THREE WORDS
Say: Listen carefully. I am going to say three words. You say them back after I stop.
Ready? Here they are . . . PONY (wait 1 second), QUARTER (wait 1 second), OR-
ANGE (wait 1 second). What were those words?
_____ (1)
_____ (1)
_____ (1)
Give 1 point for each correct answer, then repeat them until the patient learns all three.

5 ( )   SERIAL 7s AS A TEST OF ATTENTION AND CALCULATION
Ask: Subtract 7 from 100 and continue to subtract 7 from each subsequent remain-
der until I tell you to stop. What is 100 take away 7? _____ (1)
Say:
Keep going _____ (1), _____ (1),
_____ (1), _____ (1).

3 ( )   RECALL OF THREE WORDS
Ask:
What were those three words I asked you to remember?
Give one point for each correct answer _____ (1),
_____ (1), _____ (1).

2 ( )   NAMING
Ask:
What is this? (show pencil) _____ (1).
What is this? (show watch) _____ (1).

1 ( )   REPETITION
Say:
Now I am going to ask you to repeat what I say. Ready? No ifs, ands, or buts.
Now you say that _____ (1)

For more
information or
additional copies
of this exam
call (617) 587-4215
©1975, 1998,
MiniMental, LLC

Continued

Table 14-3—cont'd

MiniMental LLC

SCORE	ITEM
3 ( )	**COMPREHENSION**

Say:

Listen carefully because I am going to ask you to do something.

Take this paper in your left hand (1), fold it in half (1), and put it on the floor.(1)

1 ( )   **READING**

Say:

Please read the following and do what it says, but do not say it aloud. (1)

Close your eyes

1 ( )   **WRITING**

Say:

Please write a sentence. If patient does not respond, say: Write about the weather. (1)

_____

_____

1 ( )   **DRAWING**

Say: Please copy this design.

TOTAL SCORE _____   Assess level of consciousness along a continuum

Alert	Drowsy	Stupor	Coma

	YES	NO		YES	NO	FUNCTION BY PROXY
						Please record date when patient was last able to perform the following tasks.
Cooperative:	☐	☐	Deterioration from			Ask caregiver if patient independently handles:
Depressed:	☐	☐	previous level of			
Anxious:	☐	☐	functioning:	☐	☐	
Poor Vision:	☐	☐	Family History of Dementia:	☐	☐	Money/Bills:
Poor Hearing:	☐	☐	Head Trauma:	☐	☐	Medication:
Native Language:			Stroke:	☐	☐	Transportation:
			Alcohol Abuse:	☐	☐	Telephone:
_____			Thyroid Diseasee:	☐	☐	

FUNCTION BY PROXY:

	YES	NO	DATE
Money/Bills:	☐	☐	_____
Medication:	☐	☐	_____
Transportation:	☐	☐	_____
Telephone:	☐	☐	_____

From Mini-Mental State: A Practical Method for Grading the Cognitive State of Patients for the Clinician. *Journal of Psychiatric Research* 12(3):189-198, 1975, Copyright 1975. 1998, MiniMental LLC.

Box 14-7   ZUNG SELF-RATING DEPRESSION SCALE

1. (−) I feel down-hearted and blue.
2. (+) Morning is when I feel the best.
3. (−) I have crying spells or feel like it.
4. (−) I have trouble sleeping at night.
5. (+) I eat as much as I used to.
6. (+) I still enjoy sex.
7. (−) I notice that I am losing weight.
8. (−) I have trouble with constipation.
9. (−) My heart beats faster than usual.
10. (−) I get tired for no reason.
11. (+) My mind is as clear as it used to be.
12. (+) I find it easy to do the things I used to.
13. (−) I am restless and can't keep still.
14. (+) I feel hopeful about the future.
15. (−) I am more irritable than usual.
16. (+) I find it easy to make decisions.
17. (+) I feel that I am useful and needed.
18. (+) My life is pretty full.
19. (−) I feel that others would be better off if I were dead.
20. (+) I still enjoy the things I used to do.

From Zung W: Self-rating depression scale, *Arch Gen Psychiatry* 12:65, 1965.

There are six gradations on which the score is based: not present (score 1), very much (score 2), mild (score 3), moderate (score 4), severe (score 5), and very severe (score 6). This assessment tool is very useful for assessing the impact of depression on the quality of life, not the degree of depression that might be present.

Integrated Assessments

Multidimensional Functional Assessment of the Older American's Resources and Services (OARS)

The Multidimensional Functional Assessment of the Older American's Resources and Services (OARS) organization is a lengthy and comprehensive tool designed to evaluate ability, disability, and the capacity level at which the aged person is able to function. Five dimensions are considered for assessment: social resources, economic resources, physical health, mental health, and ADLs. Each component uses a quantitative rating scale: 1—excellent, 2—good, 3—mildly impaired, 4—moderately impaired, 5—severely impaired, and 6—completely impaired. At the conclusion of the assessment a cumulative impairment score (CIS) is established, which can range from the most fit (6) to total disability (30). This aids in establishing the degree of need. Information considered in each domain includes the following.

Social resources. The social resources dimension evaluates the social skills and the ability to negotiate and make friends (the number of times friends are seen, the number of telephone conversations). In the assessment interview is the aged person able to ask for things from friends, family, and strangers? Is there a caregiver around in case of need? Who is it, and how long is the person available? Does the individual belong to any social network or group, such as a special interest or church group?

Economic resources. Data about monthly income and sources (Social Security, Supplemental Security Income, pensions, and income generated from capital) are needed to determine the adequacy of income compared with the cost of living and food, shelter, clothing, medications, and small luxury items. This information can provide insight into the client's relative standard of living and point out areas of need that might be alleviated by use of additional resources unknown to the aged person.

Mental health. Consideration is given to intellectual function, the presence or absence of psychiatric symptoms, and the amount of enjoyment and interaction the aged person gets from life.

Physical health. Diagnosis of major and common diseases of older persons, the type of prescribed and over-the-counter medications the person is taking, and the aged person's perception of his or her health status are the basis of evaluation. Excellent physical health includes participation in regular vigorous activity, such as walking, dancing, or biking at least twice a week. Seriously impaired physical health is determined by the presence of one or more illnesses or disabilities that may be severely painful, may be life threatening, or require intensive care.

Activities of daily living. The ADLs are divided into two parts for assessment: (1) care of the body, which involves such activities as walking, getting in and out of bed, bathing, combing hair, shaving, dressing, eating, and getting to the bathroom on time by oneself, and (2) IADLs, such as dialing the telephone, driving a car, hanging up clothes, obtaining groceries, taking medication, and having correct knowledge of the dosage.

• • •

Box 14-8   GERIATRIC DEPRESSION SCALE

Patient _____ Examiner _____ Date _____

Directions to patient: Please choose the best answer for how you have felt over the past week.
Directions to examiner: Present questions VERBALLY. Circle answer given by patient. Do not show to patient.

1. Are you basically satisfied with your life?	yes	**no** (1)
2. Have you dropped many of your activities and interests?	**yes** (1)	no
3. Do you feel that your life is empty?	**yes** (1)	no
4. Do you often get bored?	**yes** (1)	no
5. Are you hopeful about the future?	yes	**no** (1)
6. Are you bothered by thoughts you can't get out of your head?	**yes** (1)	no
7. Are you in good spirits most of the time?	yes	**no** (1)
8. Are you afraid that something bad is going to happen to you?	**yes** (1)	no
9. Do you feel happy most of the time?	yes	**no** (1)
10. Do you often feel helpless?	**yes** (1)	no
11. Do you often get restless and fidgety?	**yes** (1)	no
12. Do you prefer to stay at home rather than go out and do things?	**yes** (1)	no
13. Do you frequently worry about the future?	**yes** (1)	no
14. Do you feel you have more problems with memory than most?	**yes** (1)	no
15. Do you think it is wonderful to be alive now?	yes	**no** (1)
16. Do you feel downhearted and blue?	**yes** (1)	no
17. Do you feel pretty worthless the way you are now?	**yes** (1)	no
18. Do you worry a lot about the past?	**yes** (1)	no
19. Do you find life very exciting?	yes	**no** (1)
20. Is it hard for you to get started on new projects?	**yes** (1)	no
21. Do you feel full of energy?	yes	**no** (1)
22. Do you feel that your situation is hopeless?	**yes** (1)	no
23. Do you think that most people are better off than you are?	**yes** (1)	no
24. Do you frequently get upset over little things?	**yes** (1)	no
25. Do you frequently feel like crying?	**yes** (1)	no
26. Do you have trouble concentrating?	**yes** (1)	no
27. Do you enjoy getting up in the morning?	yes	**no** (1)
28. Do you prefer to avoid social occasions?	**yes** (1)	no
29. Is it easy for you to make decisions?	yes	**no** (1)
30. Is your mind as clear as it used to be?	yes	**no** (1)

total: Please sum all bolded answers (worth one point) for a total score. _____

Scores: 0-10 Normal   11-20 Moderate depression   21-30 Severe depression

Format modified slightly from original. From Yesavage et al: Development and validation of a geriatric depression screening scale: a preliminary report, *J Psychiatr Res* 17:37-49, 1983.

The OARS assessment tool is designed so that each component can be used individually. This enables it to be added to or integrated into self-designed tools. Other comprehensive assessment instruments include PACE (Patient Appraisal and Care Evaluation) and CARE (Comprehensive Assessment and Referral Evaluation) (Kane, Kane, 1981). These methods of appraisal are also very lengthy.

SPICES Tool

A relatively new tool (SPICES) developed by Fulmer and Wallace (1991) has proved reliable and valid in use with the elder population whether they are healthy or frail; in acute, skilled nursing, or long-term care facilities, or at home. The acronym *SPICES* assesses six common syndromes of the elderly that require nursing interventions: *S*leep disorders, *P*roblems with eating or

Box 14-9	ITEMS FROM THE SCALED U.S. VERSION OF THE GENERAL HEALTH QUESTIONNAIRE

A. Somatic symptoms

A1. Been feeling in need of some medicine to pick you up?
A2. Been feeling in need of a good tonic?
A3. Been feeling run down and out of sorts?
A4. Felt that you are ill?
A5. Been getting any pains in your head?
A6. Been getting a feeling of tightness or pressure in your head?
A7. Been having hot or cold spells?

B. Anxiety and insomnia

B1. Lost much sleep over worry?
B2. Had difficulty staying asleep?
B3. Felt constantly under strain?
B4. Been getting edgy and bad-tempered?
B5. Been getting scared or panicky for no reason?
B6. Found everything getting on top of you?
B7. Been feeling nervous and uptight all the time?

C. Social dysfunction

C1. Been managing to keep yourself busy and occupied?
C2. Been taking longer over the things you do?
C3. Felt on the whole you were doing things well?
C4. Been satisfied with the way you have carried out your tasks?
C5. Felt that you are playing a useful part in things?
C6. Felt capable of making decisions about things?
C7. Been able to enjoy your normal dry to day activities?

D. Depression

D1. Been thinking of yourself as a worthless person?
D2. Felt that life is entirely hopeless?
D3. Felt that life isn't worth living?
D4. Thought of the possibility that you might do away with yourself?
D5. Found at times you couldn't do anything because your nerves were too bad?
D6. Found yourself wishing you were dead and away from it all?
D7. Found that the idea of taking your own life kept coming into your mind?

From *Psychological Medicine*, Copyright © 1979, Cambridge University Press.

Box 14-10	SOCIAL DYSFUNCTION RATING SCALE

Self-Esteem

1. Low self-concept (feelings of inadequacy, not measuring up to self-ideal)
2. Goallessness (lack of inner motivation and sense of future orientation)
3. Lack of a satisfying philosophy or meaning of life (a conceptual framework for integrating past and present experiences)
4. Self-health concern (preoccupation with physical health, somatic concerns)

Interpersonal System

5. Emotional withdrawal (degree of deficiency in relating to others)
6. Hostility (degree of aggression toward others)
7. Manipulation (exploiting of environment, controlling at other's expense)
8. Overdependency (degree of parasitic attachment to others)
9. Anxiety (degree of feeling of uneasiness, impending doom)
10. Suspiciousness (degree of distrust or paranoid ideation)

Performance System

11. Lack of satisfying relationships with significant persons (spouse, children, kin, significant persons serving in a family role)
12. Lack of friends, social contacts
13. Expressed need for more friends, social contacts
14. Lack of work (remunerative or nonremuerative, productive work activities that normally give a sense of usefulness, status, confidence)
15. Lack of satisfaction from work
16. Lack of leisure time activities
17. Expressed need for more leisure, self-enhancing, and satisfying activities
18. Lack of participation in community activities
19. Lack of interest in community affairs and activities that influence others
20. Financial insecurity
21. Adaptive rigidity (lack of complex coping patterns to stress)

From Linn MW et al: A social dysfunction rating scale, *J Psychiatr Res* 6:300, 1969. Copyright © 1969, Pergamon Journals Ltd.

Patient Name:_____   Date_____

Spices	Evidence
Sleep disorders	
Problems with eating or feeding	
Incontinence	
Confusion	
Evidence of falls	
Skin breakdown	

Fig. 14-1   SPICES. (From Fulmer SPICES: an overall assessment tool of older adults. Developed by Meredith Wallace and Terry Fulmer, Hartford Institute for Geriatric Nursing, New York University, New York.)

feeding, *I*ncontinence, *C*onfusion, *E*vidence of falls, and *S*kin breakdown. Nurses are encouraged to make a 3 × 5 card with this acronym on it and carry it with them to use as a reference when caring for the older adult (Fig. 14-1). It is a system for alerting the nurse of the most common issues that occur in the health and well-being of the older adult, particularly those who have one or more medical conditions.

Assessment of Social Supports

Assessment of social supports looks at an individual's surrounding network of intimates, friends, and family. It is an important aspect of one's life and provides the sustenance and comfort often needed to surmount adversity such as a disability resulting from medical conditions. The screening tools focus attention on specific qualities of social support networks. These questions may facilitate discussion of important support issues with the elder and the elder's caregiver.

Family APGAR
The Family APGAR explores five specific family functions: *A*daptation, *P*artnership, *G*rowth, *A*ffection, and *R*esolution. A score of less than 3 points out of a possible 10 points indicates a highly dysfunctional family (at least as perceived by the person). A 4- to 6-point score

suggests moderate family dysfunction. These results alone should not be considered definitive for family dysfunction. The APGAR tool is useful in the following situations:

Interviewing a new patient
Interviewing a person who will be caring for a chronically ill family member
Following adverse events (death, diagnosis of cancer, etc.)
When the patient history suggests family dysfunction

If an elder has more intimate social relationships with friends than with the spouse or family or is without family or spouse, the Friend APGAR should be used. The questions are the same as in the Family APGAR, but with the word *friend* substituted for *family.*

An additional value of these instruments is the ability to assess the caregiver's perception of emotional support and social supports with a new diagnosis of Alzheimer's disease of a relative (Table 14-4).

Spirituality Assessment

Spirituality, or *spiritual well-being,* is defined as "the affirmation of life in a relationship with God, self, community, and environment that nurtures and celebrates wholeness" (National Interfaith Coalition on Aging,

Table 14-4

The Family APGAR

The following questions have been designed to help us better understand you and your friends. Friends are non-relatives from your school or community with whom you have a sharing relationship.

Comment space should be used if you wish to give additional information or if you wish to discuss the way the question applies to your friends. Please try to answer all questions.

The following questions have been designed to help us better understand you and your family. You should feel free to ask questions about any item in the questionnaire.

Comment space should be used if you wish to give additional information or if you wish to discuss the way the question applies to your family. Please try to answer all questions.

"Family" is the individual(s) with whom you usually live. If you live alone, consider family as those with whom you now have the strongest emotional ties.

For each question, check only one box

	Almost always	Some of the time	Hardly ever		Almost always	Some of the time	Hardly ever
I am satisfied that I can turn to my friends for help when something is troubling me. Comments:	☐	☐	☐	I am satisfied that I can turn to my family for help when something is troubling me. Comments:	☐	☐	☐
I am satisfied with the way my friends talk over things with me and share problems with me. Comments:	☐	☐	☐	I am satisfied with the way my family talks over things with me and shares problems with me. Comments:	☐	☐	☐
I am satisfied that my friends accept and support my wishes to take on new activities or directions. Comments:	☐	☐	☐	I am satisfied that my family accepts and supports my wishes to take on new activities or directions. Comments:	☐	☐	☐
I am satisfied with the way my friends express affection, and respond to my emotions, such as anger, sorrow, or love. Comments:	☐	☐	☐	I am satisfied with the way my family expresses affection, and responds to my emotions, such as anger, sorrow, or love. Comments:	☐	☐	☐
I am satisfied with the way my friends and I share time together. Comments:	☐	☐	☐	I am satisfied with the way my family and I share time together. Comments:	☐	☐	☐

Who lives in your home?* List by relationship (e.g., spouse, significant other,† child, or friend).

Please check below the column that best describes how you now get along with each member of the family listed.

Relationship	Age	Sex	Well	Fairly	Poorly
_____	____	____	☐	☐	☐
_____	____	____	☐	☐	☐
_____	____	____	☐	☐	☐

If you don't live with your own family, please list below the individuals to whom you turn for help most frequently. List by relationship (e.g., family member, friend, associate at work, or neighbor).

Please check below the column that best describes how you now get along with each person listed.

Relationship	Age	Sex	Well	Fairly	Poorly
_____	____	____	☐	☐	☐
_____	____	____	☐	☐	☐
_____	____	____	☐	☐	☐

From Smilkstein G, Ashworth C, Montano, D: Validity and reliability of the Family APGAR as a test of family function, *J Fam Pract* 15:303-311, 1982.

*If you have established your own family, consider home to be the place where you live with your spouse, children, or significant other; otherwise, consider home as your place of origin (e.g., the place where your parents or those who raised you live).

†"Significant other" is the partner you live with in a physically and emotionally nurturing relationship, but to whom you are not married.

Table 14-5

Jarel Spiritual Well-Being Scale

DIRECTIONS: Please circle the choice that *best* describes how much you agree with each statement. Circle only *one* answer for each statement. There is no right or wrong answer.

	Strongly agree	Moderately agree	Agree	Disagree	Moderately disagree	Strongly disagree
1. Prayer is an important part of my life.	SA	MA	A	D	MD	SD
2. I believe I have spiritual well-being.	SA	MA	A	D	MD	SD
3. As I grow older, I find myself more tolerant of others' beliefs.	SA	MA	A	D	MD	SD
4. I find meaning and purpose in my life.	SA	MA	A	D	MD	SD
5. I feel there is a close relationship between my spiritual beliefs and what I do.	SA	MA	A	D	MD	SD
6. I believe in an afterlife.	SA	MA	A	D	MD	SD
7. When I am sick I have less spiritual well-being.	SA	MA	A	D	MD	SD
8. I believe in a supreme power.	SA	MA	A	D	MD	SD
9. I am able to receive and give love to others.	SA	MA	A	D	MD	SD
10. I am satisfied with my life.	SA	MA	A	D	MD	SD
11. I set goals for myself.	SA	MA	A	D	MD	SD
12. God has little meaning in my life.	SA	MA	A	D	MD	SD
13. I am satisfied with the way I am using my abilities.	SA	MA	A	D	MD	SD
14. Prayer does not help me in making decisions.	SA	MA	A	D	MD	SD
15. I am able to appreciate differences in others.	SA	MA	A	D	MD	SD
16. I am pretty well put together.	SA	MA	A	D	MD	SD
17. I prefer that others make decisions for me.	SA	MA	A	D	MD	SD
18. I find it hard to forgive others.	SA	MA	A	D	MD	SD
19. I accept my life situations.	SA	MA	A	D	MD	SD
20. Belief in a supreme being has no part in my life.	SA	MA	A	D	MD	SD
21. I cannot accept change in my life.	SA	MA	A	D	MD	SD

FACTOR I: FAITH/BELIEF DIMENSION

(Scoring: SA = 6; SD = 1)

Item 1 _____
Item 2 _____
Item 3 _____
Item 4 _____
Item 5 _____
Item 6 _____
Item 8 _____   Subscore _____

From Hungelmann J, Kenkel-Rossi E, Klassen L, Stollenwerk R, Marquette University College of Nursing, 1987, Milwaukee, Wis. (Copyright.)

Continued

Table 14-5—cont'd

Jarel Spiritual Well-Being Scale

	Strongly agree	Moderately agree	Agree	Disagree	Moderately disagree	Strongly disagree
FACTOR II: LIFE/SELF RESPONSIBILITY						
(Reverse Scoring: SA = 1; SD = 6)						
Item 7 _____						
Item 12 _____						
Item 14 _____						
Item 17 _____						
Item 18 _____						
Item 20 _____						
Item 21 _____ Subscore _____						
FACTOR III: LIFE SATISFACTION/SELF-ACTUALIZATION						
(Scoring: SA = 6; SD = 1)						
Item 9 _____						
Item 10 _____						
Item 11 _____						
Item 13 _____						
Item 15 _____						
Item 16 _____						
Item 19 _____ Subscore _____ Total score _____						

1975). Spiritual needs are broader and more personal than religion. They transcend the physical and psychosocial elements of the person. Nurses tend not to deal with spiritual needs of patients because they are thought to be too personal. Yet, if nurses are to care for the whole person, spiritual needs must be part of the assessment process. Spirituality helps elders' adaptive capacity. The Jarel Spiritual Well-being Scale can help the nurse identify areas of spiritual strength and distress (Table 14-5).

Environmental and Safety Assessment

Safety issues become a major environmental concern for the older adult who is frail and living at home, as well as for the elderly in various assisted care environments. Altered mobility, sensory function, and health conditions all can create an unsafe situation, whether as a single-factor problem or as multiple factors. Issues of neighborhood safety, lighting, types of floor coverings (e.g., scatter rugs), use of electric or gas appliances, stairs, inadvertent food poisoning or medication errors, as well as many other potential or real situations, should be assessed by the nurse. A variety of checklists

are available for assessing different environments. Box 14-11 presents assessment and intervention of the home environment for older persons.

Fig. 14-2, p. 286, gives guidelines for a home safety assessment, Box 14-12, p. 287, presents guidelines and resources for providing a safe and accessible environment, and Box 14-13, p. 288, provides a community assessment guide.

• • •

All of the assessment tools presented here are screening tools and are not for definitive diagnoses. They are resources for nurses to use that can alert them to real or potential problems for which subsequent action needs to be taken. Health assessment is an appraisal of health status in an attempt to identify latent and obscure conditions, to serve as a screening process, to serve as a follow-up on health care plans, and to serve as the initial establishment of a health baseline. The aim is to help the aged remain as independent and functional as possible at their highest level of wellness, regardless of their place of residence—in acute or long-term care institutional settings or in their own home.

Box 14-11 **ASSESSMENT AND INTERVENTION OF THE HOME ENVIRONMENT FOR OLDER PERSONS**

Area or Activity	Problem	Intervention
Bathroom	Getting on/off toilet	Raised seat; side bars; grab bars
	Getting in/out tub	Bath bench; transfer bench; handheld shower nozzle; rubber mat; hydraulic lift bath seat
	Slippery or wet floors	Nonskid rugs or mats
	Hot water burns	Check water temperature before bath; set hot water thermostat to 120° or less
		Use bath thermometer
	Doorway too narrow	Remove door and use curtain; leave wheel chair at door and use walker
Bedroom	Rolling beds	Remove wheels; block against wall
	Bed too low	Leg extensions; blocks; second mattress; adjustable-height hospital bed
	Lighting	Bedside light; night light; flashlight attached to walker or cane
	Sliding rugs	Remove; tack down; rubber back; two-sided tape
	Slippery floor	Nonskid wax; no wax; rubber-sole footwear; indoor-outdoor carpet
	Thick rug edge/doorsill	Metal strip at edge; remove doorsill; tack tape down edge
	Night-time calls	Bedside phone; cordless phone; intercom; buzzer; lifeline
Kitchen	Open flames and burners	Substitute microwave; electric toaster oven
	Access items	Place commonly used items in easy-to-reach areas; adjustable-height counters, cupboards, and drawers
	Hard-to-open refrigerator	Foot lever
	Difficulty seeing	Adequate lighting; utensils with brightly colored handles
Livingroom	Soft, low chair	Board under cushion; pillow or folded blanket to raise seat; blocks or platform under legs; good armrests to push up on; back and seat cushions
	Swivel and rocking chairs	Block motion
	Obstructing furniture	Relocate or remove to clear paths
	Extension cords	Run along walls; eliminate unnecessary cords; place under sturdy furniture; use power strips with breakers
Telephone	Difficult to reach	Cordless phone; inform friends to let phone ring 10 times; clear path; answering machine and call back
	Difficult to hear ring	Headset; speaker phone; adapted handles
	Difficult to dial numbers	Preset numbers; large button and numbers; voice-activated dialing
Steps	Cannot handle	Stair glide; lift; elevator; ramp (permanent, portable, or removable)
	No handrails	Install at least one side
	Loose rugs	Remove or nail down to wooden steps
	Difficult to see	Adequate lighting; mark edge of steps with bright-colored tape
	Unable to use walker on stairs	Keep second walker or wheel chair at top or bottom of stairs

Modified from Rehabilitation Engineering Research Center on Aging (RERC-Aging), Center for Assistive Technology, University at Buffalo.

Box 14-11	ASSESSMENT AND INTERVENTION OF THE HOME ENVIRONMENT FOR OLDER PERSONS—cont'd	

Home Management	Laundry	Easy to access; sit on stool to access clothes in dryer; good lighting; fold laundry sitting at table; carry laundry in bag on stairs; use cart; use laundry service
	Mail	Easy-to-access mailbox; mail basket on door
	Housekeeping	Assess safety and manageability; no-bend dust pan; lightweight all-surface sweeper; provide with resources for assistance if needed
	Controlling thermostat	Mount in accessible location; large-print numbers; remote-controlled thermostat
Safety	Difficulty locking doors	Remote-controlled door lock; door wedge; hook and chain locks
	Difficulty opening door and knowing who is there	Automatic door openers; level doorknob handles; intercom at door
	Opening/closing windows	Lever and crank handles
	Cannot hear alarms	Blinking lights; vibrating surfaces
	Lighting	Illumination 1-2 feet from object being viewed; change bulbs when dim; adequate lighting in stairways and hallways; night lights
Leisure	Cannot hear television	Personal listening device with amplifier; closed captioning
	Complicated remote control	Simple remote with large buttons; universal remote control; voice-activated remote control; clapper
	Cannot read small print	Magnifying glass; large-print books
	Book too heavy	Read at table; sit with book resting on lap pillow
	Glare when reading	Place light source to right or left; avoid glossy paper for reading material; black ink instead of blue ink or pencil
	Computers keys too small	Replace keyboard with one with larger keys

SPECIAL PROBLEMS AFFECTING ASSESSMENT OF THE OLDER ADULT

A number of factors complicate assessment of the older adult. These include differentiating the effects of aging from those originating from disease, the coexistence of multiple diseases, the underreporting of symptoms by older adults, atypical presentation or nonspecific presentation of illness, and the increase in iatrogenic illnesses.

Overdiagnosis or underdiagnosis occurs when the normal age changes are not considered; these include both physical changes and biochemical changes (such as laboratory values). Box 14-14, p. 289, lists the laboratory values that do and do not change with age and that

if the nurse is not aware of age differences, could lead to an overdiagnosis or missed diagnosis. Underdiagnosis is more common in the care of the aged. Many symptoms or complaints are ascribed to normal aging rather than to a disease entity that may be developing. Difficulty in assessing the older adult with multiple chronic conditions is also a challenge. Symptoms of one condition can exacerbate or mask symptoms of another.

Underreporting of symptoms by the older adult also complicates assessment. Past experiences of older adults, their culture or educational background, ageism, fear, depression, and cognitive dysfunction are some of the issues that hinder them from seeking assessment and treatment of medical problems. Older adults also think that some of their problems are a normal part of

	Okay (y/n)	Plan to improve	
Basic Structure			
Intact roof			
Solid floors and stairs			
Functioning toilet (or outhouse)			
Source of fresh water			
Wheelchair ramp			
Temperature Control			
Fan/air conditioner			
Proper use of heating pads			
Proper hot water heater temperature			
Adequate heat/insulation			
Nutrition			
Kitchen condition/food storage			
Evidence of alcohol use			
Pests			
Fire Prevention and Response			
Use of kerosene heaters			
Use of open gas burners on stove for heat			
Smoking in bed			
Use of oxygen			
Dangerous electrical wiring			
Smoke alarms			
Exit plans in case of fire			
Self-Injury/Violence Prevention			
Locks			
Method of calling for help			
Proximity of neighbors			
Surrounding criminal activity			
Emergency phone numbers by telephone			
Loaded guns/knives			
Household toxins			
Water/bathtub			
Power tools			
Medication Management			
Duplicate medicines, outdated drugs, pill box			
Correct labeling			
Storage safety, accessibility, refrigeration			
Caregiver familiarity			
Wandering Control (for confused patients)			
Doortap latches, special locks			
Fenced yards with hidden latches			
Identification bracelets			
Electronic wandering alarms			

Use for:
— client
X clinician

Client's signature _____

Clinician's signature _____

RESIDENCE

Date _____

Fig. 14-2 Guidelines for home safety assessment. (Modified from Yoshikawa TT, Cobbs EL, Brummel-Smith K: *Ambulatory geriatric care,* St Louis, 1993, Mosby.)

Box 14-12   GUIDELINES AND RESOURCES FOR PROVIDING A SAFE AND ACCESSIBLE ENVIRONMENT

Guidelines for New or Adapted Housing*

1. Public use and common-use portions be readily accessible to and usable by individuals with handicaps
2. The doors be wide enough to allow passage into and within the premises by handicapped in wheelchairs
3. All premises contain an accessible route into and through the building
4. Light switches, electrical outlets, and other environmental controls be placed in accessible location
5. Reinforcements be built into walls to allow later installations of grab bars
6. Kitchens and bathrooms be usable by people in wheelchairs

Steps in Adapting a Residence

1. Assess the residence for safety, accessibility, and usability.
2. Determine what assistive devices, repairs, and/or modifications are needed. Contact local Center for Independent Living, Community Development Department, Area on Aging, or similar agency to obtain advice and referrals. Follow the telephone trail!
3. If renting, work with landlord or management company to do the work. Obtain approval or denial in writing. Contact Fair Housing Act agency if management will not permit tenant to make modifications at his or her own expense.
4. Obtain referrals for contractors to modify or repair housing.
5. Obtain estimates for necessary work or costs of assistive devices.
6. Determine available financial resources:
   a. Obtain prescription of medical necessity for assistive devices. Determine whether cost will be covered by private insurer, Medicare, Medicaid.
   b. Contact public housing authority to determine if there is low-income assistance for housing modifications. Funds from the Older Americans Act Title III often can be used to modify and repair homes.
   c. Contact the welfare and energy departments for help with weatherization of the home or costs of energy. Funds are available for low-income elders.
   d. Contact local Community Development Department, Center for Independent Living, Area on Aging for funding sources and referrals. Programs such as Community Development and Social Service Block Grants, the Farmer's Home Administration, and the Older Americans Act provide funds for ramps, security (e.g., new locks), and general repairs. Follow the telephone trail. Be patient.

For More Information

1. ABLEDATA: database including consumer guides, a directory of manufacturers, commercially available products, noncommercial prototypes, customized products, and one-of-a-kind products:
   ABLEDATA
   8455 Colesville Road
   Suite 935, Silver Spring, MD 20910
   1-800-227-0216
   Website: http://www.abledata.com
2. http://www.blvd.com   Commercially available assistive products
3. http://www.microsoft.com/enable/   Accessibility products from Microsoft and others
4. *Project Link* (Links persons with disabilities and the elderly to commercially available assistive products.) Can be reached at:
   Center for Assistive Technology
   515 Kimball Tower
   University at Buffalo
   3435 Main Street
   Buffalo, NY 14214-9980
   (800) 628-2281 (Voice/TTY)
5. The Tech Act Program automatically routes your call to the nearest Technical Assistance Center and can be reached at: (800) 949-4232.

*Fair Housing Amendment Act of 1988 (PL 100-430)

Box 14-13 COMMUNITY ASSESSMENT GUIDE

Overall Features
Climate
Location
Topography
Roadways
Open space
Distribution of buildings
Noise level
Economic state
Community planning

Population Characteristics
Overall age, sex, ethnic distribution
Proportion of elderly in population
Ethnic/socioeconomic characteristics of elderly
Intergenerational relations

Service Facilities
Shopping/basic service
Food, drug, clothing stores
Dry cleaners
Shoe repair
Restaurants
Banks
Post office

Educational
Public library
Adult education programs

Transportation
Private cars
Taxis
Subways and/or buses

Health care
Ambulance service
Clinics
Hospitals
Physicians
Dentists
Home care services
Pharmacists
Folk healers

Social/recreational
Places of worship
Outdoor parks
Indoor facilities:
    The "Y"
    Cinemas
    Bowling
    Private clubs

Social services
Social Security office
Welfare office
Senior citizens' programs:
    Senior centers, clubs, nutrition programs, outreach
        services

Environmental/Safety Conditions
Pavements/curbs
Crosswalks
Street lighting
Air quality
Sanitation services
Unleashed animals
Police department (crime rate)
Fire department (fire, arson rate)

From Rauckhorst LM et al: Community and home assessment, *J Gerontol Nurs* 6:321, 1980.

aging and dismiss symptoms as inevitable. Confusion, weakness, and functional decline are all rather broad and common symptoms but may in fact be the atypical presentation of illness for an older adult. Often confusion may be precipitated by a myocardial, urinary tract, or respiratory tract infection without the classic symptomatology nurses usually expect to find. Fatigue can be precipitated by depression, congestive heart failure, anemia, or hypothyroidism. Insomnia can be caused by age-related changes in sleep patterns, anxiety, delirium, fecal impaction, or immobility. Many times, the basic causes of these atypical and nonspecific symptoms are not even considered.

Iatrogenic illness is common among the aged adult. This, too, can complicate assessment. Drugs can have a paradoxical effect; a drug with the purpose of calming an individual can instead excite the individual or result in bizarre behavior. Many times, symptoms of adverse drug reactions can be nonspecific and mimic those of other illnesses, go unrecognized, or be ignored. It is therefore vitally important that the nurse be aware of the inherent obstacles of assessing the older adult.

Box 14-14   SUMMARY OF LABORATORY VALUES FOR THE OLDER ADULT

Values That Change With Age

Alkaline phosphatase ↑
Serum albumin ↓
Uric acid ↑
Total cholesterol ↑
   High-density lipoprotein (HDL)
      Male ↑
      Female ↓
   Triglycerides ↑
Serum B_{12} ↓
Serum magnesium ↓
Partial pressure arterial oxygen (Pao_2) ↓
Triiodothyronine (T_3) ↓
Fasting blood sugar (FBS) ↑
1-hour postprandial blood sugar ↑
2-hour postprandial blood sugar ↑
White blood cell counter ↓

Unchanged Values With Age

Serum bilirubin
Aspartate transaminase (AST)
Alanine aminotransferase (ALT)
Gamma-glutamyl transpeptidase (GGTP)
Prothrombin time (PT)
Partial thromboplastin time (PTT)
Serum electrolytes
Total protein
Calcium
Phosphorus
Serum folate
pH
Arterial carbon dioxide tension ($Paco_2$)
Serum creatinine
Thyroxine (T_4)
Red blood cell indexes
Platelets

Ordinarily Different From Younger Adults

Serum alkaline phosphatase ↑ 2.5 times normal
FBS up to 135 to 150 mg/dl
Postprandial glucose of oral glucose tolerance test ↑
   10 mg/dl above normal per decade of age
Normal serum creatinine with existence of markedly ↓ creatinine clearance
High erythrocyte sedimentation rate (up to 40 mm/hr)
Hemaglobin (lowest acceptable level)
   Women 11.0 g/dl
   Men 11.5 g/dl
Blood urea nitrogen ↑ to 28 to 35 mg/dl

Modified from Cavalieri T, Chopra A, Bryman P: When outside the norm is normal: interpreting lab data in aged, *Geriatrics* 47(5):66, 1992; and Kelso T: Laboratory values in the elderly: are they different? *Emerg Med Clin North Am* 8(2):241, 1990.

▶ KEY CONCEPTS

- Assessment of the physical, cognitive, psychosocial, and environmental status is essential to meeting the specific needs of the older adult and implementing appropriate interventions.
- Knowledge of how to administer a particular geriatric assessment tool is needed to achieve accurate information.
- Co-morbidity of many older adults complicates obtaining and interpreting assessment data.

▶ Activities and Discussion Questions

1. What is the importance of BADLs and IADLs?
2. For each BADL, develop a plan of interventions that you would institute to compensate for BADL deficits and still foster an elder's independence as much as is realistic.
3. What makes an assessment tool effective?
4. What tool(s) would be most appropriate for assessing an elder in the community, in the hospital, in long-term care, or in day care? Give your rationale for the choices.

RESOURCES

Handbook of Geriatric Assessment, 3rd edition, by J.J. Gallo, W. Reichel, and L.M. Anderson (1998, Aspen).

"A New Scale for Clinical Assessments in Geriatric Populations." Journal article by R.I. Shader, J.S. Harmatz, and C. Salzman. *J Am Geriatr Soc* 42:107-113, 1994.

Tests: A Comprehensive Reference for Assessments in Psychology, Education, and Business, 4th edition, 1997, edited by Todd JC, Maddox G. Available from Pro Ed, 8700 Shoal Creek Boulevard, Austin, TX 78757-6897.

REFERENCES

Benner P: *From novice to expert,* Menlo Park, Calif, 1984, Addison-Wesley.

Bennett JA: Activities of daily living: old-fashioned or still useful? *J Gerontol Nurs* 25(5):22, 1999.

Covinsky K: Depressive symptoms and disability progression, *Pepper Rev* 3(3):4, 1996.

Crum R et al: Population-based norms for the Mini-Mental Status Exam by age and education level, *JAMA* 269:2386, 1993.

Data on file, Pfizer, Inc., New York.

Fulmer T, Wallace M: SPICES, Hartford Institute for Geriatric Nursing, New York, 1991, New York University.

Gallo JJ, Reichel W, Andersen L, editors: *Handbook of geriatric assessment,* ed 2, Gaithersburg, Md, 1995, Aspen.

Ham RJ: Assessment. In Ham RJ, Sloane PD, editors: *Primary care geriatrics: a case-based approach,* ed 3, St Louis, 1996, Mosby.

Hays A, Borger F: A list in time, *Am J Nurs* 85(12):1107, 1985.

Healthy People 2000: US Department of Health and Human Services, Public Health Service, Washington, DC, 1991, US Government Printing Office.

Kane RA, Kane RL: *Assessing the elderly: a practical guide to measurement,* Lexington, Mass, 1981, Lexington Books.

Katz S et al: Studies of illness in the aged: the index of ADL, *JAMA* 185:914, 1963.

Katz S et al: Progress in the development of the index of ADL, *Gerontologist* 10:20-30, 1970.

King C: Guidelines for improving assessment skills, *Generations* 21(1):73, 1997.

Kleinman A: *Patient and healers in the context of culture: an exploration of the borderland between anthropology, medicine, and psychiatry,* Berkeley, 1980, University of California Press.

Mendez MF, Ala T, Underwood KL: Development of scoring criteria for the Clock Drawing Task in Alzheimer's disease, *J Am Geriatr Soc* 40:1095-1099, 1992.

Moore et al: A functional dementia scale, *J Fam Pract* 16:499, 1983.

National Interfaith Coalition on Aging: *Spiritual well-being,* Washington, DC, 1975, The Coalition.

Nolan KA, Mohs RC: Screening for dementia in family practice. In Richter RW, Blass JP, editors: *Alzheimer's disease: a guide to practical management,* part II, St Louis, 1994, Mosby.

Pfeiffer E: *Physical and mental assessment—OARS.* Workshop Intensive, Western Gerontological Society, San Francisco, April 28, 1979.

Pfeifferling JH: A cultural prescription for mediocentrism. In Eisenberg L, Kleinman A, editors: *The relevance of social science for medicine,* Boston, 1981, Reidel.

Podsiadlo D, Richardson S: Timéd "up and go": test of basic functional mobility for frail elder persons, *J Am Geriatr Soc* 39:142, 1991.

Ravohorst LM et al: Community and home assessment, *J Gerontol Nurs* 6:321, 1980.

Tappan RM: Development of the refined ADL assessment scale for patients with Alzheimer's and related disorders, *J Gerontol Nurs* 20(6):30, 1994.

Tuokko H et al: The clock test: a sensitive measure to differentiate normal elderly from those with Alzheimer disease, *J Am Geriatr Soc* 40:579-584, 1992.

Wallace M, Fulmer T: SPICES: an overall assessment tool of older adults, *Try this:* best practice in nursing care to older adults, New York, *The Hartford Institute for Geriatric Nursing* 1(1) Aug 1998.

Williams M: *Functional assessment.* Presented at Gerontological Nursing, Contemporary Forums, San Francisco, May 7-13, 1995.

Yesavage JA et al: Development and validation of a geriatric depression screening scale: a preliminary report, *J Psychiatr Res* 17:37-49, 1983.

Zarit SH: Brief measures of depression and cognitive function, *Generations* 21(1):41, 1997.

Zung W: Self-rating depression scale, *Arch Gen Psychiatry* 12:65, 1965.

15

Medication Use and Management

Upon completion of this chapter, the reader will be able to:

- Explain age-related pharmacokinetic changes.
- Discuss potential use of chronotherapy for the older adult.
- Describe drug use patterns and their implications for the older adult.
- Explain the role of elder, caregiver, and social network in ensuring medication adherence.
- List interventions that can help promote medication adherence by the elder.
- Identify diagnoses or symptoms for which psychotropic drugs are prescribed.
- Discuss issues concerning psychotropic medication management in the elderly population.
- Identify several neurotransmitters and their influence on mental illness and mental health.
- Discuss the Omnibus Budget Reconciliation Act (OBRA) guidelines for psychotropic medication use in institutionalized patients.
- Develop a nursing care plan for patients prescribed psychoactive medications.

Adverse reaction A harmful, unintended reaction to a drug administered in a normal dose (e.g., confusion).

Akathisia Restlessness and uncontrollable muscular movements.

Anorgasmy Inability to achieve an orgasm.

Anticholinergic A group of drugs that reduce spasms of certain smooth muscles; relax the iris; and decrease gastric, bronchial, and salivary secretions through the blocking of vagal impulses.

Antipsychotics A substance or procedure that counteracts or diminishes symptoms of psychoses.

Anxiolytics A sedative or minor tranquilizer used to treat episodes of anxiety.

Bioavailability The amount of drug that becomes available for activity in target tissues.

Biotransformation A series of chemical alterations of a drug occurring in the body.

Bradykinesia An abnormal condition resulting in slowness of speech and movement; associated with parkinsonism and extrapyramidal disorders.

Chronotherapy Adjustment of medications to coincide with the biologic rhythm of the body for therapeutic effect.

Degradation Decrease in amount and strength of a drug by the action of body processes.

Dystonia Any impairment of muscle tone; commonly involves the head, neck, and tongue.

Extrapyramidal disease Pertaining to the tissues and structures outside the cerebrospinal pyramidal tracts of the brain, resulting in involuntary movements, as well as changes in muscle tone and posture.

Half-life The time it takes to excrete half of a drug. This is dependent on the degree of kidney function.

Idiosyncratic reaction An abnormal susceptibility to a drug that is peculiar to that individual; hypersensitivity to a particular drug (i.e., an allergy).

Neuroleptic A substance that alters consciousness, creating indifference to surroundings and reducing motor activity and anxiety.

Neurotransmitters Any of numerous chemicals produced in the brain that activate transmission of nerve impulses.

Pharmacodynamics The study of the mechanism of action of a drug and the biochemical and physiologic effect.

Pharmacokinetics Absorption, distribution, metabolism, and excretion of a drug in the body.

Polydipsia Excessive thirst.

Polyuria Excessive frequency and volume of urination.

Psychotropic Describes drugs that have a special action on the psyche.

Regimen A systematic course of treatment or behaviors.
Side effect A consequence other than that for which the drug is used (e.g., dry mouth).
Tardive dyskinesia Involuntary rhythmic movements of the tongue, jaw, or extremities developed in association with neuroleptic medications.

Target tissue Tissue or organ intended to receive the greatest concentration of a drug or to be most affected by the drug.
Titration As used in this chapter, to ascertain the amount of a medication to produce the desired effect.

▶THE LIVED EXPERIENCE

It is so hard to keep track of my medications. I try arranging them in little cups to take with each meal, but then there are the ones that I take at odd times. Those are the easiest to forget. I get really confused and think sometimes I have taken them twice. I really wish I didn't have to take so many pills, but I'm not sure what would happen if I stopped any of them. I don't even know why I'm taking most of them.

Gerald, hypertensive, diabetic, and having cardiac problems

Well, I have talked to Dad about all the pills he takes. I'm sure that he makes mistakes about taking them, but I just can't be there watching all the time. Maybe I should get him one of those dispensers I've seen in the pharmacy, but first I think I will help him gather them all up and take them to the doctor. Maybe he can discontinue some of them. But then, he has three doctors. I guess I'll ask the pharmacist what I should do. And, I have to find out if those over-the-counter things Dad buys are safe with all the other things he is taking.

Gerald's daughter

*T*here has been a virtual explosion of new drugs in the past 15 years. Newer cardiovascular drugs for hypertension and dysrhythmias have resulted in better control of these conditions. A proliferation of nonsteroidal antiinflammatory drugs (NSAIDs) has provided the beginning of greater relief for arthritic conditions and pain. Therapy to combat gastrointestinal (GI) disorders, such as peptic and gastric ulcers, hyperacidity, and esophageal reflux, and to counteract the GI effects of NSAIDs has expanded the number of drug choices. Less sedating and safer antihistamines and many new rapid-acting psychotropic drugs, particularly for depression, have appeared and are readily used. New forms of old drugs have also come forth with increasing frequency. Transdermal patches for the delivery of pain relief, hormone replacement, angina, and hypertension control are now part of a number of medication regimens. The introduction of recombinant deoxyribonucleic acid (DNA) technology with preparations such as human insulin (Humulin), a hepatitis B vaccine, and tissue plasminogen activator (t-PA) is revolutionizing medication development. Finally, the conversion of prescription drugs to the over-the-counter (OTC) (nonprescription) drug market continues (Todd, 1990), and these drugs are appearing on pharmacy and supermarket shelves.

Although such advances in drug therapy are desirable, they bring with them concern about the effect of these new and improved drugs on the older person. Many nonspecialist physicians still do not realize that older patients are vulnerable to drugs. Many new drugs differ only in subtle ways from older, less expensive therapeutic agents and have the potential for use by a relatively small group of patients. As new drugs are introduced, their advantages draw attention, and their potential side effects and other limitations or hazards are obscured. At issue, too, is the tendency to think that new is better, causing physicians to prescribe newer, more expensive medications for older persons, sometimes unnecessarily.

The world population of individuals 65 years of age in the year 2000 is approximately 600 million people. In the United States 16% of adults are over 60 years of age and take nearly 40% of the medications prescribed, the average being 4.5 drugs per person. A comparable number of elders, in addition to their prescription drugs, use between 40% and 50% of the OTC medications, with an average of two medications per person. Elders who reside in long-term care facilities take an average of four to seven different medications (Hogstel, 1992). The trend of multiple drug use will continue as research produces more sophisticated therapies. A survey by the Pharmaceutical Manufacturers Association found 221 drugs at various stages of clinical development for 23 common diseases of the elderly (Stewart et al, 1991). The fast pace of drug research and development and the use of such drugs by elderly persons despite the lack of sufficient research with aged subjects require an understanding of the changes in pharmacokinetic and pharmacodynamic effects in the aged. From a Maslovian perspective, drugs impinge on many levels of needs. When they are used appropriately, drugs can enhance; when they are used inappropriately, they threaten all levels of the hierarchy of needs. At times, even when drugs are used appropriately, they may impinge on the elder's health.

PHARMACOKINETICS AND PHARMACODYNAMICS

The term *pharmacokinetics* refers to those aspects of a drug involved in the distribution of the drug in the body from the point of administration through absorption, metabolism, and excretion (Vestal, Dawson, 1985; Roberts, Tumer, 1988; DeMaagd, 1995). The term *pharmacodynamics* refers to the processes involved in the interaction between a drug and the effector organ, ending in a response of the organ (Roberts, Tumer, 1988; DeMaagd, 1995).

Absorption

Absorption time is the time required for a medication introduced into the body by the oral, parenteral, or rectal route to enter the general circulation. Drug bioavailability, the amount of drug in the blood, depends on this (Cusack, Vestal, 1986; Demaagd, 1995; Lee, 1996).

The small intestine is the organ in which maximal absorption occurs when medications are given by mouth. Parenteral routes of administration enter the circulation either immediately by intravenous administration or at a steady rate through intramuscular injection. Drug absorption depends on two independent aspects of the process: the rate of absorption, which determines the time of onset, and the extent of absorption (the amount of drug that passes through the absorbing surface into the body). This differs from bioavailability, which is the fraction of an administered drug that enters the systemic circulation.

In the aged there does not seem to be conclusive evidence that there is an appreciable change in the absorption process. Changes in GI motility seem to be the one factor that might influence absorption, and that is only in the time it takes the medication to pass into the small intestine. This is significant because the increase or decrease in motility may enhance or interfere with the action of the drug. Delayed stomach emptying and delivery of the drug to the vast absorption surface of the small intestine may diminish or negate the effectiveness of short-lived drugs. Some enteric-coated medications, which are specifically meant to bypass stomach acidity, may be delayed so long that their action begins in the stomach and may produce undesirable effects such as gastric irritation or nausea. Increased motility of the small intestine lessens the drug contact time and diminishes the effect of the drug. Conversely, slowed intestinal motility can increase the contact time and increase drug efficiency because of prolonged absorption or can cause adverse reactions to occur.

Antispasmodic drugs, if taken as part of a multiple medication regimen, have the propensity to slow gastric and intestinal motility. In some instances this drug action may be useful, but when there are other medications involved, it is necessary to consider the problem of drug absorption. Impaired or slow mesenteric (splanchnic) blood flow definitely interferes with absorption. Sluggish blood flow lengthens the absorption time and increases the amount of drug absorbed. However, many authorities agree that the quality of the absorption process is unchanged even though it may be slowed (Cusack, Vestal, 1986; Demaagd, 1995; Lee, 1996). Diminished gastric pH in the aged will retard the action of acid-dependent drugs. Antacids or iron preparations affect the availability of some drugs for absorption by binding the drug with elements and forming compounds.

Distribution

Distribution, or transport, depends on the adequacy of the circulatory system. The largest portion of cardiac output and drug concentrations go to the heart, brain, kidneys, and liver, with lesser amounts directed to the muscles, bone, and fat (Cusack, Vestel, 1986; Lee, 1996). Altered cardiac output and sluggish circulation delay the arrival of medication at the target receptors and retard the release of a drug, or its by-products, from the body. In addition, distribution influences the amount of free and bound drug in the circulation system. This facet of distribution depends on the availability of plasma protein. In the younger adult, adequate quantities of plasma albumin are present to bind with drugs. In the aged, the amount of plasma albumin available for binding with drugs diminishes. This means that more free (unbound) active drug circulates in the aged person's blood and becomes a contributing factor in overdose and toxicity (Lee, 1996). The pharmacologic effect perceived originates from the free drug. Unbound, or free, drugs circulate and can be filtered through cell and organ membranes, excreted unchanged by the kidney, or metabolized to a less active, inert form. Drug bound to plasma albumin (protein) is in an inactive state and cannot travel through the body because of this inactivation (Leventhal, 1999).

Changes in body composition during aging influence drug distribution. Total body water decreases, altering cellular distribution of drugs that are water soluble, such as cimetidine, digoxin, and ethanol. These drugs will be reflected in a higher-than-usual blood level in the elderly. Adipose tissue, or the fat content of the body, nearly doubles in older men and increases by one half in older women. Drugs that are highly lipid soluble may be stored in the fatty tissue, thus extending and possibly elevating the drug effect (Vestal, Dawson, 1985; Vestal, 1990; Lee, 1996). This potentially occurs in such drugs as lorazepam, diazepam, chlorpromazine, phenobarbital, and haloperidol (Haldol). These medications can be stored in fatty tissue, which can increase and prolong their effect.

Free drug concentration is an important factor in the distribution and elimination of a drug. Serum albumin is not significantly lower in the aged except when there is chronic illness or poor nutrition. Distribution of the drug may be altered by changes in the plasma protein concentration, red blood cells, and other body tissue. When drugs are being prescribed, attention should be given to whether the patient is young or old, frail or chronically ill, fat or lean, male or female. All of these factors have a marked influence on drug action.

Metabolism

The microsomal enzyme system of the liver is the primary site of drug metabolism (biotransformation). There is a consensus that there is a decreased blood flow to the liver, whether from disease or normal aging or both. This results in decreased hepatic clearance (Lamy, 1990; Vestal, 1990); thus the half-life* of a drug increases as a result of a diminished rate of metabolism in the aged.

The duration of drug action is determined by the metabolic rate. Slow metabolism suggests that the drug will remain in the body longer and produce a prolonged half-life. Sensitivity of the central nervous system alters receptor activity and produces greater receptor variation because of physiologic decline in autonomic nervous function, such as exaggerated or idiosyncratic reactions to hypotensive drugs or a hypothermic effect from phenothiazines.

A drug has specific affinity for receptor sites, which are designated areas inside or outside particular cells. When the drug reaches the receptor, it is translated into a chemical action that affects the body. This alteration at the receptor site is called *pharmacodynamics*.

Excretion

Under normal circumstances when a drug is taken by mouth, it is absorbed throughout the walls of the GI tract into the bloodstream, which facilitates distribution to various tissues of the body. Degradation, breakdown of the drug into intermediate compounds, may occur with some drugs to produce a more excretable form. Elimination is primarily effected through the kidneys in urine; some of the drug, however, is eliminated through bile, the GI tract, feces, sweat, and saliva. Administration, supervision, evaluation, and education of the patient depend in part on this knowledge. Fig. 15-1 illustrates the intricate relationship between physiologic age changes and the pharmacokinetics/pharmacodynamics of drugs with the aged population. These interrelated processes are the basis for many of the positive and adverse responses of the aged to medications. Only a brief discussion of important issues is presented here. Specific and more detailed information on the pharmacokinetics and pharmacodynamics of drugs can be found in numerous pharmacology textbooks.

The biologic half-life, the time required for half of the drug to be excreted, is affected by the degree of kidney function. Altered filtration and decreased plasma volume, which occur in dehydration, are common in the aged. These prolong and elevate blood levels of drugs, as can occur with penicillin. In some instances this situation can be beneficial, but with drugs such as streptomycin and vancomycin, toxic effects can overshadow the therapeutic value. Other drugs are ineffective in the presence of a low creatinine clearance.

---

*Half-life (also called t½) is the time required for plasma concentration of a drug to be reduced by half.

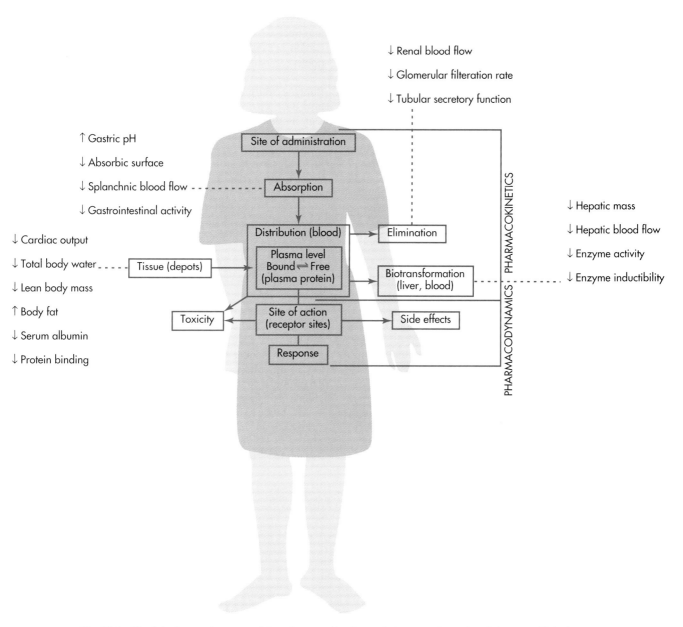

Fig. 15-1   Physiologic age changes and the pharmacokinetics and pharmacodynamics of drug use. (Data from Vestal RE, Dawson GW: Pharmacology and aging. In Finch CE, Schneider EL, editors: *Handbook of biology and aging,* New York 1985, Van Nostrand Reinhold; Roberts J, Tumer N: Pharmacodynamic basis for altered drug reaction in the elderly, *Clin Geriatr Med* 4[1]:127, 1988; Lamy PP: Hazards of drug use in the elderly, *Postgrad Med* 76[1]:50, 1982; Kane RL, Ouslander JG, Abrass IB: *Essentials of clinical geriatrics,* New York, 1984, McGraw-Hill; Montatmat SC, Cusack BJ, Vestal RE: Management of drug therapy in the elderly, *N Engl J Med* 321[5]: 303, 1989.)

Nurses need to be cognizant of kidney function in the aged, specifically urine creatinine clearance, which is a better index of renal function for the elderly than serum creatinine. Calculation of creatinine clearance in elderly women is obtained using the same formula as for men and multiplying the answer by 0.85. A well elder usually has a creatinine clearance of 70 ml/min. Disease conditions may reduce this level of kidney function. When the creatinine clearance falls below 30 ml/min, the excretion of the drug eliminated by the kidney decreases, greatly increasing the risk of drug accumulation or, in the case of a nephrotoxic drug, the risk of renal damage (Lee, 1996; Leventhal, 1999). The nurse should always check for a creatinine clearance level. If there is none, an accurate one can be calculated (see Chapter 7).

Pharmacologic Chronobiology

Chronobiology is a developing science that may lead to more effective drug therapy. The best time to administer medications based on biorhythms of various physiologic processes is now being considered for therapeutic and toxic effects. With a new discipline or science, new terminology appears; Box 15-1 lists and defines chronobiologic terms.

Biorhythms exert a major impact on body processes involved in drug therapy. An awareness of biorhythmic influences on disease can have an effect on the care of the aged. For example, the aged individual with slow or altered physiologic processes of aging and/or disease may receive a therapeutic or toxic effect from a medication because of the timing of the drug administration.

Pharmacokinetics, Pharmacodynamics, and Biorhythms

Our biorhythms strongly influence pharmacokinetics and pharmacodynamics. Absorption is dependent on gastric acid pH, emptying of the GI tract, and blood flow. All have been shown to have biorhythmic variations. Distribution of protein-bound drugs depends on albumin and glycoproteins produced by the liver. During the day, albumin levels are high, but they are low in the early-morning hours. Drug metabolism also is influenced by biorhythmic activity. Oxidation, hydrolysis, decarboxylation, and demethylation by liver enzymes demonstrate rhythm variations. Renal elimination depends on kidney perfusion, glomerular filtration, and urine acidity. These also have shown variations in circadian rhythm. The brain, heart, and blood cells have also been found to have varied rhythmicity, resulting in a cyclic response for beta-blockers, calcium channel blockers, angiotensin-converting enzyme (ACE) inhibitors, nitrates, and other similar drugs. These are among the frequently prescribed drugs that elders take for chronic cardiac conditions (Turkoski, 1998). Table 15-1 shows the rhythmic influence on diseases and physiologic processes.

Box 15-1	COMMON CHRONOBIOLOGIC TERMS
Chronobiology	The study of mechanisms of biologic time structure
Chronopharmacology	The study of interactions of biologic rhythms with medication
Chronotherapeutics	Pharmacotherapy using drug delivery schedules or technologies based on biorhythms (predicted and/or individual)
Chronothesy	Administration time differences in the effects of medications
Chronotolerance	Rhythm-dependent changes in tolerance to medication
Chronotoxicity	Adverse drug reactions as a function of biorhythms
Circadian cycle	The approximately 24-hour biorhythms in living organisms
Circamensual cycle	Biologic rhythms with a frequency of about 1 month
Circannual cycle	Biologic rhythms with a frequency of 1 year ±3 months
Circaseptan cycle	Biologic rhythms with a frequency of about a week
Ultradian cycle	Biologic rhythms with a frequency of more than 28 hours
Oscillation	One cycle (remains constant regardless of length of cycle)
Infradian cycle	Biologic rhythms of less than 20 hours

From Turkoski BB: Medication timing for the elderly: the impact of biorhythms on effectiveness, *Geriatr Nurs* 19(3):146-151, 1998.

Implications of Chronopharmacologic Therapy

The potential for decreasing the dose of medications and/or the frequency of administration for elders is the primary benefit of chronopharmacologic therapy. Both decreases may ultimately improve the therapeutic effect and decrease toxic effects for elders, as well as the general population, and they may improve patient adherence to a medication regimen. In addition, chronotherapeutics may provide financial benefit to the patient by reducing the overall medication expense because fewer administrations are needed to achieve a therapeutic effect.

Nurse's Role

The nurse's role is an important one. Nurses have a degree of discretion over drug administration. In the institutional setting, this discretion may occur as part of the nursing care plan; however, institutions still have rigid time schedules for medication administration that can negate the effectiveness of therapy by not timing the administration with body processes for the best therapeutic effect. In the home care setting, there is a greater latitude for adjusting medication time schedules and explaining to the patient what medication is to be taken at a certain time.

The nurse needs to become a member of the therapeutics committee to help make a change in medication administration timing. The nurse can also consult with the pharmacist. Finally, the nurse can begin to bring research on chronotherapy to the attention of physicians and co-workers (Turkoski, 1998).

Instituting chronotherapy at an agency might begin with one classification of drugs, using chronopharmacologic standards from pharmacologic literature. When the staff has become comfortable with the chronotherapy of this one classification of drugs, additional medications should be added one by one on a regular basis (Turkoski, 1998). Box 15-2 provides guidelines for application of chronotherapy.

Drugs designed to alter dose and frequency in accordance with biorhythms are already beginning to appear on the market. Among the first are antihypertensive drugs.

Table 15-1

Rhythmic Influences on Disease and Physiologic Processes

Disease/process	Rhythmic influence
Allergic rhinitis	Symptoms worse in the morning
Arterial BP	Circadian surge—morning hours
Asthma	Greatest respiratory distress overnight (during sleeping)
	Symptoms peak in early morning (4:00-5:00)
Blood plasma	Plasma volume falls at night = hematocrit increases
Cancer	Tumor cells proliferate when normal cell miosis is low
Cardiac disease	Angina, myocardial infarction, thrombolytic stroke occur in the first 4 hours after waking (peak 9:00) (through 22:00)
	(Prinzmetal angina—during sleep)
Catecholamines	Increase in early morning
Fibrinolytic activity	
Platelet activation	
Endogenous depression	May result from abnormality in circadian rhythm, which affects cortisol levels, body temperature, sleep/wake cycle
Gastric system	Gastric acid secretion peaks every morning (2:00-4:00); circannual variability—incidence of gastric ulcers > winter
Osteoarthritis	Pain more severe in morning
Potassium excretion	Lowest in morning/highest in late afternoon
Rheumatoid arthritis	Pain more severe in late afternoon
Systemic insulin	Highest in afternoon

From Turkoski BB: Medication timing for the elderly: the impact of biorhythms on effectiveness, *Geriatr Nurs* 19(3):146-151, 1998.
BP, Blood pressure.

Box 15-2   APPLICATIONS OF CHRONOPHARMACOLOGY*

Allergic rhinitis	H_1 receptor antagonists	Once daily/evening dose
Angina	Beta-agonists/theophyllines	Once daily at night or $^2/_3$ night, $^1/_3$ morning
	Corticosteroids	Morning or $^2/_3$ morning $^1/_3$ late in day
	Respiratory treatment	Early evening
Duodenal ulcers	H_2 receptor antagonists	Once daily dose—evening
	Prophylactic	Once daily dose—morning
Edema	Furosemide	Once daily—morning
Hypertension	Infusion antihypertensives	
Ischemic activity	Long-acting beta-blockers	Once daily at night
Osteoarthritis	NSAIDs	Once daily—morning
Platelet coagulation	Aspirin	Once daily—morning
	Plasminogen activators	Between noon and midnight
Rheumatoid arthritis	NSAIDs	Once daily—evening
Unstable diabetes mellitus	NPH Insulin	Bedtime dose

From Turkoski BB: Medication timing for the elderly: the impact of biorhythms on effectiveness, *Geriatr Nurs* 19(3):146-151, 1998.
NSAIDs, Nonsteroidal antiinflammatory drugs.
*General guidelines must be adjusted for individual clients.

DRUG INTERACTIONS

Drug interactions are a result of two or more medications given simultaneously or in close sequence with an outcome response of drug potentiation, drug antagonism, or drug synergism; the last-mentioned response is rare. Interactions may be precipitated by drug-drug, drug-nutrient, drug-disease, and social or psychologic factors that influence drug response.

The interactions can occur within or outside the body. Many of the interactions are a result of pharmacokinetic activity. A variety of interactions can occur. Within the body, absorption can be delayed by drugs exerting an anticholinergic effect. Tricyclic drugs (antidepressants) act in this manner to decrease GI motility and interfere with the absorption of other drugs. Several drugs compete to simultaneously bind and occupy the binding sites needed by the other drug, creating a varied bioavailability of one or both of the drugs. Interaction may be blocked at the receptor site, preventing the drug from reaching the cells. Interference with enzyme activity may alter metabolism and cause drug deficiencies, or toxic and adverse responses may develop from altered tubular function. Outside the body, interactions can occur any time that two medications are mixed before administration. An example of this is the improper preparation of more than one type of insulin for injection. Appendix 15-A indicates medications that should or should not be prescribed or used by the older adult.

Concern with the elderly's total response to drug therapy and its effect on the ability to perform activities of daily living and on functional capacities such as vision, hearing, memory, and mobility is a substantial reason for the nurse to do a drug assessment of each aged person.

Adverse Reactions

Drug use and misuse are a combination of many factors and create a geriatric health problem, not exclusively the fault of the aged or their physicians. It is clear that as the person ages, altered biodegradability, altered nutritional and fluid status, inadequate assessment before prescribing (treating the symptoms rather than the underlying cause), polypharmacy, and compliance factors result in a three- to four-times-higher rate of adverse drug reactions in the elderly than in the remainder of the population. At least 6 million elders are at risk for adverse drug reactions that may affect their development, adaptation, and social supports (Carruth, Boss, 1990; Wilcox et al, 1994). An estimated 40% of the elderly in the community experienced adverse drug reactions, 80% of which occurred with well-known drugs given at usual dosages (Lamy, 1986a, 1990). Geriatric admissions to the hospital attributable to adverse drug reactions are estimated to be 10% to 16% (Nolan, O'Malley, 1989; Col et al, 1990).

Wilcox et al (1994) found 20 potentially inappropriate drugs prescribed for elders; these included three controversial cardiovascular agents (propranolol, methyldopa, and reserpine). Among the most common drugs that produce adverse reactions are warfarin, digoxin, prednisone, diuretics, antihypertensives, insulin, aspirin, and antidepressants (Nolan, O'Malley, 1989; Hogstel, 1992; Lepkowsky, 1992; Wilcox et al, 1994). The most common reactions have been identified as sedation, lethargy, confusion, and falls (Palmieri, 1991; Hogstel, 1992).

Confusion perhaps is the most striking reaction. The increase in confusion of a demented patient is often considered to be further decompensation resulting from the person's present illness and is treated by increasing the medication dose, when in fact the medication may have been causing the response. Confusion in any individual who previously has not been confused may be interpreted as a new symptom of some disease yet unidentified, and a new medication is inappropriately prescribed. In the classic work of Wolanin and Phillips (1981), drug intoxication and confusion are discussed in detail. Lethargy can also be misinterpreted as a symptom connected with cardiac, respiratory, or neurologic conditions rather than a medication response.

Polypharmacy (multiple medication use) with several psychoactive drugs exerting anticholinergic action is perhaps the greatest precipitator of the adverse reaction of confusion. In addition, although the potential for an adverse drug reaction or interaction is only 6% when two drugs are taken, it rises to 50% when five drugs are ingested and to 100% when eight or more medications are taken together (Shaughnessy, 1992). Box 15-3 lists drugs that can lead to intellectual impairment; these are also cited by DeMaagd (1995). Box 15-4 presents the effects of systemic drugs on vision. Although they are not detailed here, more than 200 medications interfere with or contribute to sexual dysfunction for adults of any age (Butler et al, 1994; Miller, 1995). The categories that are most responsible for sexual dysfunction are cardiovascular drugs (antihypertensives and ACE inhibitors) and psychotropic drugs (antidepressants and phenothiazines).

Drug Toxicity

Drug toxicity is a major concern in the care of the elderly. Drug toxicity is a condition that occurs when the amount of a drug in the body exceeds the amount necessary to bring about a therapeutic effect, exceeds the therapeutic level, or becomes a harmful agent in the body, producing adverse effects (Weitzel, 1991) (Box 15-5). A drug that has a cumulative effect has the potential for drug toxicity. Other drugs may produce drug

Box 15-3	DRUGS WITH THE POTENTIAL TO CAUSE INTELLECTUAL IMPAIRMENT

Alcohol
Analgesics
Anticholinergics
Antidepressants
Antipsychotics
Antihistamines
Antiparkinsonian agents
Beta-blockers
Cimetidine
Digitalis
Diuretics
Hypnotics
Muscle relaxants
Sedatives
Sudden withdrawal of benzodiazapines

Data from Nolan L, O'Malley K: Prescribing for the elderly. I. Sensitivity of the elderly to adverse drug reactions, *Am Geriatr Soc* 36(2):142, 1988; Lamy PP: Drug reactions and the elderly, *J Gerontol Nurs,* 12(2):36, 1986; and Lamy PP: Adverse drug effects, *Clin Geriatr Med* 6(2):293, 1990.

toxicity under such circumstances as polypharmacy, slowed metabolism, altered excretion, dehydration, drug overdose because of self-medication errors, or excessive prescribed dosage. Table 15-2, p. 301, presents specific drugs commonly prescribed for the elderly that may result in toxicity. Appendix 15-B briefly describes side effects of drugs used by the elderly.

Nursing Interventions

The nurse is a key person in the prevention of drug toxicity and in the education of clients on the safe use and administration of medications. As part of an interdisciplinary approach, the nurse works with the physician, pharmacist, and dietitian to teach, monitor, and promote the actions necessary to prevent drugs from becoming toxic and to treat toxicity promptly should it occur.

Monitoring

The most effective way to prevent or minimize drug effects is by monitoring the client. The nurse's role includes knowledge of defining characteristics (signs and symptoms) indicative of toxicity and education of the elderly about drugs, dosage, and therapeutic and nontherapeutic indicators (see Table 15-2).

Box 15-4   EFFECTS OF SYSTEMIC DRUGS ON VISION

Drug	Effect
Furosemide (Lasix)	Blurred vision, decreased tolerance to contact lenses, photophobia, allergic reactions to eyelids and conjunctivae
Propranolol (Inderal)	Transient blurred vision with diplopia, decreased accommodation
Dimetapp (antihistamine and anticholinergic effect)	Mydriasis (contraindicated in angle-closure glaucoma), blurred vision, intolerance to contact lenses
Diazepam (Valium)	Allergic conjunctivitis
Digoxin (Lanoxin)	Diplopia, blurred vision, changes in color perception (warnings of toxicity)

Modified from Osis M: Drugs and vision, *Gerontion* 1(5):15, 1986.

Box 15-5   GENERAL PHYSIOLOGIC SYSTEM CHARACTERISTICS OF DRUG TOXICITY

Cardiovascular

Dysrhythmias
Tachycardias
Palpitations
Hypotension
Congestive heart failure
Hypertension
Bone marrow depression
   Leukopenia
   Thrombocytopenia
   Anemia
   Agranulocytosis

Central Nervous System

Confusion
Gait changes
Insomnia
Drowsiness
Blurred vision or visual changes
Slurred speech
Ototoxicity
Tremors
Irritability
Problems with temperature control
Anticholinergic effects
Seizures

Hepatic Changes

Jaundice
Clotting problems
Decreased liver function

Gastrointestinal (GI)

Anorexia
Nausea and vomiting
Diarrhea
GI bleeding
Pancreatitis

Renal

Electrolyte imbalance
Polyuria
Urinary retention
Fluid retention

Respiratory

Dyspnea
Asthmatic reactions

Skin

Rash
Urticaria
Pruritus
Photosensitivity

Advocacy Role

An awareness of the elder's overall functioning is needed in the nurse advocacy role for the nurse to influence the plan of treatment, clarify the treatment goals, and coordinate the activities of physicians and other clinicians to keep them focused on the goals of the client and family. For some drugs it may be wise to do a periodic blood level determination to establish that the elder is remaining within the therapeutic parameters.

Table 15-2

Toxic Characteristics of Specific Drugs Prescribed for the Elderly

Drugs	Signs and symptoms

Benzodiazepines
  Diazepam (Valium)
  Flurazepam (Dalmane)
  Lorazepam (Ativan)
	Ataxia, restlessness, confusion, depression, anticholinergic effect

Cimetidine (Tagamet)	Confusion, depression
Digitalis	Confusion, headache, anorexia, vomiting, dysrhythmias, blurred vision or visual changes (halos, frost on objects, color blindness), paresthesia
Furosemide (Lasix)	Electrolyte imbalance, hepatic changes, pancreatitis, leukopenia, thrombocytopenia
Gentamycin (Garamycin)	Ototoxicity (impaired hearing and/or balance), nephrotoxicity
Levodopa (L-Dopa)	Muscle and eye twitching, disorientation, asterixis, hallucinations, dyskinetic movements, grimacing, depression, delirium, ataxia
Lithium (Eskalith, Lithane)	Confusion, diarrhea, drowsiness, anorexia, slurred speech, tremors, blurred vision, unsteadiness, polyuria, seizures, muscle weakness
Methyldopa (Aldomet)	Hepatic changes, mental depression, fever, bradycardia, nightmares, tremors, edema
Nonsteroidal antiinflammatory drugs (NSAIDs)	
Ibuprofen (Advil, Motrin, Nuprin, Rufen)	Photosensitivity, fluid retention, anemia, nephrotoxicity, visual changes
Indomethacin (Indocin) Fenoprofen (Nalfon)	

Phenylbutazone (Butazolidin)
  Piroxicam (Feldene)
  Sulindac (Clinoril)
  Tolmetin (Tolectin)
	Confusion plus all of the above

Phenothiazide tranquilizers	Tachycardia, dysrhythmias, dyspnea, hyperthermia, postural hypotension, restlessness, anticholinergic effects
Phenytoin (Dilantin)	Ataxia, slurred speech, confusion, nystagmus, diplopia, nausea, vomiting
Procainamide (Pronestyl, Procan, Promine)	Dysrhythmias, depression, hypotension, SLE syndrome, dyspnea, skin rash, nausea, vomiting
Ranitidine (Zantac)	Liver dysfunction, blood dyscrasias

Sulfonylureas—1st generation
  Chlorpropamide (Diabinese)
  Tolbutamide (Orinase)
	Hypoglycemia, hepatic changes, HF, bone marrow depression, jaundice

Theophylline (Theo-Dur, Elixophyllin, Slo-Bid)	Anorexia, nausea, vomiting, GI bleeding, tachycardia, dysrhythmias, irritability, insomnia, seizures, muscle twitching
Tricyclic antidepressants Amitriptyline (Elavil, Endep, Amitril); doxepin (Sinequan, Adapin); imipramine (Tofranil)	Confusion, dysrhythmias, seizures, agitation, tachycardia, jaundice, hallucinations, postural hypotension, anticholinergic effects

Data from Skidmore-Roth L: *Nursing drug reference,* St Louis, 1992, Mosby; *Physician's desk reference,* Oradell, NJ, 1992, Medical Economics; Salzman C: Basic principles of psychotropic drug prescriptions for the elderly, *Hosp Community Psychiatry* 33:133, 1982; and Todd B: Identifying drug toxicity, *Geriatr Nurs* 4:231, 1985.
SLE, Systemic lupus erythematosus; *HF,* heart failure; *GI,* gastrointestinal.

Drug Holidays

Another intervention that may be used to decrease the potential of drug toxicity is a "drug holiday," which is a planned omission of a specific drug or drugs for one or more days or weeks. The benefits of such an option were identified by Keenan (1983) in the institutional setting, but these might be extrapolated to elders in the community. They include increased alertness of the individual, a decreased use of medications and subsequent reduction in overall medication cost, and easier scheduling of activities that may be restricted when certain medications are taken (e.g., an individual taking a diuretic might not be able to leave home until noon for fear that there will be no toilet accessible or that he or she will not be able to find one in time).

Although a drug holiday may be beneficial, questions arise regarding the length of time of the drug holiday. A variety of drugs taken by the elderly accumulate in body fat and take much longer than other drugs to be depleted below therapeutic levels. For those medications, a 1- or 2-day holiday may be ineffective. Perhaps rather than a drug holiday, reducing the number of medications prescribed and implementing a drug holiday in some situations would be more appropriate. Whatever the approach, the nurse assumes the major intervention role.

PATTERNS OF DRUG USE

Individuals over the age of 65 are the largest users of prescription and OTC medications. It is estimated that people over the age of 60 constitute 16% of the population in the United States and take almost 40% of the prescribed medications (Hogstel, 1992). Although there is limited information about the number of OTC medications used by the aged, the number is thought to be as great or greater.

Darnell et al (1986) noted that 90% of the elderly took an average of three OTC drugs and five prescription drugs daily. DeMaagd (1995) cites the figure of at least two OTC drugs at any given time. The most commonly prescribed and used drugs are cardiovascular drugs, antiinfectives, antipsychotic drugs, antidepressants, and diuretics (Baum et al, 1988; Hogstel, 1992; DeMaagd, 1995). Analgesics, laxatives, and antacids are the most-used OTC drugs, followed by cough products, acetaminophen, nonsteroidal topical preparations, milk of magnesia, Pepto-Bismol, eye washes, and vitamins (Hogstel, 1992). Now, with the conversion of prescription drugs to OTCs, additional categories may appear (Miller, 1996).

Polypharmacy

Polypharmacy is a major problem among older adults. The elderly often have multiple health problems or chronic conditions that are treated with multiple drugs. Because of this, they are prone to excessive drug use. The polypharmacy that occurs is an attempt to treat several disorders simultaneously, creating high risks for interactions and adverse drug reactions. Polypharmacy stems from multichronicity, the prescribing methods of physicians, the beliefs and practices of the aged, and the ever-increasing practice of seeing more than one primary care provider, each of whom prescribes the same class of drugs.

Self-Prescribing of Medications

The cost of medications continues to rise. Physician reimbursement for patient visits is low, and the number of physicians who will accept Medicare as total reimbursement continues to decrease markedly; also, Medicare does not adequately reimburse the patient for medications. As a result, elders do not seek or get medical assistance because of the out-of-pocket cost or do not want to bother the physician unless they are very ill. They medicate themselves with former prescriptions, prescriptions borrowed from friends, or OTC drugs.

Symptoms experienced by the aged such as pain, constipation, insomnia, and indigestion are amenable to OTC self-treatment. The use of OTC drugs often enables elders to gain relief from symptoms less expensively than through prescription drugs and to obtain sufficient comfort to continue their activities of daily living (Cameron, 1996).

Many OTC preparations have active ingredients that in large amounts would require a prescription; thus some drugs contain potentially dangerous substances. The elderly also use traditional medications such as folk medicine, herbs, and homeopathic remedies.

Today, with the frequent concurrent use of multiple medications, including prescribed and OTC drugs, the nurse needs to be aware of medications that the aged person is taking and the possible interactions among them.

Over-the-Counter Medications

OTC preparations number over 300,000 products (SRx senior mini-class curriculum, 1988) and are increasing in number yearly as prescription drugs are released by the Food and Drug Administration to the OTC category. In the past few years over 600 prescription drugs have become available as OTC medications. Although self-medication is an important part of our health care, the individual has the responsibility to be educated on the safe and wise use of these products. These products are just as much medications as those prescribed by physicians. OTC drugs are used by 75% of the aged to relieve symptoms of minor discomfort, illness, or injury and are stocked on supermarket, pharmacy, and drug emporium shelves. Undesirable effects can occur from these drugs, as well as from prescription drugs.

Misuse of Drugs

Drug misuse is a problem for both the health profession and the elderly. Health, medical care, and personal habits of the aged foster the ingestion of a wide variety of drugs. The overwhelming majority of the aged have minimal supervision of their medications. Some of the misuse stems from the fact that physicians prescribe doses that have guidelines based on mature adults rather than the older adult. Normal age changes in the elderly create a difference in their ability to handle standard doses of drugs (see Fig. 15-1).

Forms of misuse include overuse, underuse, erratic use, and contraindicated use. Most misuse is a result of inadequate physician training in geriatric pharmacology and inadequate assessment, as evidenced by treatment of a symptom rather than the cause of a symptom. An example of this is leg edema. This is generally associated with congestive heart failure, but in fact it may be just venous stasis resulting from immobility. Prescribing a diuretic would be inappropriate, but if the assessment is inadequate, the likelihood of just such a prescription is highly probable. Nurses, too, have a responsibility to be knowledgeable about drugs and doses appropriate for elders and to question when a drug seems inappropriate.

Misuse of drugs by the aged may be deliberate. Personality response may be such that under stress, oral intake may become either excessive or deficient, resulting in overuse or underuse of drugs (prescribed or OTC). Misuse may also be an individual's means of asking for help. One cannot negate the self-destructive motive (including the response to alienation or low social status), as well as the fact that drug misuse may be a manifestation of certain psychopathologic states. Often, however, drug misuse by the aged is unintentional and based on inadequate knowledge. Even so, it is frequently judged as noncompliance regardless of the reason for misuse.

Noncompliance/Nonadherence

Another major problem for the older adult is adherence to a medication regimen. Noncompliance is often considered deliberate misuse of medication. Seventy-five percent of elders intentionally do not adhere to their drug regimen but, instead, alter the dose, either because they think the drug is ineffective or because of the uncomfortable side effects. Others stop the drug or drugs because they think the medications are not needed anymore (Lamy, 1986a, 1986b) or because of their high cost. The nurse and other health care personnel become exasperated and angry at the individual because of noncompliance with the established medical program or treatment plan.

Nonadherence, although semantically the same as *noncompliance,* is a less harsh and less accusatory term when addressing why elders do not follow a suggested or prescribed plan of treatment. In an attempt to help and do what they think is best for the patient, the nurse and other care providers tend to forget or ignore that one cannot and will not comply with a prescription or treatment plan when there are incompatibilities that interfere with the practicalities of life or are distressful to the individual's well-being, or when actual misinformation or disability prevents compliance. For example, the aged individual cannot take medication three times a day with meals if he or she eats only two meals a day, and the aged person may not continue to take a medication if it brings about lethargy and inability to participate in social activities. Nonadherence includes not only the person for whom the medication is prescribed, but also the provider of care and the social support network (Kutzik, Spiers, 1993; Spiers, Kutzik, 1995).

The aged person has been repeatedly blamed for noncompliance, but how can anyone comply if the directions are unclear or are presented in a rapid-fire fashion in medical jargon? It is common to give discharge medication instructions when the person is leaving the hospital. It is also common to explain the treatment and give directions concerning medications when the patient is physically uncomfortable, to explain in English and not in the patient's primary language if that language is other than English, and to explain in a noisy or busy place. It is no wonder that a problem of adherence occurs under such circumstances. One tends to forget that it takes longer for the aged to process information and that visual and hearing impairments and cultural or language barriers can interfere with adequate communication of important instructions.

Confusion about the frequency of taking medication and the identification of the medication to take is extremely common. Unintentional errors are made by the elderly because of too-rapid or poor explanations, which are often given at times of high anxiety, fear, or physical distress. The elderly have been known to omit drugs by not purchasing them because of the expense or to alter the dosage in an attempt to stretch the medication over a longer period of time. When the person begins to feel better, drugs are sometimes stopped. Persons with little educational background and those in economic difficulty are more likely not to adhere to therapies they do not understand or cannot afford, including medication. It should be noted that regardless of the setting, the elderly, whether experiencing failing sight (fewer than 15% of elders have 20/20 vision), hearing difficulties (by age 80, two thirds of the population have impaired hearing) (Shimp, Ascione, 1988), or memory lapses, can be educated if difficulties are compensated for rather than merely considered insurmountable hurdles.

Multidimensional Framework

Kutzik and Spiers (1993) developed and revised (Spiers, Kutzik, 1995) a multidimensional framework for medication adherence that looks at the barriers to adherence by elders. The framework suggests that there is a simultaneous branching out between the three stages—initial instruction, regimen establishment, and self-management—and the three levels—individual, provider-treatment, and social support network. The integration of the stages and levels provides a reasonable approach to understanding the dynamics of elder adherence (Table 15-3).

The individual must first comprehend and be committed to the treatment. The care provider must be able to communicate the information in a form(s) necessary to compensate for physical-sensory and cognitive changes so that the individual understands and is willing to follow the treatment plan.

The elder must be able to use what has been learned so as to operationalize this information (obtain the medication, apply instructions, adjust to the regimen). The influence of the health professional is relatively strong to this point. Social context has a less direct influence on the drug regimen. However, it is affected by medical knowledge in the elder's cultural/belief system.

Finally, strong social network factors are more important because of the shrinking network that elders have available to them. Success at this level depends on the number of persons in the elder's support network who are able to assist the elder, if necessary, with the integration and/or reintegration of the regimen and the monitoring of adherence.

Strategies for improving patient adherence in hospital settings require the caregiver to assess the patient's ability to open childproof caps (a request can be made for easily removable caps), to take prescribed medications (sufficient motor skills), and to read labels and accompanying instructions. The caregiver also needs to provide written legible directions and to teach and supervise self-administration of medications during the hospital stay.

In any setting the caregiver needs to be alert to assess the accuracy of comprehension of instructions and to reinforce the directions as needed. Placing the medications in view when giving directions to the client and using a variety of teaching aids, such as individualized teaching with demonstration and feedback or audiovisual aids, are helpful strategies. It is important to adjust teaching to those with hearing and visual deficits. If the individual has a hearing aid, make sure it is in place and working. If glasses are used, make certain they are on, the lenses are clean, and lighting is adequate. Individualized regimens that are consistent with the patient's routine and life-style provide better opportunities to facilitate compliance. Other methods to improve adherence include providing bold, large black-lettered information in the client's language and at the client's reading level, and when possible, enlisting the participation of a significant other.

Memory aids to remind the aged person to take daily medication include a weekly calendar with pockets for medications indicating the day, time, and date and a daily tear-off calendar. Larger calendars are helpful when multiple drugs must be taken; a check can be placed in the date square each time a medication is taken. Transparent envelopes or sandwich bags containing the medication can be affixed to the dated square. Each envelope or bag should state the name of the drug, dose, and times that the medication is to be taken that day. In addition to a calendar, commercial drug caddies can be tried. These containers are available for single or multiple doses for a day, week, or month. Other methods include color coding the tops of the medication containers, circling the hours on a clock face affixed to the container, and setting an alarm clock to remind the elder when to take the medication. There are also electronic pill containers that audibly let the person know when it is time to take his or her medication; however, they may be too expensive for some elders' limited resources. These methods can be of tremendous assistance to the aged person who is having difficulty managing medications.

Memory failures associated with nonadherence to medication regimens are of two general types: forget-

Table 15-3

A Multidimensional Framework for Medication Adherence

	Individual	Provider-treatment	Social support network
STAGE 1 INITIAL INSTRUCTIONS	Comprehension Commitment to treatment	Communication effectiveness Number of providers	Community medical education Cultural beliefs
STAGE 2 REGIMEN ESTABLISHMENT Attaining medications	Mobility Finances Beliefs (e.g., medication sharing) Motivation	Medication cost Number of medica- tions needed	Accessibility to pharmacies Financial aid
Application	Ability to reconstruct in- structions Regimen strategy	Complexity of regimen Container design Label readability	Administration aid
Adjustment	Perception of effectiveness Self-manipulation of dosage/regimen	Rx manipulation Rx monitoring	Level of emotional/ functional support
STAGE 3 SELF-MANAGEMENT Integration/reintegration	Emotional adjustment to long-term medication dependence Regimen routinization and synthesis Response to challenges/ change	Life-style change re- quired by regular medication taking Regimen changes	Response to individual change Stability of support net- work/living situation
Monitoring	Ability to self-monitor for change	Degree of compre- hensive Rx review	Support network vigilance

From Spiers MV, Kutzik DM: *A multidimensional framework for understanding medication adherence in the elderly: prescription for re-thinking,* Unpublished paper, 1995.

ting the way to correctly take medications and "prospective" recall failure (failure to remember to take medication at the correct times) (Leirer et al, 1991). This latter type of nonadherence was reported to increase with the number of different prescriptions taken. The use of voice mail that telephones the elder each time a medication is to be taken to remind him or her of the type and amount of medication can reduce nonadherence to as low as 2.1% (Leirer et al, 1991). Voice mail reminders are thought to reduce nonadherence in three ways: (1) improve accuracy of the exact time elders remember to take their medication, (2) reduce the frequency of completely forgetting to take medication, and (3) reduce the frequency of self-overmedication.

For the individual who may not adhere because of low literacy, the use of matching colored dots on the drug container and a calendar or voice mail may be of value. Allow the individual to decide his or her own schedule and tailor it around his or her life-style. The use of cueing (i.e., choosing daily events such as brushing teeth or dentures or watching a daily television program) is also useful in facilitating compliance by those individuals who have very limited literacy ability (Hussey, 1991).

One should not forget to ask if the individual has had any "bad reactions" (adverse drug reactions) to any drugs and, if so, what occurred, the length of the reaction, and whether it was necessary to see a physician if the drug was used after that time.

The caregiver will find that questions about medications the aged person ingests are perceived as very personal and almost as sensitive an issue as asking him or her to reveal a secret. It is important to be aware of this and to ask questions in a nonthreatening, nonjudgmental manner. It is helpful to use open-ended questions, as well as some specific direct questions. For example, if you are trying to ascertain whether the patient has missed any doses of a medication, rather than asking how many times the doses were missed, it would be better and less threatening for the nurse to say, "It is quite common to forget to take your medication once in a while. How many times this month would you say you forgot to take your digoxin (or other specific drug)?" Many aged persons feel threatened by an authoritative manner and hesitate to reveal how they have been taking medications for fear that the caregiver will find fault and reprimand them.

Box 15-6   SUGGESTIONS TO IMPROVE MEDICATION ADHERENCE

Simplify the Medication Administration Process*
Memory aids
    Calendars
    Day, week, month pill containers
    Voice-mail reminders
Convenient medication refills
Easy-to-open medication containers
Reduce number of doses daily when possible
Reduce number of medications when possible
Reduce frequency per day by grouping compatible medications together
Tailor medication regimen to life-style

Disseminate Drug Information
Audiovisual information
Individual or group instruction (including family, caregiver, significant other)
Written instructions
    Information sheets, leaflets in bold type
    Reasonably large print
Periodic review of drug information

Teach Proper Medication Management Skills
Medication administration and training program
Self-care instruction

*Use lay terms: *twice a day* instead of *bid.*

Two issues remain when one discusses or considers elders and adherence to medication regimens (or to any therapy): (1) medication management is a complex activity that bears little resemblance to the simplistic notion of compliance (Conn et al, 1995) and (2) health professionals are frequently younger than their aged patients and have little concept of how patients define their own quality of life or the quality of their therapy (Tobias, 1994). It is important, then, that the health professional listen to elders and start asking them about their perspective on their drug therapy to accomplish as smooth a regimen as is realistically feasible for the elder. Box 15-6 offers suggestions for medication adherence that the nurse can institute to help older adults follow their medication regimen.

DRUG USE ASSESSMENT AND INTERVENTIONS

The major issues of polypharmacy—adherence to a drug regimen and varying effects of drugs on the aging process—point to the need for an adequate medication history. This should be the initial step in helping the aged to achieve safe drug use and to gather the information necessary to establish an individualized approach to medication management. A comprehensive drug history should help maintain a therapeutic medication regimen, assist in identifying missing knowledge necessary to take medication correctly, eliminate unnecessary medications, and reduce the risk of adverse drug reactions.

Usually it is the role of the pharmacist to obtain a medication history. When there is no pharmacist, however, the nurse should be prepared to do so. One should start by asking, "What prescription medications are you taking?" A systematic way to gather information is to do a 24-hour medication history. If using the review of systems, the nurse may ask what medications are routinely used for headache, eye problems, ear problems, and endocrine problems (e.g., thyroid, insulin). Additional information about drug management can be gathered: as the medication is named, the individual is asked to describe the dose, frequency of administration, and purpose.

Open-ended questions such as "What do you take for headaches?" or "What do you use for indigestion or bowel problems?" should be asked. These provide information about the elder's motivation and beliefs concerning the taking of medications; current prescriptions and OTC preparations; current administration schedule;

current medication status; knowledge about his or her medications; medication-related problems such as side effects or nonadherence; number of prescription drugs he or she is taking; frequency of visits to the physician or primary care practitioner; level of sensory, memory, and physical disability; ability to pay for prescription medications; and level of use of social drugs such as alcohol and caffeine (Ascione, Shimp, 1988; Ascione, 1994; Higbee, 1994).

Information about "street" drugs (opiates, marijuana, and cocaine) should be discussed, and specifics regarding "back fence" drug use (drugs that are obtained from friends and relatives) should be identified. Use of vitamins, herbal preparations, homeopathic remedies, and home remedies should also be noted. Many OTC preparations contain traces or lower doses of drugs that in higher dosage would require a prescription. Herbal preparations such as *Ginkgo biloba* (used to increase cerebral circulation) may cause increased blood pressure or headache. The interaction of nonprescription preparations with prescription drugs may precipitate a prescribed drug to reach toxic levels if an individual is taking several preparations that contain the same ingredients. Because many drugs take 2 to 4 weeks to be completely excreted, recently discontinued drugs, as well as the reason for their discontinuation, may be significant.

When the aged person does not remember all that he or she is taking, ask that all medications be put in a paper bag and brought in for evaluation. Garner as much information as possible from the individual regarding the amount, frequency, and reason for taking each drug. There are many forms of medication assessment tools that can be used, or nurses can adapt or generate one of their own to obtain the needed information.

Once the medication history is obtained, problem areas can be identified. Answers to the following questions should serve as a guide to definitive interventions:

1. Is the drug necessary? Many elderly persons continue to take medication indefinitely or have had a large prescription that they did not want to waste, or the physician never told them to stop taking the drug. Some aged persons are taking drugs because of behavioral changes or symptoms that are a consequence of unrecognized toxicity from other medications. Often the elderly do better without medication or may be able to follow a regimen when there are only one or two medications. The nurse should think about consolidating medications if there are medications with the same active chemicals that directly or indirectly accomplish the same end. For example, an individual who is taking a hypnotic and a tricyclic medication can perhaps achieve better sleep with the tricyclic administered at bedtime, since a side effect of the tricyclic is drowsiness. This would mean taking one medication (the tricyclic) instead of two and would avoid other side effects such as hangover and daytime drowsiness caused by taking the hypnotic as well.

2. Does the drug have undesirable side effects? The greatest lack of information by the aged is in the area of side effects. The nurse should know specific side effects before caring for a person. Aged individuals should be alerted to the possible side effects of drugs they are receiving. The nurse should also tap as a resource the clinical pharmacist. Either with or without the assistance of the clinical pharmacist, when side effects exist, the nurse should assess what they are and if they interfere with the individual's ability to function fully. For example, sleeping pills trigger confusion, hallucinations, and excitation; excessive use of vitamin A can produce joint problems, headaches, blurred vision, night blindness, or loss of hair. All anticholinergic drugs, many of which are common to the pharmacopoeia of the aged, exacerbate some of the common problems of aging, such as dry mouth, blurred vision, and anorexia. A helpful tip for nurses is to never allow an elder to have lenses changed on glasses until medication routines are well established. Medication changes often produce temporary visual changes (see Box 15-5). Another peculiarity of medication reaction among the aged is a tendency toward amnesic periods when taking benzodiazepines, especially lorazepam (Ativan). Haloperidol (Haldol), a psychotropic drug frequently used for behavioral control, is notorious for stimulating tardive dyskinesia in the aged. These few examples are meant to alert the nurse to observe carefully when instituting any new medication regimen. Not all of the possible adverse reactions will be found in textbooks; geropharmacology is an area ripe for clinical research by nurses who are in a prime position to observe reactions over time.

3. When more than one drug is involved, are interactions occurring? If interactions are evident, are they detrimental? An account of OTC drugs should also be obtained to establish if these drugs have an independent or collective effect when taken with prescription medications that will produce interactions or interfere with the pharmacokinetics.

4. Do the drugs induce malnutrition? Many drugs leach vitamins and minerals from the body. The aged have a history of poor nutritional status and thus are more vulnerable to this problem. Box 15-7 indicates drug-induced nutritional deficiencies. Depending on the degree of medication used, it might be helpful to the prescribing physician to pinpoint what vitamin and mineral supplements are necessary.

At the time of the drug assessment or any time the client visits the physician or the hospital, clinic, or office, he or she should bring all prescribed medications. If this is not possible, the aged person should carry a current list of medications. It is a good idea for the nurse to initiate this if the aged person does not have a record of his or her drugs. The nurse should make a list for reference, for agency records, and for the aged person to carry in a wallet or change purse.

| Box 15-7 | DRUGS INTERFERING WITH NUTRITIONAL STATUS THROUGH MALABSORPTION AND/OR MINERAL DEPLETION |

Antacids
Vitamins B_6, B_1; iron

Antibiotics
Folic acid; vitamins B_1, B_2, B_3, B_6, B_{12}, C; iron

Anticonvulsants
Vitamins B_1, B_6, B_{12}, D, K; calcium

Antilipemics
Folic acid; vitamins A, B_{12}, D, K

Diuretics
Vitamins B_1, B_2, B_{12}; potassium; zinc; calcium; magnesium

Laxatives
Vitamins A, D, E, K; sodium; potassium

Pencillamine*
Zinc

Data from Ebersole P, Hess P: *Toward healthy aging: human needs and nursing response,* ed 5, St Louis, 1998, Mosby; and Klar AV: Nutritional assessment in older Americans, *Clin Lett Nurse Pract* 3(6):6, 1999.
*Used in chelation.

LeSage and Stauffacher (1988) asked the following four questions to identify active or potential drug use or misuse: (1) What drug therapy or regimen is the older adult or caregiver actually following? (2) What is the older adult's or caregiver's knowledge base underlying decision making related to drug therapy? (3) Has the defined therapeutic outcome been achieved? (4) Does the person taking the drug have signs and symptoms that are commonly associated with adverse effects of drug therapy in older persons?

Patient Education

The area in which nurses have the biggest impact on medication use is patient education. The elderly have problems understanding how and when medications should be taken. Language barriers, either because of poor vocabulary or because the aged person speaks a language other than English, have a direct bearing on the adequacy of explanations. To minimize this kind of problem, the nurse should provide the patient with an adequate oral explanation supplemented by written instructions. Even with good directions, the elderly can become easily confused when more than one medication is involved. The better informed the aged are about their medications, the better they will be able to respond to their prescribed regimen.

Two strategies for helping elders use medications safely are discussed here. One strategy focuses on the dissemination of information about medications that the elder is taking. The objectives are to provide the necessary knowledge so that the elder can take the medication appropriately, understand the reasons for taking the medication, minimize the harmful effects, and avoid practices that would aggravate the drug effect. These objectives can be accomplished by the use of oral instructions in language that matches the elder's level of understanding and that are delivered in a slow, deliberate, and paced manner. Written information provides reinforcement and can be in the form of graphics, information sheets, prescription labels, and booklets. One must be careful not to overload the individual with too much information or input at one time (Ascione, Shimp, 1988).

The second strategy focuses on proper management of medications. This can be accomplished by reducing the number of medications and developing a schedule appropriate to or compatible with the individual's lifestyle. If one medication duplicates the action of another, consolidation of medications is appropriate (Mastrangelo, 1994).

It is important to remember that using one type of intervention on one occasion is insufficient to accomplish the goals of proper medication use or long-term compliance. A combination of interventions over an extended period of time has been shown to be the most effective approach (Haynes et al, 1987).

Education of the aged in the safe use of drugs can be accomplished on an individual basis or in small groups. The elderly should be taught to exercise their right to question and know what they are taking, how it will affect them, and the alternatives open to them (Higbee, 1994; Delong, 1995). Pamphlets and booklets written in lay terms and in appropriate language should be available to the aged. If there are none that are appropriate, the nurse should be creative and develop a booklet or information sheet that will meet the drug information needs of the aged patient, taking into account sight and memory changes. Information is best presented in numbered line fashion rather than in paragraph form (Morrow et al, 1988). Written information should be in large, boldface type. Audiovisual aids are available for health teaching, but if they are too expensive, the nurse should consider devising some.

Dispensing Procedures

Containers and container labels are another problem area in which the nurse can be of assistance. Most childproof containers continue to be "geriatric proof." For individuals who have arthritic hands or must open the container quickly, it is a frustrating, nearly impossible task. It is now possible for the aged person to ask that the medication be placed in a screw- or flip-top container. Nurses in the hospital, clinic, or physician's office who are responsible for ordering medications from the pharmacy should intercede and make such a request for the patient.

On most labels, much information is typed in a very small space. Not only are the patient's name and the directions for administration on the label, but the label also includes the physician's name; the prescription number; the name, address, and phone number of the pharmacy; and, at times, warning labels. So much in such a little space is difficult for the average adult to decode.

Current prescription labels should be reevaluated with geriatric patients in mind. Larger labels should be used to accommodate all information in readable form (and appropriate language) and to facilitate easier hand/finger movement coordination. There are also colored labels on prescriptions that warn about taking medications with or without food, that the medication "may make you drowsy," etc. Some kind of international color coding (like the international signs and symbols used to identify buildings for restrooms and other needs) could be developed for medication categories, which would appear on the bottle cap; for example, a red heart for heart preparations, perhaps purple for antihypertensive drugs, and other colors for other classifications may be effective. Since no standardized system of this nature currently exists, the nurse may need to devise a color system for patients and a color key that would be kept with the medications to avoid confusion.

Braille labels for the blind and visually impaired are available. The braille label, which is a clear piece of material affixed over the regular label, is embossed with the drug name, strength, and prescription numbers (Braille Labels for Drugs, 1983).

Computers are now being widely used in supermarket and chain-store pharmacies to review and monitor safe drug usage of customers. This increases information exchange between physicians and pharmacists in the surveillance of drug compatibilities. Although this is effective in most cases, one drawback is that unless medications are consistently purchased from a particular pharmacy, an accurate drug profile or surveillance cannot be maintained.

Most medications are taken orally. Many of the tablets and capsules are difficult to swallow because of their size or because they stick to the buccal mucosa. Administration of a drug in liquid form is sometimes preferable and allows flexibility; concentrations can be varied so that quantities of solution can be prepared and taken by the teaspoon, tablespoon, or ounce. For the aged person at home, these are simply and commonly used measurements. When using liquid preparations, it is the nurse's responsibility to ascertain that the client is using an appropriate measure. Crushing tablets or emptying the powder from capsules into fluid or food should not be done unless specified by the pharmaceutical company or approved by a pharmacist, because it may interfere with the effectiveness of the drug (either underdose or toxicity) or create problems in administration, as well as injure the mouth or GI tract.

Enteric coatings are used to protect the stomach against irritating substances or to protect certain drugs from breakdown by the stomach acid. Some pharmaceutical companies coat the drug beads in extended-action capsules with different types of coatings to al-

Box 15-8   MEDICATIONS THAT SHOULD NOT BE CHEWED OR CRUSHED

Type	Rationale
Enteric-coated tablets	Prevent destruction of drug in stomach
	Prevent irritation in stomach to achieve a prolonged action
Timed-release tablets	
Slow-release core	Give prolonged release
Mixed-release granules	Immediate and prolonged release
Multilayer tablets	One-layer immediate dose; each layer released to maintain blood level of medication
Porous inert carriers	Slow release into gastric fluid
Soluble matrix	Wax matrix provides slow release into gastric fluid; prevents high concentration of drug in local area; prevents gastric upset

Box 15-9   GUIDELINES FOR TRANSDERMAL DELIVERY SYSTEMS

Proper Administration

1. Know the proper place for administration (some require specific anatomic placement).
2. Place on clean surface (if hairy, should be shaved).
3. Press firmly for 10 seconds for secure contact (no wrinkles or raised edges).
4. Wash hands after contact with patch.
5. DO NOT cut patch in half to decrease dose (this can cause evaporation or spill out of medication, and decrease adherence to skin).

Site Rotation

1. Do not reapply to same area for at least 7 days.

Rash Management

1. Rash is most common side effect (occurs in about 50% of patients because of active ingredient or adhesive).
2. Apply topical corticosteroid to site as a pretreatment or after patch is removed.

Proper Disposal

1. Fold sticky edges together.
2. Dispose down toilet or in a closed garbage can to keep away from pets or children.

Modified from Fischer RG, Clark N: Skin contact: a clinical review of transdermal drug delivery systems, *Adv Nurs Pract* 2(10):15, 1994.

low some of the medication to be released immediately and the remainder at predetermined intervals. Some tablets are made of an inert porous plastic matrix that is impregnated with the active drug. As the drug passes through the GI tract, it is slowly leached out and absorbed by the body, which is a timed-release effect. Coated beads, plastic matrix tablets, and layered tablets should not be crushed, since all of the medication would be released at one time or inactivated by stomach acid. This is tantamount to administering higher doses of medication than prescribed or none at all (Box 15-8).

Placing capsules on the front of the tongue facilitates swallowing. Capsules are lighter than tablets and will float to the back of the buccal cavity when fluid is consumed, which thus washes them back and, it is hoped, down. Tablets are pushed down the gullet as a surge of fluid is swallowed.

The transdermal patch, also called the transdermal delivery system (TDDS) (Fischer, Clark, 1994), is one of the newer approaches to medication administration. Drug administration is limited to certain medications at present (7 to 10 medications). The TDDS provides for a more constant rate of drug administration and eliminates concern for GI absorption variation, GI tolerance, and drug interaction. In addition, lower doses are needed and compliance is better because of the need for less frequent administration. It also provides for rapid drug therapy termination when necessary. Box 15-9 provides guidelines for the TDDS.

The drug regimen of nursing home patients consumes much of the time of professional nursing staff as they administer, record, and evaluate. Rovner (1987) showed that two simple changes could reduce costs and

Box 15-10 MASTER

*M*inimize the number of medications needed. (Is there still a need for the medication?)

*A*lternate drugs (if possible). (Is there a drug as effective that has fewer side effects or that can be taken less frequently?)

*S*tart with a low dose and go slow if dose has to be increased. (The lowest possible dose should be used.)

*T*itrate therapy to the individual patient. (Is the dose appropriate for age, weight, liver, and kidney function? Adjust drug accordingly.)

*E*ducate the patient. (Education should include the name, dosage, frequency, side effects, and length of time the patient should continue medication therapy.)

*R*eview regularly. (Consider all of the above, as well as whether the elder sees any difficulty with the medication therapy.)

release nurses to perform other functions. He recommended the following:

- Reduce the number of times per day a medication is given, considering its known pharmacokinetics.
- Reorganize the dose-interval schedule of the drugs making up the total drug regimen.

The nurse has enormous responsibility in the administration of medications to the elderly and in the education of the aged about drug use. A brief discussion of inhalers and medication associated with diabetes can be found in Chapters 20 and 18, respectively.

Outcomes

Reassessment of the elder will determine the outcomes of medication use. Observation of the aged client should be an ongoing process to determine if physical and/or mental changes have occurred, as well as whether the therapeutic goal or response has been achieved. Listen to the elderly when they describe how they feel or changes that they notice after they have begun a new medication, have had a dose adjustment, or even when they continue to take several medications. Periodically check blood levels of such drugs that have a cumulative effect or are enhanced or diminished by interaction with other medication, such as warfarin (Coumadin), digitalis preparations, quinidine, theophylline, phenytoin (Dilantin), carbamazepine (Tegretol), and various antibiotics Appendix 15-C provides special considerations of drugs admin-

istered to the older adult. The mnemonic *MASTER* should always be kept in mind when administering medications to elders. It is one way to be alert to and prevent unnecessary medication use and adverse side effects in elder care. The components are spelled out in Box 15-10.

PSYCHOTROPIC MEDICATIONS

Psychotropic medications are drugs that alter brain chemistry, emotions, and behavior. They include antipsychotics or neuroleptics, antidepressants, mood stabilizers, antianxiety agents, and sedative/hypnotics. This section of the chapter provides an overview of psychotropic medications used to treat symptoms that occur in disorders of behavior, cognition, arousal, and mood in the geriatric population. A section is devoted to treating the movement disorders that may occur as a side effect from the use of neuroleptics. Because each individual experiences symptoms in a unique way, several types of drugs are frequently prescribed in different patients for any particular illness. In other words, medications are used to target specific troublesome symptoms. Nursing care of patients taking psychotropic medications is discussed.

Many older patients are ambivalent about medications, believing that they must take them while simultaneously resenting and welcoming them. The patient's understanding about his or her psychiatric disorder and the rapport established with the health care provider will influence reactions to medications, including behaviors about taking them. Resistance may occur when a person is fearful that a psychoactive medication is prescribed for "craziness" or that the medication is addictive. A psychotherapeutic approach to care of the emotionally disturbed client should include both medication and psychotherapy. In practice, psychotherapy for elders is limited by reimbursement policies and personnel limitations.

A patient should be prescribed a psychotropic medication only after thorough medical, psychologic, and social assessments are done. Nursing assessment before medication intervention contributes knowledge and baseline information that can optimize the patient's medical and psychologic improvement. Issues to consider include the patient's medical status (and other medications that might interact with psychotropics), mental status, ability to carry out activities of daily living, and ability to conduct social activities and satisfying relationships with others, as well as the potential for patient or caregiver compliance with any pharmacologic or nonpharmacologic recommendations (Keltner, Folks, 1993).

General guidelines for nurses to consider include the questions in Box 15-11. The information generated from these questions should be shared with the patient to improve patient understanding and safety.

Antipsychotics

Psychosis covers a range of thinking and behavioral characteristics that are based on responses of the ill person to a private reality—a reality that is distressing and problematic for the patient and those around him or her. Characteristically, psychosis occurs in schizophrenia but can also occur in mania, depression, delirium, dementia, and paranoid states. Psychosis manifests itself as delusional thinking and hallucinations, both of which can cause extreme anxiety and bizarre behavior.

Antipsychotics, formerly known as *major tranquilizers* and frequently known as *neuroleptics,* are drugs

used to treat psychotic symptoms. (Originally given in high doses, these drugs produced loss of initiative, blunted affect, lethargy, somnolence, and movement disorders; hence the name *major tranquilizers.* In contrast, antianxiety agents have been called *minor tranquilizers*—these are usually benzodiazepines, which produce only sedation without most of the effects of the major tranquilizers. The development of newer drugs with different effects has made obsolete the terms "major" and "minor" tranquilizers.)

The underlying cause of symptoms must be carefully considered. The need for staff to medicate a patient because of loudness or other agitated behaviors must be evaluated in light of the context of conditions influencing the patient. Who is complaining and in what circumstance?

Medical, psychologic, social, and environmental influences can cause thinking and behavioral changes that result in psychic disturbances. Behavior changes can also occur suddenly from reversible causes such as infection, fever, electrolyte imbalance, addition of a new drug to an established regimen, or stress.

Biochemical processes in the brain influence all activities, including behavior, emotion, mood, cognition, and motor movement. Categorizing drugs by their receptor activities assists in identifying side-effect profiles. Boxes 15-12 and 15-13 illustrate potential side effects with the different receptors. Since most psy-

---

Box 15-11   QUESTIONS TO CONSIDER ABOUT THE DRUG AND THE SPECIFIC PATIENT

1. Is the drug working to improve the patient's symptoms?
   a. What are the therapeutic effects of the drug? (What symptoms are targeted?)
   b. What is the time frame for the therapeutic effects?
   c. Have the appropriate drug and dose been prescribed?
   d. Has the appropriate time been tried for therapeutic effects?
2. Is the drug harming the patient?
   a. What physiologic changes are occurring?
   b. What laboratory values are changing?
   c. What mental status changes are occurring?
   d. What functional changes are occurring?
   e. Is the patient experiencing side effects?
   f. Is the drug interacting with any other medication?
3. Does the patient understand the following?
   a. Why he or she is taking the drug?
   b. How the drug is supposed to be taken?
   c. How to identify side effects and drug interactions?
   d. How to reduce or manage side effects?
   e. Limitations imposed by taking the drug (sedative effects)?

Box 15-12   POTENTIAL ADVERSE EFFECTS CAUSED BY BLOCKADE OF MUSCARINIC ACETYLCHOLINE RECEPTORS

Blurred vision
Constipation
Decreased salivation
Decreased sweating
Delirium
Hyperthermia
Memory problems
Narrow-angle glaucoma
Photophobia
Sinus tachycardia
Urinary retention

Modified from Kaplan HI, Sadock BJ: *Pocket handbook of psychiatric drug treatment,* ed 2, Baltimore, 1996, Williams & Wilkins.

chotherapeutic agents do not affect a single neurotransmitter system, a wide range of side effects or adverse effects may result. Unidentified neurotransmitters may be the cause of some adverse effects. Simple side effects are considered unpleasant consequences of taking drugs, but adverse effects are usually more serious. Both types of effects can be cause for discontinuing the drug.

An important consideration for the geriatric patient is selection of the best medication for the individual. The side-effect profile influences selection. There are different classes and potencies of antipsychotics. Strong antipsychotics (high potency), such as haloperidol, are less sedating but cause more extrapyramidal reactions. The elderly are susceptible to developing extrapyramidal reactions, particularly neuroleptic-induced parkinsonian symptoms. Weak antipsychotics (low potency), such as chlorpromazine, are sedating and cause orthostatic hypotension, thereby precipitating falls. Furthermore, the anticholinergic properties in

the weaker antipsychotics can cause dry mouth, constipation, urinary retention, hypotension, and confusion. Table 15-4 illustrates comparisons of sedative, extrapyramidal, anticholinergic, and cardiovascular side effects of the different potencies of antipsychotics. Careful nursing observation is essential for monitoring side effects and drug interactions whenever any of these medications are given.

Response to treatment is the most important consideration when geriatric patients are taking psychotropics. Subjective patient comments about feelings and symptoms and objective observations about the patient's behavior are important data for evaluating the effectiveness of a drug. The nurse should ask patients about their feelings, symptoms, and side effects. Generally, calmness is the first noticeable beneficial sign. Hallucinations may or may not respond to medication, and delusions do not usually respond. However, the patient's calmness and improved restfulness will change perceptions about the hallucinations and delusions; usually these symptoms become less distressing. Although side effects are the usual reason for changing to another class of drug, an adequate trial of a drug cannot be assessed until time has been allowed for a therapeutic response to occur. Such a response can vary from 24 hours to 5 days or longer in individuals. The general rule for safety, comfort, and minimization of side effects—particularly in the elderly—is to "start low and go slow."

Geriatric Dosing

The Health Care Finance Administration and the Congressional Omnibus Budget Reconciliation Act (OBRA) of 1987 mandated that the elderly in long-term care settings receive psychotropic drugs for specific diseases or symptoms and that the use be monitored, reduced, or eliminated when possible (OBRA, 1987). Behaviors requiring neuroleptic use are listed in Box 15-14. *Organic mental syndromes* refer to behaviors such as agitation associated with dementia but not diagnosed as psychotic-psychiatric disorders. OBRA guidelines also delineate the recommended dosages. Physicians may exceed the recommended doses if documentation reasonably explains the rationale for the benefit of the higher dose in restoring function and/or preventing dangerous behavior (Stoudemire, Smith, 1996). Likewise, there are guidelines for dosage reduction, behavioral interventions for reducing or eliminating the medications, and directions for documentation about adequacy of treatment for symptom reduction.

Box 15-13   POTENTIAL ADVERSE SIDE EFFECTS OF PSYCHOTHERAPEUTIC DRUGS AND ASSOCIATED NEUROTRANSMITTER SYSTEMS

Dopamine Blockade
Endocrine dysfunction
   Hyperprolactinemia
   Sexual dysfunction

Movement Disorders
Dystonia
Parkinsonism
Tardive dyskinesia

Norepinephrine Blockade (Alpha₁)
Dizziness
Postural hypotension
Reflex tachycardia
Delayed or retrograde ejaculation

Histamine Blockade
Sedation
Weight gain

Modified from Kaplan HI, Sadock BJ: *Pocket handbook od psychiatric drug treatment,* ed 2, Baltimore, 1996, Williams & Wilkins.

Table 15-4

Comparison of Side Effects of Antipsychotics

Generic name	Side effects			
	Sedative	Anticholinergic	Extrapyramidal	Hypotensive
LOW POTENCY				
Chlorpromazine	High	High	Low	IM: High PO: Low
Thioridazine	High	High	Low	Moderate
INTERMEDIATE POTENCY				
Perphenazine	Moderate	Moderate	Moderate	Low
Loxapine succinate	Moderate	Moderate	Moderate	Low
Molindone HCl	Moderate	Moderate	Moderate	—
HIGH POTENCY				
Haloperidol	Low	Low	High	Low
Thiothixene	Low	Low	High	Moderate
Fluphenazine HCl	Low	Low	High	Low
Trifluoperazine HCl	Moderate	Low	Moderate	Low
NEWER ANTIPSYCHOTICS				
Risperidone	Low	Low	Dose related	Low
Clozapine	High	High	Low	High
Olanzapine	Moderate	Moderate	Low	Moderate

Modified from Bloom HG, Shlom EA: *Drug prescribing for the elderly,* New York, 1993, Raven; Jenike MA: *Geriatric psychiatry and psychopharmacology: a clinical approach,* St Louis, 1989, Mosby; and Semla TP, Beizer JL, Higbee MD: *Geriatric dosage handbook,* ed 3, Cleveland, 1998, Lexi-Comp.

Movement Disorders

Movement disorders are neurologic side effects of many antipsychotic medications and are referred to as *extrapyramidal syndrome (EPS)* reactions. These include acute dystonia, akathisia, parkinsonian symptoms, tardive dyskinesia, and neuroleptic malignant syndrome.

Acute dystonia. An acute dystonic reaction may occur hours or days following antipsychotic medication administration or after dosage increases and may last minutes to hours. An acute dystonic reaction is an abnormal involuntary movement consisting of a slow and continuous muscular contraction or spasm. Involuntary muscular contractions of the mouth, jaw, face, and neck are common. The jaw may lock (trismus), the tongue may roll back and block the throat, the neck may arch backward (opisthotonos), or the eyes may close. In an oculogyric crisis, the eyes are fixed in one position. Often this creates a feeling of needing to look up constantly without the ability to make the eyes come down. Dystonias can be painful and frightening.

Caregivers or others unfamiliar with these EPS reactions become alarmed. Although frightening, these incidents are not usually dangerous. They are quickly responsive to anticholinergic medication, such as benztropine (Cogentin), trihexyphenidyl (Artane), or diphenhydramine (Benadryl), providing relief within minutes if given intravenously, within 10 to 15 minutes if given intramuscularly, and within 30 minutes if given orally. These medications should be readily available to treat an EPS reaction and are usually given for a brief time following a reaction. After several weeks without an EPS reaction, these medications should be tapered off. Especially in the elderly, the anticholinergic properties of some of these medications are not desirable. Anticholinergics and amantadine (Symmetrel), a dopamine agonist, are useful in preventing dystonic reactions, but because of slow onset of action, they should not be used for acute treatment.

| Box 15-14 | BEHAVIORS FOR APPROPRIATE AND INAPPROPRIATE USE OF NEUROLEPTICS |

Unnecessary drugs; each resident's drug regimen must be free from unnecessary drugs.

Antipsychotic drugs are given *only as necessary* therapy to treat the following specific conditions as diagnosed and documented in the clinical record:
Schizophrenia
Schizoaffective disorder
Delusional disorder
Psychotic mood disorder (mania, depression with psychotic features)
Acute psychotic episode
Brief reactive psychosis
Tourette's disorder
Huntington's disorder
Organic mental syndromes (dementia and delirium included) with associated psychotic and/or agitated behaviors
Short-term (7 days) symptomatic treatment of hiccups, nausea, vomiting, or pruritus

Behaviors for which antipsychotic medication *is* appropriate:
Agitated psychosis (biting, kicking, hitting, scratching, assaultive and belligerent behavior, sexual aggressiveness) presenting a danger to self or care providers or interfering with ability to provide care
Hallucinations, delusions, paranoia
Continuous crying out and screaming

Behaviors less responsive to antipsychotics: antipsychotic therapy should *not* be used if one or more of the following is/are the *only* indication:
Repetitive, bothersome behavior (pacing, wandering, repetitious statements or words, calling out, fidgeting)
Poor self-care
Unsociability
Indifference to surroundings
Uncooperativeness
Restlessness
Impaired memory
Anxiety
Depression (without psychotic features)
Insomnia
Agitated behaviors that *do not* represent danger to the patient or others

Data from Semla TP, Beizer JL, Higbee MD: *Geriatric dosage handbook,* ed 3, Cleveland, 1998, Lexi-Comp; US Statutes, Omnibus Budget Reconciliation Act (OBRA) of 1987, 101 Stat 1330-160, US Health Care Financing Administration: Medicare and Medicaid: (requirements for long-term care facilities, *Federal Register* 54(21):5316-5373, 1989; Stoudemire A, Smith DA: OBRA regulations and the use of psychotropic drugs in long-term care facilities: impact and implications for geropsychiatric care, *Gen Hosp Psychiatry* 18:77-94, 1996.

Akathisia. Akathisia refers to the compulsion to be in motion. Patients describe feeling restless, being unable to be still, having an unrelenting desire to move, and feeling "like crawling out of my skin." Often this symptom is mistaken for worsening psychosis. Pacing, aimless walking, fidgeting, shifting weight from one leg to the other, and marked restlessness are characteristic behaviors for a person experiencing akathisia. Akathisia may occur at any time during therapy.

Treatment response is variable. Usually, approaches include lowering the antipsychotic dose, changing to a less potent drug, or adding a drug to counteract the akathisia. Although results are less successful than in treating acute dystonias, the same drugs are tried: anticholinergics, antiparkinsonians, antihistamines, and benzodiazepines (lorazepam). Propranolol and clonidine have also been used and do improve the subjective complaints of akathisia. However, hypotension and sedation are often unacceptable side effects and can be dangerous in the elderly.

Parkinsonian symptoms. In neuroleptic-induced Parkinson syndrome, a bilateral tremor (as opposed to a unilateral tremor) is often seen. More commonly, bradykinesia and rigidity are seen, which may progress to akinesia. Rigidity is the most common symptom associated with drug-induced parkinsonism. The patient may have an inflexible facial expression and, with the slow movements also occurring, appear bored and apathetic and be mistakenly diagnosed as depressed.

More common with the higher-potency antipsychotics, parkinsonian symptoms may occur within weeks to months of initiation of antipsychotic therapy. Women and the elderly are more frequently affected by this syndrome, and some become tolerant to the effects, whereas others need ongoing treatment (Gelenberg, Katz, 1993).

Tardive dyskinesia. Exposure to neuroleptics continuously for at least 3 to 6 months raises the risk of developing the delayed dyskinetic side effect known as *tardive dyskinesia.* Both low- and high-potency agents are implicated. Tardive symptoms usually appear first as wormlike movements of the tongue, and other facial movements include grimacing, blinking, and frowning. Slow, maintained, involuntary twisting movements of the limbs, trunk, neck, face, and eyes (involuntary eye closure) have been reported (Burke et al, 1982). Per-

---

Box 15-15   RISK FACTORS FOR TARDIVE DYSKINESIA

Advanced age
Length and amount of neuroleptic exposure
Medical conditions
  Edentulousness
  Decreased estrogen
Female gender
Mood disorder
History of extrapyramidal syndrome (EPS) reactions
Treatment with antidepressants or anticholinergics
Use of depot neuroleptics (intramuscular [IM] administration, slow-release drug over 10 days to 2 weeks; not commonly used in elderly persons)
History of drug interruptions ("drug holidays")
Smoking
Dementia
Brain damage
Mental retardation

Modified from Lohr JB et al: Treatment of disordered behavior. In Salzman C, editor: *Clinical geriatric psychopharmacology,* ed 2, Baltimore, 1992, Williams & Wilkins.

---

haps newer drugs, lower doses, and faster detection may promote less of this disturbing side effect. Lohr et al (1992) describe risk factors, which are outlined in Box 15-15.

Treatment is based on prevention, early detection, and medication manipulation. Antipsychotic use in the nonpsychotic patient should be avoided and used only for brief periods if absolutely necessary.

The Abnormal Involuntary Movement Scale (AIMS), which was designed by the National Institute of Mental Health (NIMH, 1976), should be used before therapy and after initiation of therapy. For monitoring movement disorders see Barnes Rating Scale for Drug-Induced Akathisia (Appendix 15-D), Simpson-Angus Rating Scale for EPS (Appendix 15-E), and the Abnormal Involuntary Movement Scale (AIMS) (Appendix 15-F). Always, the benefit of the drug must be weighed in relation to the intensity and seriousness of the psychotic symptoms.

Neuroleptic malignant syndrome. Antipsychotics impair the body's hypothalamic dopaminergic thermoregulatory pathways. Hence, patients taking neuroleptics cannot tolerate excess environmental heat. Even mild elevations of core temperature can result in liver damage. The problem is more likely to occur during hot weather. The nurse or caregiver must protect the elder from hyperthermia by making sure the environment is cool enough. Appropriate interventions include adequate hydration, relocation to a cooler area away from direct sunlight, and use of a fan or sponge bath. The patient may or may not share his or her discomfort about the heat, so assessment of body temperature is essential. Any circumstance resulting in dehydration greatly increases the risk of heatstroke. Diuretics, coffee, alcohol, lithium, and uncontrolled diabetes may decrease vascular volume, thereby decreasing the body's ability to sweat. Anticholinergics inhibit the sweating and lead to further heat retention (Lazarus, 1989). Heatstroke in old age is associated with very high mortality and morbidity rates.

Antidepressants

Antidepressants, as their name implies, are drugs that counter depression. In the treatment of mild to moderate major depression, all antidepressants are efficacious. In the treatment of severe, major depression with melancholia, tricyclic antidepressants (TCAs) and venlafaxine are superior to selective serotonin reuptake inhibitors (SSRIs). SSRIs are generally better tolerated and have fewer serious side effects than TCAs. The classes of antidepressants that are available in the United States and their side effects are listed in Table 15-5.

Depression and Target Symptoms

Target symptoms include depressed mood, lack of energy, fatigue, lack of interest in usual activities, inability to concentrate, loss of appetite, weight changes, sleep problems (difficulty falling asleep or staying asleep or early morning awakening), feelings of worthlessness, and suicidal thoughts.

Once a diagnosis of depression is made, medication selection requires careful consideration. Prior treatment responses will indicate whether a drug should be tried for subsequent depressive episodes. The elderly are more sensitive to anticholinergic and cardiovascular properties of drugs. Dosing low and slowly titrating medication increases are important.

Medical conditions and the type and number of medications currently taken are considerations in selecting an antidepressant medication. For example, a person with glaucoma or with benign prostatic hypertrophy should not be taking medications with anticholinergic effects; hence, the TCAs should be avoided in these persons.

The drugs that least interfere with the elderly person's quality of life should be considered. Many sexually active men and women may be concerned about the negative impact that SSRIs have on their sex lives but may be unable or unwilling to discuss their concerns. Letting them know that sexual dysfunction (primarily anorgasmy and ejaculatory delay) can occur and can be treated may give patients the permission they need to talk about their concerns.

Side Effects of Antidepressants

The side-effect profiles differ between the classes of drugs and are summarized in Table 15-5. Generally, the side effects of the TCAs include dry mouth, constipation, urinary retention, dysrhythmias, tachycardia, cardiac conduction defects, blurred vision, sedation, dizziness, and weight gain. Many of these problems are common to older persons and become increasingly troublesome when exacerbated by medication. TCAs are contraindicated in persons with heart block or heart disease.

Table 15-5

Classes and Side Effects of Antidepressants Available in the United States

Class	Examples	Side effects
Tricyclic antidepressants (TCAs)	Amitriptyline, doxepin, imipramine, clomipramine Nortriptyline, desipramine	Dry mouth, constipation, urinary retention, orthostasis, sedation Less of above side effects
Selective serotonin reuptake inhibitors (SSRIs)	Fluoxetine, sertraline, paroxetine, fluvoxamine	Nausea, vomiting, dry mouth, headache, sedation, nervousness, anxiety, dizziness, insomnia, sweating, ejaculatory/orgasmic dysfunction
Atypical blockers (phenethylamine type)	Bupropion, venlafaxine	Nausea, dry mouth, headache, dizziness, nervousness
Serotonin-2 antagonists/serotonin reuptake inhibitors	Trazodone, nefazodone	Sedation, orthostasis, nausea, dizziness, headache
Monoamine oxidase inhibitors (MAOIs)	Phenelzine, tranylcypromine	Orthostasis, weight gain, sexual dysfunction (anorgasmia), edema, insomnia

Data from Kaplan HI, Sadock BJ: *Pocket handbook of psychiatric drug treatment,* ed 2, Baltimore, 1996, Williams & Wilkins; Schatzberg AF: Course of depression in adults: treatment options, *Psychiatr Ann* 26(6):336-341, 1996; and Semla TP, Beizer JL, Higbee MD: *Geriatric dosage handbook,* ed 3, Cleveland, 1998, Lexi-Comp.

Dangers of Overdose

Suicidal feelings and impulsivity pose safety concerns when the TCAs are prescribed. That is, an overdose can produce QRS (quinidine-like) dysrhythmias, tachycardia, and hypotension that are all unresponsive to treatment. The average lethal dose of imipramine is 30 mg/kg (Kaplan, Sadock, 1996). Overdose with the monoamine oxidase inhibitors (MAOIs) is fatal with single doses of 1.75 to 7 g (Kaplan, Sadock, 1996). Lethal doses of the SSRIs have not been established. They are generally considered safer than the TCAs.

Decisions regarding treatment for depression must go beyond the decision of which medication is best. Actual situational adjustments that create depression must be dealt with as grieving processes that have healing properties if dealt with supportively. For a discussion of depression from the psychosocial perspective, see Chapter 25.

Treatment With Stimulants

Patients who suffer from depressive symptoms (but are not clinically depressed) might demonstrate apathy or disinterest in their surroundings, lack of energy, and withdrawal. These symptoms in the elderly respond to central nervous system stimulants such as amphetamine or methylphenidate. These agents are effective in chronically medically ill elderly persons who have become demoralized and refuse participation in rehabilitation. These stimulants are not antidepressants.

Methylphenidate (Ritalin) and *d*-amphetamine (Dexedrine) should be given only in the morning and early afternoon to prevent insomnia at night. Like all psychotropic medications, dosing should start low (2.5 to 5 mg/day) and titrate slowly, increasing every 2 or 3 days (by 2.5 to 5 mg) until a total of 20 mg/day is reached (Lohr et al, 1992). Side effects are tachycardia, mild blood pressure increases, agitation, restlessness, and confusion. Methamphetamine (Desoxyn) has similar effects. Patients taking these medications should be encouraged to resume all daily activities. Responses should include motivation, interest, attention, and a sense of well-being.

Mood Stabilizers

Mood stabilizers are the group of agents used for the treatment of mania associated with bipolar disorders. Particular features are prominent in the elderly who suffer from mania. That is, the person may demonstrate confusion, paranoia, labile affect, pressured speech and flight of ideas, morbid or depressive content of thought, increased psychomotor activity resembling agitated depression, a long period between the depressive episode and the appearance of mania, and altered orientation and attention span (Liptzin, 1992). Geriatric dosing, side effects, and nursing actions are listed for drugs commonly used in the treatment of mania: lithium, carbamazepine, and valproic acid (Table 15-6).

Issues for Older Persons

The safe use of lithium requires pretreatment medical workup. Baseline thyroid function tests should be performed. Although the evaluation should focus on cardiac, renal, and thyroid functions, mental status is another important assessment. Some authors suggest an electroencephalogram before and during treatment to determine the baseline and to observe for lithium-related changes in the brain. Evaluating for evidence of dementia, memory loss, or confusion is essential because lithium can cause these changes. Likewise, the patient should be evaluated for tremor or lack of coordination. A baseline creatinine level should be obtained because lithium may cause an elevated level in the elderly; this may not mean that renal function is impaired but may indicate an age-related skeletal muscle tissue breakdown. Further evaluation is indicated if levels are elevated.

Evaluation should include a list of medications and an assessment of the type of diet. Lithium interacts with other medications and certain foods. For example, a low-salt diet will elevate the lithium level, and a high-salt diet will decrease it. Likewise, thiazide diuretics and NSAIDs will elevate the serum lithium level.

Dosing

The starting dose for the elderly manic patient should be 300 mg twice daily. The dose may be increased weekly in increments of 300 mg/day to achieve a maximum dose of 900 to 1200 mg/day (Semla et al, 1998). Serum concentration and clinical response determine the proper dose. Serum concentrations must be monitored frequently, with an interval of 12 hours after the last dose before blood can be drawn. Therapeutic effects in acute mania may be seen in the elderly when the level is 0.6 to 1.2 mEq/L (Semla et al, 1998). Maintenance for relapse prevention can be achieved with lower levels of 0.6 to 0.8 mEq/L. Although this is a low level in younger persons, it is therapeutic for the elderly if symptoms of mania are improved. The patient needs to learn symptoms of minor toxicity (nausea, vomiting, weakness, diarrhea, drowsiness). Also the patient needs to maintain adequate hydration.

Table 15-6

Antimanic Medications: Dosages, Side Effects, and Nursing Actions

Drug	Geriatric dose	Side effects	Nursing actions
Lithium	300 mg twice daily initially; increase by 300-mg increments weekly according to clinical state and therapeutic serum range; maximum dose of 900-1200 mg/day in divided doses Serum concentration 0.6-1.2 mEq/L for therapeutic effects Serum concentration 0.6-0.8 mEq/L for maintenance	Confusion Polyuria Polydipsia Nausea Vomiting Diarrhea Tremor Ataxia Thyroid changes Renal changes (narrow margin between therapeutic and toxic blood levels)	Take drug with food. Monitor mental status. Monitor fluid intake and output. Monitor salt intake. Monitor weight gain/loss. Avoid excess caffeine. Observe for electrolyte imbalance. Observe for resting tremor and coarseness. Observe motor coordination; ensure safety in case of fall. Monitor blood level frequently (weekly, then monthly). Teach patient symptoms of toxicity.
Carbamazepine	200 mg twice daily initially, with meals; increase by 200 mg/day at 2- to 3-week intervals; maximum dose for acute mania of 800-1200 mg/day in divided doses or 7-15 mg/kg/day to attain therapeutic blood level Blood level of 6-12 μg/ml is therapeutic	Confusion Memory loss Ataxia Hepatotoxicity Impaired water excretion Depression of bone marrow—leukopenia	Take drug with food. Monitor mental status. Observe for oversedation. Monitor motor coordination; ensure safety in case of fall. Monitor fluid intake and output. Observe for infection. Monitor blood levels weekly for 6 weeks, then monthly.
Valproic acid, divalproex	125 mg/day initially; increase as tolerated and as necessary Research in elderly limited; maintenance dose for anticonvulsant action of 30-60 mg/kg/day in divided doses Blood level of 50 to 100 μg/ml recommended	Gastrointestinal (GI) symptoms (anorexia, nausea, vomiting, dyspepsia, diarrhea) Neurologic symptoms (tremor, sedation, ataxia) Alopecia Increased appetite Weight gain Hepatotoxicity Decreased platelets	Take drug with food (except divalproex). Monitor for side effects. Monitor liver function tests and platelets. Avoid in patients with liver dysfunction. Do not crush enteric-coated drug (divalproex) or capsules. Watch for signs of bruising or bleeding.

Modified from Liptzin B: Treatment of mania. In Salzman C, editor: *Clinical geriatric psychopharmacology,* Baltimore, 1992, Williams & Wilkins; Semla TP, Beizer JL, Higbee MD: *Geriatric dosage handbook,* ed 3, Cleveland, 1998, Lexi-Comp.

Side Effects

Side effects are the same for the young and old in spite of the use of lower dosage and serum levels in the geriatric population. Although toxicity is not usually a problem, those at risk for serious side effects include the physically ill, the very old, the frail, the cognitively impaired, and those taking multiple medications. Side effects include the following: confusion, disorientation, and memory loss; flattening of T waves on the electrocardiogram; polyuria and polydipsia; nausea, vomiting, and diarrhea; fine resting tremor; benign goiter; and ataxia. Lithium-induced hypothyroidism, more common in women than in men, may resemble dementia or depression. Thyroid levels should be checked every 3 to 6 months. Fortunately, careful monitoring can prevent toxic reactions. At toxic concentrations, the lithium level is elevated (>2 mEq/L) and all of the symptoms mentioned previously worsen. For example, resting tremor becomes a gross tremor.

Anxiolytics

Drugs used to treat anxiety are referred to as *anxiolytics* or *antianxiety agents,* or sometimes as *sedatives.* These agents include benzodiazepines, buspirone, beta-blockers, and antihistaminics. The decision to treat anxiety pharmacologically must be based on the person's degree of impairment, extent of preoccupation, inability to perform activities of daily living, and subjective feelings of discomfort.

Benzodiazepines

Although benzodiazepines have been available for almost 30 years, only minimal research has been done in the elderly. What is evident, however, is that there are toxic effects in the elderly. Specifically, the toxic effects include sedation, unsteady gait, confusion, disorientation, cognitive impairment, memory impairment, agitation, and wandering. Because these symptoms resemble dementia, elderly persons can easily be misdiagnosed once they start taking benzodiazepines. Another danger about this class of drugs is the central nervous system depression that results when they are combined with alcohol, hypnotics, analgesics, narcotics, and some antidepressants and neuroleptics. Unsteady gait can lead to risk of falls and hip fractures.

If possible, the benzodiazepines should be avoided. If necessary, lorazepam can be prescribed in doses of up to 1 mg; these doses have been shown to have negligible effects on memory.

Side effects. Although there are various short, intermediate, and long-acting benzodiazepines, the side effects are similar. The most common side effect is drowsiness. Other effects include dizziness, ataxia, mild cognitive deficits, and memory impairment. Since toxicity develops easily in the elderly, only short-term treatment is recommended with agents with relatively short half-lives. Some authors recommend against using the following specific benzodiazepines in the elderly: chlordiazepoxide, clorazepate, diazepam, prazepam, flurazepam, and quazepam (Semla et al, 1998). Lorazepam, which has a short half-life and no active metabolites, is a safe choice in the elderly.

Diphenhydramine

Diphenhydramine (Benadryl) is an antihistamine that is useful for its antianxiety properties. It is sedating but has anticholinergic properties. By itself, diphenhydramine can produce dry mouth, blurred vision, urinary retention, and constipation. (As discussed in the antipsychotic and antidepressant sections previously, anticholinergics in the elderly can be cumulative and produce confusion, disorientation, oversedation, agitation, and delirium.)

NURSING CONSIDERATIONS

All of the medications presented in this chapter have indications, side effects, interactions, and individual patient reactions. The nurse's advocacy role includes education for the patient and family or caregiver. Furthermore, the nurse must determine whether side effects are minimal and tolerable or serious. Asking the patient produces subjective data, and observing the patient's interactions, behavior, mood, emotional responses, and daily habits provides objective data. From this compilation of data, patient problems can be delineated, nursing diagnoses developed, outcome criteria planned, and interventions initiated. Nursing actions for the side effects associated with each drug class are presented in Table 15-7. These actions will help guide care planning for individual elderly persons.

Medications occupy a central place in the lives of many older persons: cost, acceptability, interactions, untoward side effects, and the need to schedule medications appropriately all combine to create many difficulties. Although nurses, with the exception of advance practice nurses, do not prescribe medications, we believe that a full understanding of medications is needed by nurses working with elders.

Table 15-7

Nursing Interventions for Side Effects of Psychotropic Medications

Type of drug	Common side effects	Nursing interventions
Antipsychotic	Sedation	Reassure patient/family that this side effect subsides in 5-10 days; prevent falls; avoid work requiring alertness, such as driving; dosing only at hour of sleep (hs) may decrease sedation during day.
	Orthostatic hypotension (more pronounced with low-potency medications)	Teach patient to dangle feet at bedside for 1-2 minutes before rising; rise slowly; support stockings may be helpful; prevent falling or tripping on obstacles.
	Photosensitivity Photophobia	Protect skin from sun with clothing and sunscreen; sunglasses may be more comfortable because of dilated pupils.
	Hyperthermia	Maintain adequately cool environment; teach patient to avoid hot temperatures and to increase water intake; ensure adequate hydration.
	Weight gain	Discuss with patient/family that this is a side effect; consult with dietitian for dietary planning; encourage avoidance of fattening foods; sweets may be craved to counteract sedation.
	Acute dystonic reactions (more common with some high-potency medications)	Simpson-Angus testing at regular times of day; Cogentin 0.5 mg IM for immediate relief (may repeat if 0.5 mg ineffective); observe for confusion associated with anticholinergic properties of Cogentin; reassure patient of immediate and full recovery with injection; for prevention thereafter, use amantadine; monitor for repeat EPS reactions; assess need for changing medication; assess patient compliance related to EPS.
	Parkinsonism	Same as above; may give benztropine (Cogentin) PO; reassurance needed.
	Tardive dyskinesia (may occur after 3-6 months of continuous treatment)	Assess for signs using AIMS test; observe for tongue movements and involuntary movement early in treatment; decrease dose of medication, change drug, consider vitamin E; if antipsychotic discontinued, tardive dyskinesia will get worse; if given Cogentin, tardive dyskinesia will appear worse. Much support is needed, because this is not always reversible.
	Akathisia	Assess for signs using Barnes scale; decrease dose, change drug, consider propranolol. Reassure patient that this is a side effect and will subside; difficult and uncomfortable to tolerate; monitor for safety and impulsive behavior related to anxiety and distress.
Anticholinergic effects of antipsychotics, antidepressants, antiparkinson agents	Blurred vision	Encourage use of magnifying glass and adequate lighting; reassure that the side effect subsides (up to 2 weeks); refer to physician if continues.

Data from Keltner NL, Schwecke LH, Bostrom CE: *Psychiatric nursing: a psychotherapeutic approach,* St Louis, 1991, Mosby.
IM, Intramuscularly; *EPS,* extrapyramidal syndrome; *PO,* orally; *TCAs,* tricyclic antidepressants; *CNS,* central nervous system; *GI,* gastrointestinal.   *Continued*

Table 15-7—cont'd

Nursing Interventions for Side Effects of Psychotropic Medications

Type of drug	Common side effects	Nursing interventions
Anticholinergic effects of antipsychotics, antidepressants, antiparkinson agents—cont'd	Urinary hesitancy (particularly in elderly men with benign prostatic hypertrophy)	Consider less anticholinergic drug; encourage patient to report this symptom; provide privacy; run water in the sink, warm water over perineum.
	Urinary retention	Encourage frequent voiding, whenever urge exists; teach patient to monitor output; catheterization may be indicated; observe for discomfort, pain.
	Dry mouth	Give water, ice, sugar-free lozenges or candy or gum; often a disturbing side effect and may be associated with bad breath; provide materials for adequate oral hygiene; explain that this is a side effect.
	Constipation	Often a problem in elderly without medication; add fluids, fruit, vegetables to diet; prune juice at hs or in morning (patient preference); stool softener can be helpful. Monitor for bowel movement frequency and bowel sounds to prevent obstruction or ileus.
	Dizziness	Teach patient to change positions slowly, especially from stooping or sitting to standing (tying shoes, lying in bed).
	Tiredness/sedation	Teach to avoid activities requiring alertness and concentration; decrease dose or increase dose more slowly if this occurs with TCAs; give medication at hs if possible; teach patient that alcohol and other CNS depressants worsen sedative effect.
Anxiolytics	Sedation Confusion Memory loss Amnesia	Prevent accidents by teaching patient and family to avoid activities requiring alertness; keep patient oriented to environment; assess level of confusion by checking mental status daily; use drug with short half-life and no active metabolites (lorazepam); teach patient that sedative effects are worsened with alcohol or other CNS depressants.
Lithium	GI effects	Take medication in divided doses with food; observe for worsening of diarrhea (fluid loss).
	Polydipsia	Explain side effect; tendency is to overhydrate; teach patient to maintain adequate hydration (particular vigilance needed if patient exercises vigorously); encourage fluids up to 3000 ml daily.
	Polyuria	Observe for diabetes insipidus; teach patient that frequent urination is a side effect.
	Tremors	Small tremor may be harmless; observe for worsening tremor; can determine whether increased salt intake (lowers lithium level) improves tremor.

▶ KEY CONCEPTS

- Individuals over 75 years old cannot be expected to react to medication in the way they did when they were 25 years old.
- Any medication has side effects. The therapeutic goal is to reduce the targeted symptoms without undesirable side effects. Drug-drug and drug-food incompatibilities are an increasing problem of which nurses must be aware.
- Polypharmacy reactions are one of the most serious problems of elders today and are usually the first area to investigate when untoward physiologic events occur.
- Drug misuse may be triggered by physician practices, individual self-medication, physiologic idiosyncrasies, altered biodegradability, nutritional and fluid states, and inadequate assessment before prescribing.

NANDA and Wellness Diagnoses

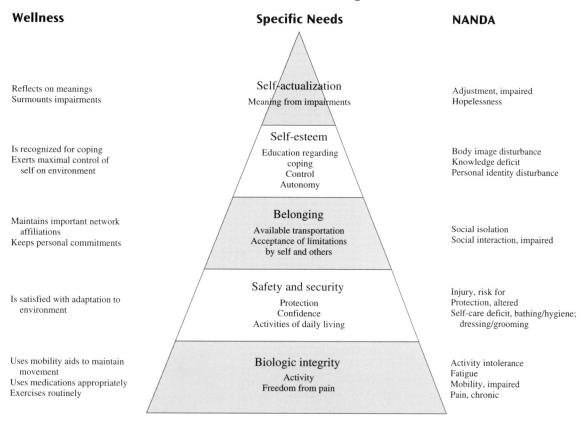

Wellness	Specific Needs	NANDA

Wellness

Reflects on meanings
Surmounts impairments

Is recognized for coping
Exerts maximal control of
    self on environment

Maintains important network
    affiliations
Keeps personal commitments

Is satisfied with adaptation to
    environment

Uses mobility aids to maintain
    movement
Uses medications appropriately
Exercises routinely

Specific Needs

Self-actualization
Meaning from impairments

Self-esteem
Education regarding
coping
Control
Autonomy

Belonging
Available transportation
Acceptance of limitations
by self and others

Safety and security
Protection
Confidence
Activities of daily living

Biologic integrity
Activity
Freedom from pain

NANDA

Adjustment, impaired
Hopelessness

Body image disturbance
Knowledge deficit
Personal identity disturbance

Social isolation
Social interaction, impaired

Injury, risk for
Protection, altered
Self-care deficit, bathing/hygiene;
    dressing/grooming

Activity intolerance
Fatigue
Mobility, impaired
Pain, chronic

These are not all of the possible wellness or NANDA diagnoses that may be identified. The above are frequent examples of nursing diagnoses that should be considered when planning care for the older adult in whatever setting.

- Nurses must investigate drugs immediately if confusion is observed in an individual who is normally alert and aware. Many drugs cause temporary cognitive impairment in older persons. These should be discontinued, or if that is not possible, the individual needs to be informed to forestall fears of Alzheimer's disease.
- Nonadherence of clients with medication regimens is a constant concern among health professionals. Look for possible reasons. One cannot comply with a prescription or treatment when there are incompatibilities that interfere with the practicalities of life or are distressful to the individual's well-being or when actual misinformation or disability prevents compliance.
- Chronotherapy that uses biorhythms of the body for most effective medication therapy is relatively new. It has the potential to decrease dose, frequency, and cost of medication regimens and to improve adherence to drug therapy.
- Biochemical processes in the brain influence all activities, including behavior, emotion, mood, cognition, and movement.
- Neurotransmitters, of which there are many yet only partially identified or understood, are the chemicals that stimulate these processes.
- The side effects of psychotropic medications vary significantly; thus these medications must be selected with care when prescribed for the aged.
- The response of the elder to treatment with psychotropic medications should show reduced distress, clearer thinking, and more appropriate behavior.
- Newer drugs should be prescribed for the elderly with caution because the long-term effects, side effects, and efficacy may vary significantly with the aged.

- The aged are particularly vulnerable to developing movement disorders (extrapyramidal symptoms, parkinsonism symptoms, akathisia, dystonias).
- The Health Care Financing Administration and the Congressional Omnibus Budget Reconciliation Act (OBRA) have severely restricted the use of psychotropic drugs for the elderly unless they are truly needed for specific disorders. Then they must be carefully monitored.
- Antidepressant medications must be tailored to the elder with careful observation for side effects.
- Dosage levels must be carefully titrated for elders, and their responses accurately and consistently recorded.

► Activities and Discussion Questions

1. What are the age-related changes that occur in pharmacokinetics of the older adult?
2. What is meant by *chronotherapeutics* and how applicable is it to elders? Explain your answer.
3. What are the drug use patterns of the elderly, and what can be done to correct or improve them?
4. Explain the role of the elder, the care provider, and the social network in medication adherence.
5. List a variety of measures that the nurse can suggest to assist older adults with their medication use and adherence to a medication regimen.
6. Develop a nursing care plan using wellness and NANDA diagnoses.
7. What are the most troublesome side effects of antipsychotic medications?
8. Discuss several reasons why tricyclic antidepressants might not be advisable for certain elders.
9. Provide a description of the type of antidepressant you think would be most dangerous to an elder who is feeling suicidal.
10. Develop a teaching plan for an elder with a bipolar disorder who has recently begun taking lithium.
11. Mrs. J. is calling out repeatedly for a nurse; other patients are complaining, and you simply cannot be available for long periods to quiet her. Considering the setting and the OBRA guidelines, what would you do to manage the situation?
12. When you discover that Mr. L. has not been taking his psychoactive medications (but has been hiding them), what will be your nursing intervention?

RESOURCES

Food and Drug Interactions. (Large-size print.) Originally published by *FDA Consumer Magazine.* Send postcard to FDA, HEF-88, 5600 Fisher Lane, Rockville, MD 20857.

National Institute on Aging, Age Pages Fact Sheet. For sale by Superintendent of Documents, U.S. Government Printing Office, Washington, DC 20402.

Team Up and Talk About Prescriptions: Prescription Medications and You: A Consumer Guide. (AHCPR Pub No 96-0056; English, Spanish versions available.) For bulk copies (more than 10 copies), contact: NCPIE, 666 11th Street NW, Suite 810, Washington, DC 20001-4542; (202) 347-6711; (202) 638-0773 (fax) ($25 per 50 copies). Booklet also available on AHCPR website: www.ahcpr.gov (click on Consumer Health).

REFERENCES

Ascione FJ: Medication compliance in the elderly, *Generations* 18(2):28, 1994.

Ascione FJ, Shimp LA: Helping patients to reduce medication misuse and errors, *Generations* 2:52, 1988.

Baum C et al: Prescription drug use and changes over time, *Medical Care* 26(2):105, 1988.

Braille labels for drugs, *AARP Bull* 24(2):27, 1983.

Burke RE et al: Tardive dystonia: late onset and persistent dystonia caused by antipsychotic drugs, *Neurology* 32:1335-1346, 1982.

Butler RN et al: Love and sex after 60: how physical changes affect intimate expression, *Geriatrics* 49(9):20, 1994.

Cameron KA: *Nonprescription medicines: new opportunities and responsibilities for self care,* Special Report 44, Washington, DC, 1996. United Seniors Health Cooperative.

Carruth AK, Boss BJ: More than they bargained for: adverse drug effects, *J Gerontol Nurs* 16(7):841, 1990.

Col N, Fannale JE, Kronholm P: The role of medication noncompliance and adverse drug reactions in hospitalization of the elderly, *Arch Intern Med* 150:1, 1990.

Conn VS, Taylor SG, Wienke JA: Managing medications: older adults and caregivers, *J Nurs Sci* 1(1-2):40, 1995.

Cusack BJ, Vestal RE: Clinical pharmacology: special considerations in the elderly. In Caulkins E, Davis PJ, Ford AB, editors: *The practice of geriatrics,* Philadelphia, 1986, Saunders.

Darnell JC et al: Medication use by ambulatory elderly: an in-home survey, *J Am Geriatr Soc* 34(1):1, 1986.

Delong MF: Caring for the elderly. IV. Medication use and abuse, *NurseWeek* 8(8):8, 1995.

DeMaagd G: High-risk drugs in the elderly population, *Geriatr Nurs* 16(5):198, 1995.

Fischer RG, Clark N: Skin contact: a clinical review of transdermal drug delivery systems, *Adv Nurs Pract* 2(10):15, 1994.

Gelenberg AJ, Katz MD: Antipsychotic agents. In Bressler R, Katz MD, editors: *Geriatric pharmacology,* New York, 1993, McGraw-Hill.

Haynes RB, Wang E, Gomez MD: A critical review of interventions to improve compliance with prescribed medications, *Patient Educ Counsel* 10:155, 1987.

Higbee MD: Consumer guidelines for using medications wisely, *Generations* 18(2):43, 1994.

Hogstel MO, editor: *Clinical manual of gerontological nursing,* St Louis, 1992, Mosby.

Hussey LC: Overcoming the clinical barriers of low literacy and medication noncompliance among the elderly, *J Gerontol Nurs* 17(3):27, 1991.

Kaplan HI, Sadock BJ: *Pocket handbook of psychiatric drug treatment,* ed 2, Baltimore, 1996, Williams & Wilkins.

Keenan R: The benefits of a drug holiday, *Geriatr Nurs* 2:103, 1983.

Keltner N, Folks DG: *Psychotropic drugs,* ed 2, St Louis, 1997, Mosby.

Kutzik D, Spiers M: *Drug therapy adherence among elderly: barriers to successful self management.* Paper presented at the Gerontological Society of America, San Francisco, Calif, Nov 21, 1993.

Lamy PP: Adverse drug reactions and the elderly: an update. In Ham RJ, editor: *Geriatric medicine annual,* Oradell, NJ, 1986a, Medical Economics.

Lamy PP: Drug reactions and the elderly, *J Gerontol Nurs* 12(2):36, 1986b.

Lamy PP: Adverse drug effects, *Clin Geriatr Med* 6(2):293, 1990.

Lazarus A: Differentiating neuroleptic-related heatstroke from neuroleptic malignant syndrome, *Psychosomatics* 30(4):454-456, 1989.

Lee M: Drugs and the elderly: do you know the risks? *Am J Nurs* 9(7):24, 1996.

Leirer VO et al: Elders' nonadherence: its assessment and medication reminding by voice mail, *Gerontologist* 31(4):514, 1991.

Lepkowski MI: General principles of drug therapy in the elderly. In Lantz J, editor: *Nursing care of the elderly,* San Diego, Calif, 1992, Western Schools.

LeSage J, Stauffacher MZ: Detection of medication misuse in elders, *Generations* 12:32, 1988.

Leventhal K, guest editor: Aging and medications, *Focus Geriatr Care Rehabil* 12(7):1, 1999.

Liptzin B: Treatment of mania. In Salzman C, editor: *Clinical geriatric psychopharmacology,* Baltimore, 1992, Williams & Wilkins.

Lohr JB et al: Treatment of disordered behavior. In Salzman C, editor: *Clinical geriatric psychopharmacology,* ed 2, Baltimore, 1992, Williams & Wilkins.

Mastrangelo R: Consolidating medications, *Adv Nurs Pract* 2(10):29, 1994.

Miller CA: Drug consult: medications and sexual functioning in older adults, *Geriatr Nurs* 16(2):94, 1995.

Miller CA: Drug consult: multiple choices in drugs, *Geriatr Nurs* 17(5) 1996.

Morrow D, Leirer VO, Sheikh J: Adherence and medication instructions, *J Am Geriatr Soc* 36(12):1147, 1988.

National Institute of Mental Health, Psychopharmacology Research Branch: Abnormal involuntary movement scale. In Guy W, editor: *ECDEU assessment manual for psychopharmacology,* revised, Rockville, Md, 1976, The Institute.

Nolan L, O'Malley K: Adverse drug reactions in the elderly, *Br J Hosp Med* 41:446, 1989.

Omnibus Budget Reconciliation Act of 1987, Washington, DC, 1987, US Government Printing Office. House of Representatives, 100th Congress, 1st Session, Report 100-391.

Palmieri DT: Cleaning up confusion: adverse effects of medication in the elderly, *J Gerontol Nurs* 17(10):32, 1991.

Roberts J, Tumer N: Pharmacodynamic basis for altered drug reaction in the elderly, *Clin Geriatr Med* 4(1):127, 1988.

Rovner B: Prevalence of mental disorders in nursing homes: health service needs and allocation of resources. In *Proceedings of the third congress of the International Psychogeriatric Association,* vol 3, Chicago, 1987.

Semla TP, Beizer JL, Higbee MD: *Geriatric dosage handbook,* ed 3, Cleveland, 1998, Lexi-Comp.

Shaughnessy AF: Common drug interactions in the elderly, *Emerg Med* 24(21):21, 1992.

Shimp LA, Ascione FJ: Causes of medication misuse and error, *Generations* 12(2):17, 1988.

Spiers MV, Kutzik DM: *A multidimensional framework for understanding medication adherence in the elderly: a prescription for rethinking,* 1995, Unpublished paper.

SRx senior mini-class curriculum, SRx Regional Program, Medication Education for Seniors, 1988.

Stewart RB et al: Changing patterns of therapeutic agents in the elderly: a ten year overview, *Age Ageing* 20(30):182, 1991.

Stoudemire A, Smith DA: OBRA regulations and the use of psychotropic drugs in long-term care facilities: impact and implications for geropsychiatric care, *Gen Hosp Psychiatry* 18:77-94, 1996.

Sunderland T: Neurotransmission in the aging central nervous system. In Salzman C, editor: *Clinical geriatric psychopharmacology,* ed 2, Baltimore, 1992, Williams & Wilkins.

Turkoski BB: Medication timing for the elderly: the impact of biorhythms on effectiveness, *Geriatr Nurs* 19(3):146-151, 1998.

Tobias DE: Ensuring and documenting the quality of drug therapy in the elderly, *Generations* 18(2):43, 1994.

Todd B: Prescription of the 90's, *Geriatr Nurs* 11(3):114, 1990.

US Statutes, Omnibus Budget Reconciliation Act (OBRA) of 1987, 101 Stat 1330-160, US Health Care Financing Administration: Medicare and Medicaid: requirements for long-term care facilities, *Federal Register* 54(21):5316-5373, 1989.

Vestal RE: Clinical pharmacology. In Hazzard W et al, editors: *Principles of geriatric medicine and gerontology,* New York, 1990, McGraw-Hill.

Vestal RE, Dawson GW: Pharmacology and aging. In Finch CE, Schneider EL, editors: *Handbook of biology and aging,* New York, 1985, Van Nostrand Reinhold.

Weitzel EA: In Maas M, Buckwalter KC, Hardy M, editors: *Nursing diagnosis and interventions for the elderly,* Redwood City, Calif, 1991, Addison-Wesley.

Wilcox SM, Himmelstein DU, Woolhandler S: Inappropriate drug prescribing for the community-dwelling elderly, *JAMA* 272(4):292, 1994.

Wolanin MO, Phillips LRF: *Confusion: prevention and care,* St Louis, 1981, Mosby.

appendix 15-a   Medications That Should and Should Not Be Used by Older Adults

Brand	Generic name	Treatment purpose	Do not use	Limited use	Okay to use
CARDIOVASCULAR MEDICATIONS					
Aldomet	Methyldopa	Mild to moderate hypertension	X		
Capoten	Captopril	Hypertension and congestive heart failure		X	
Catapres	Clonidine	Mild to moderate hypertension	X		
Cyclospasmol	Cyclandelate	Vasodilation	X		
Coumadin	Warfarin	Anticoagulation			X
Dyazide	Hydrochlorthiazide and triamterene	Potassium-sparing diuretic		X	
Inderal	Propranolol	Hypertension; angina; supraventricular tachyarrhythmias			X
Klor	Potassium	Supplement			X
Lanoxin	Digoxin	Congestive heart failure			X
Lasix	Furosemide	Diuretic		X	
Lopressor	Metoprolol	Dysrhythmias; cardiac myopathy		X	
Minipres	Prazosin	Mild to moderate hypertension			X
Nitro-Bid	Nitroglycerin	Coronary vasodilator			X
Pavabid	Papaverine	Coronary vasodilator	X		
Persantine	Dipyridamole	Decrease blood clot formation	X		
Tenormin	Atenolol	Hypertension			X
Trental	Pentoxifylline	Intermittent claudication	X		
TRANQUILIZERS AND HYPNOTICS					
Ambien	Zolpidem	Short-term insomnia			X
Ativan	Lorazepam	Anxiety	X		
Dalmane	Flurazepam	Short-term insomnia	X		
Halcion	Triazolam	Short-term insomnia	X		
Librium	Chlordiazepoxide	Anxiety	X		
Nembutal	Pentobarbital	Sedative; sleep agent	X		
Seconal	Secobarbital	Sedative; sleep agent	X		
Restoril	Temazepam	Short-term insomnia		X	
Valium	Diazepam	Anxiety	X		
Xanax	Alprazolam	Anxiety	X		
ANTIDEPRESSANTS					
Aventyl	Nortriptyline	Depression			X
Elavil	Amitriptyline	Depression	X		
Serax	Oxazepam	Anxiety		X	
Triavil	Perphenazine and amitriptyline	Depression	X		
Norpramin	Desipramine	Depression			X

ANTIPSYCHOTICS

Brand	Generic	Use				
Desyrel	Trazodone	Major depression	X			
Haldol	Haloperidol	Psychosis	X			X
Eskalith, Lithane	Lithium carbonate	Bipolar disorder	X			
Mellaril	Thioridazine	Psychosis	X			
Navane	Thiothixene	Psychosis	X			
Pamelor	Nortriptyline	Depression	X			X
Prolixin	Fluphenazine	Acute and chronic psychosis	X			
Sinequan	Doxepin	Depression and anxiety	X			
Stelazine	Trifluoperazine	Acute and chronic psychosis	X			
Thorazine	Chlorpromazine	Psychosis	X			
Tofranil	Imipramine	Depression	X			

ANALGESICS

Brand	Generic	Use				
Advil	Ibuprofen	Antiinflammatory and pain relief	X		X	
Aspirin	Acetylsalicylic acid	Antiinflammatory and pain relief	X		X	
Bufferin	Acetylsalicylic acid	Antiinflammatory and pain relief	X			
Darvon	Propoxyphene	Mild to moderate pain	X			
Darvocet	Propoxyphene and acetaminophen	Mild to moderate pain	X			
Demerol	Meperidine	Moderate to severe pain	X		X	
Dilaudid	Hydromorphone	Moderate to severe pain			X	
Bayer aspirin	Acetylsalicylic acid	Antiinflammatory and pain relief			X	
Empirin	Acetylsalicylic acid	Antiinflammatory and pain relief			X	
Feldene	Piroxicam	Antiinflammatory	X		X	
Morphine	Morphine sulfate	Severe pain			X	
Percodan	Oxycodone	Moderate to severe pain	X		X	
Talwin	Pentazocine	Moderate to severe pain			X	
Tylenol	Acetaminophen	Mild to moderate pain			X	
Vicodin	Hydrocodone	Mild to moderate pain			X	
Wygesic	Propoxyphene and acetaminophen	Mild to moderate pain	X		X	

GASTROINTESTINAL MEDICATIONS

Brand	Generic	Use				
Antivert	Meclizine	Motion sickness/antinausea	X	X		
Colace	Docusate	Prevent constipation	X			
Compazine	Prochlorperazine	Antiemetic	X	X		
Dialose Plus	Docusate and yellow phenolphthalein	Laxative	X			
Doxidan	Docusate calcium and casanthranol	Stool softener	X			

Continued

Brand	Generic name	Treatment purpose	Do not use	Limited use	Okay to use
GASTROINTESTINAL MEDICATIONS—cont'd					
Maalox	Magnesium hydroxide and aluminum hydroxide	Peptic ulcer disease			X
Metamucil	Psyllium	Simple and chronic constipation; increase fiber			X
Milk of magnesia	Magnesium hydroxide	Laxative		X	
Mylanta	Aluminum hydroxide; magnesium hydroxide and simethicone	Hyperacid secretions; peptic ulcer disease	X		
Pepcid	Famotidine	Hyperacid secretions; peptic ulcer disease			X
Phenergan	Promethazine	Nausea and vomiting; motion sickness		X	
Reglan	Metoclopramide	Gastroesophageal reflux; nausea and vomiting		X	
Tagamet	Cimetidine	Hyperacid secretions and peptic ulcer disease			X
Tigan	Trimethobenzamide	Nausea	X		
Zantac	Ranitidine	Gastroesophageal reflux; duodenal and gastric ulcers			X
ANTIINFECTIVES					
Bactrim and septra	Trimethoprim/sulfamethoxazole	Susceptible infections such as PCP, acute otitis media, chronic bronchitis, UTI			X
Cipro	Ciprofloxacin	Infections of lower respiratory tract, skin, bone and joint, urinary tract			X
Gantrisin	Sulfisoxazole	Urinary tract infection			X
Keflex	Cephalexin	Infections of skin, urinary tract, respiratory tract, bone and joint			X
Penicillin	Penicillin	Pneumonia			X
Vibramycin	Doxycycline	Unusual organisms (mycoplasmal infection, traveler's diarrhea, others)			X
NEUROLOGIC MEDICATIONS					
Artane	Trihexyphenidyl	Parkinson disease	X		
Cogentin	Benztropine	Parkinson disease	X		
Dilantin	Phenytoin	Seizures			X
Hydergine	Ergoloid mesylate	Alzheimer's dementia		X	
Neurontin	Gabapentin	Seizures			X
Sinemet	Carbidopa/levodopa	Parkinson disease			X
Tegretol	Carbamazepine	Seizures			X

NUTRITIONAL SUPPLEMENTS

Brand	Generic	Purpose			
Feosol	Calcium	Supplementation			X
Fergon	Iron	Iron supplementation for anemia			X
	Iron	Iron supplementation for anemia			X
	Niacin	Supplementation			X
	Vitamins	Supplementation			X
	Vitamin E	Supplementation		X	

MUSCULOSKELETAL MEDICATIONS

Brand	Generic	Purpose			
Flexeril	Cyclobenzaprine	Acute muscle spasms; pain		X	
Norflex	Orphenadrine	Muscle relaxant		X	
Robaxin	Methocarbamol	Acute muscle spasms		X	
Soma	Carisoprodol	Acute muscle spasms		X	

OTHERS

HORMONES

Brand	Generic	Purpose			
Premarin	Estrogen	Vasomotor symptoms of menopause	X		
Synthroid	Levothyroxine	Thyroid replacement			X

DIABETES

Brand	Generic	Purpose			
Diabinese	Chlorpropamide	Control blood glucose			X

PCP, Pneumocystis carinii pneumonia; UTI, urinary tract infection.

appendix 15-B Side Effects of Drugs Used by the Elderly

ANALGESIC (MILD; ASA)

Gastric irritant, allergic rhinitis, anticoagulant, uric acid precipitation.

ANALGESIC (STRONG)

Depress central nervous system (CNS), circulation, and respiration; some cause constipation, sedation.

ANTACIDS

Decrease nutrient absorption; interfere with absorption of some other drugs; decrease stomach acidity; decrease calcium metabolism and absorption.

ANTIARRHYTHMICS

Procainamide may cause agranulocytosis, fever, chills, and hypersensitivity; lidocaine needs careful monitoring in persons with impaired liver function; quinidine can cause tinnitus, nausea, and arrhythmias (idiosyncrasies are common); use propranolol (beta-adrenergic blocker) cautiously with the old.

ANTIARTHRITICS

Phenylbutazone and oxyphenbutazone cause numerous side effects with high risk of severe or fatal toxic reactions; corticosteroids can cause gastrointestinal problems, depression, personality disturbance, irritability, and toxic psychoses.

ANTICHOLINERGICS

Blurred vision, dry mouth, urinary retention, intraocular pressure.

ANTICOAGULANTS

Necessary to titrate to avoid internal bleeding; antibiotics and mineral oil decrease vitamin K production and thus potentiate anticoagulant effects.

ANTICONVULSANTS

Decreased folic acid activity, hypersensitivity, inhibit metabolism; primidone can cause anemia and visual hallucinations.

ANTIDEPRESSANTS

Imipramine, desipramine, amitriptyline, and nortriptyline all possess anticholinergic properties and must be used with caution in patients with glaucoma.

ANTIHISTAMINES

Drowsiness, blurred vision, and CNS depression, which is potentiated by alcohol.

ANTIHYPERTENSIVES

Thiazides and furosemide deplete potassium; triamterene or spironolactone may cause hyperkalemia; guanethidine and rauwolfia derivatives should be used together cautiously, since they may cause excessive postural hypotension, bradycardia, and mental depression; hydralazine causes headaches, angina, and an arthritis-like syndrome.

ANTIINFECTIVES

Hypersensitivity, gastrointestinal disturbance, pruritus, deafness, hepatic dysfunction, aplastic anemia; effects vary with the particular drug.

ANTIPARKINSONIANS

Levodopa may cause nausea, hypotension, dyskinesia, agitation, restlessness and insomnia, cardiac and gastrointestinal effects; use with caution in patients with bronchial asthma or emphysema.

ANTIPSYCHOTICS

In various degrees depending on the drug, all phenothiazines can cause photosensitivity, blood dyscrasias, agranulocytosis, and extrapyramidal effects (seen in 90% of patients after 10 weeks of therapy); haloperidol causes lethargy, decreased thirst, and jaundice (dosage should be considerably reduced for geriatric patient); lithium carbonate has toxic level close to therapeutic level; side effects are diarrhea, vomiting, tremors, sodium depletion, and muscular weakness; adequate salt and water intake is essential.

COUGH AND COLD PREPARATIONS

Over-the-counter (OTC) cough and cold preparations contain antihistamines and adrenergic decongestants; drugs with anticholinergic effects can contribute to a variety of drug interactions when taken with prescription drugs.

DIGITALIS

Therapeutic and toxic levels are close; frequent toxicity produces nausea, arrhythmias, hazy, yellow vision, and weight loss; potassium depletion sensitizes myocardium to digitalis and may also prolong toxicity, resulting in confusion and hallucinations.

DIURETICS

Thiazides can cause photosensitivity, pancreatitis, sodium and potassium depletion, and precipitate uric acid; ethacrynic acid can cause potassium depletion, vertigo, gastrointestinal problems, and hearing impairment; furosemide has similar side effects and may also alter color vision; spironolactone is potassium sparing but may cause hyperkalemia and drowsiness.

ESTROGENS

Titrate dosage; use for 3 weeks with 1-week rest.

HYPNOTICS

Barbiturates cause daytime drowsiness and hangover, aggravate cerebral anoxia, hypotension, delirium, and depress respiratory function; may cause decrease in REM sleep and rebound on withdrawal; chloral hydrate causes gastrointestinal irritation; dalmane may cause an arthritic-like allergic reaction.

HYPOGLYCEMICS

Action altered by other drugs; avoid alcohol; oral preparations have numerous adverse side effects; some persons allergic to pork and/or beef insulin.

LAXATIVES

Phenolphthalein may cause cardiac and respiratory distress in susceptible individuals.

PSYCHOTROPICS

Antianxiety drugs cause CNS depression and ataxia and may be habit forming with a definite withdrawal syndrome; benzodiazepines cause drowsiness, vivid dreams, ataxia, and convulsions on withdrawal; alcohol should be avoided.

VITAMINS

Ascorbic acids in dose of 1 g/day can cause diarrhea and precipitation of oxalic and uric acid crystals; vitamin D in large doses produces hypercalcemia, weakness, fatigue, headache, nausea, vomiting, and diarrhea.

appendix 15-c   *Special Drug Considerations for the Elderly*

Drug	Special considerations
ANALGESIC AGENTS	
Acetaminophen (APAP) (Tylenol, Datril)	Acetaminophen is the preferred analgesic agent with noninflammatory pain and is as effective as propoxyphene and codeine. Chronic daily ingestion of more than 4 to 5 g can lead to liver damage.
Aspirin (ASA)	Aspirin is the least expensive and is preferred over acetaminophen in inflammatory pain.
	It is as effective as propoxyphene and codeine.
	Gastrointestinal blood loss occurs in three fourths of those who take it and is of concern to patients with borderline anemia; concomitant liquid antacid minimizes. Antiplatelet effect may be of benefit in prevention of recurrent myocardial infarction and transient ischemic attack.
Propoxyphene and propoxyphene combinations (Darvocet-N 100 and Darvon compounds)	Single-ingredient propoxyphene is not as effective as aspirin or acetaminophen. Confusional reactions are increased. Avoid long-term full-dose use.
Codeine and codeine combinations (Tylenol No. 1-4)	Codeine has equal potency with aspirin and acetaminophen. Combination has greater potency. Nausea, vomiting, and constipation are more common.
Pentazocine (Talwin)	Pentazocine is less effective than aspirin and is prone to causing confusional reactions.
Phenacetin	Never use phenacetin chronically, because both prescription and over-the-counter (OTC) medications will lead to analgesic nephropathy, especially in combination analgesics.
Meperidine (Demerol), morphine, hydromorphone (Dilaudid)	Use one-third to one-half usual adult dose, since much more potent. No side effect differences in equal analgesic doses, but incidence increases with age.
ANTIINFLAMMATORY ANALGESIC AGENTS	
Phenylbutazone (Azolid, Butazolidin) and oxyphenbutazone (Tandearil)	Both have longer half-life and higher incidence of gastrointestinal upset and severe toxic reactions in older patients; therefore give with meals and/or liquid antacid to minimize gastrointestinal effect. These are not recommended in those over 60 years old by some authorities. Phenylbutazone and oxyphenylbutazone cause fluid retention, blood dyscrasias, and increased oral anticoagulant effect. Do not give full dose for more than 7 to 14 days.
Tolmetin (Tolectin), fenoprofen (Nalfon), sulindac (Clinoril), ibuprofen (Motrin), naproxen (Naprosyn)	All nonsteroidal antiinflammatory analgesics are less effective than aspirin in inflammatory disease but lower incidence of gastrointestinal side effects. These are much more expensive than aspirin.

Modified from Deverau MO, Andrus L, Scott C: *Elder care,* New York, 1981, Grune & Stratton.

Continued

Drug	Special considerations
ANTIDIABETIC AGENTS	Weight reduction and dietary measures control up to 70% of maturity-onset diabetes. Oral agents may increase cardiovascular morbidity. Hypoglycemic signs of tremor, sweating, and tachycardia are not as readily discernible.
	Chlorpropamide (Diabinese) has an active metabolite and prolonged half-life.
CARDIOVASCULAR DRUGS	
Digitalis preparations	Digoxin (Lanoxin) is the preferred glycoside. Avoid digitoxin and digitalis leaf (long hepatic and renal half-lives). Although beneficial in low-output failure and atrial fibrillation, digitalis preparations are successfully withdrawn in up to three fourths of patients. Subacute toxicity of anorexia with weight loss is more common than initial signs of gastrointestinal or cardiovascular effects. Baseline and follow-up electrocardiograms are essential. Dose is based on lean body weight and creatinine clearance with attention to electrolyte and thyroid status.
	One third to one half of patients are noncompliant.
Quinidine	Quinidine has higher serum levels if used concurrently with both drugs and digoxin. Half-life is prolonged. Cinchonism (gastrointestinal effects, light-headedness, tinnitus) occurrence is more common with low body weight. Decrease loading dose by one third in patients with significant heart failure.
Propranolol (Inderal)	Toxic effects are more common, as is reduced beta-blocking responsiveness in older patients. Propranolol aggravates bronchospastic tendency in chronic obstructive pulmonary disease and can precipitate heart failure. Propranolol also affects diabetic control at higher doses, and there is increased tendency of "cold limb" effect in lower extremities in those with peripheral vascular or vasospastic diseases.
Nitroglycerin tablets (Nitrostat)	Nitrostat is the most stable form. Patient must sit down before sublingual dose placement. Beware of orthostatic effect of all vasodilators.
Nitroglycerin ointment (Nitrol)	Never rub into skin. Headache may be relieved with aspirin or acetaminophen.
Long-acting nitrates (isosorbic [Isordil, Sorbitrate] and pentaerythritol tetranitrate [Peritrate])	Long-acting nitrates are variably effective. Be careful about blood pressure-lowering effect.
ANTIHYPERTENSIVE AGENTS	
Diuretics	All diuretics increase incontinence.
Thiazides (many; no significant difference; use hydrochlorothiazide generic)	Start with lowest possible dose. Patient must drink sufficient liquids. Watch volume, serum electrolyte, urate, and glucose effect.
Furosemide (Lasix)	Furosemide is most potent diuretic and should be held until thiazides no longer effective. It promotes calcium excretion and profoundly depletes sodium, potassium, and chloride. Cautious use of potassium supplements and salt substitutes is necessary because the elderly tend to have lower total body potassium with decreased muscle mass.
Spironolactone (Aldactone)	Spironolactone is potassium-sparing diuretic often used in combination with thiazide (Aldactazide). Special caution is necessary if concurrent potassium supplement or salt substitute is used. Fatal hyperkalemia has been reported.

Continued

Drug	Special considerations
ANTIHYPERTENSIVE AGENTS—cont'd	
Triamterene (Dyrenium)	Traimeterene is a potassium-sparing diuretic most often used in combination with thiazide (Dyazide) with similar precaution and with spironolactone.
SYMPATHOLYTIC ANTIHYPERTENSIVE AGENTS	Beware of continued blood pressure below 120/70, orthostatic effects, impaired male sexual function, and drowsiness or sedation.
Methyldopa (Aldomet)	Reduce dosage when methyldopa is given in combinations with thiazide (Aldoril). Sodium retention is seen when diuretic is not used. Daily dose at bedtime may take advantage of sedative effect, with therapeutic effect equivalent to multiple daily doses.
Propranolol (Inderal)	Propranolol is the only sympatholytic agent not requiring diuretic to prevent sodium retention. See cardiovascular section. If pulse is less than 50 to 60 beats/min, drug is poorly tolerated.
Guanethidine (Ismelin)	Guanethidine is a profound sympatholytic agent with long second-phase half-life. Use in small doses. Tricyclic antidepressants can interfere with antihypertensive effect.
Reserpine	Avoid giving reserpine to those with depression, sinusitis, peptic ulcer disease, and history of breast cancer.
ANTICOAGULANT AGENTS	
Heparin	Heparin increases risk of bleeding with age, especially in women over 60 years old.
Warfarin (Coumadin)	Warfarin increases risk of bleeding with age because of altered sensitivity with genetic, nutritional, and liver factors. Carefully evaluate use, and do serial prothrombin times. Beware of risk of hemorrhage, especially with possible hemorrhagic stroke, peptic ulcer disease, hiatal hernia, and diverticulosis or any bleeding diathesis. Concurrent aspirin usage is not possible except with heart valve prostheses.
SEDATIVE-HYPNOTICS AND MINOR TRANQUILIZERS	
Barbiturates (butabarbital [Butisol]; pentobarbital [Nembutal]; phenobarbital; secobarbital [Seconal]; amobarbital [Amytol])	With the exception of phenobarbital as an anticonvulsant, continued use of other barbiturates is irrational because of prolonged half-lives, paradoxic excitation in some, and tolerance and sleep pattern aberrations in all.
Benzodiazepines, chlordiazepoxide (Librium), diazepam (Valium), clorazepate (Tranxene), lorazepam (Ativan), oxazepam (Serax), and flurazepam (Dalmane)	Prolonged half-lives and cumulation of benzodiazepines have been reported with all except Ativan and Serax. Prolonged daily sedative (1 to 3 months) or hypnotic (7 to 14 days) use is not recommended because of depression of normal sleep pattern and resultant confusion, delirium, and psychologic changes. Serax is best choice because of short half-life. No hypnotic should be used nightly longer than 14 days; instead skip to every third night.
Chloral hydrate (Noctec)	Chloral hydrate is an excellent hypnotic in patients with no liver disease.
ANTIHISTAMINES	
Diphenhydramine (Benadryl), hydroxyzine (Atarax, Vistaril), phenylephrine (Dimetane), and chlorpheniramine (Chlor-Trimeton)	Antihistamines may be used for intercurrent use as needed for sedation and hypnotic effect. Beware of anticholinergic and tolerance effect with long-term use.

Continued

Drug	Special considerations
NONBARBITURATE HYPNOTIC AGENTS	
Ethinamate (Valmid), methazualone (Quaalude), methyprylon (Noludar), and ethchlorvynol (Placidyl)	None of these are recommended because of same types of problems as in barbiturates.
MAJOR TRANQUILIZERS—ANTIPSYCHOTIC AGENTS	
Phenothiazines, thioridazine (Mellaril), trifluoperazine hydrochloride (Stelazine), trifluopromazine (Vesprin), and fluphenazine (Prolixin)	Use lowest possible dose and titrate approximately. Increased incidence of extrapyramidal symptoms in elderly. Postural (orthostatic) hypotension is a problem. Temperature control and tardive dyskinesia are more common with higher doses.
Butyrophenones (haloperidol [Haldol] and thioxanthene [Navane])	Highest incidence of extrapyramidal symptoms occurs with these drugs. These are potent antipsychotic agents with low order of side effects and create episodes of amnesia and confusion.
ANTIDEPRESSANT AGENTS	Antidepressants are useful only in endogeneous depression in up to one-half usual dosage.
Amitriptyline (Elavil), nortriptyline (Aventyl), imipramine (Tofranil), desipramine (Pertofrane), protriptyline (Vivactil), and doxepin (Sinequan)	These drugs can exacerbate tremors, psychosis, constipation, postural hypotension, benign prostatic hypertrophy, delayed micturition, and dysrhythmias. Because of prolonged half-life, use caution in full-dose bedtime use, especially with Elavil and Tofranil.
ANTIPARKINSONIAN AGENTS	
Trihexyphenidyl (Artane), procyclidine (Kemadrin), benztropine (Cogentin), and diphenhydramine (Benadryl)	Prophylactic use with antipsychotic agents is generally not recommended. When extrapyramidal symptoms appear, 1- to 3-month use may be beneficial. Watch for constipation, tremors, and delirium resulting from prolonged use, especially with Cogentin.
Carbidopa-levodopa (Sinemet)	Carbidopa-levodopa is generally better tolerated than levodopa alone, with less side effects (hypotension, syncope, anorexia, nausea, and emesis).

appendix 15-D   *Barnes Rating Scale for Drug-Induced Akathisia*

For each item circle the number identifying the response which best characterizes the patient:

Patients should be observed while engaged in neutral conversation while they are seated, and then standing (for a minimum of two minutes in each position). Symptoms observed in other situations, e.g., engaged in activity on the ward, may also be rated. Subsequently, the subjective phenomena should be elicited by direct questioning.

OBJECTIVE

0   Normal, occasional fidgety movements of the limbs.
1   Presence of characteristic restless movements: shuffling or tramping movements of the legs/feet, or swinging of one leg, while sitting, and/or rocking from foot to foot or "walking-on-the-spot" when standing, BUT movements present for less than half the time observed.
2   Observed phenomena, as described in (1) above, which are present for at least half the observation period.
3   The patient is constantly engaged in characteristic restless movements and/or has the inability to remain seated or standing without walking or pacing during the time observed.

SUBJECTIVE

Awareness of restlessness

0   Absence of inner restlessness.
1   Nonspecific sense of inner restlessness.
2   The patient is aware of an inability to keep the legs still, or a desire to move the legs, and/or complains of inner restlessness aggravated specifically by being required to stand still.
3   Awareness of an intense compulsion to move most of the time and/or reports a strong desire to walk or pace most of the time.

DISTRESS RELATED TO RESTLESSNESS

0   No distress
1   Mild
2   Moderate
3   Severe

From Barnes TRE: A rating scale for drug-induced akathisia, *Br J Psychiatry* 154:672–676, 1989.

GLOBAL CLINICAL ASSESSMENT OF AKATHISIA

0 Absent

No evidence of awareness of restlessness. Observation of characteristic movements of akathisia in the absence of a subjective report of inner restlessness or compulsive desire to move the legs should be classified as pseudoakathisia.

1 Questionable

Nonspecific inner tension and fidgety movements.

2 Mild akathisia

Awareness of restlessness in the legs and/or inner restlessness worse when required to stand still. Fidgety movements present but characteristic restless movements of akathisia not necessarily observed. Condition causes little or no distress.

3 Moderate akathisia

Awareness of restlessness as described for mild akathisia above, combined with characteristic restless movements such as rocking from foot to foot when standing. Patient finds the condition distressing.

4 Marked akathisia

Subjective experience of restlessness includes a compulsive desire to walk or pace. However, the patient is able to remain seated for short periods of at least 5 minutes. The condition is obviously distressing.

5 Severe akathisia

The patient reports a strong compulsion to pace up and down most of the time. Unable to sit or lie down for more than a few minutes. Constant restlessness, which is associated with intense distress and insomnia.

appendix 15-E   *Simpson-Angus Rating Scale*

For each item circle the number identifying the response which best characterizes the patient:	
1. Gait: The patient is examined as he or she walks into the examining room—his gait. The swing of the arms, the general posture all form the basis for an overall score for this item.	0 = Normal 1 = Mild diminution in swing while patient is walking 2 = Obvious diminution in swing suggesting shoulder rigidity 3 = Stiff gait with little or no arm swing noticeable 4 = Rigid gait with arms slightly pronated; this would also include stooped, shuffling gait with propulsion and repropulsion
2. Arm dropping: The patient and the examiner both raise their arms to shoulder height and let them fall to their sides. In a normal subject, a stout slap is heard as the arms hit the sides. In the patient with extreme Parkinson syndrome, the arms fall very slowly.	0 = Normal, free fall with loud slap and rebound 1 = Fall slowed slightly with less audible contact and little rebound 2 = Fall slowed, no rebound 3 = Marked slowing, no stop at all 4 = Arms fall as though against resistance, as though through glue
Cogwheel rigidity may be palpated when the examination is carried out for items 3, 4, 5, and 6. It is not rated separately and is merely another way to detect rigidity. It would indicate that a minimum score of 1 would be mandatory.	
3. Shoulder shaking: The patient's arms are bent at a right angle at the elbow and are taken one at a time by the examiner, who grasps one hand and also clasps the other around the patient's elbow.	0 = Normal 1 = Slight stiffness and resistance 2 = Moderate stiffness and resistance 3 = Marked rigidity with difficulty in passive movement 4 = Extreme stiffness and rigidity with almost a frozen joint
4. Elbow rigidity: The elbow joints are separately bent at right angles and passively extended and flexed with the patient's biceps observed and simultaneously palpated. The resistance to this procedure is rated.	0 = Normal 1 = Slight stiffness and resistance 2 = Moderate stiffness and resistance 3 = Marked rigidity with difficulty in passive movement 4 = Extreme stiffness and rigidity with almost a frozen joint
5. Wrist rigidity: The wrist is held in one hand and the fingers held by the examiner's other hand with the wrist moved to extension, flexion, and ulnar and radial deviation, or the extended wrist is allowed to fall under its own weight, or the arm can be grasped above the wrist and shaken to and fro. A zero score would be a hand that extends easily, falls loosely, or flaps easily upwards and downwards.	0 = Normal 1 = Slight stiffness and resistance 2 = Moderate stiffness and resistance 3 = Marked rigidity with difficulty in passive movement 4 = Extreme stiffness and rigidity with almost a frozen wrist

From Simpson GM, Angus JWS: A rating scale for extrapyramidal side effects, *Acta Psychiatr Scand* 212:11-18, 1970.

6. Head rotation: The patient sits or stands and is told that you are going to move his or her head from side to side; that it will not hurt and that he or she should try to relax. (Questions about pain in the cervical area or difficulty in moving the head should be obtained to avoid causing any pain.) Clasp the patient's head between the two hands with the fingers on the back of the neck. Gently rotate the head in a circular motion three times and evaluate the muscular resistance to this movement.	0 = Loose, no resistance 1 = Slight resistance to movement although the time to rotate may be normal 2 = Resistance is apparent and the time of rotation is shortened 3 = Resistance is obvious and rotation is slowed 4 = Head appears still and rotation is difficult to carry out
7. Glabellar tap: Patient is told to open eyes wide and not to blink. The globular region is tapped at a steady, rapid speed. The number of times the patient blinks in succession is noted. Care should be taken to stand behind the subject so that he or she does not observe the movement of the tapping finger. A full blink is frequently not observed; more often there will be contraction of the infraorbital muscle producing a twitch each time a stimulus is delivered. Variations in the speed of tapping ensures that the muscle contraction is related to the tap.	0 = 0-5 blinks 1 = 6-10 blinks 2 = 11-15 blinks 3 = 16-20 blinks 4 = 21 or more blinks
8. Tremor: Patient is observed walking into examining room and then is reexamined for this item with arms extended at right angles to the body and the fingers spread out as far as possible.	0 = Normal 1 = Mild finger tremor, obvious to sight and touch 2 = Tremor of hand or arm occurring spasmodically 3 = Persistent tremor of one or more limbs 4 = Whole body tremor
9. Salivation: Patient is observed while talking and then asked to open the mouth and elevate the tongue. (Once the patient has received antiparkinson agents, this sign is unlikely to be present.)	0 = Normal 1 = Excess salivation to the extent that pooling takes place 2 = Excess salivation is present and might occasionally result in difficulty in speaking 3 = Speaking with difficulty because of excess salivation 4 = Frank drooling
10. Akathisia: Patient is observed for the presence of observable restlessness. After a determination of observable restlessness is made, the patient should be assessed by asking, "Do you feel restless or jittery inside; is it difficult to sit still?"	0 = No restlessness reported or observed 1 = Mild restlessness observed during the exam; e.g., occasional jiggling of the foot occurs during the sitting part of the exam 2 = Moderate restlessness observed; e.g., on several occasions, jiggles foot, crosses and uncrosses legs, or twists a part of the body 3 = Restlessness is frequently observed during the exam; e.g., the foot or legs move most of the time 4 = Restlessness persistently observed during the exam; the patient cannot sit still and may get up and walk

appendix 15-F   *Abnormal Involuntary Movement Scale (AIMS)*

Instructions: MOVEMENT RATINGS:	Complete Examination Procedure before making ratings. Rate highest severity observed. Rate movements that occur upon activation one value less than these observed spontaneously.	Code for #1-7
		0 = None 1 = Minimal, may be extreme normal 2 = Mild 3 = Moderate 4 = Severe

FACIAL AND ORAL MOVEMENTS	1. Muscles of facial expression, e.g., movements of forehead, eyebrows, periorbital area, cheeks; including frowning, blinking, smiling, grimacing.	☐
	2. Lips and perioral area, e.g., puckering, pouting, smacking.	☐
	3. Jaw, e.g., biting, clenching, chewing, mouth opening, lateral movement.	☐
	4. Tongue rate only increases in movement both in and out of mouth. NOT inability to sustain movement.	☐
EXTREMITY MOVEMENTS	5. Upper (arms, wrists, fingers) Include choreic movements (i.e., rapid, objectively purposeless, irregular, spontaneous) and athetoid movements (i.e., slow, irregular, complex, serpentine). Do NOT include tremor (i.e., repetitive, regular, rhythmic).	☐
	6. Lower (legs, knees, ankles, toes), e.g., lateral knee movement, foot tapping, heel dropping, foot squirming, inversion and aversion of foot.	☐
TRUNK MOVEMENTS	7. Neck, shoulders, hips, e.g., rocking, twisting, squirming, pelvic gyrations.	☐
GLOBAL JUDGEMENTS	8. Severity of abnormal movements: Mark one [0] None [1] Minimal [2] Mild [3] Moderate [4] Severe	
	9. Incapacitation due to abnormal movements: Mark one [0] None [1] Minimal [2] Mild [3] Moderate [4] Severe	
	10. Patient's awareness of abnormal movements (Rate only patient's report) [0] No Awareness [1] Aware, No Distress [2] Aware, Mild Distress [3] Aware, Moderate Distress [4] Aware, Severe Distress	
DENTAL STATUS	11. Current problems with teeth and/or dentures	Yes = 1 No = 0 ☐
	12. Does patient usually wear dentures?	Yes = 1 No = 0 ☐

From Guy W, editor: *ECDEU assessment manual for psychopharmacology, revised,* Rockville, Md, 1976, National Institute of Mental Health.

AIMS EXAMINATION INSTRUCTION

Step 1:   Ask the patient whether there is anything in his or her mouth (such as gum or candy), and if there is, to remove it.

Step 2:   Ask about the current condition of the patient's teeth. Ask if he or she wears dentures. Ask whether teeth or dentures bother the patient now.

Step 3:   Ask whether the patient notices any movements in his or her mouth, face, hands, or feet. If the answer is yes, ask the patient to describe the movements and to what extent they currently bother the patient or interfere with activities.

Step 4:   Have the patient sit in a chair with hands on knees, legs slightly apart, and feet flat on the floor. (Look at the entire body for movements while the patient is in this position.)

Step 5:   Ask the patient to sit with hands hanging unsupported for a male patient, hands hanging between legs, and for a female patient wearing a dress, hands hanging over her knees. (Observe hands and other body areas.)

Step 6:   Ask the patient to open his or her mouth. Observe the tongue at rest within the mouth. Do this twice.

Step 7:   Ask the patient to protrude his or her tongue. (Observe abnormalities of tongue movement.) Do this twice.

Step 8:   Ask the patient to tap his or her thumb with each finger, as rapidly as possible for ten to fifteen seconds, first with the fingers of the right hand, then with the left hand. (Observe facial and leg movements.)

Step 9:   Flex and extend both arms out in front, with palms down. (Observe trunk, legs, and mouth.)

Step 10:   Ask the patient to stand up. (Observe the patient in profile. Observe all bodily areas again, hips included.)

Step 11:   Ask the patient to extend both arms out in front, with palm down. (Observe trunk, legs, and mouth.)

Step 12:   Have the patient walk a few paces, turn, and walk back to the chair. (Observe hands and gait.) Do this twice.

chapter 16

Coping With Chronic Disorders

►LEARNING OBJECTIVES

Upon completion of this chapter, the reader will be able to:

- Describe various patterns of chronic illness.
- Relate strategies that have been used successfully to maintain maximal function and comfort in the client with a chronic disorder.
- Name the special considerations that influence the experience of chronic illness.
- Describe the essential activities of daily living and the instrumental activities of daily living.
- Discuss strategies that increase an individual's ability for self-care.
- Explain the concept of wellness in chronic illness.

►GLOSSARY

Accoutrements Equipment necessary to function effectively; originally referring to military equipment.
Beneficience Acts of kindness that are beneficial; used to describe one of the ethical positions.
Biorhythms Cyclic, biologic events such as sleep, menstrual, or respiratory cycles.
Chronotherapy Therapy that is given according to physiologic cyclic body processes.

Circadian Patterns based on a 24-hour cycle.
Exorbitant Exceeding that which is usual or proper.
Rehabilitation The restoration of normal or near-normal function after a disabling disorder.
Restorative Pertaining to the restoration or renewal of a normal state of health or consciousness.
Trajectory The path followed by a body or an event moved along by the action of certain forces.

►THE LIVED EXPERIENCE

In living with a chronic illness, one is always in danger of a major flare-up over some minor change. Because of this vulnerability, older people become obsessed with everything that might trigger an exacerbation and consequently relate their concerns to anyone who will listen. They become boring and thus are shunned at a time when they most need someone. I have to continually try not to let my disabilities define me, not to present them to others as my identity. It is almost instinctual to use them to seek sympathy. I avoid groups that will continually remind me of my disabilities rather than my remaining abilities.

Fred, age 88

I sure don't look forward to getting really old and being all crippled up. I know there will be inevitable changes, but being unable to get around well would be just too much. I'm just in awe of Fred and the courage he has to face his physical problems with so few complaints.

Cheryl, a 27-year-old community health nurse

342

CHRONIC ILLNESS

"Chronic illness is the irreversible presence, accumulation, or latency of disease states or impairments that involve the total human environment for supportive care and self-care, maintenance of function and prevention of further disability" (Lubkin, 1995, p. 8).

Most of the disorders of aging are chronic ones that must be treated within a framework of life-style changes, living situation adaptations, and attention to the whole person coping with a disorder (Burggraf, Barry, 1996). Those who are now coping with chronic illness need support, assistance, accoutrements, and comforts to enjoy the extended life span that is more and more possible for the aging population. This text and particularly this chapter are devoted to those issues.

Chronic disorders and acute illness cannot really be separated, because so many conditions are intricately intertwined; acute disorders have chronic sequelae, and many of the commonly identified chronic disorders tend to intermittently flare up into acute problems requiring hospitalization. Many elders have several chronic disorders simultaneously and have great difficulty managing the complexity of the overlapping and often contradictory demands and incompatible medications.

Physical disabilities are often multiple and serious but need not kill the spirit or define the person. Hwu (1995) noted that psychologic functioning was often more affected than physical or social functioning. The diagnosis, duration of the disease, and economic status were the factors most influential in psychologic adjustment. The challenge to the aged individual with multiple disabilities and chronic problems may simply become overwhelming. Heidrich (1996) found that women with arthritis were as psychologically distressed as those with breast cancer and that strong social networks had more positive effects on both conditions than any other factors. In addition, Hwu (1995) found that social functioning may mediate psychologic adjustment, but that is largely dependent on education and occupation, as well as age, sex, marital status, and economic status. In Hwu's study, the least affected aspects of a patient's functioning were related to performing activities of daily living (ADLs).

The things nurses "do" and the order in which they are done is probably far less important in chronic disease management than how they are done and with what attitude. As an example, a home health nurse knelt on the carpet while applying dressings to open, non-healing leg wounds that were a result of impaired circulation in an elder. She laughed and chatted, sharing some of her own interests and concerns as she worked. She had brought a book of hummingbird photographs for the client to enjoy. She said, "I practice down on my knees." This, from our perspective, is nursing in its highest sense. It is symbolic of much of our practice with elders: conducted "down on our knees," pleading to powers beyond our understanding to maintain the highest levels of health and function.

Chronic Illness and Aging

Chronic illness is the hallmark of aging. It is the accrual of life's earnings, sometimes self-generated and often inherent or a result of imposed life-styles and environmental hazards. Too often, the result of treating acute disorders is a chronic residual disability. The thought has been, "It's a small price to pay for staying alive." Also, for years, individuals with strokes or intractable pain of arthritis were simply told, "You must just learn to live with it." But, finally, chronic disorders are being taken seriously as we confront the individual, social, and economic costs of chronic impairment. The development of geriatric nursing has been largely based on caring for those with persistent disorders that kill slowly while eroding joy and function.

Scope of the Problem

There is a growing recognition that chronic illness is a major area of health concern and that health care professionals and the lay public have inadequate knowledge of chronic illness, its management, and the priorities and economics that have dictated inadequate policies and services.

Although the prevalence of chronic diseases continues to rise with the lengthening of the life span of the frail aged and with highly technical medical care, the federal and state health care dollars devoted to chronic diseases are very limited. Declines in mortality result in increased morbidity and numbers of individuals with multiple chronic disorders. At times, the aggressive treatment of one disorder results in the emergence of additional disabilities that are iatrogenically induced.

Dr. Robert Butler, director of the International Longevity Center, predicts, "We won't get a solution until angry families demand services they haven't had. There'll be a whale of a splash when the baby boomers hit Golden Pond, starting in 2011. Then you wouldn't be elected dog-catcher if you didn't respond to chronic care needs" (Ingram, 1996, p. 7).

The average Medicare enrollee will spend about $3000 annually out-of-pocket on chronic disorders. Medicare stringently limits home care support for chronic disorders. Verbrugge and Patrick (1995) analyzed seven chronic conditions—three nonfatal (arthritis, visual impairment, and hearing impairment) and four fatal (ischemic heart disease, chronic obstructive pulmonary disease, diabetes mellitus, and malignant neoplasms)—for their impact on activity levels and use of medical services. The nonfatal conditions limited functioning considerably more than the fatal conditions did but received far fewer health services.

Chronic illnesses tend to be composed of multiple diseases; are long term, unpredictable, and expensive; intrude into the life course and self-concept; and require extensive palliative care. The incidence of chronic illness triples after 45 years of age but is thought to decrease markedly in relation to higher socioeconomic status. However, Reed et al (1995) studied a large sample of affluent elderly persons in Marin County, California, to obtain information about the health status of an advantaged population. They found few differences in health and function from those with less socioeconomic advantage. Although death was somewhat postponed in the advantaged group, the prevalence of disease and disability was not.

The most prevalent chronic conditions in individuals over 65 years of age can be seen in Table 16-1 (US Bureau of the Census, 1998). As is evident, the longer one lives, the greater is the accumulation of chronic disorders and gender differences. Of course, one must consider the population predominance of women over the age of 75 and the possibility that only the hardier men survive beyond age 75. Interestingly, individuals between 65 and 74 years old have a higher incidence of dermatitis, sinusitis, ulcers, and asthma than those over 75.

Even with devoted family caretakers, it is highly likely that a very old woman, at some point, will require care in a nursing home as a result of numerous, ongoing chronic problems that have become devastatingly disabling. Less than 10% as many old men will need a nursing home. It is also likely that resources of the family and individual will by then have become exhausted. Elders and others with disabilities make up 27% of Medicaid beneficiaries but account for 59% of the total Medicaid spending, most of it being on long-term care (Riley, 1996). Recent figures show that annual spending of Medicaid dollars per capita for elders averages $9293. This leaves many recipients extremely vulnerable to legislation that is quite rapidly shifting responsibility entirely to states.

Transition From Health to Illness

Recognition of and adaptation to a chronic illness are likely to be a transition required of an aged person. For example, the move from being a "healthy" elder to being an elderly "diabetic" requires changes in life-style, self-concept, and relationships. There is a constant struggle between focusing on the well self and being defined by disabilities (and presenting them to others as one's identity). It is almost instinctual to use disabilities to seek sympathy. Some elders become obsessed with everything that might trigger an exacerbation of their condition and consequently relate their concerns to anyone who will listen. They become boring and thus are shunned at a time when they most need someone. Adapting one's identity and self-perception to incorporate an illness that will be a life companion is very taxing.

The nurse's greatest challenge in working with the chronically ill is to help them to maintain hope, to sustain interest in their own welfare, and to develop the capacity to view the restrictions imposed by the disorder as having the potential for personal enrichment. Sacks's work (1995) with the neurologically disabled provides insight into a humanistic and expansive manner of dealing with chronic deficits: ". . . I am sometimes moved to wonder whether it may be necessary to redefine the very concepts of 'health' and 'disease,' to see these in terms of the ability of the organism to create a new organization and order, one that fits its special, altered disposition and needs, rather than in the terms of a rigidly defined 'norm'" (p. xviii).

Nurses must resist the urge to "educate" the client. The giving of information by one who has not experienced the particular condition and does not know the outcome or the subjective resources of the individual is presumptuous at best and often insulting. The good and helpful intentions of the nurse must be in the direction of supplementing, and enhancing when possible, the individual's knowledge of resources, both objective and subjective. Knowledge of the client and caring about the client are crucial, and in the case of chronic disorders the client must educate the nurse before a plan of care can be developed.

Chronic Illness Trajectory

In considering an appropriate conceptual framework for the study of chronic illness, we have tried to blend Corbin and Strauss with Maslow. The trajectory model of chronic illness, originally conceptualized by Anselm Strauss (Strauss, Glaser, 1975), has helped health care

Table 16-1

Prevalence of Selected Chronic Conditions, by Age and Sex: 1995*

		Rate†							
		Male				**Female**			
Chronic condition	Conditions (1000)	Under 45 years old	45 to 64 years old	65 to 74 years old	75 years old and over	Under 45 years old	45 to 64 years old	65 to 74 years old	75 years old and over
Arthritis	32,663	22.4	176.7	385.5	437.0	36.0	285.4	498.2	616.1
Dermatitis, including eczema	9,333	33.3	25.1	23.6‡	31.8‡	40.5	45.8	34.2	23.8‡
Trouble with—									
Dry (itching) skin	6,440	16.0	26.8	38.0	50.1	21.9	33.4	49.1	53.6
Ingrown nails	5,371	15.6	20.4	20.8‡	44.0	15.0	36.9	39.9	43.2
Corns and calluses	4,347	5.7	15.5	21.4‡	33.4‡	11.0	41.0	42.8	74.1
Visual impairments	8,511	27.7	60.3	68.7	135.6	12.8	37.1	43.1	88.7
Cataracts	6,256	1.8‡	16.8	72.1	214.0	1.1‡	21.6	132.1	247.0
Hearing impairments	22,465	41.4	203.6	332.8	423.5	26.3	89.7	159.0	307.3
Tinnitus	6,805	13.2	66.3	94.2	68.8	7.3	44.1	55.3	56.7
Deformities or orthopedic impairments	31,784	90.0	186.6	167.1	163.9	101.3	165.2	168.0	210.5
Ulcer	4,297	10.4	29.9	19.9‡	17.9‡	12.0	27.7	38.7	19.6‡
Hernia of abdominal cavity	4,664	9.2	29.1	67.0	53.6	5.0	35.4	44.6	56.1
Frequent constipation	3,644	2.7	7.2‡	9.4‡	43.0‡	14.5	26.4	33.0	72.6
Diabetes	8,693	6.2	62.1	131.4	110.6	9.7	65.4	134.3	121.1
Migraine	11,897	21.8	31.7	15.2‡	13.8‡	70.7	82.6	35.2	10.1‡
Heart conditions	21,114	24.0	143.1	316.3	439.4	34.0	100.0	229.3	318.0
High blood pressure (Hypertension)	29,954	34.0	233.2	352.0	344.5	30.3	212.9	423.8	465.3
Varicose veins of lower extremities	7,398	4.1	17.1	46.9	41.1‡	23.3	73.4	101.6	115.0
Hemorrhoids	9,077	20.9	63.8	49.0	58.2	24.2	63.4	58.4	57.7
Chronic bronchitis	14,533	44.2	37.4	58.1	45.6	58.9	88.7	72.4	70.9
Asthma	14,878	60.7	31.4	47.8	16.9‡	61.0	73.6	44.3	40.0
Hay fever, allergic rhinitis without asthma	25,730	96.0	96.4	76.1	61.7	99.5	133.0	84.8	61.2

From US National Center for Health Statistics, *Vital and Health Statistics*, Series 10, No 193, and earlier reports; and unpublished data.

*Covers civilian noninstitutional population. Conditions classified according to ninth revision of International Classification of Diseases. Based on National Health Interview Survey.

†Conditions per 1000 persons.

‡Figure does not meet standards of reliability or precision.

Table 16-2

Definitions of Phases and Goals

Phase	Definition
Pretrajectory	Before the illness course begins; the preventive phase; no signs or symptoms present
Trajectory onset	Signs and symptoms are present, includes diagnostic period
Crisis	Life-threatening situation
Acute	Active illness or complications that require hospitalization for management
Stable	Illness course/symptoms controlled by regimen
Unstable	Illness course/symptoms not controlled by regimen but not requiring hospitalization
Downward	Progressive deterioration in physical/mental status characterized by increasing disability/symptoms
Dying	Immediate weeks, days, hours preceding death

From Woog P: *The chronic illness trajectory framework: the Corbin and Strauss nursing model,* New York, 1992, Springer.

providers to better understand the realities of chronic illness. Later, Corbin and Strauss (1988) presented a view of chronic illness as a trajectory that traces a course of illness through eight phases, which may be upward, downward, or plateaued. In its entirety, a chronic illness may include a preventive phase, a definitive phase, a crisis phase, an acute phase, a comeback, a stable phase, an unstable phase, deterioration, and death. Phases of chronic illness are seen in Table 16-2.

Maslow's concept of five major levels of need that affect function and self-perception fit well with the Corbin/Strauss model (Fig. 16-1). The patient's perceptions of needs met and basic biologic functional limitations are paramount to predicting movement within the illness trajectory (Woog, 1992). In this respect, our wellness approach largely hinges on assisting the elder in meeting as many of Maslow's defined needs as possible at any given time. These efforts enhance the individual's potential for remaining on a plateau or gaining ground in any of the trajectory phases.

It is significant to note that Corbin and Strauss (1988) focused a great deal of attention on the impact of chronic illness on self-concept and self-esteem. There ". . . are a host of biographical consequences, which in turn cycle back to affect to some degree the trajectory work and the illness itself. These include the changing relationships of body, self, and sense of biographical time" (Corbin, Strauss, 1988, p. 2). The trajectory of chronic illness varies with the individual and the disorder. It may progress slowly, relentlessly, or unpredictably through exacerbations and remissions, or the superimposition of other disorders and treatments may change the projected course of the disability. It is being found that the diagnosis itself is significant in coping. Women with arthritis perceived their illness to be more severe and less controllable than those with breast cancer, and this had profound effects on their psychologic well-being (Heidrich, 1996).

In 1988 Strauss and Corbin emphasized the changing nature of health care needed for an aging population in which chronic disorders are by far the most prevalent form of illness. The incidence of chronic disease is increasing in proportion to lifesaving technologies. Until the late 1930s, prevailing illnesses were predominantly caused by bacteria or parasites. With the advent of antibiotics and immunizations these diseases decreased markedly in the industrialized nations. Instead, cancers, arthritis, and cardiovascular conditions have become the most common health problems. Recently, cancers and cardiovascular conditions have decreased somewhat, and infectious diseases are returning with a vengeance. Since the publication of the fifth edition of *Toward Healthy Aging: Human Needs and Nursing Response,* we have seen enormous restructuring of the health care system in ways that are beginning to more realistically serve the large numbers of chronically ill persons. In many ways, the acquired immunodeficiency syndrome (AIDS) epidemic has been the catalyst for change. As society becomes more unhealthy in terms of environment, diet, infectious agents, and stress inducers, more attention is being paid to seeking a healthy life-style. Strauss, a pioneer in conceptualizing chronic illness, died in September 1996. We believe he accomplished much toward achieving some of the goals of understanding chronic illness that we are advancing toward at present.

Perceived Uncertainty of the Illness Trajectory

Wineman et al (1996), grounded in the theories of illness trajectory, have proposed that there is a relationship between effectiveness of coping and the degree of

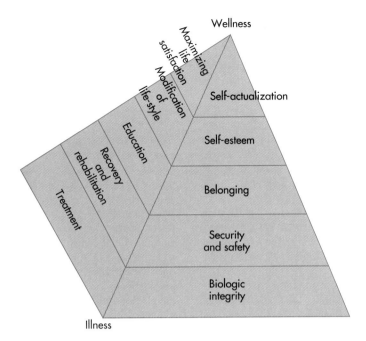

Fig. 16-1   Correlation between illness-wellness continuum and Maslow's hierarchy of needs. (Developed by Patricia Hess.)

perceived uncertainty in chronic disease and functional disability. They have shown in previous research that the types and quality of social supports and the perception of purpose in life influence one's adaptation to chronic disorders (Mishel, Braden, 1988). Although research is progressing in untangling and understanding the relationships among these apparently critical factors, nurses are the most likely health care providers to be cognizant of these issues and to encourage clients' expression of perceptions related to the uncertainty, quality, and durability of support networks and to their purpose in life. Given the uncertainty of future resources and the numerous concerns about the stability of the health care system, uncertainty is pervasive even in the best of circumstances.

Knowledge of disease processes may help in coping with even those diseases that have an unpredictable course. Many disabilities require organizing and maintaining physical and social arrangements involving space, time, work, and other persons. Knowledge of personal strengths and needs and careful monitoring of body signs must guide an individual's decisions. Symptoms are signposts. Assisting clients in becoming alert to subtle bodily signs and symptom changes can be extremely beneficial in reaching a healthier level of exis-

tence. Body awareness and management of symptoms that cause acute distress are essential in the process. The comeback phase of illness is a period of rehabilitation that is an uphill course. It may be long and difficult with small setbacks, periods of improvement, and plateaus of unpredictable duration. During this period the client raises many questions that may not have answers:

- How reversible is this illness?
- Which of my previous activities will I be able to pursue?
- How long will I remain on a plateau?
- How much will my actions affect the outcome, and what actions should I take?
- Will the fluctuations in function always be a part of my life?

The nurse's function is to encourage the client to express these questions and, together, seek answers and resources.

Special Considerations

Regardless of the nature of chronic problems, there are special considerations that almost universally need attention and must be addressed actively by nurses. It is not sufficient to wait until the client brings up the topic.

Gender and Chronic Illness

Because women typically live longer than men and more frequently live alone, the issues of management of chronic disorders have a large gender component. Several studies have shown that older women are treated less promptly and less aggressively than older men for several acute disorders (Coronary Heart Disease, 1994; Pittman, Kirkpatrick, 1994; Blumenthal, 1995; Nease et al, 1995; O'Connor et al, 1996). Whether there is also an unconscious discriminatory practice in chronic care and home care is unknown. Under the guidance of Bernadine Healy, appointed in 1990 to head the National Institutes of Health, some of the "vast knowledge gap" related to women's health care is being closed. More serious even than the knowledge gap is the lack of caregivers for numerous old women. This is currently not addressed in any systematic way.

Fatigue From Living With Chronic Disorders

Fatigue from living with chronic disorders is seldom considered in its full significance. It is a variable and unpredictable condition that is often ignored or relegated to an insignificant and incidental aspect of growing old. It may occur in the presence or absence of any other disorder but cannot be ignored. The lassitude that one experiences is often evidence of depression, as well as chronic illness. The zest for life is gone, and every action seems to involve an inordinate amount of energy that is hardly worth the effort. Nurses confronted by this attitude tend to become either impatient or caught up in the feeling of futility. The most important intervention is undoubtedly to validate the reality and debilitating effects of the disorder. Discussing patterns of fatigue and identifying the precipitants are important. If the elder can be engaged in keeping a log of the low points of energy, it may prove useful. It is also helpful to emphasize the wisdom of the body and the assumption that it is presently necessary for the individual to move in "low gear." Permission to rest periodically and engage in brief periods of mild activity may reassure elders that they can indeed cope with this overwhelming inertia. Individuals should be encouraged to expend their energy in ways that improve their quality of life rather than to please others.

When caregivers work with the aged who have disabling chronic conditions, the concept of time is important. More time is required. A slower pace of activity and large segments of time for direct care are needed. The slower movements of the aged and the response to physiologic stress require more time for care activities with rest periods in between.

Pain and Chronic Illness

The reader is advised to review Chapter 17 thoroughly while keeping in mind that chronic disorders usually involve not only certain painful physical impairments but also frequently depressed moods that exacerbate pain perception. Often an antidepressant is needed in combination with analgesics. However, our attachment to the belief that only Western medicine really works and that all else is adjunctive has limited our thinking about pain management. "Alternative" strategies can be extremely effective, especially when sought and managed by the individual. We do not suggest that they are always effective, but in many cases therapeutic benefits are obtained from a combination of scientifically undefined qualities, personal idiosyncrasies, placebo effects, and individual control.

However, chronic conditions can and often do produce penetrating pain. Most adjunctive therapies are not adequate for management of extreme pain without medication as well. Chronicity and pain often go hand in hand, and one of the major management issues is the control of pain.

Many elders attempt, some quite successfully, to manage their disorders with over-the-counter medication combinations, alcohol, and "physician shopping" to acquire multiple prescriptions. Any of these methods can result in addiction and leave the elder vulnerable.

Sexuality and Chronic Illness

Sexual problems and misinformation are pervasive in society in spite of generally high levels of exposure to knowledge about sex and the near-toxic exposure to sexuality in the media, schools, and politics. In spite of this, little attention is paid to those who are living daily with chronic disorders that interfere with sexual satisfaction and the fundamental feelings of sexual attractiveness. In addition, individuals with chronic disorders are not immune to the sexual problems that occasionally beset most individuals. Various disorders may produce mechanical problems, erectile problems, decreased libido, and decreased lubrication. Certain disorders involving ostomies and incontinence may produce revulsion in the partner and sexual anxiety in the afflicted. Discussing and assessing medication regimens, the expected dysfunctions that accompany particular diseases, and the individual's expectations are all important. A sexual history may provide important clues regarding the individual's needs and desires. The nurse's responsibility is toward an open, accepting discussion of the patient's sexuality and the provision of information and resources appropriate to the client's situation. The acronym *PLISST* is helpful in reminding us of a useful format for discussing sexuality (Box 16-1). Refer to Chapter 25 for additional discussion of sexuality.

Grieving the Lost Self

Grieving the loss of appearance, function, independence, and comfort may occupy much of one's time initially when adapting to a chronic disorder, particularly if the onset has been abrupt and the loss interferes directly with a major source of one's pleasure. As the mother with a handicapped newborn mourns the loss of the visualized "perfect" infant, the elder may begin to memorialize the "perfect" self that no longer exists. In fact, the perfection of the earlier image of the self may grow far beyond the reality that existed. The nurse's function is to encourage verbalization, talk with the elder about the lost self, and recognize the stages of grief that may be occurring. Clearly, grief reactions will be highly individual, depending on the significance of the loss to the individual and the number of additional losses with which the individual is attempting to cope. The number and recency of other losses in the life of the individual may have depleted psychic reserves.

There often seems to be a subversive sense of failure or weakness in individuals who have developed a chronic disorder, as if they could will it away by strength of mind, determination, and courage. Suffering a chronic illness is compounded by a sense of responsibility for remaining healthy, especially in the current wellness climate (Benner et al, 1994). There is often the persistent thought that hard work and adherence to a strict treatment regimen will bring about cure, and when that does not occur, a sense of shame develops and the person wishes to hide from others (Doolittle, 1994). This is a serious problem that is deeply rooted in the work ethic that has been so cultivated in the older generation.

Given these tendencies, it is imperative that the nurse not overtly or covertly reinforce the client's sense of personal failure. It is not helpful to suggest, "Well, have you tried . . ." Living with a chronic illness is a process that is continually changing as one adapts to the grief of the lost self and learns to embrace the needs of the emerging self. Unfortunately, health care providers often reinforce the notion that the individual is responsible for the illness and is in some way defective in allowing it to occur.

ASSESSMENT

Assessment of the elder with chronic disorders involves selection of appropriate tools, repeated testing, careful observation, periodic monitoring, alert watchfulness, and, most important, discussion and corroboration with elders about their perceptions and the meaning their illness has for them. In the case of chronic illness and the great variability in presentation and impact on individual life-style, thorough biopsychosocial assessment is critical.

Activities of Daily Living

Chronic disorders and the qualification for home care are defined by the degree of impairment in activities of daily living (ADLs) such as eating, toileting, dressing, bathing, and transferring. The more complex and higher-level functions are categorized as instrumental activities of daily living (IADLs) and include activities such as using the telephone, using transportation, paying bills, planning meals, and managing medications. It is apparent that ADLs are largely mechanical, and IADLs are largely cognitive. To qualify for Medicare coverage of home care, one must be homebound, be expected to improve with treatment, have a signed order from a physician, and require the services of a professional. Impairment in ADLs is not sufficient to receive Medicare reimbursement (Rice, Rappl, 1996). However, it is useful to assess the level of ability of an individual for self-care. There are many tools designed to accomplish this. One of the simplest and most used is the Barthel index. The scale, which measures ADLs and IADLs with values weighted toward difficulty or complexity, is a useful assessment of a person's capacity to manage with or without assistance. Another tool for assessing self-care is the Lawton, Brody IADL index. See Chapter 14 for assessment tools.

Box 16-1	PLISST

*P*ermission to masturbate, fantasize, and claim feelings
*L*imited *I*nformation related to problem being experienced
*S*pecific *S*uggestions—only when nurse is clear about the problem
Intensive *T*herapy—referral to professional with advanced training if necessary

Assessing Biorhythms

Chronotherapy is an idea that has been around for a long time but only recently has been approached in relation to the effect of biorhythms on function. Little real attention was given to it until 4 or 5 years ago. It is now considered an integral aspect of medication management. In this chapter we suggest that it should be given more consideration in terms of chronic care management in general. When is the individual functioning at peak level? When are some treatments and activities most acceptable (Fig. 16-2)? Circadian rhythms are the most easily recognized, but lunar rhythms, seasonal rhythms, and many other micropulses and macropulses affect each of us at all times. Although at this time we understand little about them, we must be cognizant of the variances we are likely to encounter in metabolism and function. Presently biorhythms are particularly recognized in relation to steroid administration, asthmatic attacks, cardiac disorders, cardiac event vulnerability, cancer chemotherapy treatments, and diabetic management (Long, 1996).

Maintaining a Health Diary

The health diary has multiple purposes in the assessment and management of chronic disorders. Its most important function is probably to serve as a mechanism by which an elder may develop self-awareness regarding perception and management of a chronic disorder. It has no recommended form or structure and is thus designed according to individual preference. The entries may be lengthy, with much embellishment, or brief, precise descriptions of daily activities and body responses. Some persons make daily entries, whereas others make entries only occasionally. Kept over time, the health diary reveals progression or remission of the condition and provides concrete longitudinal assessment data that may long since have been forgotten by the diarist. It also reveals something of the individual's personality style in the way perceptions are recorded, and it serves as a coping mechanism. A diarist is able to convey, at will, any thoughts or feelings and has full freedom of expression. The act of expressing brings control and solace. The intended, or unintended, recipient of the information be-

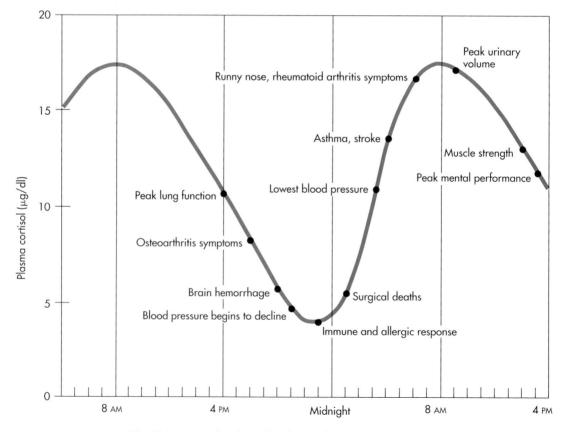

Fig. 16-2   Twenty-four-hour circadian rhythm of cortisol secretion.

comes incidental to the process when it is considered as a therapeutic mode of self-care, personal integration, and release. Gerontic nurses might encourage clients with prolonged disorders to keep a health diary. It is extremely useful in many ways, the most important being the acute awareness in the nurse of the true meaning of "wellness" and courage.

INTERVENTIONS

Interventions in the care of the chronically ill must take into consideration the client's emotional responses, individual needs, motivation for self-care, supports from family and friends, and available resources, as well as the trajectory experience.

Caring

Caring, continuity, commitment, competence . . . a litany of *C*'s have historically formed the foundation of nursing care. Today, in the face of information overload, pandemics, media irresponsibility, ethical confusion, and the ever-growing capability to technologically accomplish things that are humanely questionable, caring may be fundamental to the continuance of civilization. Caring and compassion form the difference between civilization and corruption. Compassion has been seen as a distinguishing aspect of being human. Although caring forms a cornerstone of nursing, it could be found as an entry in the index of only two current nursing texts (Benner et al, 1994; Lubkin, 1995), and compassion was not found in any.

Numerous definitions of *caring* in relation to nursing have been presented in the past. A recent and commonly accepted one is Watson's: "The moral idea of nursing consists of transpersonal human-to-human attempts to protect, enhance, and preserve humanity" (1988, p. 54). In our present system, "caring time" is a rare commodity. Milne and McWilliam (1996) surveyed physicians, nurses, and nurse managers and found that they understood *caring* primarily to be "spending time with," "being with," and "doing for." They concluded that there was insufficient time for caring and that they must take leadership roles in achieving promotion and allocation of "caring time" within each of their agencies.

Self-Care

In chronic care, self-care is of the greatest importance and must be cultivated beyond all else. The very nature of chronicity demands it. It is important in understanding the self-care movement to know its origins. As it became more apparent that the present system was incapable of providing ongoing care for most of the conditions of elders, self-care as an idea grew in popularity. McElmurry et al (1994) help us understand that the self-care movement is rooted not only in the economic imperative but also in the primacy of the biomedical ethical principle of respect for autonomy and self-governance. This has been a radical change in perspective. Less than 20 years ago the prevailing ethical principle was that of beneficience, conferring good on others—sometimes against their desires. Orem's self-care movement (1980) in nursing has grown popular partially because of increasing awareness of the individual's direct impact on disease and the impotence of nursing and/or medicine to effect positive change in a depressed, declining individual who no longer cares.

Alternative Practices in Self-Care

Interestingly, many of the largest health maintenance organization (HMO) providers are now offering reimbursement for alternative medicine therapies such as massage, touch therapy, acupuncture, chiropractic, biofeedback, homeopathy, and naturopathy (HMOs, 1996). This trend arises from studies showing that alternative medicine is less expensive, demands fewer hospitalizations, and tends to be used by individuals who are more concerned about managing their own health in a holistic manner. Now it is possible for individuals to direct their own care, order their own special supplies without physician approval (see Resources at the end of this chapter), and in many cases purchase their medications over the counter. Although this is an important trend, it places even greater responsibility on the client for making wise decisions, sometimes with insufficient information or education. Nursing will be more often called on to assist clients in obtaining background information and sorting out options in health management.

Small-Group Approaches to Chronic Illness

Early affiliation with a group confronting similar issues will usually assist in the adaptation to the altered role requirements and provide shared strategies for coping. Group meetings are among the most effective and economic ways of assisting clients in meeting informational and psychosocial needs. They can also be designed to provide family support and counseling. Self-help groups can be seen as support systems, consumer participant systems, expressive-social influence groups, or homogeneously identified therapeutic groups. Facilitating adjustment to new roles and activities and facilitating redefinition of self and meanings constitute a large part of working with the physically challenged in groups.

The first meeting should set the tone and expectations for the group and also make clear any necessary ground rules. It is important to involve the group in identifying topics and issues that they wish to focus on during the groups. These ideally should be planned sufficiently in advance to allow the group facilitator to gather information, brochures, and other resources that may be valuable to the group members. In addition to information, there are many psychologic issues to be addressed, such as the following:

1. Fears about incapacitation, pain, abandonment, isolation, and death
2. Expressions of low self-esteem and loss of confidence
3. Feelings of helplessness and uselessness; a desire to be whole and well again
4. A desire to fit into the family system once again
5. Willingness to redefine role relationships with significant others
6. A desire to face and handle public situations without fear or embarrassment

Adaptive and Assistive Devices

For the majority of those coping with disabilities, the goal is not just survival but maintaining a quality of life that is gratifying and prolonging independence as long as possible. Disabilities that interfere with the valued activities of one's life must be compensated for to the greatest extent desirable by personal or equipment assistance.

Assistive devices include mobility aids; vehicle modifications; aids for vision, speech, and hearing impairments; prosthetics and orthotics; bathing devices; environmental control systems; computer access devices; and many others. High technology has been used to provide assistive devices, computerized training programs, programmed pill containers, distance monitoring of patients, and robotic aids for the handicapped. Voice-activated computer programs are now highly developed and can assist elders who are completely disabled in accomplishing many things. Many varieties of adaptive feeding and homemaking devices are available to compensate for deficits in function.

As the effects of computer applications impact the delivery of care for the elderly, new difficulties are cre-

ated. Computer-assisted retraining can be applied to rehabilitation of patients with stroke, aphasia, or cognitive impairment. Speech synthesis and telecommunication devices are available for the verbally and orally handicapped. Electronic monitoring of the status, activity, and location of hospital and nursing home clients is increasingly feasible. Pocket-sized computer notebooks would be useful for the mildly memory impaired. Electronic monitors can locate the wandering individual. The many potential applications of computer technology must be surveyed and correctly applied for maximal benefit. Given the possibilities, it is imperative that health care providers become educated regarding potentials and serve as advocates for the elderly who could benefit from assistive devices (Pousada, 1995).

Each year, more training is required for families and professionals simply to use the equipment; in addition, as equipment becomes more sophisticated, it often becomes too expensive for most elders. The challenge of the future is to use computer advances to enhance the quality of life for the elderly while lowering the ultimate cost. At this time, the challenge is to provide some of the many assistive devices that should be made generally available. Arras and Dubler (1995) note that we must begin to focus on the ethical and social implications of these developments and ask how high-tech home care can best serve "the needs of a compassionate but prudent society" (p. 30). Assistive devices seldom qualify for reimbursement. Health insurance and managed care tend to cover only those things that directly affect morbidity or mortality (Torres-Gil, 1995). Table 16-3 lists the assistive devices most used by elders. An occupational therapist should be contacted for assistance in solving individual adaptive needs. At present, this is a highly specialized field.

Prevention of Iatrogenic Disturbances

In this era of rapid patient turnaround and numerous treatments compressed into a few days, nurses are well aware of the deleterious iatrogenic effects of hospitalization superimposed on the acute illness that required treatment (Box 16-2). Hospitalized individuals with some functional disabilities often rapidly regress into a helpless state. Simple interventions, noted time and again, have actually proved helpful in retaining functional status during episodic illness (Wanich et al, 1992). A geriatric clinical specialist, noted in the Wanich study, facilitated the following interventions that were found most helpful: staff education regarding special needs of the hospitalized elder; daily orientation cues for the patient and reassurance regarding the probability of transient delirium; getting the patient up and out of the room at least once daily; use of speech, physical, and occupational therapy daily for particular therapeutic exercises; environmental modifications and personalization of the environment; minimal use of medications; and interdisciplinary discharge planning with frequent revisions. For those individuals with frequent exacerbations of chronic disorders, a consistent follow-up telephone link to the primary provider for general discussion and problem solving is an excellent idea.

Table 16-3

Persons Using Assistive Technology Devices, by Age: 1994*

Assistive device	Total	Under 45 years old	45 to 64 years old	65 years old and over
Any anatomical device†	**4565**	**2491**	**1325**	**748**
Rate per 1000 persons	17.6	14.0	26.3	24.1
Back brace	1688	795	614	279
Neck brace	168	76	78	13‡
Hand brace	332	171	119	42
Arm brace	320	209	86	25‡
Leg brace	596	266	138	192
Foot brace	282	191	59	31
Knee brace	989	694	199	96
Other brace	399	239	104	56
Any artificial limb	199	69	59	70
Artificial leg or foot	173	58	50	65
Any mobility device†	**7394**	**1151**	**1699**	**4544**
Crutch	575	227	188	160
Cane	4762	434	1116	3212
Walker	1799	109	295	1395
Medical shoes	677	248	226	203
Wheelchair	1564	335	365	863
Scooter	140	12	53	75
Any hearing device†	**4484**	**439**	**969**	**3076**
Hearing aid	4156	370	849	2938
Amplified telephone	675	73	175	427
TDD/TTY§	104	58	25‡	21‡
Closed caption television	141	66	32‡	43
Listening device	106	26‡	22‡	58
Signaling device	95	37‡	23‡	35
Interpreter	57	27‡	21‡	9‡
Any vision device†	**527**	**123**	**135**	**268**
Telescopic lenses	158	40	49	70
Braille	59	28‡	23‡	8‡
Readers	68	15‡	14‡	39
White cane	130	35‡	48	47

From US National Center for Health Statistics, *Advance Data,* No 292, Nov 13, 1997; and US Bureau of the Census: *Statistical abstract of the United States: 1998,* ed 118, Washington, DC, 1998.
*In thousands, except as indicated. For the civilian noninstitutionalized population. Based on the National Health Interview Survey.
†Numbers do not add to totals because a person could have used more than one device.
‡Figure does not meet standards of reliability or precision.
§TDD/TTY is a typewriter-like device for the deaf that communicates over telephone lines using text.

Box 16-2	COMMON IATROGENIC DISORDERS OF THE OLD CAUSED BY HOSPITALIZATION

Loss of mobility caused by insufficient ambulation

Temporary incontinence caused by inattention when needed, sometimes becoming a permanent problem

Confusion caused by medications, treatments, anesthesias, translocation

Pressure sores caused by infrequent changes of position

Dehydration caused by limited access to fluids

Fluid overload caused by improper use of intravenous fluids

Nosocomial infections caused by infectious agents in surroundings

Urinary tract infections caused by improper pericare and catheter usage

Upper respiratory tract infections caused by immobility and shallow breathing; pneumonia

Fluid and electrolyte imbalances caused by medications, treatments

Falls caused by unfamiliar environment and instability

Impaired sleep caused by treatments and environment

Malnutrition caused by anorexia, insufficient assistance in eating

REHABILITATION AND RESTORATIVE CARE

Restorative care is rehabilitative care within a humanistic framework provided under the guiding assumption that the care and services are thoughtfully designed to capitalize on the individual client's needs and strengths in a manner that will help him or her achieve the "highest practicable level of function" (Klusch, 1995).

Considerations in Planning Rehabilitation Care

Rehabilitation is long term, but plans for rehabilitation should begin during hospitalization for acute care. The following issues are important to consider:

1. The client is in a crisis when admitted to the hospital, and personal strengths are not always visible or easily assessed.
2. Client anxiety impairs learning during hospitalizations, yet clients are more motivated toward change when physical status is threatened.

3. Early discharge to home or a nursing home may impede continuation of rehabilitative efforts.
4. Multidisciplinary discharge planning must begin on admission, and a nurse/case manager should be assigned to each client who will need rehabilitation.
5. Twenty-four-hour rehabilitative focus is necessary; it is insufficient to consider physical therapy two or three times per day as "rehabilitation."

Medicare requirements influence inpatient hospital stays for rehabilitative care. A client's medical or surgical needs alone may not warrant inpatient hospital care, but hospitalization may nevertheless be necessary because of the client's need for rehabilitative services. A hospital level of care is required by a client needing rehabilitative services if that client needs a relatively intense program that requires a multidisciplinary coordinated team approach to upgrade ability to function. There are two basic requirements that must be met for inpatient hospital stays for rehabilitation care to be covered by Medicare:

1. The services must be reasonable and necessary (in terms of efficacy, duration, frequency, and amount) for the client's condition.
2. It must be reasonable and necessary to furnish the care on an inpatient hospital basis rather than in a less intensive facility, such as a skilled nursing facility, or on an outpatient basis.

Preadmission screening requires a review of the client's condition and previous medical record to establish that significant benefit can be gained from an intensive hospital program or extensive inpatient evaluation. Inpatient assessment of an individual's status and potential for rehabilitation is essential. Assessment is not merely a paperwork review but includes an on-site professional review of the client's condition by all of the necessary disciplines. Inpatient assessment conducted by a rehabilitation team through examination of the client usually requires 3 to 10 days; during this time the client is also receiving therapies in addition to screening.

Comprehensive nursing assessment is critical. Nursing assessment includes a comprehensive biopsychosocial history and a client care plan with long- and short-term goals. Weekly interdisciplinary team conferences are held to evaluate client progress and revision of goals. Discharge goals and family conferences are a part of these weekly conferences. The following services should be available to patients in acute rehabilitation programs:

1. Rehabilitation nursing
2. Physical therapy
3. Occupational therapy

4. Speech therapy
5. Social services
6. Discharge planning
7. Psychologic services
8. Prosthetic and orthotic services
9. Audiology
10. Physician services
11. Consultation with vocational rehabilitation specialists

Rice and Rappl (1996) explain that when assessing individual needs, it is important to focus on loss of function rather than the specific disease because therapeutic treatments will be designed to improve function. They provide a list of conditions and diagnoses appropriate for home health rehabilitation referrals.

The best of the geriatric rehabilitation units being developed now under various funding mechanisms are specifically designed to foster function and teach individuals how to influence their environment to adapt to whatever their disability may be. These are also the units where health care providers become most acutely aware of the need for interdisciplinary teamwork and planning. Resnick (1993) reports on a "supportive care unit" developed by the Department of Medicine at the University of Maryland that is designed to bridge the gap between acute care and home care. In the 6 years of the unit's existence, orthopedic procedures have been the major reason for admission to the unit. Individuals with joint replacements, fractures, stroke, amputations, and arthritis make up most of the clientele. More than 86% of the individuals are discharged to home, and 80% of those are able to remain there for 2 years or longer.

Problems in Rehabilitation

Staff members who have worked intensively with the aged in acute rehabilitation settings have noted the following problems occurring frequently (Highland Hospital Nursing Staff, 1988):

- The aged are reluctant to engage in activities using objects that are childish or in activities that are seemingly irrelevant to daily tasks.
- Individuals suffering traumatic injury early in life are now living until old age; however, the problems they experience are exacerbated by the normal changes related to aging, such as bowel and bladder atonia. This subject has been addressed thoroughly by Treichsmann (1987).
- Frustration, agitation, and irritation are often the overt expressions of the functionally impaired. Rather than focusing entirely on the visible symptoms, it may be more productive to establish groups

to teach ways to enhance function. Memory training, sensorimotor skill training, and physical therapy are some of the methods of restoring maximal potential of impaired persons. Remodeling of the environment for ease of adaptation and function should also be considered (Lapp, 1987).

Rehabilitation and the Future

The agenda for rehabilitation into the twenty-first century includes increased numbers of rehabilitation hospitals, more consistent reimbursement, and available rehabilitation educational programs.

Nurses advocating for the needs of the aged and disabled, armed with clinical examples, anecdotal evidence, and empirical research findings, have the power to affect the character of legislation proposed in the U.S. House of Representatives and Senate, as has been shown by the responsiveness of Congress to the lobbying power of nurses in Washington, D.C. (Schumacher, 1996). Cost-effectiveness is the strongest argument in today's political climate. An extremely important issue involves the increased numbers of disabled elders who will be alive because of technologic advances but will require decades of rehabilitative services. How will their care be financed, and will services generally be available? What will happen to Medicare after 2010, and will exorbitant home care costs be sustainable? Numerous questions need answers very soon.

•   •   •

In summary, we suggest the following points that practitioners must consider in planning rehabilitative care:

1. Chronic illness must be seen through the eyes of the persons experiencing it.
2. The illness is often a lifelong course that passes through many phases.
3. Biographic, medical, spiritual, and everyday needs must be considered.
4. Collaborative rather than purely professional relationships may be most effective.
5. Lifelong support may be necessary, although the type, amount, and intensity of such support will vary.

EFFECTS OF CHRONIC ILLNESS ON THE INDIVIDUAL AND FAMILY

Often the ill individual feels like a burden to the family and engages in numerous compensatory behaviors to reduce this feeling of guilt. Home care is inconsistently provided and financed, and caregiver burdens are enormous. These have been explored and described endlessly (see Chapter 23 for additional discussion). Most often, families are found to extend themselves far beyond their limits in attempting to deal with a member with a chronic disorder.

Management of chronic problems of the aged becomes an issue of the individual and the family. Nurses are resource persons, advisors, teachers, and at times assistants, but the individual is in control of his or her adaptation. Nurses will assist by performing the following functions:

- Identifying and stating strengths that the individual demonstrates
- Discussing healthy life-style modifications
- Encouraging the reduction of risk factors in the environment
- Helping the individual to devise methods of improving function, halting disabilities, and adapting life-style to reasonable expectations of self
- Providing access to resources when possible
- Referring appropriately and when needed
- Organizing interdisciplinary case conferences
- Informing the individual of insights gained in management of disorders

The goal of care of the chronically ill may be to slow decline, relieve discomfort, and support the preferred life-style with as few restrictions as possible (Strauss, Glaser, 1975). Not all chronic conditions require nursing service. The ability of the aged individual and the family to manage and cope with the problems encountered determines the need. It is necessary for those who care for the aged with chronic conditions to be reoriented and resocialized to care norms and to recognize a different system of rewards. The basics of the care process emphasize improving function; managing the existing illness; preventing secondary complications; delaying deterioration and disability; and facilitating death with peace, comfort, and dignity (Wells, 1986). Progress is not measured in attempts to achieve cure but, rather, in maintenance of a steady state or regression of the condition while remembering that the condition does not define the person. This thinking is essential if realistic expectations for the caregiver and the aged are to be achieved. Beyond that, the individual will in some manner seek to understand the meaning of the intrusive nonself of ongoing impairment and struggle to incorporate it in some manner into the perceived total self. The nurse's involvement in this process is to ask about the meanings of the illness and to listen and learn.

WELLNESS IN CHRONIC ILLNESS

The aged with one or more chronic conditions can be supported toward the achievement of wellness and maximization of life satisfaction by caregivers who ascribe to a holistic philosophy that incorporates efforts directed toward the maintenance of the elderly person's self-care and self-esteem. Fig. 16-1 shows how the wellness continuum and Maslow's hierarchy of needs can complement each other in the attainment of wellness and self-actualization. It is clear that a reorganization of thinking is needed by the aged and those associated with them: kin, friends, and caregivers. Physical manifestations of chronic illness should not be the sole determining factor in the establishment of the elder's state of health or wellness. The greatest factor in establishing wellness is adaptation. To achieve maximization of life satisfaction, adaptation of life-style is necessary.

What is wellness in the face of chronic illness? This produced a lively, contentious discussion among a group of assertive elders. Comments such as "Let's get real!" "I'm like the old one-hoss shay . . . losing a little something every day. Someday, I'll wake up and find that nothing works." Elders do not graciously accept their chronic disorders—they mourn their losses. They talk about them, but not to the exclusion of other events and interests in their lives. They believe that competition and conviction undergird their remarkable survival capacity and will always remain important. They also believe in being responsible and responsive to their community. They are an elite group with plenty of past laurels, but it is doubtful that they will ever believe it is time to sit back and rest on them. Although they argue about wellness in illness, we believe they are the epitome of wellness.

• • •

In this chapter we have considered ways in which nurses may assist their clients toward an enriched capacity for living in the shadow of chronic disabilities, so many of which are common to the aged. Arthritis is almost universal, but it is more troublesome for some than for others; often there is some mild to severe cardiovascular problem; breathing becomes more difficult; digestive disorders and nutritional problems go hand in hand, often including elimination problems; and diabetes is common and sometimes out of control, creating many other problems. Several of these disorders may intermingle to put a damper on the vitality of all but the most mentally robust. However, a state of wellness may be achieved and maintained quite consistently if the individual feels capable of and motivated to manage the problems, with or without assistance.

KEY CONCEPTS

- Lubkin (1995) states: "Chronic illness is the irreversible presence, accumulation, or latency of disease states or impairments that involve the total human environment for supportive care and self-care, maintenance of function and prevention of further disability." Declines in mortality, increasing medical expertise, and sophisticated technologic developments have resulted in a great increase in the survival of the very old with multiple chronic disorders.

- Statistics regarding the extent of chronic disease are suspect because they often reflect only those who have come for medical care. In addition, decreased function without incapacitation is rarely reported.

- Women live longer than men and for that and other unknown reasons tend to have a higher incidence of chronic disease.

- One of the most difficult aspects of chronic disease is the unpredictability of the trajectory.

- The management in the home by the family, self, or significant other is central to care and should not be considered peripheral to medical management.

NANDA and Wellness Diagnoses

Wellness	Specific Needs	NANDA
Maximizes life satisfaction Seeks meaning in disorder	**Self-actualization** Meanings	Spiritual distress
Modifies life-style appropriately Seeks education regarding condition	**Self-esteem** Education	Fear (of future) Self-esteem, chronic low
Maintains social activities	**Belonging** Tenderness Acceptance Sexuality	Body image disturbance Sexual dysfunction Social isolation
Accepts limitations Uses adaptive equipment	**Safety and security** Protection Problem solving Functional activities of daily living	Adjustment, impaired
Seeks treatment Modifies activities appropriately	**Biologic integrity** Freedom from pain Activity Rest/sleep	Activity intolerance Pain, chronic Fatigue

These are not all of the possible wellness or NANDA diagnoses that may be identified. The above are frequent examples of nursing diagnoses that should be considered when planning care for the older adult in whatever setting.

- Adaptations and assistance with activities of daily living (ADLs) and instrumental activities of daily living (IADLs) are the crux of chronic disease management.
- The most prevalent chronic problems of the aged are arthritis, hearing impairment, heart conditions, and hypertension.
- The most frequent assistance needed by those with chronic disorders is with bathing, dressing, and ambulation.
- The goals of rehabilitation for the aged are to ensure opportunity for optimal personal development and function. Although rehabilitation legislation is chiefly designed to return individuals to productive employment, this is not at this time a goal for most of the aged.

▶ ## Activities and Discussion Questions

1. What are some of the patterns of chronic illness that cause great distress?
2. Discuss ways that one might modify a living situation to accommodate an individual with limited energy as a result of chronic disorders.
3. What are the special considerations that nurses should address when counseling an individual with a chronic disorder? Practice or role-play various ways that these issues can be addressed.
4. What do you think would be the most devastating loss in activities of daily living?
5. How would you encourage an individual toward maximal participation in self-care?
6. What would be the measures of wellness during chronic illness?

RESOURCES

Rehabilitation Therapy Catalog. Available from Briggs Corporation, PO Box 1698, Des Moines, IA 50306-1698; www.BriggsCorp.com.

Association of Rehabilitation Nurses
    4700 West Lake Road
    Glenview, IL 60025-1485
    (800) 229-7530 or (708) 375-4710

Rehabilitation Institute of Chicago
    345 Superior Street
    Chicago, IL 60611
    (312) 908-6000

REFERENCES

Arras JD, Dubler NN: Ethical and social implications of high tech home care. In Arras JD, editor: *Bringing the hospital home: ethical and social implications of high tech home care,* Baltimore, 1995, Johns Hopkins Press.

Benner P et al: Moral dimensions of living with a chronic illness: autonomy, responsibility, and the limits of control. In Benner P, editor: *Interpretive phenomenology: embodiment, caring and ethics in health and illness,* Thousand Oaks, Calif, 1994, Sage.

Blumenthal SJ: *Older women's health fact sheet,* Washington, DC, April 28, 1995, US Department of Health and Human Services, Public Health Service, Office on Women's Health.

Burggraf V, Barry R: *Gerontological nursing: current practice and research,* Thorofare, NJ, 1996, Slack.

Corbin JM, Strauss A: *Unending work and care: managing chronic illness at home,* San Francisco, 1988, Jossey-Bass.

Coronary heart disease, *Harvard Women's Health Watch* 1(6):1, 1994.

Doolittle ND: A clinical ethnography of stroke recovery. In Benner P, editor: *Interpretive phenomenology: embodiment, caring and ethics in health and illness,* Thousand Oaks, Calif, 1994, Sage.

Heidrich SM: Mechanisms related to psychological well-being in older women with chronic illnesses: age and disease comparisons, *Res Nurs Health* 19(3):225, 1996.

Highland Hospital Nursing Staff: Personal communication, 1988.

HMOs are starting to offer alternative medicine coverage, *San Francisco Chronicle,* p A7, Oct 7, 1996.

Hwu YJ: The impact of chronic illness on patients, *Rehabil Nurs* 20(4):221, 1995.

Ingram D: New data reveal national cost of chronic conditions, *Aging Today* 17(5):1, 1996.

Klusch L: *Solutions in restorative caregiving,* Des Moines, 1995, Briggs Health Care Products.

Lapp D: *Practical demonstration of cognitive training techniques.* Proceedings of the third congress of the International Psychogeriatric Association, Chicago, 1987 (abstract).

Long K: Perfect timing: an overview of chronotherapy, *Nurse Pract Forum* 7(1):7, 1996.

Lubkin IM: *Chronic illness: impact and interventions,* ed 3, Boston, 1995, Jones & Bartlett.

McElmurry BJ et al: Nursing ethics and chronic illness. In Benner P et al: Moral dimensions of living with a chronic illness: autonomy, responsibility, and the limits of control. In Benner P, editor: *Interpretive phenomenology: embodiment, caring and ethics in health and illness,* Thousand Oaks, Calif, 1994, Sage.

Milne HA, McWilliam CL: Considering nursing resource as "caring time," *J Adv Nurs* 23(4):809, 1996.

Mishel M, Braden C: Finding meaning: antecedents of uncertainty in illness, *Nurs Res* 37:98, 1988.

Nease RF et al: Variation in patient utilities for outcomes of the management of chronic stable angina: implications for clinical practice guidelines, *JAMA* 273(15):1185, 1995.

O'Connor GT et al: A regional intervention to improve the hospital mortality associated with coronary artery bypass graft surgery, *JAMA* 275(11):841, 1996.

Orem D: *Nursing: concepts of practice,* ed 2, New York, 1980, McGraw-Hill.

Pittman DA, Kirkpatrick M: Women's health and the acute myocardial infarction, *Nurs Outlook* 42:207, 1994.

Pousada L: High-tech home care for elderly persons. In Arras J, editor: *Ethical and social implications of high tech home care,* Baltimore, 1995, Johns Hopkins University Press.

Reed D et al: Health and functioning among the elderly of Marin County, California: a glimpse of the future, *J Gerontol Med Sci* 50A(2):M61, 1995.

Resnick NM: Urinary incontinence. In Reuben DB, Wieland DL, Rubenstein LZ: Functional status assessment of older persons: concepts and limitations. In Vellas B, Albarede JL, Garry PJ, editors: *Facts and research in gerontology,* vol 7, New York, 1993, Springer.

Rice R, Rappl L: The patient receiving rehabilitation services. In Rice R, editor: *Home health nursing practice: concepts and application,* ed 2, St Louis, 1996, Mosby.

Riley T: The future of Medicaid—the states see hard choices, *Aging Today* 17(5):9,12, 1996.

Sacks O: *An anthropologist on Mars,* New York, 1995, Knopf.

Schumacher K: Rep Schroeder featured at ANA-PAC leader's luncheon, *Capital Update* 14(9):8, 1996.

Strauss A, Corbin J: *Shaping a new health care system,* San Francisco, 1988, Jossey-Bass.

Strauss A, Glaser B: *Chronic illness and the quality of life,* St Louis, 1975, Mosby.

Torres-Gil F: Disability and aging: tools design and policy, *Aging Today* 16(6):7, 1995.

Treichsmann R: *Aging with disability,* New York, 1987, Demos.

US Bureau of the Census: *Statistical abstract of the United States: 1998,* ed 118, Washington, DC, 1998, US Government Printing Office.

Verbrugge LM, Patrick DL: Seven chronic conditions: their impact on US adults' activity levels and use of medical services, *Am J Public Health* 85(2):173, 1995.

Wanich K et al: Functional status outcomes of a nursing intervention in hospitalized elderly, *Image J Nurs Sch* 24(3):201, 1992.

Watson J: *Human science and human care: a theory of nursing,* New York, 1988, National League for Nursing.

Wells TJ: Incontinence care. In Calkins E, David P, Ford A, editors: *The practice of geriatrics,* Philadelphia, 1986, Saunders.

Wineman NM et al: Relationships among illness uncertainty, stress, coping, and emotional well-being at entry into a clinical drug trial, *Appl Nurs Res* 9(2):53, 1996.

Woog P: *The chronic illness trajectory framework: the Corbin and Strauss nursing model,* New York, 1992, Springer.

chapter 17

Pain and Comfort

▶LEARNING OBJECTIVES

Upon completion of this chapter, the reader will be able to:

- Define the concept of pain.
- Differentiate acute from chronic pain.
- Identify data to include in a pain assessment.
- Discuss comfort measures.
- Discuss pharmacologic and nonpharmacologic management of pain.
- Identify factors that affect elders' pain experience.
- Discuss the goals of pain management for the elderly.
- Develop a nursing care plan for an elder in acute pain and chronic pain.

▶GLOSSARY

Adjuvant A drug that has a primary use other than pain (antidepressant, anticonvulsant) but is also analgesic for some painful conditions.

Endorphins An opiate-like substance produced naturally by the body that modulates the transmission of pain and raises the pain threshold.

Equianalgesic The dosage and route of administration of one drug that produces approximately the same degree of analgesia as the dosage of another drug.

Iatrogenic Caused by medical personnel or procedures or through exposure to the environment of a health care facility.

Intractable Having a disease or symptom that remains unrelieved by treatment.

Nocebo A negative response (like a side effect) after the administration of a placebo.

Nociceptors An afferent nerve receptor particularly sensitive to a noxious (harmful, injurious, toxic) stimulus.

Placebo A substance given as medicine that has no basic therapeutic value but relieves symptoms or helps the patient in some way because he or she believes or expects that it will.

Prodromal A symptom indicating the onset of disease.

Titration The adjustment of a given medication until the desired effect is established.

▶THE LIVED EXPERIENCE

I'm just totally flattened. Yesterday I asked the nurse to take the PCA away because I felt so good. I really didn't comprehend that I felt good because the pain was under control. This morning when the physical therapist came in to do the routine with my knee, I couldn't believe how it hurt. Maybe I wasn't thinking too clearly yesterday, only 2 days postop. Well, now I'm going to ask for something to get rid of the pain before the afternoon session of PT.

Shirley, 2 days after knee replacement surgery

It amazes me how many old people hold off until they can't stand the pain before they will ask for anything. I try to let them know they should have pain medication before the pain is severe, but I think sometimes they don't remember what I tell them. Also, I guess they have been taught to endure pain. Not me; I don't believe in pain!

Shirley's nurse

*C*omfort seems to be an intrinsic balance of the physiologic, emotional, social, and spiritual essence of the individual and can be perceived as an integral component of wellness. By definition, *comfort* is "a state of ease and satisfaction of the bodily wants and freedom from pain and anxiety."

Nurses use the word *comfort* to describe goals and outcomes to nursing measures, but the meaning remains vague and essentially abstract to the person who is the recipient of the nursing intervention. Hamilton (1989) studied the meaning and attributes of comfort from the point of view of chronically ill elderly persons who were hospitalized in a geriatric setting. The findings identified several themes: disease process (pain, bowel function, and disability); self-esteem (feelings, adjustment, independence, usefulness, faith in God); positioning (if elders could carry out activities in bed, chair, or wheelchair); approach and attitude of staff (relationships, encounters); and hospital life (surroundings and environment—feeling at home, well fed, pleasant surroundings). Table 17-1 summarizes each of these themes and includes contributors to and distractors from comfort and elders' suggestions for facilitating more comfort.

The International Association for the Study of Pain (1979, 1992) and the American Pain Society (1992) define *pain* as "an unpleasant sensory and emotional experience associated with actual or potential tissue damage, or described in terms of such damage." Hamilton (1989) explains comfort as multidimensional "and meaning many things to different people." This description parallels McCaffery's definition of pain, which states: "Pain is whatever the person experiencing pain says it is" (McCaffery, Beebe, 1989).

Pain, whatever its source, is one of the most common complaints of the elderly. It erodes personality, saps energy, and manifests itself in an ever-intensifying cycle of pain, anxiety, and anguish until the cycle is broken. Pain can evoke depression, sleep disorders, decreased socialization, impaired mobility, and increased health care costs (Sarvis, 1995). The pervasive undertreatment of pain has led the Tri-Council for Nursing, composed of the American Association of Colleges of Nursing (AACN), the American Nurses Association (ANA), and the National League for Nursing (NLN), to approve a resolution that states, "in order to reduce pain and suffering, healthcare provider should include pain along with temperature, pulse, respiration and blood

Table 17-1

Summary of Comfort Findings

Comfort themes	Contributors to comfort	Distractors to comfort	Adds to comfort
Disease process	Achieving relief from pain; regular bowel function	Physical disabilities; being in pain most of the time	Better pain management
Self-esteem	Faith in God; being independent; feeling relaxed; feeling useful	Adjust to change; being afraid	Being informed; taking part in decision making
Positioning	Individually adjusted seating; sitting correctly; independent movement in chair	Unsuitable wheelchairs; sitting too long; sliding down in chair; being in unfavorable position in bed	Return to bed when requested; better seating arrangements
Staff approach and attitudes	Friendly, kind people; empathetic nurses; reliable nurses	Lack of caring and understanding; inaccessible nurses	Caring and understanding; encouraging patients to help themselves
Hospital life	Homelike surroundings; social and family contacts; informal pastimes; occupational and physical therapy	Fragmented care; tolerate the system; boredom with activities; lack of privacy Unpleasant meal atmosphere	Staff continuity New content in activities; continuation of personal pastimes; improved patient mealtimes; some privacy

Modified from Hamilton J: Comfort and the hospitalized chronically ill, *J Gerontol Nurs* 15(4):28, 1989.

pressure as the fifth vital sign." The Department of Veterans Affairs has also seen the importance of pain as a vital sign and has included pain as a fifth vital sign as part of its new nationwide pain management strategy (Federwisch, 1999). The Joint Commission on Accreditation of Healthcare Organizations (JCAHO) has approved standards to be released in the year 2000 for pain assessment and management in hospitals, ambulatory care, and home care settings. This accrediting body expects health care settings to (1) recognize and treat pain properly, (2) make information about analgesics and nondrug interventions readily available, (3) promise patients attentive analgesic care, (4) define policies for using analgesic technology, and (5) continuously monitor and improve the quality of pain management (Pasero et al, 1999a).

The nurse has a definition or interpretation of pain, as does the patient to whom the nurse ministers. These interpretations are formulated from experiences and are influenced by the unique history of the individual and the meaning ascribed to the pain by each. Now that pain is considered the fifth vital sign, it becomes as important as the other vital signs and should receive as much attention.

Meinhart and McCaffery (1983) cite two factors that influence nurses' and other caregivers' responses to a client's pain and discomfort: (1) one's ability to sympathize with another person, which depends on one's ability to identify imaginatively with the person, and (2) whether one is responsive to hurt in individuals whom one does not know. It is also important to realize that an individual responds in a certain way to pain because he or she has been taught that this is correct and normal. Likewise, nurses and other caregivers respond on the basis of their own pain experiences. Repeated exposure to the pain of others desensitizes one and may make pain seem commonplace. Nurses, caregivers, and elders themselves persist with and act on their misconceptions of pain in the elderly. Table 17-2 enumerates misconceptions of pain as they relate to the elderly.

Ethnically diverse responses to pain based on years of social modeling, group-pressure influence on pain tolerance, and the influence of the family on pain can be observed (Bates, 1996). Thus social learning is extremely influential in the development of the meaning of and attitude toward pain, something older adults have had many years to internalize. In American culture a dichotomy exists for some: the practice of self-inflicted pain (in a sense) is seen in professional and amateur sports activities. This infliction of pain is expected and is a rite of passage, so to speak. Equally significant is that

until they experience bodily discomfort such as aches and pains, older persons do not perceive themselves as old. However, when these manifestations do occur, they become a rite of passage into perceived old age.

ACUTE AND CHRONIC PAIN

Acute, temporary pain follows tissue injury and abates when the injury heals. It also serves as a warning signal to the body. Almost everyone has experienced this type of pain and knows that it is a temporary, time-limited situation (usually less than 6 months) with attainable relief from analgesics. Chronic pain is not that simple. It has no time frame—it is continually persistent at varying levels of intensity, and it manipulates the individual and can manipulate the person attempting to give care (Portenoy, 1995; Salerno, Willens, 1996). It is pain that lasts longer than 3 months. Table 17-3 compares acute and chronic pain. Chronic pain can manifest itself as depression, eating disturbances, or sleep disturbances. This type of pain is categorized as being (1) caused by uncontrolled neoplastic disease; (2) chronic nonmalignant pain (nonneoplastic), which usually lasts longer than 6 months and is coped with adequately; and (3) intractable nonmalignant pain, which is the most common pain in elders and erodes an individual's coping ability.

Chronic pain may be due to the following:
1. Muscle and joint pain, which includes low back pain, arthritis, and bursitis
2. Causalgia, a searing type of pain, comparable to placing a lighted cigarette to the skin, that is experienced after sudden systemic shock and lasts 6 to 12 months (but 25% or more of elders experience it for longer periods of time)
3. Neuralgia arising from peripheral nerves, which is similar to the pain that occurs in conjunction with shingles (herpes zoster) and whose most devastating type is tic douloureux
4. Phantom pain, which arises from an amputated part and begins as a pins-and-needles sensation, possibly developing into cramping, burning, or shooting pains that last for years, similar in type to the sensations experienced by persons paralyzed with spinal cord injuries
5. Vascular pain, which is most dramatically evident in migraine headaches
6. Terminal cancer pain, which produces fear and anxiety in the patient and distress in the staff

Table 17-2

Pain Management in the Elderly

Misconception	Correction
Pain is a natural outcome of growing old.	It is true that the elderly are at greater risk (as much as twofold) than younger adults for many painful conditions; however, pain is not an inevitable result of aging. The illogical nature of this misconception is best illustrated by the comment of a 101-year-old male participant in a study on aging. When he stated that his left leg hurt, the physician suggested that it was to be expected at age 101. The man then asked the physician to explain why his right leg, which was also 101 years old, did not hurt a bit.
Pain perception, or sensitivity, decreases with age.	This assumption is unsafe. Although there is evidence that emotional suffering specifically related to pain may be less in older than in younger patients, no scientific basis exists for the assertion that a decrease in perception of pain occurs with age or that age dulls sensitivity to pain. Assessment and intervention for pain in the elderly should begin with the assumption that all neurophysiologic processes involved in nociception are unaltered by age.
If the elderly patient does not report pain, he or she does not have pain.	Elderly patients commonly underreport pain. Reasons include expecting to have pain with increasing age; not wanting to alarm loved ones; being fearful of losing their independence; not wanting to distract, anger, or bother caregivers; and believing caregivers know they have pain and are doing all that can be done to relieve it. The absence of a report of pain does not mean the absence of pain.
If an elderly patient appears to be occupied, asleep, or otherwise distracted from pain, he or she does not have pain.	Older patients often believe it is unacceptable to show pain and have learned to use a variety of ways to cope with it instead (e.g., many patients use distraction successfully for short periods of time). Sleeping may be a coping strategy or indicate exhaustion, not pain relief. Assumptions about the presence or absence of pain cannot be made solely on the basis of a patient's behavior.
The potential side effects of opioids make them too dangerous to use to relieve pain in the elderly.	Opioids may be used safely in the elderly. Although the opioid-naïve elderly may be more sensitive to opioids, this does not justify withholding the use of them in the management of pain in this population. The key to use of opioids in the elderly is to "start low and go slow." Potentially dangerous opioid-induced side effects can be prevented with slow titration; regular, frequent monitoring and assessment of the patient's response; and adjustment of dose and interval between doses when side effects are detected. If necessary, clinically significant respiratory depression can be reversed by an opioid antagonist drug.
Alzheimer's patients and others with cognitive impairment do not feel pain, and their reports of pain are most likely invalid.	No evidence exists that the cognitively impaired elderly experience less pain or that their reports of pain are less valid than individuals with intact cognitive function. It is probable that patients with dementia, progressive deficits of cognition, apraxias, and agnosia, particularly those in long-term care facilities, suffer significant unrelieved pain and discomfort. Assessment of pain in these patients is challenging but possible. The best approach is to accept the patient's report of pain and treat the pain as it would be treated in an individual with intact cognitive function.
Elderly patients report more pain as they age.	Even though elderly patients experience a higher incidence of painful conditions, such as arthritis, osteoporosis, peripheral vascular disease, and cancer, than younger patients, studies have shown that they underreport pain. Many elderly patients grew up valuing the ability to "grin and bear it," and, unfortunately, have been heavily influenced by the "Just Say No" to drugs campaign.

From McCaffery M, Pasero C: *Pain: clinical manual,* ed 2, St Louis, 1999, Mosby; data from Butler RN, Gastel B: Care of the aged: perspectives on pain and discomfort. In Ng LK, Bonica J, editors: *Pain, discomfort and humanitarian care,* New York, 1980, Elsevier; Harkins SW, Price DD: Assessment of pain in the elderly. In Turk DC, Melzack R, editors: *The handbook of pain assessment,* New York, 1992, Guilford; Harkins SW, Price DD: Are there special needs for pain assessment in the elderly? *APS Bull* 3:1-5, Jan/Feb 1993; and Harkins SW et al: Geriatric pain. In Wall PD, Melzack R, editors: *Textbook of pain,* London, 1994, Churchill Livingstone.

Table 17-3

Comparison of Acute and Chronic Pain

Characteristics	Acute pain	Chronic pain
Experience	An event	A situation, state of existence
Source	External agent of internal disease	Unknown, or if known, changes cannot occur or treatment is prolonged or ineffective
Onset	Usually sudden	May be sudden or develop insidiously
Duration	Transient (up to 6 months)	Prolonged (months to years)
Pain identification	Pain versus nonpain	Pain versus nonpain
	Areas generally well identified	Areas less easily differentiated
		Intensity becomes more difficult to evaluate (change in sensations)
Behavior	Typical response pattern with more visible signs:	Response patterns vary, few overt signs (adaptation):
	Facial expressions	Sleeping
	Crying, guarding	Sleep disturbances
	Guarding, moaning	Confusion
	Groaning, restlessness	Rubbing
	Clenching teeth	Stoicism
	Biting lower lip	Depression
	Tightly shut eyes	Combativeness
	Open, somber eyes	Inactivity
	Involuntary movements	
	Immobility of body part	
	Purposeless body movements	
	Rhythmic body movements, rocking, rubbing	
	Change in speech and vocal pitch (anxiety)	
	Slow monotone (severe pain)	
	Fetal position	
Clinical signs	Elevated blood pressure	No change in vital signs
	Tachycardia	
	Talking	
	Diaphoresis	
Meaning	Meaningful (informs person something is wrong)	Meaningless, person looks for meaning
Pattern	Self-limiting or readily corrected	Continuous or intermittent
		Intensity may vary or remain constant
Course	Suffering usually decreases over time	Suffering usually increases over time
Action	Leads to action to relieve pain	Leads to action to modify pain
Prognosis	Likelihood of eventual complete relief	Complete relief usually not possible

Modified from Karb V: Pain. In Phipps W, Long B, Woods N, editors: *Medical-surgical nursing: concepts and clinical practice,* ed 4, St Louis, 1991, Mosby; and Forrest J: Assessment of acute and chronic pain in older adults, *J Gerontol Nurs* 21:10, 1995.

Peripheral vascular occlusion in people with advanced diabetes often produces a constant burning pain, similar to the pain of frostbite, to the extremities. The aged person who suffers a paralyzing or weakness-inducing stroke with loss of complete sensation on the affected side often experiences deep boring or crushing sensations, or burning and cold sensations in the face, neck, trunk, leg, or generally over the entire affected side. Movement of the affected side and other sensations such as touch, sound, bright light, and air increase this kind of pain. Feeling in the affected extremity may be perceived as feeling similar to being squeezed or twisted. Often the extremity is held in a strange position by the patient.

THE PAIN PROCESS

The process of pain occurs in four phases: transduction, transmission, pain perception, and modulation (Pasero et al, 1999b). The pain process begins with damage to tissue. The damaged cells release prostaglandin (PG), bradykinin (BK), histamine (H), serotonin (5-hydroxytryptamine [5-HT]), and substance P, which activate and sensitize nociceptors and generate an action potential that changes the ion charge of sodium (Na^+) and other ions, causing their proportions to transfer either into or out of the cells. This initial process in initiating the pain response is called *transduction.*

The next phase of the pain process is *transmission.* This is the continuation of the action potential transmitting the information to the spinal cord, from which it is then relayed to the brainstem and thalamus. Substance P and other neurotransmitters are released to enable the pain impulse to cross the synaptic gap to the dorsal horn neuron. The pain impulse continues from the dorsal horn, by way of the spinothalamic tract or other tracts to the thalamus and other centers of the brain. The thalamus acts as the relay station, sending the impulse to central structures.

The *perception of pain* is the conscious experience of pain. Once perceived, neurons in the brainstem send messages to the spinal cord and release substances such as endogenous opioids, serotonin, and norepinephrine, which inhibit or block the transmission of the nociceptive impulses. It is here that pain medications are used and modulation occurs.

Pain medications are used to control and interact with or block the pain response at any of the points in the pain process (called *modulation*). Medication can block histamine and other substances released at the transduction level, reestablish the correct action potential to block disarranged ions across cell membranes, and block the actual perception of pain. When pain medication is administered, it is important to know where it is working in the pain process (Fig. 17-1). When a patient is undertreated and pain is unrelieved, the impact on many body systems can be extremely harmful. These harmful effects are listed in Box 17-1.

PAIN CONTROL

Two major types of pain require attention: nociceptive pain (traumatic stimuli), which is either somatic or visceral, and neuropathic pain. Somatic pain is an aching or throbbing sensation that is localized to an area. It stems from bone, joints, muscles, skin, and connective tissue. Visceral pain arises from organs because of tumor or obstruction of hollow areas. Organ pain is reasonably localized pain with an achy sensation. Pain associated with obstruction causes intermittent cramping and poorly localized pain.

Neuropathic pain may be centrally generated, coming from injury to either the peripheral or central nervous system (CNS). Sensations of this pain usually are described as burning, tingling, pressure, and sometimes sharp and diffuse. Dysregulation of the autonomic nervous system generates sympathetic pain. Pain sensations associated with diabetes, alcoholism, or nutritional deficiency are classified as polyneuropathies, whereas those associated with damage to a particular peripheral nerve (which generates pain, in part, along the damaged nerve path, such as in nerve root compression or impingement) is considered mononeuropathic pain. Understanding the dynamics of pain is essential to effective intervention and to meeting the challenging nature of pain control of the older adult.

Pharmacologic Pain Control

Generally, pain relief is accomplished by medication aimed at blocking or altering pain impulses as they travel to the higher brain centers. Opioids and adjuvant (nonnarcotic) agents are available for use. Adjuvant preparations are usually effective for mild to moderate pain but may be combined with opioids if necessary. Opioids are usually reserved for moderate to severe pain. General principles of pain control for the aged are the same as for the young; however, the aged require special consideration. Opiates produce a greater analgesic effect, a higher peak, and a longer duration of effect in the older adult as a result of altered absorption, distribution, metabolism, and excretion (see Chapter 15). It is recommended that an initial dose be one-half to two-thirds the usual dose given to a younger person and, as needed, increased in increments of 25% (Watt-Watson, Donovan, 1992; Portenoy, 1995; Pasero et al, 1999; Portenoy et al, 1999; Young, 1999). Opioids that can safely be used with the older adult are morphine, oxycodone, hydrocodone, hydromorphone, and trans-

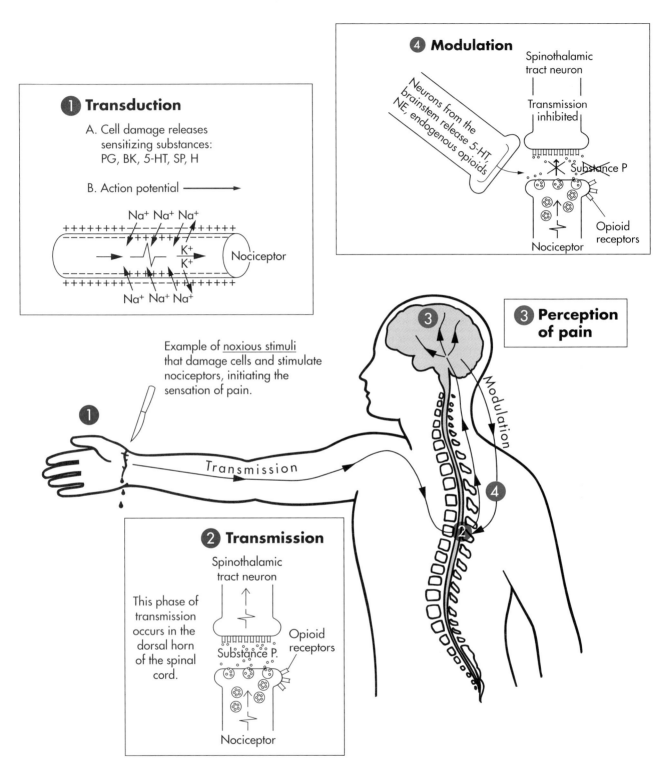

1 Transduction

A. Cell damage releases sensitizing substances: PG, BK, 5-HT, SP, H

B. Action potential ⟶

Na⁺ Na⁺ Na⁺

Nociceptor

Na⁺ Na⁺ Na⁺

4 Modulation

Spinothalamic tract neuron

Transmission inhibited

Neurons from the brainstem release 5-HT, NE, endogenous opioids

Substance P

Opioid receptors

Nociceptor

Example of <u>noxious stimuli</u> that damage cells and stimulate nociceptors, initiating the sensation of pain.

3 Perception of pain

Transmission

Modulation

2 Transmission

Spinothalamic tract neuron

This phase of transmission occurs in the dorsal horn of the spinal cord.

Substance P.

Opioid receptors

Nociceptor

Fig. 17-1 Basic mechanisms underlying the causes of pain and effects of pain. *PG,* Prostaglandin; *BK,* bradykinin, *5-HT,* 5-hydroxytryptamine; *SP,* substance P; *H,* histamine; *Na⁺,* sodium; *K⁺,* potassium; *NE,* norepinephrine. (From McCaffery M, Pasero C: *Pain: clinical manual,* ed 2, St Louis, 1999, Mosby.)

Box 17-1   HARMFUL EFFECTS OF UNRELIEVED PAIN

↑ Heart rate, ↑ cardiac output, ↑ peripheral vascular resistance, ↑ systemic vascular resistance, ↑ coronary vascular resistance, hypertension, ↑ myocardial oxygen consumption, hypercoagulation, deep vein thrombosis
Reduction in cognitive function, mental confusion
↑ Behavioral and physiologic responses to pain, altered temperaments, higher somatization, ↑ vulnerability to stress disorders, addictive behavior, and anxiety states
↑ Adrenocorticotrophic hormone (ACTH), ↑ cortisol, ↑ antidiuretic hormone (ADH), ↑ epinephrine, ↑ norepinephrine, ↑ growth hormone (GH), ↑ catecholamines, ↑ renin, ↑ angiotensin II, ↑ aldosterone, ↑ glucagon, ↑ interleukin-1, ↓ insulin, ↓ testosterone
Debilitating chronic pain syndrome: postmastectomy pain, postthoracotomy pain, phantom pain, postherpetic neuralgia
↓ Gastric and bowel motility
↓ Urinary output, urinary retention, fluid overload, hypokalemia
Depression of immune system
Glucogeneogenesis, hepatic glycogenolysis, hyperglycemia, glucose intolerance, insulin resistance, muscle protein catabolism, ↑ lipolysis
Sleeplessness, anxiety, fear, hopelessness, ↑ thoughts of suicide
↓ Flow and volumes, atelectasis, shunting, hypoxemia, ↓ cough, sputum retention, infection

Modified from McCaffery M, Pasero C: *Pain: clinical manual,* ed 2, St Louis, 1999, Mosby.

dermal fentanyl. The use of merperidine (Demerol) should be avoided with the elderly because of the toxic metabolite accumulation, as well as the long half-life of drugs such as methadone. The metabolites of Demerol can produce confusion, psychotic behavior, and seizure activity. The same can be said for pentazocine (Talwin) and methadone.

It is necessary to be aware of equianalgesic doses so that when parenteral pain medications are replaced with oral medications, or one oral medication is replaced with another, the dosage has pain relief power equivalent to the previous drug. Table 17-4 provides these equivalents.

Pain management in the elderly is fraught with many misconceptions that nurses consciously or subconsciously hold. Table 17-5, p. 370, lists and clarifies these misbeliefs.

In addition, patient's misbeliefs about pain and its control can compound the attempts to provide adequate pain control. These include the following (Watt-Watson, Donovan, 1992):
- Pain is to be expected with treatment and diagnoses such as cancer.
- I have no control over my pain.
- Surgery or a pill will fix me up.
- I should not ask for anything for pain unless I'm desperate.

Davies (1996) and Sarvis (1995) also point out that professionals may not ask the elder about their pain for the following reasons:
- The professional may assume that the individual will spontaneously report pain. However, the elder may not want to bother the physician with pain complaints, considering all the other medical problems he or she may have, and many older adults consider pain an expected part of aging.
- Clinicians are hesitant to prescribe analgesics for the elderly because of concern for troubling side effects with polypharmacy.
- Under managed care, the ability to provide appropriate pain relief is limited by removal of more effective but more costly analgesics from the hospital's formulary (Gray, 1996).
- Use of opioids causes too many problems, such as addiction and associated stigma. Other medications that the physician may prescribe for the elderly may be as effective but less problematic.

When acute pain is severe, as in postoperative recovery, it is prudent to combine a narcotic and an adjuvant preparation to achieve maximal pain relief. This combination affects pain response at both the peripheral and central nervous system levels (Fig. 17-2, p. 371).

An important point to remember is that the dose of the nonnarcotic analgesic must be sufficiently strong to work synergistically with the narcotic preparation. In addition, medication should be given at the point of beginning discomfort, not at the height of pain intensity. An around-the-clock (ATC) medicating schedule has been in the literature since about 1989. It has not been implemented in many instances. This is unfortunate because it is a viable way to provide a more stable therapeutic plasma level of drug and eliminate the extremes of overmedication and undermedication when patient-controlled analgesia (PCA) or epidural analgesia is not used. ATC pain control allows for a prn (pro re nata; as needed) dose of medication if and when breakthrough pain occurs (McCaffery, Ritchey, 1992; Sarvis, 1995; McCaffery,

Table 17-4

Equianalgesic Dose Chart

A guide to use of the equianalgesic dose chart:
- *Equinalgesic* means approximately the same pain relief.
- The chart is a guide. Doses and intervals between doses are titrated according to individual response.
- The chart is helpful when switching from one drug to another or switching from one route of administration to another.
- Dosages in this chart are not necessarily the starting dose. They suggest a ratio for comparing the analgesia of one drug with that of another.
- The longer the patient has been receiving opioids, the more conservative the starting dose of a new opioid.

Opioid	Parenteral (IM/SC/IV)	Oral (PO over 4 hours)	Duration (hours)	Half-life (hours)
AGONISTS				
Morphine	10 mg	30 mg	3-6 PO 8-12 CR 4-5 R 3-4 IV 3-4 SC 3-4 IM	2-4
Codeine	130 mg	200 mg NR	3-4 PO 3-4 SC 3-4 IM	2-4
Fentanyl	100 μg/hr parenterally and transdermally ≅ 4 mg/hr morphine parenterally; 1 μg/hr transdermally ≅ morphine 2 mg/24 hr orally	—	2-5 OT 0.5-4 IV 0.5-4 IM 48-72 TD	3-4 13-24 TD
Hydrocodone (Vicodin, Lortab)	—	30 mg NR	4-6 PO	4
Hydromorphone (Dilaudid)	1.5 mg	7.5 mg	3-4 PO 3-4 R 3-4 IV 3-4 SC 3-4 IM	2-3
Levorphanol (Levo-Dromoran)	2 mg	4 mg	4-6 PO 4-6 IV 4-6 SC 4-6 IM	12-15
Meperidine (Demerol)	75 mg	300 mg NR	2-4 PO 2-4 IV 2-4 SC 2-4 IM	2-3

Modified from Ebersole P, Hess P: *Toward healthy aging: human needs and nursing response,* ed 5, St Louis, 1998, Mosby; and McCaffery M, Pasero C: *Pain: clinical manual,* ed 2, St Louis, 1999, Mosby.
CR, Oral controlled release; *R,* rectal; *TD,* transdermal patch; *NS,* nasal spray; *OT,* oral, transmucosal; *PO,* oral; *SC,* subcutaneous; *IM,* intramuscular; *SL,* sublingual; *IV,* intravenous; *NR,* not recommended; *UK,* unknown.

Continued

Table 17-4—cont'd

Equianalgesic Dose Chart

Opioid	Parenteral (IM/SC/IV)	Oral (PO over 4 hours)	Duration (hours)	Half-life (hours)
Methadone (Dolophine)	10 mg	20 mg	4-8 PO UK SL 4-8 IV 4-8 SC 4-8 IM	12-190
Oxycodone (Percocet; Tylox)	—	20 mg	3-4 PO 8-12 CR 3-6 R	2-3 4-5 CR
Propoxyphene (Darvon)	—	—	4-6 PO	6-12
AGONIST ANTAGONISTS				
Buprenorphine (Buprenex)	0.4 mg	—	UK SL 3-4 IV 3-6 IM	2-3
Butorphanol (Stadol)	2 mg	—	3-4 NS 3-4 IV 3-4 IM	3-4
Dezocine (Dalgan)	10 mg	—	3-4 IV 3-4 IM	2-3
Nalbuphine (Nubain)	10 mg	—	3-4 IV 3-4 SC 3-4 IM	5
Pentazocine (Talwin)	60 mg	180 mg	3-4 PO 3-4 IV 3-4 SC 3-4 IM	2-3

Pasero, 1999). Narcotic use for long-term chronic pain control in the elderly should be convenient, easy to administer, and short acting for ease of dose adjustment; there is less drug accumulation in the body and a low incidence of side effects. Box 17-2, p. 372, lists preferred opioids and adjuvant medications, as well as those that are inappropriate for use with the elderly.

Mild and moderate pain relief may be achieved with adjuvant medications such as the nonsteroidal antiinflammatory drugs (NSAIDs) or acetaminophen. The NSAIDs bind with proteins and may induce toxic responses in elders if serum albumin levels are low. Other drugs that elders routinely take compete for the same protein receptor sites and may be displaced by the NSAID, creating unstable therapeutic effects. Drugs that cause CNS effects should be used with caution in elders who are sensitive to CNS effects. In addition, NSAIDs should be used with caution because of increased risk of adverse effects, especially gastrointestinal bleeding and renal impairment. Aspirin and acetaminophen use should be monitored because of reduced renal and hepatic function with aging. Refer to Box 17-2 for preferred NSAID drugs and those to be avoided for use with elders.

The following are guidelines for the selection and use of NSAIDs:
- Weigh risks versus benefits in selection.
- Start with a low dose to determine the patient's reaction (e.g., side effects). Increase gradually to a dose that relieves pain, not to exceed the maximal daily

Table 17-5

Barriers to the Assessment and Treatment of Pain

Misconception	Correction
The best judge of the existence and severity of a patient's pain is the physician or nurse caring for the patient.	The patient is the authority about his or her pain. The patient's self-report is the most reliable indicator of the existence and intensity of pain.
Clinicians should use their personal opinions and beliefs about the truthfulness of the patient to determine the patient's true pain status.	Allowing each clinician to act on personal beliefs presents the potential for different pain assessments by different clinicians, leading to different interventions from each clinician. This results in inconsistent and often inadequate pain management. It is essential to establish the patient's self-report of pain as the standard for pain assessment.
The clinician must believe what the patient says about pain.	The clinician must accept and respect the patient's report of pain and proceed with appropriate assessment and treatment. The clinician is always entitled to his or her personal opinion, but this cannot be allowed to guide professional practice.
Comparable noxious stimuli produce comparable pain in different people. The pain threshold is uniform.	Findings from numerous studies have failed to support the notion of a uniform pain threshold. Comparable stimuli do not result in the same pain in different people. After similar injuries, one person may suffer moderate pain and the other severe pain.
Patients with a low pain tolerance should make a greater effort to cope with pain and should not receive as much analgesia as they desire.	A stoic response to pain is valued in this society and many others. Research shows that clinicians often do not like patients with a low pain tolerance. However, imposing these values on the patient and withholding analgesics is inappropriate.
There is no reason for patients to hurt when no physical cause for pain can be found.	Pain is a new science, and it would be foolish of us to think that we will be able to determine the cause of all the pains that patients report.
Patients should not receive analgesics until the cause of pain is diagnosed.	Pain is no longer the clinician's primary diagnostic tool. Symptomatic relief of pain should be provided while the investigation of cause proceeds. Early use of analgesics is now advocated for patients with acute abdominal pain.
Visible signs, either physiologic or behavioral, accompany pain and can be used to verify its existence and severity.	Even with severe pain, periods of physiologic and behavioral adaptation occur, leading to periods of minimal or no signs of pain. Lack of pain expression does not necessarily mean lack of pain.
Anxiety makes pain worse.	Anxiety is often associated with pain, but the cause-and-effect relationship has not been established. Pain often causes anxiety, but it is not clear that anxiety necessarily makes pain more intense.
Patients who are knowledgeable about opioid analgesics and who make regular efforts to obtain them are "drug seeking" (addicted).	Patients with pain should be knowledgeable about their medications, and regular use of opioids for pain relief is not addiction. When a patient is accused of "drug seeking," it may be helpful to ask, "What else could this behavior mean? Might this patient be in pain?"
When the patient reports pain relief after a placebo, this means that the patient is a malingerer or that the pain is psychogenic.	About one third of patients who have obvious physical stimuli for pain (e.g., surgery) report pain relief after a placebo injection. Therefore placebos cannot be used to diagnose malingering, psychogenic pain, or any psychologic problem. Sometimes placebos relieve pain, but why this happens remains unknown.
The pain rating scale preferred for use in daily clinical practice is the VAS.	For patients who are verbal and can count from 0 to 10, the NRS pain rating scale is preferred. It is easy to explain, measure, and record, and it provides numbers for setting pain management goals.
Cognitively impaired elderly patients are unable to use pain rating scales.	When an appropriate pain rating scale (e.g., 0-5) is used and the patient is given sufficient time to process information and respond, many cognitively impaired elderly can use a pain rating scale.

From McCaffery M, Pasero C: *Pain: clinical manual*, ed 2, St Louis, 1999, Mosby.
VAS, Visual analog scale; *NRS*, numerical rating scale.

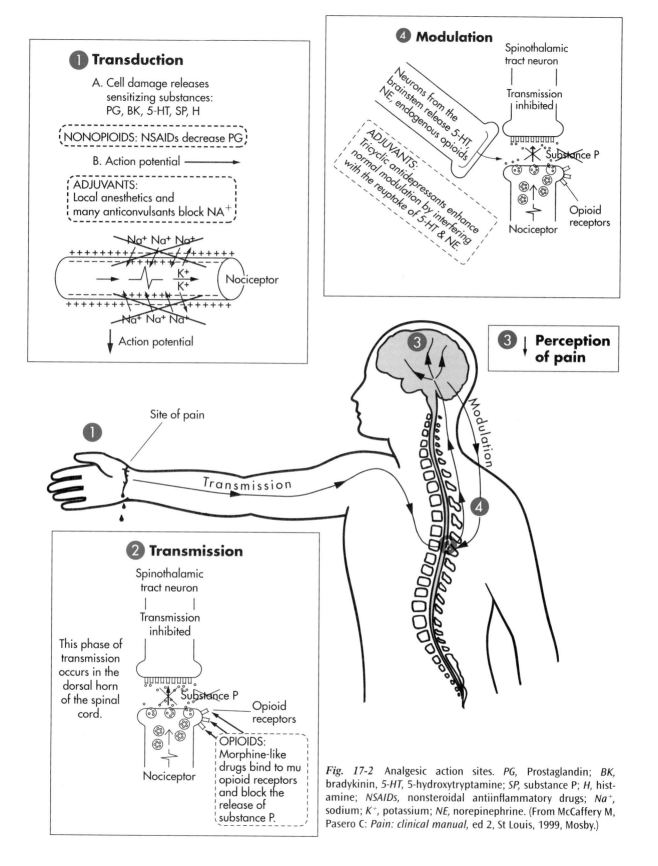

Fig. 17-2 Analgesic action sites. *PG,* Prostaglandin; *BK,* bradykinin, *5-HT,* 5-hydroxytryptamine; *SP,* substance P; *H,* histamine; *NSAIDs,* nonsteroidal antiinflammatory drugs; *Na+,* sodium; *K+,* potassium; *NE,* norepinephrine. (From McCaffery M, Pasero C: *Pain: clinical manual,* ed 2, St Louis, 1999, Mosby.)

Box 17-2	APPROPRIATE AND INAPPROPRIATE PAIN MEDICATIONS FOR THE ELDERLY

Appropriate	Inappropriate
Opioids	
Oxycodone	Meperidine (Demerol)
Hydromorphone (Dilaudid)	Propoxyphene (Darvon, Darvocet)
Tylenol with codeine	Pentazocine (Talwin)
	Methadone
Nonsteroidal Antiinflammatory drugs (NSAIDs)	
Ibuprofen	Indomethacine (Indocin)
Salicylate	Phenylbutazone
Diflunisal (Dolobid)	Aspirin
Acetaminophen	Piroxicam (Feldene)
Adjuvant medications	
Antidepressants	
Trazodone	Amitriptyline (Elavil)
Desipramine	
Fluoxetine (Prozac)	
Combined antidepressant-antipsychotic	Amitriptyline-perphenazine (Triavil)
Sedatives and hypnotics	Diazepam (Valium)
	Flurazepam (Dalmane)
	Meprobamate (Miltown, Equanil)
	Chlordiazepoxide (Limbitrol)
	Pentabarbitol (Nembutal)
	Secobarbital (Seconal)
Histamine blockers	Cimetidine (Tagamet)
	Ranitidine (Zantac)
Dementia treatment	Cyclandelate, isoxsuprine

Data from Ebersole P, Hess P: *Toward healthy aging: human needs and nursing response*, ed 5, St Louis, 1998, Mosby; and McCaffery M, Pasero C: *Pain: clinical manual*, ed 2, St Louis, 1999, Mosby.

dose. The dose may need to be increased one to two times the starting dose.
- If maximal antiinflammatory effect is desired in addition to analgesia, allow an adequate trial before discontinuing or switching. With regular doses for 1 week or longer, pain relief may increase.
- If one drug becomes ineffective but the pain is about the same, try a drug from a different chemical class.

- If the NSAID does not relieve pain when used alone, combine with oral (PO), intramuscular (IM), or intravenous (IV) narcotics for added analgesic effect (Portenoy, McCaffery, 1999).

Sharp, shooting, dull, aching, or burning pain that is not responsive to NSAIDs or narcotics may respond to adjuvant drug therapy. Some adjuvant drugs help control symptoms and signs associated with pain. Adjuvant drugs are not analgesics per se; they are anticonvulsants or antidepressants that can alter pain responses at either the transmission, pain perception, or modulation phase of the pain process. Used in combination with analgesics, they may potentiate or enhance the overall analgesic effects. Elders frequently respond well with adjuvant pain regimens. However, it is important to remember that many adjuvant drugs have a very long half-life, which increases the plasma concentration in elders. This can lead to adverse or toxic effects. Preferred adjuvant drugs and those to be avoided for elderly use are listed in Box 17-2. Some guidelines for the administration of adjuvant drugs to the elderly include the following:
- Avoid those drugs with potent anticholinergic effects. These may result in urinary retention and subsequent urinary tract infection; constipation; blurred vision, which increases the chance for injury; dry mouth, affecting the ability to eat; and confusion.
- Neuroleptics, if used, should have the least sedating, cardiotoxic, and hypotensive effects.
- Avoid drugs that precipitate or potentiate extrapyramidal symptoms.
- Tranquilizers that produce sedation and have a long half-life should be avoided. Drugs with a short half-life are more suitable.
- Drugs that can cause orthostatic hypotension should be used with caution, especially when there is a preexisting cardiac condition.
- Interactions with other drugs must be monitored carefully, since elders take many medications (polypharmacy).

The essential principles of pain control using the World Health Organization (WHO, 1990) three-step ladder approach of pharmacologic pain control are illustrated in Fig. 17-3.

Nonpharmacologic Pain Control

Nursing staff are often afraid of inducing iatrogenic addiction and thus give a less than effective dosage of pain medication. In addition to pain control through pharmacologic means, the use of various alternative

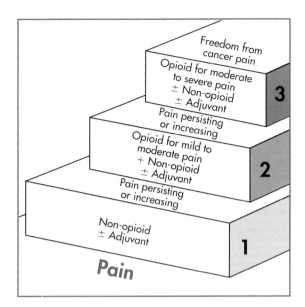

Fig. 17-3 WHO three-step analgesic ladder. (Redrawn from World Health Organization: *Cancer pain relief,* ed 2, Geneva, 1996, WHO.)

measures such as biofeedback, acupuncture or acupressure, behavior modification, hypnosis, meditation, or a combination of these modalities may help to relieve the discomfort of pain. In many instances a combination of pharmacologic and nonpharmacologic interventions is effective in relieving acute or chronic pain in the older adult.

Cutaneous Nerve Stimulation

Deep and superficial stimulation of the skin by direct, proximal, or distal application for the purpose of pain relief has been practiced for centuries. Massage, vibration, heat, cold, and ointments have been a part of nursing interventions for years. Heat is effective for musculoskeletal disorders such as rheumatic conditions. It is contraindicated with occlusive vascular disease and in the presence of cancer. In nonexpansive tissue such as bursae, heat may even increase pain. Intermittent cold packs are helpful in low back pain and radicular disturbances. They serve to negate or delay the transmission of pain impulses to the cerebral pain center. Pathophysiologic conditions should be taken into consideration when using heat and cold with the elderly. Care must be taken when applying heat and cold to the skin of the aged to prevent skin damage from extended periods of heat and cold applications.

Transcutaneous Electrical Nerve Stimulation

Another method of cutaneous stimulation is transcutaneous electrical nerve stimulation (TENS) or dorsal column nerve stimulation (DNS). Electrodes, applied and taped to the skin over the pain site or on the spine, emit a mild electrical current that is felt as a tingling, buzzing, or vibrating sensation. The patient operates the stimulator and starts the electrical impulses, which then activate the large nerve fibers that transmit impulses to block pain at the spinal cord and prevent pain signals from reaching the brain. TENS has been helpful in phantom limb pain, postherpetic neuralgia, and low back pain; however, TENS should not be used with persons who have pacemakers; nor should it be among the first choices of pain control for the aged. Those who are tape sensitive or whose skin is very friable should not use TENs or should be monitored carefully for skin irritation or breakdown (Palmieri, 1999).

Touch

Touch is a natural comfort measure, although its therapeutic properties are still not clearly understood. Sometimes considered a cutaneous stimulation technique, "therapeutic touch" used in experimental laboratory and clinical settings showed that placing hands on or near the body might result in healing or improvement (Kreiger, 1992). Relaxation and proper sensory stimulation decrease anxiety, reduce muscle tension, and help provide distraction from pain and thereby relieve pain.

Massage is a powerful modality of therapeutic touch. It can induce muscle relaxation, increase circulation, decrease swelling, soften and stretch scar tissue, reduce adhesions, and relieve pain (Kastner, 1994). Mackey (1995) suggests the use of therapeutic touch for pain relief in conjunction with pharmacologic therapy.

Acupuncture and Acupressure

Acupuncture is an alternative to electrical stimulation. Small nerve fibers are stimulated by the twirling of the needles. Acute pain is registered as pain impulses pass through the spinal cord. The acute pain registers in the brain and signals the central mechanism of the brain to return counterimpulses, which interfere with the pain impulse. Acupuncture points are located near clusters of nerve cell endings. It is thought that acupuncture stimulates these nerves and blocks the pain impulse or that it triggers the release of the body's own opiate substances: enkephalins (endorphins), a natural analgesic.

Acupressure is acupuncture without needles. Pressure applied to the traditional acupuncture points with the thumbs, tip of the index finger, or palm of the hand or by pinching and squeezing stimulates the nerves and causes the blocking of the pain impulse or, like acupuncture, triggers the release of the body's natural endorphins.

Biofeedback

An individual can learn voluntary control over some body processes and alter them by changing the physiologic correlates appropriate to them. Response to certain types of pain can be controlled. Boczkowski (1984) found that biofeedback decreased chronic pain of rheumatoid arthritis. Training and often time and equipment of some type are needed to learn how to alter one's body response. Biofeedback has produced conflicting results in regard to reducing or eliminating pain.

Distraction

Distraction lessens the perception of pain by drawing the person's attention away from pain. In some instances the individual is completely unaware of the pain. Pain messages are slower than diversional messages; therefore they can interfere with the transmission of the pain signal. Mild to moderate pain responds well to distraction. At times, if an individual concentrates intently on another subject, the acute pain may be relieved. The most common forms of distraction (Kosier et al, 1995) are listed in Box 17-3.

Relaxation, Meditation, and Imagery

Relaxation enables the quieting of the mind and muscles, providing the release of tension and anxiety and increasing pain tolerance. It may increase the effectiveness of other pain-relieving measures. Meditation and imagery are two methods of promoting relaxation.

Imagery uses the client's imagination to focus on settings full of happiness and relaxation rather than on stressful situations. Several studies suggested the use of guided imagery to decrease pain perception in foot pain and abdominal pain. The suggestion of a strong image of a pain-free state effectively alters the autonomic nervous system's responses to pain (Hamm, King, 1984; Griffin, 1986; Pearson, 1988; McCaffery, Beebe, 1989; McCaffery, Pasero, 1999).

Box 17-3   FORMS OF DISTRACTION

Visual Distraction

Reading
Watching TV
Watching a sports game
Guided imagery

Auditory Distraction

Humor
Listening to music

Tactile Distraction

Slow, rhythmic breathing
Massage
Holding or stroking a pet

Intellectual Distraction

Crossword puzzles
Card games
Hobbies

Modified from Kosier B et al: *Fundamentals of nursing,* Redwood City, Calif, 1995, Addison-Wesley.

Hypnosis

Hypnosis has been used to help alter pain perception through positive suggestions. Research has demonstrated that hypnotic analgesia reduces what are considered "overreactions" to pain when apprehension and stress are apparent.

Some people have the ability to induce self-hypnosis, and some do not. Most of the population, however, has some capacity for hypnosis and with training can increase their control in this area. There are three recognized modes of hypnosis: (1) spontaneous, which is what most of us do when we daydream; (2) the self-induced trance; and (3) formal hypnosis, which requires the services of a hypnotist.

Intense concentration is required for hypnosis. Hypnosis can be used to alter pain perception, thus blocking pain awareness; to substitute another feeling for a painful one; to displace pain sensation to a smaller body area; or to alter the meaning of pain so that it is viewed as less important and less debilitating (Thomas, 1990; Sarvis, 1995). Table 17-6 illustrates the advantages and disadvantages of specific nonpharmacologic pain relief measures.

Table 17-6

Advantages and Disadvantages of Nonpharmacologic Measures

Therapy	Advantage	Disadvantage
Cutaneous nerve stimulation	Pleasurable sensations make it popular with elders	Some elders perceive stimulation as intolerable; objectionable odors from creams and ointments such as menthol
Transcutaneous electrical nerve stimulation (TENS) Dorsal column nerve stimulation (DNS) Touch Acupuncture/acupressure	Relaxation and distraction from pain May be feasible for elders with limited income Requires limited energy expenditure Self-administration provides a sense of control Family participation for those elders unable to do for self	Improper use of heat, cold, etc., may do tissue damage
Distraction Tactile, auditory, visual, kinesthetic	Sense of control over pain Improve mood Relaxation Increase tolerance to pain	Choices may be limited by cognitive and sensory impairment
Relaxation	Decreases skeletal muscle tension Decreases anxiety Useful with chronic pain, muscle spasms, sleep loss due to pain	Must be able to understand instructions Takes time and energy to learn Ineffective with depressed or very fatigued
Biofeedback	Decreases chronic pain	Requires equipment (moderate to expensive) Takes time and energy to learn Must be cognitively intact
Imagery	Very simple, uses elders' imagination; may enhance relaxation and distraction; may feel control over pain; may perceive as an escape from pain Always available Little to no economic or social impact for the elderly	Not viewed as a credible technique Must be cognitively intact
Hypnosis	Pain relief on a long-term basis without side effects Useful for elders unable to tolerate pharmacologic measures Does not alter mental functioning (a fear of the elderly)	May not be viewed as a credible therapy Feel loss of mental control Must be cognitively intact Requires trained personnel May not be available in remote or small settings

Developed by Patricia Hess.

Placebo

When the word *placebo* is mentioned, one immediately thinks of the use of fake pills and saline injections in place of narcotic analgesics, or of an attempt to fool the patient into thinking that he or she is getting the "real thing." A placebo is defined as "any treatment or procedure that produces a response in a patient because of its intent, and not because of any actual physiologic or therapeutic properties" (McCaffery, Pasero, 1999, p. 54). Since the emphasis on patient's rights and informed consent, many professional organizations have developed position statements that specifically state that the deceptive use of placebos and the misinterpretation of the placebo response have no place in the assessment or management of patients' pain reports (American Pain Society, 1992; Acute Pain Management, 1992). The practice of using placebos is immoral and unethical; creates distrust between the patient and caregiver; and represents fraud, malpractice, breach of contract, and medical negligence (Fox, 1994). The California Board of Registered Nursing (BRN) (1997) states that "use of placebos for management of pain will not fulfill informed consent (p. 12)." It is imperative that nurses know the position statement of their individual licensing boards on the use of placebos.

Little attention has been paid to those who are placebo responders, nor has anyone until recently wondered whether these responders' pain relief mechanism was different from that of others. Patients whose pain or illness was relieved by a placebo were considered "crocks or complainers." Research has shown that approximately 36% of persons who receive placebos have a positive placebo effect. Why they work on a third of the population is unclear. Despite the fact that a placebo is generally thought to be inert and therefore harmless, reports of adverse effects such as rash, nausea, and thirst have been noted (Todd, 1987). The most common side effects are headaches, depression, or CNS stimulation. Research has shown that placebos mimic active drugs and can produce a negative placebo effect (Lavin, 1991), also considered a nocebo effect (Pain Relief, 1995).

The use of placebos is still present, and articles continue to appear in professional literature. A study by McCaffery and Ferrell (1996) indicated that one in five nurses were susceptible to being part of the use of placebos in the treatment of pain. To support nurses in their response to an order for administration of placebos, hospitals need to have written policies that address the unethical use of placebos. Nurses then can refer to these policies as a breach of patient quality of care when an order for a placebo is written. Box 17-4 presents key points about placebo use in pain management.

Pain Clinics

Pain clinic experience with elders has been limited; however, referral for elders with significant and psychologic impairment in most instances is appropriate when the usual standard measures to relieve pain (particularly chronic pain) are unsuccessful.

Pain center programs may be inpatient, outpatient, or both. Pain centers are generally one of three types:

Box 17-4   KEY POINTS ABOUT PLACEBO USE IN PAIN MANAGEMENT

1. Placebos can be effective in relieving pain, but this does not justify their use. On average, one third of patients who have obvious physical stimuli for pain (e.g., surgery) may report pain relief after administration of a placebo. However, a positive response varies between and within individuals and, therefore, cannot be predicted.
2. No medical conditions exist for which placebos are recommended as a method of assessment or treatment.
   a. Placebos cannot be used to diagnose malingering, psychogenic pain, or any psychologic problem.
   b. Use of placebos for pain relief does not prevent addiction to opioids.
   c. Placebo use deprives the patient of appropriate treatment or diagnostic measures.
3. Institutional policies that restrict the use of placebos to approved clinical trials in which informed consent is obtained are necessary not only to protect patients, but also to protect nurses and other staff from moral, ethical, and legal concerns.
   a. Placebos tend to be used in vulnerable patient populations (e.g., those with substance abuse or with pain that is difficult to diagnose or treat). This constitutes a dual standard of care.
   b. Deceitful placebo use endangers the patient's trust in caregivers and violates the patient's rights.
   c. Deceitful use of placebos violates informed consent and constitutes medical negligence, placing caregivers in a litigious position.
   d. Resorting to deceitful placebo use prevents caregivers from increasing their knowledge of more effective ways to assess and to treat pain.
   e. Deceit threatens the professional caregiver's own integrity.

From McCaffery M, Pasero C: *Pain: clinical manual,* ed 2, St Louis, 1999, Mosby.

---

syndrome oriented, modality oriented, or comprehensive. Syndrome-oriented centers focus on a specific chronic pain problem such as headache or arthritis pain. Modality-oriented centers focus on a specific treatment technique such as relaxation or acupuncture/acupressure. The comprehensive centers include many services, which begin with an initial assessment and include treatment and follow-up. Staff are usually a coordinated, multidisciplinary team of some or all of the following: physician, nurse, physical therapist, occupational therapist, massage therapist, rehabilitation specialist, and social worker.

Treatment includes a variety of approaches; medical treatment may be oral, injectable, or topical medication. Because long-term use of potent medications can be habit forming or addicting when one has chronic pain, medication adjustment is considered. Medication is used only when absolutely necessary in the management of the patient's pain. Physical methods, such as massage, heat and cold applications, exercise, and acupuncture/acupressure, to name a few, are used to reduce or alleviate chronic pain during and after the pain center program. Psychologic techniques such as biofeedback, self-hypnosis, relaxation, and behavior modification are among the methods used and taught to individuals to control the pain situation. Even though older adults may find these therapies foreign to them, they are good candidates for these treatment programs and may be able to benefit from them (Saxon, Etter, 1994).

The nurse should be familiar with the several types of clinics that exist so as to provide the patient or the family of the patient with the necessary information to make a knowledgeable decision concerning this approach and what to look for.

PAIN IN THE AGED

The prevalence of pain in community-dwelling elderly persons is known to be twice that of the young and is considered to be extremely high in the long-term care setting. Ferrell (1991), Gloth (1996), and Young (1999) suggest that the incidence of pain in the elderly who are living in the community is 25% to 50% and that it is as much as 85% in long-term care because of the presence of conditions that cause chronic pain. Box 17-5 lists common painful conditions in the elderly.

In the aged, fear and anxiety generate negative effects that emanate from thoughts that pain will result in crippling, forced dependency or that it will be of such intensity that the ability to cope will be inadequate. Pain weakens and interrupts the individual's ideas of relations to self, to others, to the environment, and in time and space.

The aged are at high risk for pain-inducing situations. They have lived longer and have a greater chance of developing degenerative and pathologic conditions through disease or injury. Several conditions may be present simultaneously, so a single pain-producing con-

---

Box 17-5   **COMMON PAINFUL CONDITIONS OF THE ELDERLY**

Musculoskeletal problems
   Rheumatoid arthritis
   Osteoarthritis
   Vertebral compression fracture
Cancer
Postherpetic neuralgia
Temporal arteritis
Traumatic injuries
Peripheral vascular disease
Myocardial ischemia
Pleuritic pain
Gastroesophageal reflux

---

dition may be overlooked in the complexity of health management. Increased susceptibility to accidents because of medications, cognitive function, or illness impacts functional abilities, which further contributes to such accidents as falls. The resultant hip fractures, sprains, and hematomas require longer periods of time to heal and prolong the pain experience. Loneliness through loss of a spouse, a job, independence, and friends and the presence of boredom and depression decrease the ability to cope with pain. These psychosocial aspects of an elder's life are rarely self-reported, because of the associated stigma.

Chronic pain experienced by a number of elders often results in dramatic life-style changes such as altered family relationships and the inability to visit friends. Ferrell and Ferrell (1990) found that of 65 elder patients studied, 54% experienced impairment of enjoyable activities, 53% experienced impaired ambulation, 49% experienced impaired posture, and 45% and 32% experienced sleep disorders and depression, respectively. In this sample it was apparent that lowered pain tolerance exists. It is not uncommon for acuity of symptoms or severity of pain to be less dramatic than in younger persons (Witt, 1984; McCaffery, Pasero, 1999). Serious abdominal and cardiac conditions that should elicit severe pain often produce little or no pain in the aged. In addition, the elderly often underreport pain because they consider it a normal part of the aging process.

Behavioral changes or manifestations such as confusion and restlessness have been cited as possible indicators of painful stimuli in the cognitively intact and cognitively impaired aged (Davis, 1997; Feldt, 1998;

Kassalaroen et al, 1998; Parke, 1998; Pasero et al, 1999c). The elderly often suffer in silence or attempt to relieve pain with inadequate measures because of the high cost of medical care, consultation, equipment, diagnostic tests, hospitalization, and medications. The perceptions of pain by others, including caregivers, influence the elder's pain (Hofland, 1992; Sarvis, 1995). Nurses must be extremely observant of subtle behavioral cues, such as guarding a part of the body, wincing, or favoring certain movements, as well as sounds and appearance, rather than internalizing and projecting their own pain experience or misconceptions on others.

Pain management and interventions for pain in the elderly often differ from those of other age-groups because of concerns regarding cognitive function and the use of such therapies as TENS, antidepressants, or relaxation techniques (Fulmer et al, 1996). In addition, medications are affected by decreases in absorption, distribution, metabolism, and elimination. The ability of elders to swallow pills easily may be impaired because of a dry mouth, ill-fitting dentures, or an impaired swallowing mechanism. Injectable medication may also be unreliable because of the inadequacy of the elder's circulation. (Refer to Chapter 15 for pharmacokinetics and pharmacodynamics of medications.) Other viable routes in providing pain relief include nebulized, transdermal, intranasal, buccal, sublingual, rectal, IV, and epidural routes. New forms of medication administration are being developed, among which is oral transmucosal (Managing Pain, 1996).

Another issue in pain management of the elderly is their fear of losing self-control and fear of addiction. The Agency For Health Care Policy and Research guidelines (Acute Pain Management, 1992) were an outstanding contribution to pain intervention, but they did not provide direction for those who care for elders who need pain relief (Fulmer et al, 1996). Box 17-6 presents principles of pain management in the care of elders.

Box 17-6   PRINCIPLES OF PAIN MANAGEMENT IN THE ELDERLY

- Always ask elderly patients about pain.
- Accept the patient's word about pain and its intensity.
- Never underestimate the potential effects of chronic pain on the patient's overall condition and quality of life.
- Be compulsive about pain assessment. An accurate diagnosis will lead to more effective treatment.
- Treat pain to facilitate diagnostic procedures. Don't wait for a diagnosis to relieve pain and needless suffering.
- Use a combination of pharmacologic and nonpharmacologic measures whenever possible.
- Give adequate amounts of drug at the appropriate frequency to control pain based on constant assessment.
- Use analgesic drugs correctly. With narcotics start with a low dosage and increase slowly. Titrate to the desired effect or to intolerable side effects.
- Anticipate and prevent side effects common in elders:
  - Give antiinflammatory drugs with food.
  - Begin bowel regimen early to prevent constipation.
  - Be prepared to give an antinausea medication with narcotic analgesic drugs.
  - Anticipate some impaired balance and cognitive function with narcotic analgesic drugs.
- Consult an equianalgesic potency table when changing medication.
- Mobilize the patient physically and psychologically. Involve the patient in his or her own care.
- Anticipate and attend to anxiety and depression.
- Reassess responses to treatment at regular intervals. Alter therapy to maximize pain relief and improve functional status and quality of life.

Modified from Ferrell BA: Pain management in elderly people, *J Am Geriatr Soc* 39:64-73, 1991; and Glickstein JK, editor: Managing chronic pain, *Focus Geriatr Care Rehabil* 10(3):6, 1996.

The Cognitively Impaired Elderly

The subjective nature of pain self-reporting has been the accepted standard for intervention and evaluation of the presence and relief of pain. However, this is not usually the case with elders who are cognitively impaired either by transient confusion or more permanent dementia. There are 2 to 5 million persons in the United States with dementia caused by various acute and chronic conditions. In the twenty-first century there will be an ever-increasing number of aged persons with

dementia. Changes in mental function greatly interfere with an individual's ability to report pain. It is important for the nurse to note if there are sensory impairments (hearing or vision), depression, aphasia, or chemical or physical restraints that may interfere with communicating pain. The nurse should not assume that those individuals who cannot verbalize their pain clearly because of cognitive impairment do not have pain or as much pain as others who are cognitively in-

Box 17-7	SOME CUES OF PAIN IN OLDER COGNITIVELY INTACT AND COGNITIVELY IMPAIRED ADULTS

Overt Behavior
Aggressive
Striking out: pinching; hitting; biting; or scratching

Physical movements
Restlessness/agitation
Drawing legs up or fetal position
Stretches
Repetitive movements
Clenched fists
Slow movements, cautious movements
Guarding
Trying to get someone's attention

Activities of daily living
Resists care
Change in appetite (decrease)
Altered sleep (decreased)

Sounds
Verbalizations
Says has pain
Antisocial behavior
  Complains
  Critical
  Blames
Silence—does not speak

Sounds—cont'd
Vocalizations
Groans
Moans
Screams
Cries
Babbles
Noisy breathing

Appearance
Facial expression
Expressionless; stares or looks past you
Winces
Pleading
Grimaces: eyes—tighten up or light up; mouth—open or pinched; brows—wrinkled or folded

Body language
Complexion—flushed look
Miserable
Tense
Lacks concentration
Perspires

Modified from Parke B: Gerontologic nurses' way of knowing, *J Gerontol Nurs* 24(6):21, 1998; and McCaffery M, Pasero C: *Pain: clinical manual,* ed 2, St Louis, 1999, Mosby.

tact but must be alert to the cues that suggest that pain and discomfort are present. One must think that if a condition causes pain in a person who can self-report the pain, the nurse must assume that the condition is painful to one who is cognitively impaired and must therefore treat the pain. Facial expressions, body movements, and activity should be assessed to determine pain and its effective relief (Box 17-7).

Nurse's Role

There is a dilemma in providing comfort. Because bureaucratic policies limit staff, the time that staff spend with patients is confined to the basic needs of treatment, medications, and physical care. The quality of physical care suffers when the paraprofessional is discouraged from taking time to fulfill comfort needs such as providing a back rub or discussing the patient's concerns. If

the caregiver could spend 5 minutes massaging and talking with the older person after a bath or treatment, anxiety, pain, and depression would be reduced. The nurse is in a very influential position to make a meaningful contribution to pain relief. It should be expected that nurses providing care to the aged would have sufficient knowledge of the pain process and the physiologic condition currently accepted by the medical community.

The ability to assess pain of another becomes complicated because of differing attitudes and the multidimensional aspects that pain projects. There are no easy answers concerning how to assess, differentiate, or judge the uniquely personal estimates of the quality and quantity of pain. Pain experiences are highly individualized, and there continues to be much yet to learn about pain.

Nurses are most familiar and comfortable with acute temporary pain because it is short-lived and amenable to expedient relief. Chronic pain presents a frustrating situation for the nurse and an intolerable situation for the patient. Nurses expect patients suffering from chronic pain to display behavior characteristics of acute discomfort; an organic basis for pain makes it legitimate. Nurses tend to undermedicate patients with chronic pain because they fear that they will foster addiction. Often nurses caring for the patient with chronic pain, especially in long-term care situations, become so familiar with the pain that they ignore it as a means of protecting themselves from feeling overwhelmed and powerless in what seems an insurmountable, futile situation. Frequently patients with chronically painful conditions are told that they must "just learn to live with it." To the individual experiencing pain, this is a dismal pronouncement and implies a withdrawal of interest and concern. In many situations of acute pain, little attention is given to the continuing chronic pain an individual may also be experiencing. An example of this situation is an older adult with acute pain of a fractured hip who also has osteoarthritis of other body joints. Treatment of the acute pain is different from that of other pain.

Assessment
Pain is undertreated in acute care, long-term care, and home care settings. Eighty percent of long-term care residents experience pain, with only 40% to 50% given analgesics. In the home care setting 50% suffer pain, the greater proportion from cancer pain (these patients are now frequently cared for at home) (Gloth, 1996). Assessment of pain in the elderly is important for several reasons: pain is the most common symptom of disease; an accurate assessment will lead to an accurate diagnosis; assessment facilitates evaluation of the effects of therapy; assessment can help differentiate acute, endangering pain from long-standing chronic pain; and successful pain management begins with an accurate assessment (Watt-Watson, Donovan, 1992). Refer to Box 17-1 for the consequences of unrelieved pain. The most prominent goal in the care of the older adult is the maintenance of functional ability. Function is compromised in the presence of pain; therefore the goal of treatment is not only appropriate and adequate pain control but also the restoration of functional ability to enable the elder to regain his or her maximal level of independence. The characteristics of pain can be described as sharp and throbbing or as sensations of pressure, dullness, and aching. Pain may or may not manifest itself in acute physical signs. Psychosocial pain or discomfort has been identified as occurring because of unkindness by caregivers or while awaiting new procedures.

A number of barriers exist to pain assessment and treatment of the older adult and are noted in Table 17-5. Accurate assessment includes asking questions about the person's pain. The accepted definition of pain is that "Pain is whatever the patient says it is" (McCaffery, Beebe, 1989; McCaffery, Pasero, 1999). Do not rely on the word *pain* alone; use other words: *discomfort, sore, ache, hurt,* and so on (Watt-Watson, Donovan, 1992). Itching is also considered a form of pain and discomfort (Jacox, 1979).

The cognitively impaired and nonverbal patient is the most difficult to assess and requires astute observation. Individuals who moan and groan may become withdrawn and quiet; disjointed verbalization may turn into an accurate description of the location of pain; the quiet and nonverbal person may be observed rapidly blinking with slight facial grimacing; and the friendly, outgoing individual might become agitated and combative. The elder who usually is involved in activities may cry easily and withdraw from activities, or the elder may rhythmically rock back and forth (Matteson et al, 1995; McCaffery, Pasero, 1999). It is important to remember that the inability to interpret or detect pain in elders who cannot and do not communicate can lead to undertreatment of pain. At present, tools for assessing pain in those who are nonverbal are not particularly satisfactory (Marzinski, 1991; Saxon, 1991); however, strides have been made to improve the assessment of pain for the cognitively impaired. Some of the present tools have been tried with the cognitively impaired and have shown that some of these elders are able to indicate their pain to the care provider. In long-term care settings, nurses who continually care for a group of cognitively impaired elders know their patients' behavior and idiosyncrasies, which helps to pick out pain cues (Parke, 1998) (see Box 17-7). Research in this area continues.

Culture and gender are additional factors that make pain assessment more difficult and complex. Box 17-8 highlights some culturally oriented responses to pain. Gender responses to pain are a relatively new area of consideration. Until recently, it has been thought by nurses and physicians that women should receive smaller doses of opioid analgesics than men. Nurses believed that gender differences affected sensitivity to pain (Ferrell et al, 1992). Gender-related variations in pain perception may be physiologic rather than psychologic differences in willingness to report pain (Vallerand, 1995; McCaffery, Pasero, 1999).

Assessment tools have been developed to help both clinicians and researchers measure, document, and

Box 17-8	CULTURALLY ORIENTED RESPONSES TO PAIN

- Minimizes pain with significant others

  or

  Uses pain to elicit sympathy and support from others
- Carefully controls the expression of pain (calm and unemotional)

  or

  Is vocal about pain (cries or moans, complains)
- Withdraws and wants to be alone when pain is severe

  or

  Seeks attention and presence of others
- Willingly accepts pain relief measures

  or

  Avoids pain relief measures in the belief that they indicate weakness
- Wants and expects quick pain relief

  or

  Accepts pain for long periods before requesting help

Modified from Bates MS: *Biocultural dimensions of chronic pain,* 1996, State University of New York Press; Kosier B et al: *Fundamentals of nursing,* Redwood City, Calif, 1995, Addison-Wesley: and Salerno E, Willens JS: *Pain management handbook,* St Louis, 1996, Mosby.

communicate clients' pain experience more accurately when patients can communicate their pain. Qualitative tools are descriptive and express the patient's pain using pain diaries, pain logs, pain graphs, and observation. The diary and graph are particularly helpful in determining adequacy of pain management. The diary or pain log is a record written and kept by the patient. For these methods to be effective, the patient needs to carry a notebook and pencil to record pain as soon as possible after the pain episode. Such items as activity, intensity, and duration of the pain during daily activities; medications taken; and when they were taken should be recorded. The diary should be reviewed with the care provider to assess the relationship between pain, medication use, and activity. The pain graph provides a visual picture of the highs and lows of the pain. The caregiver can assist in the plotting of the pain experience when necessary.

Quantitative assessment tools use pain rating, such as a numerical rating scale (NRS), to help measure pain severity. Examples are the visual analog scale (VAS) and the verbal descriptor scale (VDS). The McGill Pain Assessment Questionnaire (Melzack, 1975) is a comprehensive tool that is useful for initial intake pain as-

sessments if the client is not in acute distress. The questionnaire asks about past pain experience, medications used, other treatments tried, the current pain episode, the effect of pain on activity and work, and the quality and location of pain. The tool relies heavily on verbal descriptors and cognitive capacity and takes a long time to administer.

McCaffery and Pasero (1999) present an initial pain assessment tool that can be completed by the patient or with the help of the caregiver (Fig. 17-4). The obtained information is similar to but uses a different format than the McGill questionnaire. Several versions of the VAS can be used to quantify pain severity. One variant scale uses a 10-cm line with a zero (no pain) at the left end and 10 (worst pain) at the right end. Patients are asked to indicate where on the line they would place their pain. Another variation places the numbers 0 through 10 at 1-cm intervals along the baseline. Zero indicates no pain, 5 is labeled moderate pain, and 10 remains the worst pain. The Descriptive Pain Intensity Scale uses the same principle and graduates the description of pain from no pain to mild, moderate, severe, very severe, and worst possible pain. Elders have been found to do better with the vertical rather than the horizontal VAS scale. Fig. 17-5 illustrates the VAS scale and its variations.

A pain color scale is another approach to learning a client's degree of pain. Stewart (1977) designed a color variation for children that can be used with adults and elders as well. The scale goes from yellow-orange to red-black with verbal descriptors of no pain at the yellow end and worst pain at the black end. Providing a body outline and colored markers is another approach to learning the intensity of a client's pain. Four marker pens or crayons are used to pinpoint the pain on a body outline (Eland, 1988). Each color represents a degree of pain: none, mild, moderate, or worst pain. This is a useful tool for an individual who has difficulty with language. Using these tools, the nurse can obtain a fairly accurate idea of the degree of discomfort or pain. The existing tools for pain assessment should be adapted for the elderly as was noted with the VAS, based on their verbal, physical, and cognitive capabilities. When a person is unable to tolerate lengthy questioning, a quick assessment should be done (Box 17-9, p. 384).

Ascertain the location, quality, intensity, and chronology of the pain. Rather than ask questions, have the patient describe the pain. Leading questions often give the nurse inaccurate information. Patients frequently answer according to what they think the nurse expects to hear. Elements of a complete pain assess-

INITIAL PAIN ASSESSMENT TOOL

Date _____

Patient's name _____ Age _____ Room _____

Diagnosis _____ Physician _____

Nurse _____

I. LOCATION: Patient or nurse mark drawing.

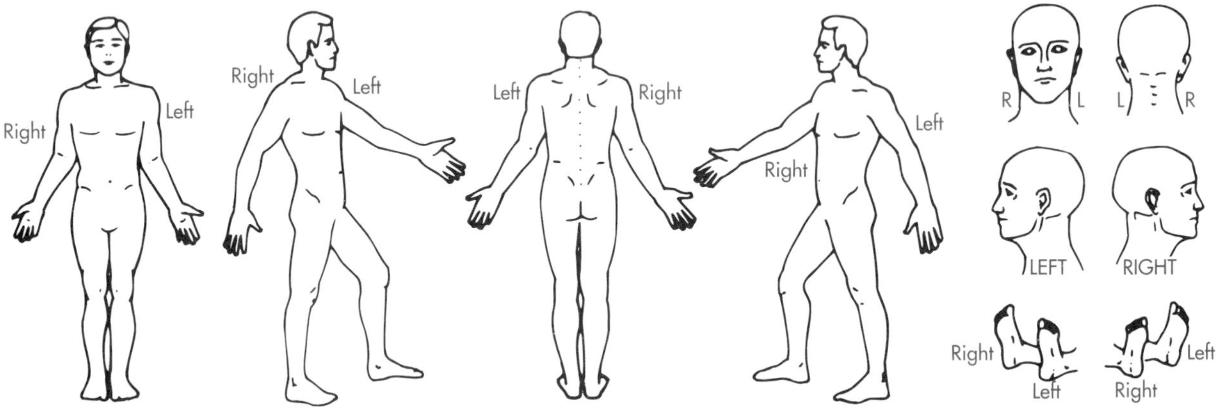

Right · Left · Right · Left · Left · Right · Left · Right · Left · Right · R · L · L · R · LEFT · RIGHT · Right · Left · Left · Right

II. INTENSITY: Patient rates the pain. Scale used _____

    Present: _____

    Worst pain gets: _____

    Best pain gets: _____

    Acceptable level of pain: _____

III. QUALITY: (Use patient's own words, e.g., *prick, ache, burn, throb, pull, sharp.*) _____

IV. ONSET, DURATION VARIATIONS, RHYTHMS: _____

V. MANNER OF EXPRESSING PAIN: _____

VI. WHAT RELIEVES THE PAIN? _____

VII. WHAT CAUSES OR INCREASES THE PAIN? _____

VIII. EFFECTS OF PAIN: (Note decreased function, decreased quality of life.) _____

    Accompanying symptoms (e.g., nausea) _____

    Sleep _____

    Appetite _____

    Physical activity _____

    Relationship with others (e.g., irritability) _____

    Emotions (e.g., anger, suicidal, crying) _____

    Concentration _____

    Other _____

IX. OTHER COMMENTS: _____

X. PLAN: _____

Fig. 17-4 Pain assessment. (From McCaffery M, Bebee A: *Pain: clinical manual of nursing practice,* St Louis, 1989, Mosby.)

Pain Distress Scales

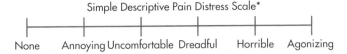

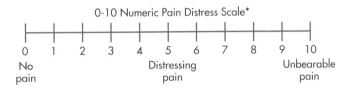

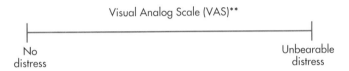

*If used as a graphic rating scale, a 10-cm baseline is recommended.
**A 10-cm baseline is recommended for VAS scales.

Fig. 17-5   Example of pain distress scale. (From *Acute pain management,* Clinical Practice Guideline, AHCPR Pub No 92-0032, Rockville, Md, 1992, US Department of Health and Human Services, Public Health Service, Agency for Health Care Policy and Research.)

ment include an accurate history, physical examination (attention to musculoskeletal and nervous systems, palpation of trigger points), functional assessment (one of several available evaluations of activities of daily living), and psychologic assessment (mini mental status examination).

Nurses must seek answers to the following questions to intervene most effectively:

- Is the elder concerned about the pain sensation itself or about the future implications of pain?
- Is the elder afraid that the pain indicates fatal illness or that the pain does or will deprive him or her of some specific pleasures of life?
- Does the elder want to be asked about the pain or not be reminded of it?
- Does the elder want to be alone for fear of showing an emotional response, or does he or she want to be alone because of having his or her own method of handling pain?
- Does the elder want visitors to share the pain or to use visitors as a distraction?

- Does the elder expect to obtain relief immediately or to suffer for a while?
- Does it matter to the elder if relief is palliative or curative?
- Does the elder believe that drugs are unnatural pain relief measures or fear the consequences of addictive drugs?
- Does crying mean that the elder wants immediate pain relief or sympathy, or is it a desire for a demonstration of technical skill?
- Does the elder view the expression of pain as natural (serving a particular purpose) or as indicative of defeat?

In addition, assessment should consider how the pain interferes with the patient's ability to meet needs of security, belonging, socialization, and self-esteem. The older adult who considers himself or herself strong and courageous may find it very humiliating to be forced to whimper or cry out with pain. What does the person want to be able to do? How does the person feel about himself or herself? Is the pain a mask for depres-

Box 17-9	QUICK ASSESSMENT IN SITUATIONS WHERE PATIENTS ARE UNABLE TO TOLERATE LENGTHY QUESTIONS

Time involved. Reading time, 5 minutes; implementation time, about 10 minutes.

Sample situation. Mr. M., 65 years old, with lung cancer and widespread metastasis, is admitted to your floor. He is not able to concentrate long enough to answer many questions. he grimaces frequently and cries out, saying, "It hurts, please give me something." His wife states that he is not swallowing anything by mouth.

Possible solution. Assess pain with minimal number of questions in order to give initial analgesic safely.

Expected outcome. Patient states he is comfortable. Further pain assessment is completed at a later time so that a detailed plan of care may be implemented.

Tell the patient that you are going to work to get him comfortable as quickly as possible but that you must get some information first:

1. Point (on his body) to where the pain is. Mr. M. points to his lower back.
2. Is this the same location for the pain over the last several days?
   Mr. M. says that this is the same area that has bothered him over the last week, but it has gotten much worse since yesterday evening.

3. On a 0 to 10 scale (0 = no pain, 10 = worst pain), what number would you give your pain right now? Mr. M. becomes very agitated and yells "It is unbearable." This is a good enough answer under the circumstances.
4. What medication were you taking at home, and did it help the pain?
   Mrs. M. tells you that her husband was taking morphine 90 mg q4h with Motrin 800 mg q6h. He has not been able to swallow anything since last night, so he has had nothing for pain since then. Prior to this, the medication was keeping the pain well controlled.

Due to Mr. M.'s condition, it was appropriate to ask only the most essential questions to initiate an analgesic regimen. The above four questions give you important baseline data and establish an initial narcotic dose.

Using a flow sheet, the immediate goal is to establish pain control quickly. Using Mr. M.'s words, ask, "Is the pain more bearable now?" Once Mr. M. is comfortable, additional questions from the initial pain assessment tool may be filled in and a long-term plan of care may be reviewed with the patient and his wife.

From McCaffery M, Bebee A: *Pain: clinical manual of nursing practice,* St Louis, 1989, Mosby.

sion, of which one is unaware? Does the person feel useless, dependent, or isolated? Has the pain changed interpersonal relationships? Finally, can you, the nurse, help control the pain so that the individual can do what is most important to him or her?

As a participant and observer in the elder's care, the nurse may not be overtly aware of the influences that the patient's pain experience has on him or her. If the elder patient is in control of the pain, it has a calming effect on the caregiver who observes and ministers. If the elder patient's pain is uncontrollable, it makes the caregiver agitated and irritated (Meinhart, McCaffery, 1983; Watt-Watson, Donovan, 1992), thus coloring the ability to accurately assess pain. Another impediment to accurate pain assessment is that the patient perceives pain as being more severe than do the caregivers, namely, physicians and nurses. Cultural expectations of the caregiver and preconceived gender expectations also affect the accuracy of assessment (Kosier et al, 1995; Vallerand, 1995; McCaffery, Pasero, 1999).

Interventions

Approximately half the adults who undergo surgery continue to have pain after surgery as a result of the common practice of prn dosing of IM opioids. Also, the nurse often refrains from giving narcotics to the elderly because of the fear of patient complications and misbeliefs about pain management (see Table 17-2 and Box 17-2). Needless suffering takes a toll physiologically and psychologically. These problems were addressed by the U.S. Department of Health and Human Services, Agency for Health Care Policy and Research, which after extensive research established national guidelines, with intervention strategies, for the management of pain. These guidelines, published in 1992, are intended to help health professionals improve the effectiveness of pain management for their patients. A brief summary of the guidelines appears in Box 17-10.

Pain can be minimized through gentle handling and touch. Use of pillows for support or body positioning, just sitting and holding the patient's hand, or allowing

From *Acute pain management,* Clinical Practice Guideline, AHCPR Pub No 920032, Rockville, Md, 1992, US Department of Health and Human Services, Public Health Service, Agency for Health Care Policy and Research.

Box 17-10   AGENCY FOR HEALTH CARE POLICY AND RESEARCH GUIDELINES

1. A collaborative, interdisciplinary approach to pain control, including all members of the health care team, and input from the patient and the patient's family, when appropriate
2. An individualized proactive pain control plan developed preoperatively by patients and practitioners (since pain is easier to prevent than to bring under control, once it has begun)
3. Assessment and frequent reassessment of the patient's pain
4. Use of both drug and nondrug therapies to control and/or prevent pain
5. A formal institutional approach to management of acute pain, with clear lines of responsibility

the individual to move at his or her own speed provides pain relief benefit.

PCA devices have not been used as extensively with elders in the acute care setting as they have with other adult patients. This may be based on criteria that require the user of a PCA device to be alert, mentally intact, and able to follow simple directions. In addition, elders with multisystem involvement are at high risk for respiratory and renal complications (Salerno, Willens, 1996). However, many elders meet the PCA criteria and still do not receive pain control with the PCA device (Matteson et al, 1995). It is therefore important that if elders are not given PCA access that they receive ATC pain control.

Activity can be helpful in several ways. Gaumer (1974) indicates that the less active an individual is, the less tolerable activity becomes. Anyone who becomes inactive will feel more aches and pain than the active person. Distraction through the use of activity may help to change the behavior of the individual who uses pain to gain attention and sympathy. It is important to identify activities that are compatible with the relief of anxiety. Use of analgesics in conjunction with activity is necessary. Administering a medication 20 to 30 minutes before a specific activity that elicits pain or giving an analgesic during activity to lessen or eliminate fear

of discomfort after activity can greatly enhance the individual's capacity for that activity. The nurse should learn the patient's body potential for coping with pain and work within those parameters.

The patient can be involved by keeping a weekly journal that includes an account of pain during the day; the times, type, and dose of medication taken; its effect; and the duration of its benefit. This type of information helps establish patterns that may be useful in improving pain management by adjusting activity, providing medications appropriately, and helping the patient feel useful and in control of some aspect of care.

The nurse's involvement in psychologic modulation of pain is in providing understanding and support for patients and in learning and practicing relaxation techniques through which the nurse can guide the patient and other psychologic practices that promote patient relaxation and coping with pain. McCaffery (1979), Meinhart and McCaffery (1983), and McCaffery and Pasero (1999) suggest guidelines for individualizing pain control measures:
1. Use a variety of pain control measures.
2. Institute pain control measures before pain becomes severe.
3. Consider patients' ideas about what they feel is most effective in controlling pain when making the nursing care plan.
4. Consider patients' ability or willingness to participate in their pain control.
5. Listen to how patients describe the severity of pain. Physical signs and perceived severity are not predictably related.
6. Be aware that patients respond differently to different pain control measures. What is effective one day may not be effective the next day.
7. Encourage patients to use a pain control method more than one time. Repeated use may prove effective. A patient's bill of rights for pain appears in Box 17-11.

Whether the pain is brief or long-standing, or the anticipated result of a diagnostic procedure or surgery, a pain plan should be initiated. This should begin with a discussion between the nurse or physician and the patient about how much pain there might be and how long it might last, along with how it will be treated and what alternatives are available if the initial treatment does not adequately relieve the pain. In addition, for those who leave the hospital with pain or who have chronic pain such as cancer, the plan should include the medications (including when, how many, how often, and how they should be taken); medications to be used if there are side effects; actions to ward off complications of medication therapy, such as constipation or nausea; any other pertinent instructions; and important numbers to call if necessary (Managing Pain, 1996; Managing Chronic Pain, 1996). One type of pain control plan appears in Box 17-12.

Evaluation

Evaluation of outcomes requires reassessment of the patient's pain status. Physical indicators may include relaxation of skeletal muscles, which during pain were tense and rigid. The individual no longer assumes a constricted pain posture. Behavior may reflect an increased activity level, a sense of self-worth, the ability to concentrate or focus better, and increased attention span. The individual is more able to rest, relax, and sleep. In fact, the individual may sleep for what might seem like excessively long periods, but this is a response to the exhaustion that pain imposes on the body.

Verbal indicators during conversation reflect the patient's referring to the decrease in pain or the absence of pain.

COMMON CAUSES OF CHRONIC PAIN IN THE ELDERLY

Nearly 90% of adults by the age of 50 have degenerative abnormalities of the lower spine. One of the most typical abnormalities is thinning of the intervertebral disks, which can eventually lead to arthritis and other painful conditions (Low Back Pain, 1989). Geriatric clients with chronic nonmalignant pain from musculoskeletal disorders have generally been treated pharmacologically without consideration of the multidimensional, multidisciplinary rehabilitation programs that are frequently offered to younger patients. For some unknown reason, many of these rehabilitation programs exclude individuals over 55 years of age. Middaugh et al (1988) debunked the bias that elderly patients do not benefit from such rehabilitation programs. The Middaugh study, using a group of young and old patients with chronic pain, showed that geriatric patients had as good, if not better, results than the younger group of patients. The study attributes some of the improvement that occurred to a high level of compliance, realistic expectations, and a lack of work-related obligations.

Osteoarthritis

Osteoarthritis is one of the most common forms of joint disease, with its prevalence increasing during the eighth decade. It is the leading cause of disability in persons 65 years of age and older (Ettinger, 1995). Joint pain and stiffness are initially intermittent and then can become constant. Pain is characterized by aching in the joints, surrounding muscles, and soft tissue; it is usually relieved by rest and exacerbated by activity. Such joints as the distal and proximal interphalangeal joints, cervical and lumbar spine, hips, knees, and toes are affected. Many older adults have other medical conditions in addition to osteoarthritis, which requires that the total picture be considered when the arthritic pain is treated. Generally, treatment consists of antiinflammatory preparations such as aspirin or other NSAIDs. Care must be taken when using antiinflammatory drugs with the older adult because they can have an adverse effect on the gastrointestinal lining. Acetaminophen, although not as effective as antiinflammatory preparations, is

Box 17-12   PAIN CONTROL PLAN

Pain Control Plan for _____

At home, I will take the following medications for pain control:

Medication	How to take	How many	How often	Comments

Medicines that I may take to help side effects:

Side effect	Medicine	How to take	How many	How often	Comments

Constipation is a very common problem when taking opioid medication. When this happens, do the following:
_____ Increase fluid intake (8 to 10 glasses of fluid per day)
_____ Exercise regularly
_____ Increase fiber in diet (bran, fresh fruit, vegetables)
_____ Use a mild laxative, such as milk of magnesia, if no nondrug pain control methods

If you do not have a bowel movement in 3 days:
_____ Take _____ every day at _____ (time) with a full glass of water.
_____ Use a glycerine suppository every morning (this may help make a bowel movement less painful).

Additional instructions:
_____
_____

Important phone numbers:
Your doctor _____   Your nurse _____
Your pharmacy _____   Emergencies _____

Call your doctor or nurse immediately if your pain increases or if you have new pain. Also call your doctor early for a refill of pain medication. Do not let your medication get below 3 or 4 days' supply.

From *Managing cancer pain,* consumer version, Clinical Practice Guideline, AHCPR Pub No 9, Rockville, Md, 1994, US Department of Health and Human Services, Public Health Service, Agency for Health Care Policy and Research.

preferred to salicylates, but consideration must be paid to the effect on liver and kidney function when it is used with the elderly. Effective pain relief can be achieved without the risk of gastric irritation or potential for gastric hemorrhage. Topical capsaicin may also reduce osteoarthritis pain. It is necessary to warn persons using capsaicin to wash their hands after application and to keep their hands away from their eyes. It is also important to tell patients to expect a strong sensation of burning. Nonpharmacologic pain management includes application of moist heat to relieve pain, spasm, and stiffness; orthotic devices such as braces and splints to support painful joints; weight reduction if the patient is overweight or obesity is a contributing factor; and oc-cupational and physical therapy. Severe arthritis with unrelieved pain and extensive disability may require local anesthetics and corticosteroid injections into joints or epidural spaces for lumbar pain or joint replacement for intractable pain.

Herpes Zoster (Shingles) and Postherpetic Neuralgia

Herpes zoster is a reactivation of the varicella virus (chickenpox), which affects mostly adults between the ages of 60 and 79. It has been estimated that about 50% of people who live to the age of 80 will have an attack of shingles (Gilchrest, 1995). Why shingles occur remains unclear, but those who are aged, immunocom-promised, have a malignancy, experience trauma, have surgery, or receive local radiation are more susceptible (Gilchrest, 1995). Shingles may also be due to a de-crease in cellular immune response to the varicella zoster antigen, which is undetected in up to 30% of pre-viously immune healthy elders over age 60. A pro-drome of itching, tingling, and aching or sharp pain oc-curs several days before the eruption of vesicles that follow a unilateral dermatome of the thorax, at the oph-thalmic nerve root of the trigeminal nerve (forehead), and at other, less common nerve roots. The herpes zoster vesicle pustules eventually rupture and crust in 10 days to 3 weeks. Until the crusting occurs, the indi-vidual is highly contagious to others who have no im-munity to chickenpox.

Treatment is essential as soon as shingles is identi-fied either in the prodromal phase, which is quite diffi-cult and often misleading, or immediately on vesicular eruption to prevent or limit postherpetic neuralgia (PHN).

PHN is experienced because of irritation of the nerve roots that leave the spinal cord. It occurs 1 to 3 months after crusting of the lesions. Age, severity of the out-break, co-morbid depression, and somatization are pre-dictors of the prevalence of the intractable pain. PHN will be experienced by 10% to 15% of patients after an acute episode of shingles has occurred (Nossel, 1996). The pain of postherpetic neuralgia has been described as a continuous deep burning, aching, bruising pain; paroxysmal (sudden) lancing pain; or pain that is elec-trical shock–like or stabbing in nature, which can last for weeks or months or, for some elderly, indefinitely. Abnormal cutaneous pain may occur outside the initial herpetic area.

Treatment for PHN includes opioids, antiviral drugs, and nerve blocks. Adjuvant therapies such as antide-pressants (desipramine is considered one of the safe tri-cyclic drugs for use with the elderly) and anticonvul-sants have been effective. Combinations of medication (antiviral medications, steroids, aspirin, and topical anesthetics for pain) have shown effectiveness but vary with the individual. The U.S. Food and Drug Adminis-tration (FDA) has approved such prescription medica-tions as acyclovir and famciclovir, which shorten the duration of chronic shingle pain, and capsaicin (Zostrix) as an over-the-counter topical anesthetic (Reyes, 1994). As in other pain control situations, med-ications should be titrated to establish the most effec-tive pain relief for the older adult. The use of cold ap-plications may provide relief, or TENS may be of value

but should be carefully used with the elderly (Portenoy, 1995; Watt-Watson, Donovan, 1992). Primary preven-tion of shingles (herpes zoster) and the subsequent PHN may be attainable in the future with widespread varicella immunization of children. For those older adults who as children endured chickenpox, a new vari-cella vaccine to prevent shingles is being tested; how-ever, it will not be available until around the year 2005 if testing proves successful (Health News, 1999). Treat-ment in the early eruption stage of herpes zoster pre-vents or limits the dissemination of vesicles and her-petic pain. This is particularly helpful for immuno-suppressed individuals.

Terminal Cancer

Terminal cancer pain requires a thorough understand-ing of the dynamics of pain management. The nurse cannot be caught in the assumption that frequent use of analgesic drugs will create iatrogenic addiction, nor should placebos ever be used for cancer pain. The es-sential issue is adequate pain relief. Key to this relief is providing medication on time without the necessity of the patient asking for pain medication. Standard nar-cotic preparations or mixtures are effective. Present-day preparations contain morphine or methadone. Ad-juvant medications are valuable additions when necessary to control pain and other symptoms produced by the disease and to decrease the level of anxiety. Un-der no circumstance is a placebo justified for use with determining or treating cancer pain (McCaffery, Ritchey, 1992; Fox, 1994; Goldstein, 1999).

In addition, invasive anesthetics and neurosurgical or neurostimulating approaches may be used. Newer in-traspinal pain relief approaches are used to relieve pain below the midthorax. This requires persons with special expertise.

Pain management entails control of not only physi-cal pain of the patient, but also emotional, psychologic, and spiritual pain. The concept of the cycle of pain, anxiety, and anguish is crucial to successful manage-ment of pain in terminal cancer. Reduction or relief of anxiety can be achieved by allowing the individual some control over the pain situation. Self-medication is an important method. Teaching the patient about his or her medication and allowing the patient to administer the medication and keep dosage records are ways of eliminating the fear that medication will not arrive on time and that the patient may have to suffer until some-one arrives to provide relief. Obviously, not all patients can administer their own medication, but the potential

Table 17-7

Management of Chronic Opioid Administration Side Effects

Constipation	Start patient on a bowel regimen containing docusate sodium 100-200 mg 2 or 3 times a day and senna (1-2 tablets at bedtime). Maintain adequate fluid intake. Provide increased roughage, if tolerated, in diet.
Respiratory depression	Not a major problem with long-term use of opioids. If respiratory depression occurs, withhold dose of opioid and stimulate patient. If opioid antagonist required, dilute 1 ampule (0.4 mg) of naloxone in 10 ml normal saline and administer slowly, titrating the drug to the patient's respiratory rate.
Sedation	Sometimes this side effect is difficult to avoid. Dextroamphetamine in doses of 2.5-5 mg twice a day may be helpful.
Nausea and vomiting	Administer antiemetics as needed.

From Miaskowski C: Current concepts in the assessment and management of cancer related pain, *Med Surg Nurs* 2(1): 113-118, 1993.

is there, and each situation must be assessed on an individual basis. The following guidelines facilitate individualized pain control regimens (see Fig. 17-3):

- Use the simplest dosage schedule and least invasive pain management modalities first.
- For mild to moderate pain, use aspirin (unless contraindicated), acetaminophen, or NSAIDs (step 1).
- When pain persists or increases, add an opioid (step 2).
- If pain continues or becomes moderate to severe, increase the opioid potency or dose (step 3).
- Schedule drugs on a regular schedule (ATC) to maintain a drug level that will help prevent recurrence of pain. (Ask the patient and family to help in establishing the effective level.)

- Administer medications for long-term cancer pain on an ATC basis with additional doses "as needed."

A flow sheet, kept by the patient or staff to rate pain on a scale of 0 to 10, provides the information to individually titrate the medication to the patient's pain need. Studies have shown that effective control of pain (attention to the psychologic, emotional, spiritual, and physical distress) in many instances has reduced the amount of medication needed.

Measures used to diminish side effects associated with long-term opioid use must be considered early in conjunction with pain management. These side effects are constipation, respiratory distress, sedation, and nausea and vomiting (Miaskowski, 1999). Table 17-7 suggests interventions to minimize these side effects.

• • •

The nurse need not look on pain with fear and trepidation. If assessment is correct and the patient is listened to and handled gently and with care, anxiety can be controlled and interventions will be more effective.

▶ KEY CONCEPTS

- The absence of pain does not necessarily imply comfort. Comfort is a state of ease and satisfaction of bodily wants, as well as freedom from pain and anxiety.
- The nurse's response to an elder's pain is influenced by the nurse's ability to imaginatively identify with another and by how well the other is known. Nurses, like others, feel less concern for a stranger than for a loved one.
- Culture, ethnicity, family, and individual characteristics all influence one's tolerance and expression of pain.
- Aged individuals with various degrees of cognitive impairment may demonstrate pain by increased levels of confusion, restlessness, or withdrawal.
- Although it is sometimes assumed, it has not been shown that pain sensitivity and perception decrease with age.
- Pain is whatever the elder says it is. The nursing goal is to assist in pain relief. Some pain medications are more appropriate than others for use with elders.

NANDA and Wellness Diagnoses

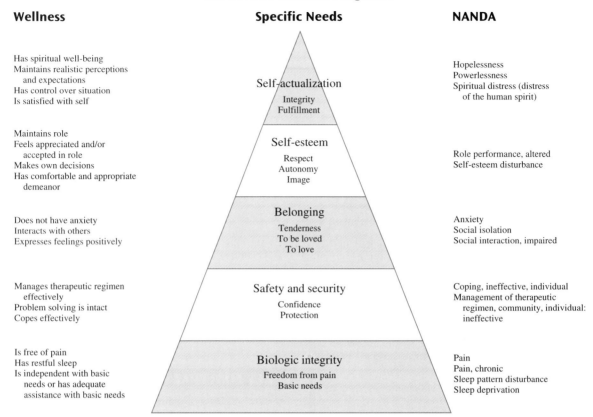

Wellness   **Specific Needs**   **NANDA**

Has spiritual well-being
Maintains realistic perceptions
  and expectations
Has control over situation
Is satisfied with self

Self-actualization
Integrity
Fulfillment

Hopelessness
Powerlessness
Spiritual distress (distress
  of the human spirit)

Maintains role
Feels appreciated and/or
  accepted in role
Makes own decisions
Has comfortable and appropriate
  demeanor

Self-esteem
Respect
Autonomy
Image

Role performance, altered
Self-esteem disturbance

Does not have anxiety
Interacts with others
Expresses feelings positively

Belonging
Tenderness
To be loved
To love

Anxiety
Social isolation
Social interaction, impaired

Manages therapeutic regimen
  effectively
Problem solving is intact
Copes effectively

Safety and security
Confidence
Protection

Coping, ineffective, individual
Management of therapeutic
  regimen, community, individual:
  ineffective

Is free of pain
Has restful sleep
Is independent with basic
  needs or has adequate
  assistance with basic needs

Biologic integrity
Freedom from pain
Basic needs

Pain
Pain, chronic
Sleep pattern disturbance
Sleep deprivation

These are not all of the possible wellness or NANDA diagnoses that may be identified. The above are frequent examples of nursing diagnoses that should be considered when planning care for the older adult in whatever setting.

- Acute pain and chronic pain require different therapeutic approaches. Chronic pain predominates in the life of the aged.
- Various combinations of pharmacologic and nonpharmacologic pain control can be effective but must be individually designed with the elder involved in the decision making.
- Giving a placebo (inert substance disguised as medication) "is never justified to determine the existence of pain" (McCaffery, Ritchy, 1992).
- Real placebo effects are a part of all successful pain management and incorporate the belief in efficacy by the elder and caregiver and the acceptability of the substance or action.

▶ Activities and Discussion Questions

1. What is pain?
2. Compare the features of acute and chronic pain.
3. List data necessary for an accurate pain assessment.
4. What are the barriers that interfere with assessment and treatment of pain?
5. What pharmacologic and nonpharmacologic therapy is available, and how can each type work with the other to relieve pain?
6. Develop a nursing care plan using wellness and NANDA diagnoses.

RESOURCES

American Chronic Pain Association
  PO Box 850
  Rocklin, CA 95677
  (916) 632-0922
American Society of Pain Management Nurses
  (404) 279-9022
National Chronic Pain Outreach Association, Inc.
  4922 Hampden Lane
  Bethesda, MD 20814
  (310) 652-4988
Acute Pain Management of Adults: Operative Procedure, Quick
  Reference Guide for Clinicians, AHCPR Pub No 92-0019.
  Available from AHCPR Publications Clearing House, PO Box
  8547, Silver Spring, MD 20907.

REFERENCES

*Acute pain management: operative or medical procedures and
  trauma,* Clinical Practice Guideline, Rockville, Md, 1992, US
  Department of Health and Human Services, Public Health
  Service, Agency for Health Care Policy and Research..

American Pain Society: *Principles of analgesic use in the treatment
  of acute and cancer pain,* ed 3, Skokie, Ill, 1992, The Society.

Bates MS: *Biocultural dimensions of chronic pain,* 1996, Albany
  State University of New York Press.

Boczkowski JA: Biofeedback training for the treatment of chronic
  pain in the elderly arthritic female, *Clin Gerontol* 2:39, 1984.

California Board of Registered Nursing (BRN): BRN focuses on
  pain management, *BRN Rep* 10(1):12, 1997.

Davies P: Pharmacological management of pain in the elderly,
  Analgesia 7(1):4, 1996.

Davis GC: Chronic pain management of older adults in residential settings, *J Gerontol Nurs* 23(6):16, 1997.

Eland JM: Pain management and comfort, *J Gerontol Nurs* 14:10,
  1988.

Ettinger HW: Joint and soft tissue disorders. In Abrams WB,
  Beers MH, Berkow R, editors: *The Merck manual of geri-
  atrics,* ed 2, Whitehouse Station, NJ, 1995, Merck Research
  Laboratories.

Federwisch A: Complete assessment: making pain the fifth vital
  sign, *NurseWeek* 12(14): 23, 1999.

Feldt KS: Examining pain in aggressive cognitively impaired
  older adults, *J Gerontol Nurs* 24(11):15, 1998.

Ferrell BA: Pain management in elderly people, *J Gerontol Soc*
  39(1):64, 1991.

Ferrell BA, McCaffrey M, Rhiner M: Does the gender gap affect
  your pain control decisions? *Nursing 92* (8):48, 1992.

Ferrell BR, Ferrell BA: Easing pain, *Geriatr Nurs* 11(5):175,
  1990.

Fox AE (pseudonym): Confronting the use of placebos for pain,
  Am J Nurs 94(9):42, 1994.

Fulmer TT et al: Pain management protocol, *Geriatr Nurs*
  17(5):222, 1996.

Gaumer WC: Psychological potentials of chronic pain, *J Psychiatr Nurs* 12:23, 1974.

Gilchrest BA: Skin changes and disorders. In Abrams WB, Beers
  MH, Berkow R, editors: *The Merck manual of geriatrics,* ed 2,
  Whitehouse Station, NJ, 1995, Merck Research Laboratories.

Gloth FM: Concerns with chronic analgesic therapy in elderly patients, *Am J Med* 101(suppl 1A):19S-24S, 1996.

Goldstein ML: Cancer-related pain. In McCaffery M, Pasero C,
  editors: *Pain: clinical manual,* ed 2, St Louis, 1999, Mosby.

Gray BB: Managed care policies affect nurses' ability to provide
  pain management, *NurseWeek* 9(3):1, 1996.

Griffin M: In the mind's eye, *Am J Nurs* 86:804, 1986.

Hamilton J: Comfort and the hospitalized chronically ill, *J Gerontol Nurs* 15(4):28, 1989.

Hamm BH, King V: A holistic approach to pain control with geriatric clients, *J Holistic Nurs* 11:32, 1984.

Health news, NBC TV, Channel 4, Aug 5, 1999.

Hofland SL: Elder beliefs: blocks and pain management, *J Gerontol Nurs* 18(6):19, 1992.

International Association for the Study of Pain: *Pain,* 6, 249,
  1979, The Association.

International Association for the Study of Pain: *Pain,* 1992, The
  Association.

Jacox AK: Assessing pain, *Am J Nurs* 79:895, 1979.

Kassalaroen S et al: Pain and cognitive status in institutionalized
  elderly, *J Gerontol Nurs* 24(8):24, 1998.

Kastner M: Researching massage as real therapy, *Massage Ther J*
  33(3):56, 1994.

Kosier B et al: *Fundamentals of nursing: comfort and pain,* Redwood City, Calif, 1995, Addison-Wesley.

Kreiger D: *The therapeutic touch: how to use your hands to help
  or heal,* New York, 1992, Prentice-Hall.

Lavin MR: Placebo effects on mind and body, *JAMA* 265:1753,
  1991.

Low back pain: Part I, *Harvard Medical School Health Letter*
  15(1):5, 1989.

Mackey RB: Discover the healing power of therapeutic touch, *Am
  J Nurs* 95(4):27, 1995.

Managing chronic pain, *Focus Geriatr Care Rehabil* 10(3):1,
  1996.

Managing pain: medical essay, *Mayo Clin Health Lett* (suppl), pp
  1-8, June 1996.

Marzinski LR: The tragedy of dementia: clinically assessing pain
  in the confused, nonverbal elderly, *J Gerontol Nurs* 17(6):25,
  1991.

Matteson MA et al: *Pain in cognitively impaired older adults,*
  48th annual scientific meeting, Gerontological Society of
  America, Los Angeles, Calif, Oct 1995.

McCaffery M: *Nursing management of the patient with pain.*
  Philadelphia, 1979, Lippincott.

McCaffery M, Beebe A: *Pain: clinical manual for nursing practice,* St Louis, 1989, Mosby.

McCaffery M, Ferrell BR: Current placebo practice and policy,
  ASPMN Pathways 5(4):1, 12, winter 1996.

McCaffery M, Pasero C: *Pain: clinical manual,* ed 2, St Louis, 1999, Mosby.

McCaffery M, Ritchey KJ: Pain assessment: debunking the myths and misconceptions, *NurseWeek* 5(16):8, 1992.

Meinhart N, McCaffery M: *Pain: a nursing approach to assessment and analysis,* East Norwalk, Conn, 1983, Appleton-Century-Crofts.

Melzack R: The McGill pain questionnaire: major properties and scoring method, *Pain* 1:277, 1975.

Middaugh SJ et al: Chronic pain: its treatment in geriatric and young patients, *Arch Phys Med Rehabil* 69(12):1021, 1988.

Miaskowski C: Pain and comfort. In Stone JT, Wyman JF, Salisbury SA, editors: *Clinical gerontological nursing: a guide to advanced practice,* ed 2, Philadelphia, 1999, Saunders.

Nossel ME: Chronic nonmalignant pain management. In Salerno E, Willens JS, editors: *Pain management handbook,* St Louis, 1996, Mosby.

Pain relief, *University of California Berkeley Wellness Letter* 5(11):4, 1995.

Palmieri RL: Using TENS for pain management, *Patient Care Nurse Pract* 2(2):43, 1999.

Parke B: Gerontological nurses' ways of knowing, *J Gerontol Nurs* 24(6):21, 1998.

Pasero C, Gordon DB, McCaffery M: Pain control: JCAHO on assessing and managing pain, *Am J Nurs* 99(7):22, 1999a.

Pasero C, Paice JA, McCaffery M: Basic mechanisms underlying the causes and effects of pain. In McCaffery M, Pasero C, editors: *Pain: clinical manual,* ed 2, St Louis, 1999b, Mosby.

Pasero C, Reed BA, McCaffery M: Pain in the elderly. In McCaffery M, Pasero C, editors: *Pain: clinical manual,* ed 2, St Louis, 1999c, Mosby.

Pearson BD: Pain control: an experiment with imagery, *Geriatr Nurs* 13:28, 1988.

Portenoy RK: Pain. In Abrams WB, Beers MH, Berkow R, editors: *The Merck manual of geriatrics,* ed 2, Whitehouse Station, NJ, 1995, Merck Research Laboratories.

Portenoy RK, McCaffery M: Adjuvant analgesics. In McCaffery M, Pasero C, editors: *Pain: clinical manual,* ed 2, St Louis, 1999, Mosby.

Portenoy RK, Pasero C, McCaffery M: Opioid analgesics. In McCaffery M, Pasero C, editors: *Pain: clinical manual,* ed 2, St Louis, 1999, Mosby.

Reyes KW: Early treatment makes shingles easier to bear, *Mod Maturity* 36(6):79, Nov/Dec 1994.

Salerno E, Willens JS: *Pain management handbook,* St Louis, 1996, Mosby.

Sarvis CM: *Pain management in the elderly,* Sacramento, Calif, 1995, CME Resources.

Saxon SV: *Pain management techniques for older adults,* Springfield, Ill, 1991, Charles C Thomas.

Saxon SV, Etter MJ: *Physical changes and aging,* ed 3, New York, 1994, Tiresia.

Stewart ML: Measurement of clinical pain. In Jacox A, editor: *Pain: a resource book for nurses and other health professionals,* Boston, 1977, Little, Brown.

Thomas BL: Elder care: pain management for the elderly—alternative interventions, part I, *AORN J* 52(6):1268, 1990.

Todd B: The placebo effect: real or imaginary, *Geriatr Nurs* 8:154, 1987.

Vallerand AH: Gender differences in pain, *Image J Nurs Sch* 27(3):235, 1995.

Watt-Watson JH, Donovan MI: *Pain management: nursing perspective,* St Louis, 1992, Mosby.

Witt JR: Relieving chronic pain, *Nurse Pract* 9(1):36, 1984.

World Health Organization (WHO), 1990. In *Management of cancer pain: adults,* Quick Reference Guide for Clinicians No 9, AHCPR Pub No 94-0593, Rockville, Md, 1994, US Department of Health and Human Services, Public Health Service, Agency for Health Care Policy and Research.

Young DM: Pain in older adults: assessment, intervention, and outcomes, *Old News, Gerontological Nursing at the University of Iowa* 1(2):5, 1999.

chapter

18

Diabetes Mellitus and the Elderly

▶LEARNING OBJECTIVES

Upon completion of this chapter, the reader will be able to:

- Explain the risks for and complications of diabetes mellitus in the older adult.
- State what assessment is necessary to screen for diabetes mellitus and how diabetes is monitored in those with the disease.
- Explain the important components of diabetes management.
- Discuss the nurse's role in diabetes management.
- Develop a nursing care plan for the elder with diabetes.

▶GLOSSARY

Cell-mediated immunity In this chapter refers to an acquired resistance to insulin produced by the pancreas.

Hgb A$_{1c}$ Glycosylated hemoglobin; a blood test that measures the amount of glucose in the hemoglobin of red blood cells. This provides an accurate evaluation of therapeutic control for the previous 1 to 3 months.

Insulin resistance Body cells are insensitive to the insulin produced by the pancreas, thus impairing glucose metabolism.

Nomogram A graph with three parallel scales graduated for different variables. When a straight line connects any two variables, a related variable may be read.

▶THE LIVED EXPERIENCE

Now I'm really scared. I thought I was doing well until the doctor told me I was developing diabetes. I know what that means! Mother had gangrene, amputations, and loss of sight. Her last years were simply miserable. Believe me, I will do everything I'm told and try to keep this thing under control. I wonder if I will end up like Mother, or if there are better ways of taking care of diabetics now.

Anna, age 65

I can see that Anna is going to need a lot of help learning to manage her diabetes. I know now that I overwhelmed her with brochures and information right off. She just looked frightened to death, and she really just has a mild elevation in blood sugar; it should be controlled with diet and exercise. I will call her tomorrow and see if she is less anxious.

Anna's geriatric clinical nurse specialist

*D*iabetes mellitus is one of the most common chronic conditions affecting the elderly. It is estimated that 10% of the population of the United States has type 2 diabetes mellitus by age 65. Diabetes is present in 40% of those over the age of 80 (Kennedy-Malone et al, 2000). Of individuals 65 years and over who have diabetes, women experience it only slightly more often than men (US Bureau of the Census, 1995). Diabetes mellitus is a complex disorder of metabolism that affects lipid and protein metabolism, as well as glucose.

The American Diabetes Association redefined the old terminology of the two major types of diabetes: insulin-dependent diabetes mellitus (IDDM) is now referred to as *type 1 diabetes,* and non-insulin-dependent diabetes mellitus (NIDDM) is now called *type 2 diabetes.* Type 1 diabetes usually occurs in early life and is a result of total destruction of the insulin-producing beta cells of the pancreas. In this type of diabetes there is an absolute insulin deficit. The hallmark is cell-mediated autoimmunity. The hallmark of type 2 diabetes is elevated glucose—a result of resistance to insulin's metabolic effect from either the presence of fewer insulin receptors on cells or a deficit in receptor binding, or impaired insulin secretion by inadequate pancreatic beta cell function (Halter, 1999). The vast majority of older adults (90%) are diagnosed with type 2 diabetes.

A number of predisposing factors account for diabetes in the older adult: age-related insulin decrease, age-related insulin resistance, obesity, decreased physical activity, drugs, genetics, and coexisting illness.

An age-related glucose intolerance or a decline in sensitivity to the metabolic effect of insulin develops. Other mechanisms such as the insulin signal mechanism that goes beyond the receptors cause the mobilization of glucose transport necessary for glucose uptake and metabolism in insulin-dependent tissue (muscle and fat) and a decrease in activity associated with insulin resistance; however, physical activity such as exercise can increase insulin sensitivity. Coexisting illness such as hypertension or hyperlipidemia is associated with a decrease in insulin sensitivity. The question remains whether diabetes is a primary or secondary event when there is a coexisting illness. Any acute illness can precipitate an elevation of glucose attributable to stress on hormones. Drugs such as diuretics, glucocorticoids, nonsteroidal antiinflammatory drugs (NSAIDs), alcohol, and a number of others may also contribute to insulin resistance.

There are many bothersome aspects to diabetes, including the destructive aspects of the secondary changes that occur system wide in response to uncontrolled or poorly controlled diabetes. Gradually and insidiously, visual, vascular, and neurologic changes occur until the end stages, when the individual is blind and is suffering from cerebrovascular accidents, often amputations of the feet or legs, renal failure, and dementia. Diabetes is truly a chronic disease that, even in the best of circumstances, slowly and unremittingly progresses.

Holding back progression of the disease is the major goal. Good control of diabetes leads to significant prevention of microvascular complications and slows the progression of the disorder (Fonseca, Wall, 1995; Hernandez, 1998). As might be expected, poor perceptions of one's health, anxiety, and depression are frequent accompaniments of a diagnosis of diabetes (Bailey, 1996), and these may dishearten and discourage the individual from consistent self-management. Social support, mas-

tery, and self-esteem have been found to be the chief ameliorators of depression and anxiety surrounding the diagnosis and living with diabetes (Bailey, 1996). A holistic, qualitative approach to diabetes and more depth and breadth in nursing practice related to the care of the diabetic patient can facilitate improved health maintenance and adherence to recommended therapies.

Diabetes often hampers sexual function or leads to impotence in men as a result of reduction in vascular flow, peripheral neuropathy, and uncontrolled circulating blood glucose. Sexual dysfunction is two to five times greater in this group than in the general population, even though interest and desire are still present. Orgasmic and ejaculatory capacity usually remain unchanged. This situation presents a considerable psychologic problem for some men. The client may need counseling regarding sexual activity modifications to provide satisfaction by alternative methods. Once the diabetes is properly controlled, impotence may disappear in some individuals. Loss of sexual function does not seem to be a problem with women who have diabetes.

ASSESSMENT

Physiologic and psychologic stressors have been given far too little attention as precipitating and fulminating factors of type 2 diabetes. Screening for diabetes by fasting and random blood glucose testing is important for early identification of potential or actual disease, and it also serves as a monitoring tool in the management of diabetes. The overall health and financial benefits of early screening could save $100 billion in direct medical costs and indirect costs of premature death and disability (Genuth et al, 1998). Two thirds of all medical costs for diabetes mellitus occur with the older adult who has the disease.

Risk factors for which elders should be screened include the following:
- Blood pressure $\geq$140/90 mm Hg
- First-degree relative (parent, sibling, child) with diabetes
- History of impaired glucose tolerance or a fasting plasma glucose level $\geq$126 mg/dl and a random plasma glucose level $\geq$200 mg/dl or an oral 2-hour glucose tolerance test of $\geq$200*
- Member of a high-risk ethnic population: black, Asian, Hispanic, or Native American

---

*The glucose tolerance test is not considered a good test for screening (Gutowski, 1999; Halter, 1999).

Box 18-1	MEDICATIONS THAT MAY AFFECT BLOOD GLUCOSE LEVELS

Increase Blood Glucose Levels

Corticosteroids
Diazoxide
Estrogens
Furosemide and thiazide diuretics
Glucagon
Lithium
Phenytoin
Rifampin
Sympathomimetics (antihistamines, decongestants, bronchodilators)
Thyroid

Decrease Blood Glucose Levels

Alcohol
Anabolic steroids
Beta-blockers (antihypertensives)
Salicylates (high doses)

Interactions With Sulfonylureas (Oral Hypoglycemics)

Increased Effects (Lower Blood Glucose Levels Further)

Allopurinol
Beta-blockers

Increased Effects (Lower Blood Glucose Levels Further)—cont'd

Clofibrate
Histamine antagonists
Imidazole antifungals
Low-dose salicylates
Monamine oxidase inhibitors
Probenecid
Tricyclic antidepressants

Drugs Not to Be Taken in Combination With Sulfonylureas

Azapropazone
Chloramphenicol
Dicumarol
Oxyphenbutazone
Phenylbutazone
Salicylates (high dose)
Sulfonamides

Decreased Effects (Hinder Hypoglycemic Action)

Barbiturates
Corticosteroids
Diuretics
Estrogens
Rifampin

Summarized from unidentified source: handout at workshop, Chronic Disorders of the Aged, sponsored by Arizona State School of Nursing, Phoenix, Ariz, Sept 1992.

- Obesity ≥120% of desirable weight or a body mass index (BMI) ≥27 kg/m^2
- Previous gestational diabetes mellitus or having had a child with a birth weight of >9 pounds
- Undesirable lipid levels: high-density lipoproteins (HDLs) ≥35 mg/dl or triglycerides ≥250 mg/dl

Although screening should begin at age 45, many elders have not been adequately screened. Those who have a normal plasma glucose level on testing should be retested at 3-year intervals. If any of the risk factors (e.g., overweight or obesity) exist, the elder should be retested every year. The older adult should also receive education about weight reduction and regular exercise and be observed for symptoms of diabetes. An impaired fasting glucose (IFG) value of 110 to 126 mg/dl also increases the older adult's risk for heart disease. Other risk factors to be considered include medications that affect blood glucose concentration (Box 18-1), hypertension, atherosclerosis, smoking, stress, diet, socioeconomic factors, a seden-

Box 18-2	PREDISPOSING FACTORS FOR DIABETES MELLITUS

Age-related insulin decrease
Age-related insulin resistance
Coexisting illness
Genetic predisposition
Medications
Obesity
Sedentary life-style

tary life-style, and being female (Meadow, 1995; Fonseca, Wall, 1995).

The risk factors for diabetes must be included in the data collected when assessing for diabetes. Box 18-2 illustrates those factors that influence the development of diabetes and that should be kept in mind when seeking the history. In addition, the history should include the

| Box 18-3 | SIGNS AND SYMPTOMS SUGGESTIVE OF DIABETES IN THE ELDERLY |

1. General symptoms such as polyphagia, polyuria, polydipsia, and weight loss
2. Recurrent infections, particularly of bacterial/fungal origin, that involve the skin, intertriginous areas, or urinary tract and sores/wounds that tend to heal slowly
3. Neurologic dysfunction, including paresthesia, dysesthesia, or hyperesthesia; muscle weakness and pain (amyotrophy); cranial nerve palsies; and autonomic dysfunction of the gastrointestinal tract (diarrhea); cardiovascular system (orthostatic hypotension, dysrhythmias); reproductive system (impotence); and bladder (atony, overflow incontinence)
4. Arterial disease (macroangiopathy) involving the cardiovascular, cerebrovascular, or peripheral vasculature structures
5. Small-vessel disease (microangiopathy) involving the kidneys (proteinuria, glomerulopathy, uremia) and eyes (macular disease, exudates, hemorrhages)
6. Lesions of the skin, such as Dupuytren contractures, facial rubeosis, and diabetic dermopathy
7. Endocrine-metabolic complications, including hyperlipidemia, obesity, and a history of thyroid or adrenal insufficiency (Schmidt syndrome)
8. A family history of type 1 or type 2 diabetes and a poor obstetric history (miscarriages, stillbirths, large babies)

Data from Andres R, Bierman E, Hazzard W: *Principles of geriatric medicine,* New York, 1985, McGraw-Hill; and Davidson MB: Diabetes mellitus and other disorders of carbohydrate metabolism. In Abrams WB, Beers MH, Berkow R, editors: *The Merck manual of geriatrics,* ed 2, Whitehouse Station, NJ, 1995, Merck Research Laboratories.

presence or absence of symptoms that for the elderly may not be the usual polydipsia, polyuria, or polyphagia, but more vague symptoms such as fatigue, weight loss, varied infection, and often cataract formation, all of which most care providers and others consider part of "old age" but that may bode trouble if not investigated (Box 18-3). Elders often have diabetes approximately 7 years before diagnosis. By then, degenerative changes in the nervous, renal, and ocular systems have begun (Kennedy-Malone et al, 2000). When there are symptoms, the duration and character of the symptoms should be described. Family history is important because of the genetic influence. Nutrition, weight, and exercise history is important to identify eating patterns, an active or sedentary life-style, and weight control

measures, all of which can provide clues for realistic adjustment and better adherence to a therapy regimen. Economic status helps establish the ability to purchase needed equipment, materials, and foods that may be suggested to maintain diabetes control. Medication history of over-the-counter and prescription drugs (see Box 18-1) and use of alcohol and tobacco are also factors that provide important information in the assessment of the elder. All have a direct or indirect effect on renal, circulatory, neurologic, and nutritional function.

The objective data, the physical examination, should include height and weight. This should be plotted on a BMI nomogram to establish whether the elder is at risk for being underweight or overweight. A BMI $\geq$27 places the individual at risk for diabetes mellitus, heart disease, and obesity ($\geq$27 is overweight; $\geq$30 is obesity). Central fat should be measured, and this can easily be done by measuring the person at his or her natural waistline and also around the hips at the superior iliac crests and then dividing the hip measurement in centimeters into the waist measurement in centimeters. The resultant number will provide an indication of central fat. A normal measurement is 0.8 for women and 0.9 for men. The greater the figure above the norm, the higher the cardiac risk for the individual. This is consistent with the apple (central fat) and pear (peripheral fat) configurations (Seidel et al, 1999).

Blood pressure should be checked to establish normotensive or hypertensive status. Examination of the eyes for visual acuity by the Snellen chart and for near vision by reading of newsprint should be done, and if the patient is being assessed by a physician or an advanced practice nurse, an ophthalmologic examination should be performed to determine the integrity of the retina, vessels, and other internal structures of the eye. The skin and feet should be meticulously inspected for any breach of skin integrity, such as corns, calluses, blisters, fissures, or fungal infections. Clinical guidelines suggest that the best means of testing neurologic and sensory intactness is the use of the Semmes-Weinstein monofilament instrument. A vibrating tuning fork is used to establish the presence or absence of vibratory sensation (Bichler, 1999; Peters, 1998). These tests should be performed at least once a year. Assessment should also be alert to complications of diabetes.

COMPLICATIONS

Complications occur over the long term of the disease and are either microvascular or macrovascular in na-

Box 18-4	SIGNS AND BEHAVIORS THAT MAY INDICATE VISION PROBLEMS

Client May Report
Pain in eyes
Difficulty seeing in darkened area
Double vision/distorted vision
Migraine headaches coupled with blurred vision
Flashes of light
Halos surrounding lights

Staff May Notice
Getting lost
Bumping into objects
Straining to read or no reading
Stumbling/falling
Spilling food on clothing
Social withdrawal
Less eye contact
Placid facial expression
TV viewing at close range
Decreased sense of balance
Mismatched clothes

Modified from McNeely E, Griffin-Shirley N, Hubbard A: Diminished vision in nursing homes, *Geriatr Nurs* 13(6):332, 1992.

Box 18-5	COMPLICATIONS OF DIABETES MELLITUS

Macrovascular Complications
Myocardial infarction
Hypertension
Stroke
Peripheral vascular disease
Neuropathy
Amputation

Microvascular Complications
Retinopathy (vision loss)
End-stage renal failure

1995). The advancement of retinopathy also correlates with neuropathy and peripheral neuropathy (Delcourt et al, 1996). Diabetes predisposes an individual to cardiac disease, hypertension, stroke, and renal failure. Box 18-5 shows the complications that occur under the umbrella of diabetes mellitus.

MANAGEMENT

Medical management of diabetes is very poor in many cases (Kerr, 1995). Johns Hopkins School of Hygiene and Public Health examined the Medicare claims records of over 100,000 elders with diabetes and found that 84% had not received proper testing for glucohemoglobin (GCH), 54% had not had a thorough eye examination, and 54% had not received adequate cholesterol monitoring. These are the three most important evaluations recommended by the American Diabetes Association. Individuals with type 2 diabetes require at least two office visits per year, lipid profiles annually, a glycosylated hemoglobin (Hgb A_{1c}) test twice yearly, and a thorough ophthalmologic examination annually. The sine qua non of good diabetes therapy is to persuade, encourage, cajole, coach, and equip elders to develop the knowledge, tenacity, courage, and optimism necessary for long-term successful management of their diabetes.

Catolico (1995) found that the barriers to self-management of diabetes among older adults included being female and having more complex management regimens, less education, and more severe complications. Those who fared the best were the older adults with high self-esteem. Management of diet, weight,

ture. However, with vigilance of the care provider and the individual himself or herself, the gradual degeneration can be slowed or delayed. Macrovascular complications include myocardial infarction, stroke, peripheral vascular disease, neuropathy, and amputation. The microvascular problems are loss of vision and end-stage renal failure.

Warning signs of foot problems include cold feet and intermittent claudication (vascular); burning, tingling, hypersensitivity, or numbness (neurologic); gradual change in shape or sudden painless change without trauma (musculoskeletal); and infections, skin color and texture changes, and slow healing, exquisitely painful or painless wounds (dermatologic) (Scardina, 1983). Subungual (under a fingernail or a toenail) hemorrhages have been observed as a first manifestation of type 2 diabetes mellitus in some previously undiagnosed cases. In addition, the neurologic vibratory and sensory status of the feet must be assessed. Another major type of problem is progressively deteriorating vision in the form of retinopathy (Box 18-4). There is also an increase in corneal epithelial fragility with the progression of diabetic retinopathy. This fragility correlates with the severity of the disease (Saini, Khandalavla, exercise, and drug therapy (if necessary) and maintaining glucose levels near normal are essential components of diabetes control. Nutrition is the cornerstone, and education is a key in the management of diabetes. Persistent elevation of blood glucose levels increases morbidity and mortality (Miller, 1996). Factors affecting diabetes control in older adults appear in Box 18-6.

The essential components of management include glucose monitoring, nutrition, exercise, education, foot care, medications, and attention to the psychologic aspects of dealing with a chronic illness.

| **Box 18-6** | **SUMMARY OF FACTORS AFFECTING DIABETES CONTROL IN OLDER ADULTS** |

1. A decline in visual acuity could affect the individual's ability to see printed educational material, medication labels, markings on a syringe, and blood glucose monitoring devices.
2. Auditory impairments could lead to difficulty hearing instructions.
3. Altered taste could affect food choices and nutritional status.
4. Poor dentition or changes in the gastrointestinal system could lead to difficulties with food ingestion and digestion.
5. Altered ability to recognize hunger and thirst may lead to weight loss, dehydration, and increased risk for hyperosmolar nonketotic syndrome.
6. Changes in hepatic or renal function could affect ability to self-administer medications.
7. Arthritis or parkinsonian tremor could affect ability to self-administer medications and use monitoring devices.
8. Polypharmacy complicates medication choices.
9. Depression affects motivation for self-management.
10. Cognitive impairment and dementia decrease self-care ability.
11. Inadequate education and poor literacy call for modifications in the method of teaching about diabetes care.
12. The level of income can affect the level of care sought or obtained.
13. Living alone without a resource person for help with management can have a negative effect on the person with diabetes.
14. A sedentary life-style and obesity can result in decreased tissue sensitivity to insulin.

Maintenance of Acceptable Blood Glucose Levels

A major goal of diabetes management is an acceptable level of blood glucose. The blood glucose levels for an older adult with diabetes should be as close to the normal range as possible (80 to 100 mg/dl). However, this may not be realistic for the older adult, because the pancreas simply does not produce as much insulin, even in those who do not have diabetes. The goal is to maintain levels that do not harm the blood vessels rather than becoming overly concerned about occasional blood glucose surges. It is recommended that glycosylated hemoglobin be monitored because it reflects the average blood glucose level over an extended period of time (Fonseca, Wall, 1995). A fasting blood glucose level of 160-200 mg/dl and an Hgb A_{1c} of <7 prevent metabolic decompensation and control the deleterious effects of complications (Halter, 1999; Blair, 1999; Terpstra, Terpstra, 1998). The American Diabetes Association has glucose guidelines for type 1 diabetes, but there is no consensus on specific glucose levels for type 2 diabetes, particularly for the aged.

Clients and their caregivers should be taught to routinely self-monitor blood glucose (SMBG). Until diabetes is controlled, the individual or the caregiver will need to monitor the blood glucose level at least four times daily (before meals and at bedtime). Too high or too low a level requires appropriate intervention. When the glucose level has been established within the range that the primary care provider has prescribed, the frequency of monitoring can be reduced to twice in 24 hours. Those testings should be rotated so that a range of blood glucose levels over time can be reviewed by the primary care provider. A log with the date, time, and glucose results should be kept and taken to each medical appointment. It is important for the older adult and the caregiver to know that when illness occurs, it is important to resume glucose testing more frequently, sometimes as much as every 2 to 3 hours, because illness causes metabolic decompensation and increases blood glucose levels. Elders also need to know that during times of illness or stress they may temporarily need insulin even though they usually may manage quite well through nutritional control.

Nutrition

Management of nutrition is complicated by age and the accompanying changes in taste. Frequently the lessened taste response causes older adults to add more salt to their food. Loss of teeth may limit the food choices available for a food plan. An initial nutrition assessment with a 24-hour recall will provide some clues to the patient's dietary habits, intake, and style of eating. If a recall is not possible, have the person bring in his or her grocery list for the past week. This, too, is a way of obtaining nutritional data. Focusing on maintaining normal ranges of weight, blood pressure, and lipids is important. A combination of guidelines from the American Diabetes Association and the American Heart Association suggests a dietary intake of approximately 55% of calories from carbohydrates, 30% from fat (10% saturated fat), and 15% from protein; foods low in cholesterol; and less than 2 g of sodium (Armetta, Molony, 1999) because of the higher risk of heart disease with diabetes. In addition, adequate vitamin and mineral intake is needed. The ideal dietary composition has not yet been determined; however, when obesity is an issue, a 10% reduction in weight often means the difference between taking oral antihyperglycemic agents or insulin and controlling the diabetes by diet and exercise alone (Heber, 1998; Armetta, Molony, 1999; Halter, 1999).

Dietary changes should be individualized to prevent malnutrition. The diet issue with elders is the degree of diet restriction versus undernourishment. Many elders become undernourished when placed on reduction diets. Frequently, the older adult is referred to a nutritionist or registered dietitian for specific dietary modifications that are realistic and prevent undernourshiment.

It is part of the nurse's responsibility to learn if there is difficulty with access to food, including food preparation and shopping for food. Working with elders' dietary habits that have been formed over a lifetime and through their cultural association may be modified if there is caregiver support. Taste and oral care may limit the adaptation to a prescribed diet. Also, it is important to be aware that periodontal disease is frequently exacerbated by diabetes.

Exercise

Exercise is an important aspect of therapy for type 2 diabetes because exercise increases insulin production. Walking is an inexpensive and beneficial way to obtain exercise. Walking 15 to 20 minutes at least three times a week is a good beginning and in conjunction with an appropriate diet is often sufficient to maintain blood glucose levels within normal levels. Some authorities believe that walking is not sufficient exercise and that a more vigorous program should be encouraged (Halter, 1999). Embarking on a more intensive exercise program should not be started until the older adult has had

a physical examination, including a stress test and electrocardiogram (ECG). Results should govern the type and extent of an exercise program that would be most beneficial and would be performed for 30 minutes at least three times a week to achieve the benefit of increased carbohydrate metabolism, increased insulin sensitivity, prevention of cardiovascular disease, decreased triglyceride levels, weight loss or maintenance, and lowered blood pressure. Those who have limited mobility can still do chair exercises or if possible use exercise machines that enable sitting and holding on for support. The pace of exercise is slower for most older adults than it is for the younger person.

Medications

Antihyperglycemics include oral and parenteral agents. Oral medications are prescribed according to the insulin deficit identified: no secretion of insulin, insulin resistance, or inadequate secretion of insulin. Table 18-1 describes the action of various oral antihyperglycemic agents used in the treatment of diabetes mellitus. These agents may be use alone or in combination to achieve the desired blood glucose control. Insulin may be used as a primary agent or to maintain effective control for type 2 diabetes when an older adult with diabetes is hospitalized during an acute illness or during a perioperative period when oral antihyperglycemic agents are not appropriate. Insulin that has been used to treat diabetes for many years has many advantages and some disadvantages as an antihyperglycemic agent. Box 18-7 lists the advantages and disadvantages of this drug.

Education

Experiential teaching, encouragement, and reinforcement of mastery are important factors that promote successful self-management. Konen et al (1996) found that symptoms of depression, anxiety, panic, and forgetfulness were unexpectedly common among elder diabetic patients and affected their ability to comply with therapy. These findings should alert nurses to the need to recognize these deterrents when attempting to teach diabetes management. Questions that the nurse should ask to help determine if elders are able to manage their own diabetes care are given in Box 18-8.

The older patient and the caregiver require thorough education, which requires time, repetition, and periodic return demonstrations of some of the material taught. The many facets of diabetes education include knowledge and explanation of the disease; the necessity to achieve good blood glucose control, as well as a list of the long-term complications if glucose remains uncon-

Table 18-1

Oral Agents in Diabetes Management

Generic name	Brand name	Purpose
SULFONYLUREAS		
Chlorpropamide	Diabinese	Enhance insulin secretion
Glimepiride	Amaryl	
Glipizide	Glucotrol	
Glyburide	Micronase	
Glyburide, micronized	Glynase	
ALPHA-GLUCOSIDASE INHIBITOR		
Acarbose	Precose	Decreases glucose absorption
BIGUANIDE		
Metformin	Glucophage	Decreases hepatic glucose production
THIAZOLIDINEDIONES		
Rosiglitazone	Avandia	Enhance insulin sensitivity
Pioglitazone	Actos	

Box 18-7 ADVANTAGES AND DISADVANTAGES OF INSULIN THERAPY

Advantages

- Hormone replacement
- No known drug interaction
- Proven effective for 75 years
- Safe for patients with renal and hepatic insufficiency who cannot eat during major illness
- Relatively inexpensive (however, the necessary equipment that must be used makes it an expensive treatment)
- Encourages self-care
- Can lower glucose in any patient in sufficient dosage and has the potential for normalizing circulating glucose levels if regimen is sufficient

Disadvantages

- Injections necessary
- Hypoglycemia a risk
- Treatment program can be complex

trolled; the relationship of diet and exercise to achieving an acceptable blood glucose level; the potential benefits of exercise; and the identification of the signs and symptoms of hyperglycemia and hypoglycemia and the actions needed to alleviate their effects. It will be necessary for the older patient and the caregiver to verbalize what hyperglycemic and hypoglycemic symptoms are and what treatment is needed. Demonstration of techniques for self–glucose monitoring include teaching how to obtain a blood sample, use of the glucose monitoring equipment, troubleshooting when there are false results, and recording the values from the machine. The patient must understand the importance of bringing the results to each medical visit. The patient must also know and be willing to accept the goals of blood glucose control. Where appropriate, demonstration and return demonstration should be given for drawing up insulin, selecting the injection site, injecting and storing insulin, and disposing of the used needle and syringes. Transporting insulin for travel is also important (Brown et al, 1999).

Medications, if prescribed for the older adult, must be carefully reviewed. The effects of drugs on blood glucose must be given serious consideration in the management of diabetes because a number of medications commonly used for elders affect blood glucose levels in adverse ways. Therefore older adults should be advised to ask if the particular drug prescribed affects their therapy and should check with their primary care provider before taking any over-the-counter medications.

Foot Care

Daily foot care and foot examination should be discussed and demonstrated for the older adult. Often the elder is not particularly flexible and will have difficulty reaching and inspecting his or her feet. A caregiver may need to do this. Regardless, the older adult should also know what a foot examination and daily care entail. Box 18-9 details essential daily foot care and the reduction of amputation risk (Peters, 1999; Umeh et al, 1999).

Long-term incidence of lower extremity amputation in the diabetic elder is over 7% and is higher in

---

Box 18-8   QUESTIONS TO ASCERTAIN ABILITY OF ELDERS FOR DIABETES SELF-MANAGEMENT

1. What is the individual's life-style?
2. How will diabetes impact his or her life-style?
3. What is the individual's functional status? How well can he or she perform ADLs, IADLs, and activities involved in glucose monitoring and in preparing and giving self-injections?
4. What is the individual's mental and psychosocial status?
5. What is the overall health status?

ADLs, Activities of daily living; *IADLs,* instrumental activities of daily living.

Box 18-9   ESSENTIALS OF DAILY DIABETES FOOT CARE AND REDUCTION OF AMPUTATION RISK

- Inspect the feet daily for blisters, cuts, reddened areas, and scratches. Use a magnifying glass or mirror to inspect the feet or have someone else do it, if cannot reach or see well enough.
- Wash feet daily but *do not* soak feet daily (causes excessive dryness).
- Blot dry rather than rub dry to avoid injury to sensitive skin. Pay particular attention to between the toes.
- Use emollient lotion, cocoa butter, lanolin lotion, mineral oil, or vegetable oil to soften dry skin to help retain moisture and prevent cracking. *Do not* put between toes; it may contribute to fungal infections.
- Dust lightly with nonscented powder between toes (can prevent excessive perspiration).
- Have a podiatrist cut toenails if they are too thick to be cut or if unable to do alone. If do own nails, soak toenails 10 to 15 minutes to soften before cutting. Cut straight across using toenail clipper. *Do not* cut corns and calluses; have the podiatrist treat them. *Do not* apply harsh chemicals or corn or wart products to toes or feet. These can remove skin, as well as the corn or wart. *Do not* apply heating pads—chemical or battery operated—to feet.
- Wear clean socks, hose, or stockings daily. Cotton socks absorb perspiration for feet that sweat. Keep feet warm

with thick fleecy insoles inside slippers to protect from cold or wear cotton socks with comfortable slippers.
- *Do not* walk barefooted at any time. Sandals for the beach protect feet from hot sand, sharp objects, etc. At home or in a care facility, wear shoes or slippers, even at night when going to the bathroom.
- Wear comfortable, well-fitting shoe with broad toe space and low heels. Good-quality athletic shoes, although expensive, outlast regular shoes and are less expensive in the long run. Carefully break in new shoes. Begin by wearing shoes an hour a day, gradually increasing the time worn.
- Shake out shoes before putting them on to remove foreign objects that might cause injury.
- *Do not* pop blisters. Infection can occur. See physician immediately.
- Avoid wearing tight-fitting hose, tight stockings, or stockings with garters; *do not* sit with legs crossed. All of these things constrict blood flow to the lower extremities.
- Stop smoking. Smoking constricts blood vessels, reducing blood flow to the lower extremities.
- Call physician for any problems such as tenderness, redness, warmth, drainage, an ingrown toenail, athlete's foot, or pain in the feet or calf.

Modified from Jarvik L, Small G: *Parent care,* New York, 1988, Crown; Helfand AE, issue editor: The aging foot, *Focus Geriatr Care Rehabil* 2(10):1, 1989; Dellasega C, Yonushonis MEH: Diabetes mellitus in the elderly. In Stanley M, Beare PG: *Gerontological nursing,* Philadelphia, 1995, Davis; and Patient education, 10 things you can do to reduce your risk of amputation, *Nurse Pract* 24(8):69, 1999.

Table 18-2

Warning Signs and Symptoms of Diabetic Foot Problems

Signs	Symptoms
VASCULAR	
Absence of pedal, popliteal, or femoral pulses	Cold feet
Femoral bruits	Intermittent claudication involving calf or foot
Dependent rubor, plantar pallor on elevation	Pain at rest, especially nocturnal, relieved by dependency
Prolonged capillary filling time >3-4 seconds	
Decreased skin temperature	
NEUROLOGIC	
Sensory: deficits in perception of vibration, proprioception, pain, and temperature	
MUSCULOSKELETAL	
Claw toes on feet	Gradual change in foot shape
Foot drop	Sudden, painless change in foot shape, with swelling, without history of trauma
"Rocker bottom" foot (Charcot joint)	
Neuropathic arthropathy	
DERMATOLOGIC	
Abnormal dryness	
Chronic tinea infections	
Keratotic lesions with or without hemorrhage (plantar or digital)	
Trophic ulcer	
Hair diminished or absent	
Nails: trophic changes	
Onchomycosis	
Subungual ulceration or abscess	
Ingrown nails with paronychia	

those who have a history of leg ulcers, high diastolic pressure, elevation of Hgb A_{1c}, proteinuria, and a 10-year history of diabetes (Moss et al, 1996). In one study of over 300 people, 43% of elders with diabetes

had peripheral neuropathy (impaired sensation), which could result in unknowing foot injury. Nurses are well aware of the need for routine examination and care of the feet of diabetic patients. Turner (1996) found that some nurses are reluctant to provide foot care regardless of the patient's condition. Plummer and Albert (1996) say that any individual, with or without diabetes, who has foot deformities, peripheral vascular disease, or peripheral neuropathy should be followed routinely by a foot care specialist. One study (Eckman et al, 1995) suggests that physicians should débride the foot and institute a course of oral antibiotics for any individual with type 2 diabetes who appears to be developing osteomyelitis of the foot. Table 18-2 presents warning signs and symptoms of diabetic foot problems.

There are many questions about the management of the ongoing and complex needs of the elder diabetic patient in our present health care system. It appears from one study that it matters little in terms of outcomes whether type 2 diabetes is managed by a private physician or a managed care group. However, outcomes regarding foot ulcers and infections were better when treated by an endocrinologist (Greenfield et al, 1995).

Nurse's Role in Diabetes Management

The elements of diabetes management in which the nurse has a major role include educating the older adult and caregiver about diabetes; supervising, monitoring, or performing glucose monitoring; supporting the diabetic patient's diet and exercise program; supervising the use of or administering antihyperglycemic agents; teaching or carrying out foot care; and emphasizing the advantages of following the appropriate treatment regimen. It is also the nurse's role to promote health by ensuring that the older adult receives a yearly cholesterol check and ophthalmologic examination and obtains an Hgb A_{1c} measurement at least twice a year.

Standards of Care for Patients With Diabetes Mellitus

Meticulous management of the diabetic patient is needed to reduce the risk of long-term complications and avert acute problems. The following evaluation is recommended:

- The history should include dietary habits, weight patterns, previous treatment programs, the current treatment regimen, exercise and activity levels, infections, illnesses, and complications of diabetes.

- Physical examination should include blood pressure measurement; eye ground examination; thyroid palpation; auscultation of pulses; foot, periodontal, and skin examination; and neurologic examination.
- Laboratory tests should include fasting plasma glucose values; glycosylated hemoglobin; a fasting lipid profile; serum creatinine if proteinuria is present; and urinalysis, including microalbuminuria, urine culture, thyroid function (thyroxine [T_4] or thyroid-stimulating hormone [TSH]), and an ECG.

Long-Term Care and the Elder With Diabetes

Assessment of whether elders in a long-term care facility can participate in their care depends on the degree of the disease burden, the degree of disability, and the amount of life expectancy remaining (Halter, 1999). Under these circumstances, the goals and treatment may need to be modified. Basic diabetes care should include a diet according to need. It is important to monitor for undernutrition: a consistent

NANDA and Wellness Diagnoses

Wellness	Specific Needs	NANDA
Considers disease as a part of life and adapts to it Accepts life as meaningful Expresses self appropriately	**Self-actualization** Fulfillment Values Integrity	Adjustment, impaired Coping, defensive Personal identity disturbance
Maintains sexuality Accepts altered body function or appearance	Self-esteem Image Autonomy Control	Body image disturbance Self-care deficit, grooming Noncompliance Sexual dysfunction Self-esteem disturbance
Maintains sexuality	**Belonging** Acceptance Sexuality Belonging	Sexual dysfunction
Manages therapeutic regimen Is knowledgeable about disease Does health maintenance	Safety and security Education Protection	Injury, risk for Management of therapeutic regimen, families: ineffective Management of therapeutic regimen, individuals: ineffective Knowledge deficit
Has intact skin Does adequate health maintenance Maintains adequate nutrition	Biologic integrity Skin integrity Health maintenance Nutrition Freedom from pain Activity	Skin integrity, impaired, risk for Tissue integrity, impaired Tissue perfusion, altered Sensory/perceptual alterations (visual/tactile) Peripheral neurovascular dysfunction, risk for Health maintenance, altered Nutrition, altered: more than body requirements

These are not all of the possible wellness or NANDA diagnoses that may be identified. The above are frequent examples of nursing diagnoses that should be considered when planning care for the older adult in whatever setting.

caloric intake is necessary for someone taking insulin. Limiting cardiovascular complications, at this point, is unwarranted (Halter, 1999). Skin and foot care remain important and should be assessed and carried out daily. Constructive leisure activities should be provided rather than exercise. Glucose monitoring should be continued, and signs and symptoms of hypoglycemia and hyperglycemia should be watched for. Attention should be given to toileting to decrease incontinence if this is present secondary to bladder dysfunction from autonomic neuropathy. Checking for urinary tract infections that develop more frequently in older diabetic patients is also important (Halter, 1999).

The goals of nursing care are to maintain the older adult with diabetes in the best health that is realistically possible. Maintaining the older adult's health is a team effort. The nurse as part of the team serves as an educator, care provider, advocate, supporter, and guide for the older person.

► KEY CONCEPTS

- Signs and symptoms of diabetes in the older adult may be vague or suggestive of other medical conditions or as part of "old age" rather than being the usual expected symptoms of polyuria, polydipsia, and polyphagia.
- Close monitoring of blood glucose levels is the most effective way to prevent, delay, or slow the progression of macrovascular, microvascular, and neurologic complications of the disease.
- Management of diabetes is a comprehensive team effort and should include the elder as much as he or she can realistically participate as part of the team. If this is not possible, the caregiver, if not the nurse, will need to ensure that the medical regimen is effective.
- Daily preventive foot care is essential for prevention of the possibility of future amputation.

► Activities and Discussion Questions

1. What are the risks and complications of diabetes for the older adult?
2. State the components of diabetes management, and explain what each component requires.
3. Describe the nurse's role in the management of diabetes.
4. Develop a nursing care plan for an elder in the community, in an acute care hospital, and in long-term care, using wellness and NANDA diagnoses.

RESOURCES

AFTER (Rehabilitation and Training Center for Limb Deficiencies and Amputation)
2559 Fairway Island Drive
West Palm Beach, FL 33414-7045
American Diabetes Association
National Center
PO Box 25757
1660 Duke Street
Arlington, VA 22314-3427
Amputee Shoe and Glove Exchange
PO Box 27067
Houston, TX 77227

REFERENCES

Armetta M, Molony SL: Topics in endocrine and hematologic care. In Molony SL et al, editors: *Gerontological nursing: an advanced practice approach,* Stamford, Conn, 1999, Appleton-Lange.

Bailey BJ: Mediators of depression in adults with diabetes, *Clin Nutr Res* 5(1):28, 1996.

Bichler LM: Foot ulcers in diabetes, *Adv Nurse Pract* 7(1):49, 1999.

Blair EM: Diabetes in the older adult, *Adv Nurse Pract* 7(7):33, 1999.

Brown JB, Bedford NK, White SJ: *Gerontological protocols for nurse practitioners,* Philadelphia, 1999, Lippincott.

Catolico JT: *Assessment of barriers to diabetes self-management in older adults.* Thesis submitted to Faculty, School of Nursing, San Francisco State University, July, 1995.

Delcourt C et al: Clinical correlates of advanced retinopathy in type II diabetic patients: implications for screening, *J Clin Epidemiol* 49(6):679, 1996.

Eckman MH, Greenfield S, Mackey WC: Foot infections in diabetic patients: decision and cost-effectiveness analysis, *JAMA* 273(9):712, 1995.

Fonseca V, Wall J: Diet and diabetes in the elderly, *Nutr Aging Age Depend Dis* 11(4):613, 1995.

Genuth S, Palmer J, Zimmerman BR: Diabetes: new criteria for diagnosis, screening, and classification, *Patient Care Nurse Pract* 1(1):12, 1998.

Greenfield D, Rogers W, Mangotich M: Outcomes of patients with hypertension and non-insulin-dependent diabetes mellitus treated by different systems and specialists, *JAMA* 274(18):1436, 1995.

Gutowski C: Understanding new pharmacologic therapy for type 2 diabetes, *Nurse Pract* 24(6):15, 1999.

Halter JB: Diabetes mellitus. In Hazzard WR et al, editors: *Principles of geriatric medicine and gerontology,* ed 4, New York, 1999, McGraw-Hill.

Heber D: *Statement,* Los Angeles, 1998, University of California, Los Angeles, Center for Human Nutrition, Innovative Research, Education, Nutritional Medicine, Public Health and International Nutrition.

Hernandez D: Microvascular complications of diabetes, *Am J Nutr* 98(6):26, 1998.

Kennedy-Malone L, Fletcher KR, Plank LM: Endocrine, metabolic, and nutritional disorders. In *Management guidelines for gerontological nurse practitioners,* Philadelphia, 2000, Davis.

Kerr CP: Management of diabetes, *J Fam Pract* 40(1):63, 1995.

Konen JC, Curtis LG, Summerson JH: Symptoms and complications of adult diabetic patients in a family practice, *Arch Fam Med* 5(3):135, 1996.

Meadow P: Variations of diabetes mellitus prevalence in general practice and its relation to deprivation, *Diabet Med* 12(8):696, 1995.

Miller CA: *Essentials of gerontological nursing: adaptation and the aging process,* Philadelphia, 1996, Lippincott.

Moss SE, Klein R, Klein BE: Long-term incidence of lower-extremity amputations in a diabetic population, *Arch Fam Med* 5(7):391, 1996.

Peters S: Diabetic foot ulcers, *Adv Nurse Pract* 6(6):59, 1998.

Plummer TS, Albert SG: Focused assessment of foot care in older adults, *J Am Geriatr Soc* 44(3):310, 1996.

Saini JS, Khandalavla B: Corneal epithelial fragility in diabetes mellitus, *Can J Ophthalmol* 30(3):142, 1995.

Scardina RJ: Diabetic foot problems: assessment and prevention, *Clin Diabet* 1(2):42, 1983.

Seidel HM et al: *Mosby's guide to physical examination,* ed 4, St Louis, 1999, Mosby.

Terpstra TL, Terpstra TL: The elderly type 2 diabetic: a treatment challenge, *Geriatr Nurs* 19(5):253, 1998.

Turner C: Nurses' knowledge, assessment skills, experience and confidence in toenail management of elderly people, *Geriatr Nurs* 17(6):273, 1996.

Umeh L, Wallhagen M, Nicoloff N: Identifying diabetic patients at high risk for amputation, *Nurse Pract* 24(8):56, 1999.

US Bureau of the Census: *Statistical abstract of the United States,* ed 115, Washington, DC, 1995, US Government Printing Office.

chapter 19

Living With Bone and Joint Problems

Upon completion of this chapter, the reader will be able to:

- Describe age-related changes in bones, joints, and muscles.
- Recognize postural changes that indicate the presence of osteoporosis.
- Discuss the factors that lead to osteoporosis.
- Explain some effective ways of preventing or slowing the progression of osteoporosis.
- Relate the differences in osteoarthritis and rheumatoid arthritis.
- Name several methods of dealing with pain and disability resulting from joint and bone disorders.

▶GLOSSARY

Arthrodesis Fixation of a joint caused by destruction of cartilage or a surgically induced fixation.

Arthroplasty Surgical reconstruction or replacement of a painful, degenerated joint.

Chondrocytes The cells that form the cartilage of the body.

Iatrogenic A condition caused by treatment or diagnostic procedures.

Nightshade The name applied to various plants of the genus *Solanum* that produce adverse reactions in certain individuals.

Nulliparous Never having given birth.

Prostaglandins Hormonelike unsaturated fatty acids produced in small amounts by the body but having a large array of significant effects on muscle and vasomotor tone, as well as platelet aggregation and endocrine and nervous system integrity.

Resorption The loss of substance or bone by physiologic or pathologic means.

Synovectomy Removal of the synovial membrane of a joint.

Synovitis Inflammation of the synovial membrane of a joint as a result of an aseptic wound or traumatic injury.

Tendinitis Inflammation of a tendon, usually resulting from strain.

Trabecular Spongy bone formed by a network of intersecting plates sensitive to biochemical changes.

▶THE LIVED EXPERIENCE

It is so discouraging to wake up feeling so stiff and sore every morning. Just getting out of bed seems like a real effort, but I usually feel better after I have moved around a bit. I was always so athletic, I can't understand how I have become so crippled up. And now I know that what my grandmother used to say about the weather affecting her rheumatism is really true. I can feel it when a storm is coming.

Mabel, age 80

I don't know how these folks with arthritis can stand being uncomfortable so much of the time. I know Mabel takes medications, but she still seems to be in a lot of pain and has so much trouble moving about. I'll try to be as gentle as possible when I help her bathe.

Elva, student nurse

MUSCULOSKELETAL SYSTEM

The musculoskeletal system, necessary for the ability to carry out the most basic activities of daily living, often shows the wear and tear of the years. Thus as many as 90% of people over 70 years of age have muscle, tendon, joint, and ligament problems and bone deterioration sufficient to cause pain and hinder movement. Tendons and ligaments are composed of dense connective tissue that attaches muscle to bone and bone to bone. Ligaments stabilize the joint, and tendons control the flexion and extension limits of the muscles. The general decline in range of motion that tends to occur in aging is thought to result from changes in these structures, earlier injuries, disease, and disuse. These are the most common chronic problems of aged individuals and the leading cause of functional impairment. However, these problems are not purely a result of aging but may also be effects of early traumas, disuse, disease, and time-related degeneration of tissue (Hazzard et al, 1999). These common conditions that accompany the normal changes of aging, as well as the chronic disorders that occur more frequently in the elderly, merit special attention.

Orthopedic impairments significantly impede the aged and interfere with quality of life. Rheumatoid arthritis, osteoarthritis, osteopenia, and osteoporosis markedly affect movement and functional capacities. Added to this, the slow muscle wasting and decline in strength (sarcopenia) that occur in aging further affect the ability to function with these disorders.

Articular Cartilage

The cartilage that cushions the bone articulations is composed of chondrocytes that are firm in consistency, have little or no vascularity, and tolerate extreme pressure (Copstead, 1995). During aging there is a loss of cartilage matrix and some calcification, resulting in less cushion and less resilience in the joints and thus symptoms of osteoarthritis (Fig. 19-1). Knees and shoulders are commonly affected. Some individuals have impairment of one or more joints, bilaterally or unilaterally. The problems are most severe in the joints (particularly the knees, hips, and spine) that have been subjected to the most pressure or repetitive motion.

Osteopenia and Osteoporosis

Normally, there is a gradual continual loss of cortical and trabecular bone in both men and women as they age. Osteopenia (which can lead to osteoporosis) and osteoporosis are both conditions in which a loss of bony tissue results in porous and brittle bones that fracture easily. *Osteopenia* is defined as bone mineral density 1 to 2.5 standard deviations below that of the normal young adult female; *osteoporosis* is bone mineral loss that exceeds that amount. Fifty percent of women over age 50 have osteopenia; this increases to 57% for women 70 to 79 years of age but decreases to 45% for women over 80 (Ezzati et al, 1994; Looker et al, 1995). This seems to indicate that those who survive beyond age 80 may be generally of sturdier bone density. To determine the factors that contribute to osteopenia, Bauer

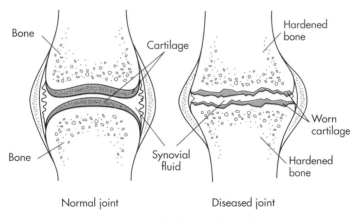

Fig. 19-1   Normal joint and diseased joint.

(1993) evaluated a group of nearly 10,000 elderly community-residing women in Maryland, Minnesota, Oregon, and Pennsylvania. He found that greater bone mass was present in individuals with the associated variables listed in Box 19-1.

The dynamics of osteoporosis are complex, involving the interrelationship of dietary mineral metabolism, vitamin D, and hormone activity. The development of osteoporosis can be compared with a savings account (bone mass), with its assets (input of calcium for added bone density) and debits (the loss of calcium with the loss of bone density). As long as there is calcium intake in proportion to the other mechanisms, bone mass and density will be maintained and osteoporosis will not occur. When there is a deficiency of calcium, or a decrease in hormone levels that impair the absorption of calcium, there will be a greater loss than input of calcium. The result is less dense bone and the gradual development of osteoporotic manifestations. Gastrointestinal age-related changes and the inadequacy of dietary calcium of older adults are among the factors that leave elders prone to osteoporosis.

Toufexis (1994) reports genetic studies that indicate a gene that heightens the risk of osteoporosis by hampering the uptake of vitamin D. According to this research, the risk of osteoporosis depends heavily on whether one inherits the low–bone density (B) form or the high–bone density (b) form of this gene. Obviously, a person who inherits the low-density gene from both parents (BB) would be at high risk. Of 311 women studied, those with BB had serious fracture potential 18 years after menopause, those with Bb had fracture potential 22 years after menopause, and women with bb were not at the fracture threshold until 29 years after menopause. Compared with women at age 50, the incidence of osteoporosis increases exponentially with every decade of life. Vertebrae, wrists, and femoral neck bones lose the greatest proportion of trabecular tissue and are thus most fragile and likely to break with unusual pressure.

Bone Mass

Bone density is determined about 75% by heredity and 25% by environmental factors (Toufexis, 1994). Risk factors are well known and include being female, white or Asian, postmenopausal, nulliparous, small, lean, and sedentary; having low intake of calcium and vitamin D and high intake of nicotine, caffeine, alcohol, and phosphate; heredity; and advancing age. At this time there is equivocal evidence regarding alcohol intake and its effects on osteoporosis. A study using data from the Framingham Heart Study found that moderate consumption of alcohol increased bone density in both men and women (Felson et al, 1995).

Osteoporosis can also result from prolonged steroid therapy and other medications such as thyroid, heparin, furosemide, tetracycline, anticonvulsants, and aluminum-containing antacids; endocrine disorders (notably Cushing syndrome, parathyroidism, hyperthyroidism, premature menopause, and hyperadrenocorticism); gastrointestinal disorders such as malabsorption syndrome, peptic ulcer, and lactase deficiency; and subtotal gastrectomy. Infection, injury, and synovitis may cause localized bone loss in affected areas.

Men with low levels of testosterone and hypogonadism have been found to be predisposed to osteoporosis and fractures (Kessenich, 1996). This suggests that osteoporosis prevention for older men may have been neglected because it has largely been considered a problem of postmenopausal women.

Assessment

Outward signs of osteoporosis are a loss of height, "dowager's hump," and fractures of vertebrae (Fig. 19-2). Ideally, it should be diagnosed by the use of a

---

Box 19-1	**VARIABLES ASSOCIATED WITH BONE MASS IN AGED FEMALES**

Variables Listed in Descending Order of Association With Bone Mass Preservation

Estrogen use
Type 2 diabetes
Thiazide use
Increased weight
Greater muscle strength
Later age at menopause
Greater height

Variables Associated With Bone Mass Loss

Alcohol use
Decreased physical activity
Calcium deficiency
Pregnancies
History of breast-feeding
Parental nationality (European)
Hair color (blond, red)

Data from Bauer DC: Factors associated with appendicular bone mass in older women, *Ann Intern Med* 118:657, 1993.

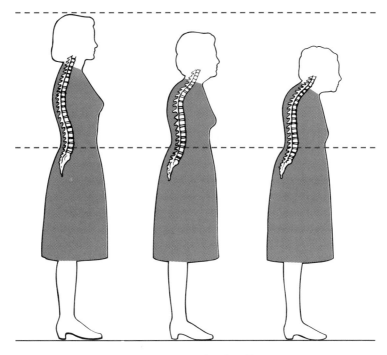

Fig. 19-2   Osteoporosis spine alignment.

bone densitometer before becoming so grossly visible (Mastrangelo, 1994). Osteoporosis is considered a "silent thief" and seldom comes to anyone's attention until there is a fracture of the hip or vertebrae (Galsworthy, Wilson, 1996). Watts (1991) contends that primary physicians have the responsibility for identifying patients at risk and instituting appropriate preventive measures.

Measuring the rate of bone resorption is a sophisticated and complex procedure best accomplished by measuring the urinary excretion of cross-linked peptides (Gertz et al, 1994). Standard x-ray examinations cannot reliably detect bone loss until the disease is advanced to at least 30% bone tissue loss. There is no simple, reliable, and risk-free diagnostic technique, although a recently approved blood test (Tandem-R Ostase) measures a blood marker, known as ostase, that gauges the rate of bone turnover (Mann, 1996). Preliminary trials of this method are encouraging. Presently, the most accurate technique is bone density measurement. This can be done through dual-photon absorptiometry (DPA), quantitative computerized tomography (QCT), or dual-energy x-ray absorptiometry (DEXA) (Watts, 1991). The DEXA is the most widely used and reliable method. The most common

skeletal sites of bone density measurements are the lumbar spine, proximal femur (hip), and distal radius (wrist joint) (Hazzard et al, 1999). Ultrasound examination of the patella is useful to identify women who have osteoporotic fractures. Although this procedure is less expensive and has considerably lower risk, it is revealing only for women with substantial bone loss. Most of the procedures are expensive and involve some degree of radiation exposure.

A major problem is the lack of attention to prevention or medical management of this common disorder (Lindsay, 1995). Few women seeing their family physician discuss risk factors, and even fewer are assessed for risk of osteoporosis. In fact, many receive medications and medical interventions that would directly increase their osteoporosis risk. Even osteoporotic bone pain, a common and excruciating result of vertebral collapse, is often virtually ignored by professionals.

In assessing osteoporosis, the measure of disability is important. Helmes et al (1995) developed the Osteoporosis Functional Disability Questionnaire (OFDQ) to assess disability in persons with osteoporosis and back pain secondary to vertebral fractures. It appears to be a reliable instrument that correlates well with objective measures of spinal osteoporosis.

Screening for risk factors of osteoporosis is an important aspect of the nurse's role and requires that the nurse be knowledgeable about the risk factors and the disease itself. The risk factors are listed in Table 19-1 for types I and II osteoporosis. Type I osteoporosis is related to personal characteristics, life-style, and disease. Type II osteoporosis is iatrogenically induced. If risk factors are identified, the nurse should obtain further data and refer the person to a physician so that further appraisal can be done and treatment begun if necessary.

Prevention and Treatment

Measures to prevent osteoporosis progression include physical activity, nutrition, exercise, weight bearing, adequate calcium intake, and life-style changes that reduce risk factors (Ali, Twibell, 1994). Education, fall prevention, and possibly estrogen replacement therapy (ERT) must be considered.

Physical activity plays an essential role in prevention of osteoporosis by maintaining bone mass. Weight-bearing activity such as brisk walking 20 minutes or more daily is excellent. It provides not only mechanical force and spinal and long bone movement, but also sunlight exposure and vitamin D.

Exercise for those with osteoporosis provides increased muscle support of bones and improves flexibility and balance elements, which are extremely valuable in preventing fractures associated with the disease, as well as in maintaining general health. Postural exercises should be done to minimize the curvature and to maintain good posture. Physical activities such as dancing, walking, and swimming are very beneficial and a safe way for individuals with osteoporosis to remain active. An osteopathic physician or physical therapist is the best person from whom to seek an exercise program suited to individual condition and needs.

Muscle-building exercises help to maintain skeletal architecture by improving muscle strength and flexibility. Some evidence indicates that muscle building also helps build bone (Osteoporosis Research, Education and Health Promotion, 1990). Participation in a variety of exercises that include all parts of the body is important to prevent boredom and promote continued interest in maintaining a program. Research is underway into mechanical stress exercise applied to specific portions of the skeleton and the effect on bone strength in those sites. Ginsburg (1994) reports that weight training with professional trainers has helped develop muscle and bone strength in women who were thought to be too fragile for such activity.

Table 19-1

Risk Factors for Types I and II Osteoporosis

General factors	Specifics
TYPE I	
Genetic background	Predominantly white women
	Northwestern European
	Fair skin
Body characteristics	Small
	Slender
Activity level	Immobile
	Inactive
Diseases	Hyperparathyroidism
	Hyperthyroidism
	Cushing syndrome
	Kidney disease
	Rheumatoid arthritis
	Advanced alcoholism
	Liver cirrhosis
	Diabetes mellitus
	Chronic obstructive pulmonary disease
TYPE II	
Drugs	Corticosteroids
	Isoniazid
	Tetracycline
	Some anticonvulsants
	Thyroid supplements
	Furosemide
	Heparin
Other	Gonadal hormone deficiencies
	Smoking

Data from Jennings J, Baylink D: Osteoporosis. In Calkins E, Davis PJ, Ford AB, editors: *The practice of geriatrics,* Philadelphia, 1986, Saunders; Miller G: Osteoporosis: is it inevitable? *J Gerontol Nurs* 11:10, 1985; and Spencer H et al: Disorders of the skeletal system. In Rossman I, editor: *Clinical geriatrics,* ed 3, Philadelphia, 1986, Lippincott.

Life-style changes are necessary for those with osteoporosis, especially when there is evidence of eating and drinking patterns of excessive alcohol, protein, salt, and caffeine. Reduction of cigarette smoking is another change that becomes necessary. All of these excesses cause bone to lose calcium.

Education or knowledge is perhaps the most important issue in prevention and treatment of osteoporosis.

Knowledge about the sites most vulnerable to fracture through accidents, falls, back strain, and poor posture should be provided. Explanation should be given about changes in the upper spine that occur when vertebrae are weakened and about the pain that results from strain on the lower spine to compensate for balance and height changes attributable to alteration of the upper spine.

Personal safety should be addressed for those with osteoporosis to avoid falls. Shoes with good support should be worn. Handrails should be used, and walking in poorly lighted areas should be avoided. Basic body mechanics such as not bending or lifting heavy objects should be learned. Use of step stools or chairs for reaching things in high places should be discouraged. Home safety should include good lighting, railings, and other aids as needed. Walkways should be kept free of obstacles; loose rugs and electrical cords should be arranged so that they do not cause falls.

Actual prevention of osteoporosis must begin in the teenage years. As women are increasingly living into their 80s and 90s, the treatment of osteoporosis is becoming big business. At this time osteoporotic damage cannot be repaired, but prevention of resorption of bone with various pharmaceuticals is an important goal that is generating much research.

Sodium fluoride has been thought to be useful in strengthening bone mass. Slow-release sodium fluoride and calcium citrate administered for 4 years have been shown to inhibit vertebral fractures (Pak et al, 1995); however, Sogaard et al (1995) found increasing reduction in bone strength and quality during long-term ingestion of sodium fluoride. Clearly, more study of sodium fluoride will be necessary.

The pharmacologic treatments now available are by prescription only: hormone replacement therapy, calcitonin, alendronate sodium (Fosamax), and raloxifene hydrochloride (Evista). The standard treatment for osteoporosis has been estrogen (Prestwood et al, 1994) and calcium supplementation, along with recommendations for increased exercise and weight bearing. Long-term use of calcium supplementation, 5 years or more, reduces the lifetime fracture rate at all sites and by 50% at the hip (US Department of Health and Human Services, 1995). However, the public is becoming more cautious because the incidence of breast cancer has risen in tandem with the use of artificial hormones. Several longitudinal studies of women have demonstrated the efficacy of ERT in slowing the rate of bone resorption in women (National Osteoporosis Foundation, 1996).

Raloxifene hydrochloride is the first in a class of selective estrogen receptor modulators (SERMs) that is being marketed as an osteoporosis preventive and a drug that also decreases risk of breast cancer (Cummings, 1999).

One must be cautious, particularly with very old women, because long-range effects of none of these medications are known. Simple, effective, and risk-free diagnostic or treatment methods are not available at this time.

Nursing Interventions
Intervention, like prevention, should be directed toward educating clients about their medical regimen, assisting them in adapting to their disease, and preventing disease progression. Medical interventions of which the nurse should be knowledgeable include the various types of therapies used in the treatment of osteoporosis (Fig. 19-3). Therapy includes the use of several drugs or combinations of drugs, some of which have not yet received Food and Drug Administration (FDA) approval. ERT for women who are in menopause or who have had surgical removal of their ovaries retards bone loss.

Nursing interventions for the individual with osteoporosis who is not hospitalized should focus on teaching and assisting the individual in maintaining a positive approach toward the disease and prevention of its progression or complications. Interventions include the following:

1. Teaching about nutritionally balanced calcium-rich diets that include milk or milk substitutes for those who are lactose intolerant (see Chapter 10)
2. Teaching the client to take 1500 mg of calcium daily through diet and/or calcium supplements
3. Teaching about the factors that inhibit calcium absorption, such as excess protein or salt, and excretion enhancers, such as caffeine; excess fiber; phosphorus in meats, sodas, and preserved foods; and the influence of the body's response to stress (decreased calcium absorption and increased excretion of calcium in the urine)
4. Discussing the pros and cons of ERT
5. Ensuring understanding of medication and adjunct regimens
6. Encouraging women to maintain a daily schedule or alternate-day schedule of weight-bearing exercises such as walking, low-impact aerobics, workout machines, swimming, or a combination of activities

Much remains to be done in preventing osteoporosis. Young women must be taught preventive measures to forestall the development of osteoporosis and reduce

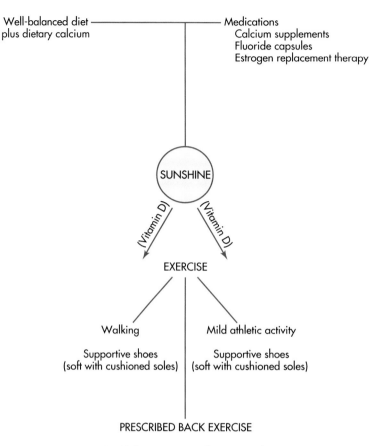

Fig. 19-3   Treatment of osteoporosis.

the enormous cost of osteoporotic fractures and the painful disability and discomfort to the individual.

DEGENERATIVE JOINT DISORDERS

Degenerative arthritic and rheumatic disorders are the most common of the afflictions that disable elders. It is estimated that there are 120 types of these problems that arise from various combinations of overuse, obesity, enzyme imbalances, and infections. They affect up to 37 million individuals in the United States, young as well as old (Dalton, 1995), and include disorders of joints and connective tissue throughout the body. These disorders create pain, depression, immobility, and functional and self-concept disturbances. Arthritis, although the most prevalent disorder of aging, is by no means equally distributed throughout the elderly population by age, gender, or geography. At age 65 more than 385

per 1000 of these are men and 498 per 1000 are women. By age 65 this increases to 437 and 616, respectively (US Bureau of the Census, 1998).

Osteoarthritis

Osteoarthritis (OA), a "wear and tear" noninflammatory joint disorder that affects at least 16 million Americans, is characterized by the deterioration of articular cartilage, which continues to slowly progress. It is the most common of the arthritic disorders, and 90% of elders show some evidence of these changes on x-ray examination, although they are not necessarily aware of arthritic changes. Elderly persons with OA experience joint deterioration more often than younger persons because joint-protective mechanisms such as neuromuscular response and muscle conditioning are impaired in elders (Felson, 1993). Excess weight and other factors exacerbate the problems (Box 19-2). Many find move-

Box 19-2	FACTORS CONTRIBUTING TO THE DEVELOPMENT OF OSTEOARTHRITIS
Age	Gender
Obesity	Climate
Overuse of joints	Injury/trauma of joints
Hyperuricemia/hypertension	

From Kee C et al: Perspectives on the nursing management of osteoarthritis, *Geriatr Nurs* 19(1):19-27, 1998.

ment restricted and joints hypertrophied, stiff, and painful. Discomfort tends to be worse in the morning after a night of inactivity, after excessive use, and when there is a change in the weather. Major areas affected are the hands, knees, hips, lumbar spine, and cervical spine. One may hear a grinding or grating sound, particularly in the neck, when moving. This crepitation is an indication of the deterioration of the synovial covering of the joint.

About 85% of people over 70 years of age have varying degrees of neck pain as a result of OA (Mayo Foundation for Medical Education and Research, 1994). OA of the knee occurs in about 10% of individuals over age 65 and accounts for considerable pain, disability, and costly care. Most total knee replacements are done because of OA (Galanos, 1992). OA of the hip is the most prevalent form of arthritis in the United States. Persons with OA of the hip experience pain, localized to the groin and anterior or lateral thigh, morning stiffness, and gel phenomenon (feeling that the joint is frozen in one position) (Hochberg et al, 1995). Although not as frequent, OA of the hand may be particularly troublesome because so much of our daily life depends on object manipulation. Characteristically, it limits movement at the base of the thumb and at the end joints of the fingers (Best Ways, 1993).

Assessment

When assessing the musculoskeletal system, the nurse must examine the joints for tenderness, swelling, warmth, redness, subluxation (partial dislocation of a joint), and crepitus (a crackling sound as of rubbing rough edges together). Various assessment tools have been devised to measure joint movement limitations. Grip and the pinch gauge measure strength. Range of motion (ROM) and pain in the hands and fingers demonstrate movement limitations. Overhead lift of

weight and shoulder rotation test strength and ROM of the shoulder. Knee extensor and hip flexion measure ROM, strength, and discomfort (Guralnik et al, 1995). In addition, there may be Heberden nodes visible on the distal joints of fingers, as well as Bouchard nodes on the proximal joints of the fingers and toes. These are often accompanied by deformities in the flexion of these joints.

Determine both the active and passive range of joint motion. How far can the person reach and bend all joints without assistance, and what is the reach, flexion, and extension with assistance? The testing of passive range of motion must go only to the point of discomfort and never to induce pain. Test the functional ability of the arms by asking the person to touch the back of the head with both hands. Test the flexibility of the hands by surveying the movements as the individual uses eating utensils.

Interventions

The goals of intervention and management of OA are to control pain, to minimize disability, and to educate the client (Hochberg et al, 1995). It is clear that obesity aggravates the symptoms of OA of the knee. Therefore the first positive action an individual might take is weight reduction. Cowan and Galanos (1992) describe a supervised fitness walking regimen for OA of the knees designed to maintain mobility and functional status. They found that when carefully supervised, walking for short periods was successful in reducing pain and increasing walking capacity. There is still disagreement in the literature about the wisdom of walking any more than necessary with an osteoarthritic knee. The value of walking, if these findings can be replicated, may be in morale and weight control, as well as in weight bearing and movement. We reiterate: the client must be the judge of whether walking for fitness increases or reduces the discomfort and limitations.

Medical management may include sodium hyaluronate, a natural chemical found in synovial fluid, particularly in that of the knee joint. A course of five injections of purified natural sodium hyaluronate has been found to relieve pain in the majority of patients for 6 months or longer (Sanofi Pharmaceuticals, 1998). Medical management guidelines for patients with osteoarthritis of the hip can be seen in Table 19-2.

Particular guidelines for the best ways to relieve OA of the hand can be seen in Box 19-3. General principles for all types of OA are intermittent rest periods interspersed with periods of mild activity; cold applications to ease pain and warmth to relax muscles (applications not to exceed 20 minutes for each); in some cases immobilization with braces when pain is aggravated by movement; and nonsteroidal antiinflammatory drugs (NSAIDs) judiciously used and never on an empty stomach (Mayo, 1994). Arthroscopy, or surgery through a thin telescope inserted directly into the joint, is sometimes helpful but is not suitable for everyone. Table 19-3 provides guidelines for nursing interventions, and Kee has summarized studies to validate the effectiveness of various interventions (Kee et al, 1998) (Table 19-4).

Surgical interventions. Surgical interventions are largely successful and are recommended for even the very old. The importance of immediate and ongoing physical therapy cannot be overstated. The acute post-surgical care is designed to restore the physiologic functions following any extensive surgery: maintaining fluids, movement, and nutritional adequacy. Pain man-

agement is critical to ensure that the individual will move about as necessary and is essential to achievement of maximal recovery. With the increasing efficiency and advances in surgery, it is quite miraculous to see the rapid recovery of even the very old. It cannot be overstated that ongoing therapy from accredited physical therapists is essential for restoration of full movement. During the recovery period weight loss (if the client is overweight) and muscle building are highly recommended. In many cases the increased ease and enhancement of the activities of daily living become highly motivating.

Surgical total joint arthroplasty (replacement of hips and knees) brings relief from pain and functional limitations. Consideration must be given to the potential for wound healing, rehabilitation, and psychosocial factors. Changes in synovium, cartilage, and soft tissues must be assessed before opting for surgical procedures such as synovectomy, arthroplasty, arthrodesis, and bone grafting. Outcomes depend on the timing of

---

Table 19-2

Medical Management of Patients With Osteoarthritis of the Hip*

NONPHARMACOLOGIC THERAPY

Patient education
  Self-management programs (e.g., Arthritis Self-
    Help Course)
  Health professional social support via telephone
    contact
  Weight loss (if overweight)
  Physical therapy
    Range-of-motion exercises
    Strengthening exercises
    Assistive devices for ambulation
  Occupational therapy
    Joint protection and energy conservation
    Assistive devices for ADLs and IADLs
  Aerobic aquatic exercise programs

PHARMACOLOGIC THERAPY

  Nonopioid analgesics (e.g., acetaminophen)
  Nonsteroidal antiinflammatory drugs
  Opioid analgesics (e.g., propoxyphene, codeine,
    oxycodone)

From Hochberg MC et al: Guidelines for the medical management of osteoarthritis. I. Osteoarthritis of the hip, *Arthritis Rheum* 38:1535, 1995.
**ADLs,* Activities of daily living; *IADLs,* instrumental activities of daily living.

Box 19-3 ACTIVITIES FOR MANAGEMENT OF ARTHRITIS OF THE HANDS

Start exercising slowly with no more than four or five repetitions one or two times daily.
Consider consultation with an occupational therapist for individually designed exercises.
Use one hand to gently massage the other from knuckle joints to fingertips, and then reverse the process; then do the same with the other hand.
Stretch wrist in circular motion, then bend backward as far as possible without discomfort.
Stretch muscles and ligaments in forearm by resting arm with palm down and rotating lower arm until palm faces upward.
Avoid overuse of any set of muscles.
Avoid repetitious movements.
Lift objects with both hands.
Press on plunger-type spray bottles with both hands.
Rise from armchair by pushing down on both palms (do not push with knuckle pressure).
Hold a coffee mug with both hands wrapped around the mug.

Modified from The best ways to relieve osteoarthritis of the hand, *Johns Hopkins Med Lett* 5(8):3, 1993.

surgery; the number of procedures that the surgeon and the hospital have to their credit; and the patient's medical status, perioperative and postoperative management, and rehabilitation (Hochberg et al, 1995). Nearly twice as many women as men have joint replacements, and over 60% of all joint replacements are in individuals over 65 years of age (US Bureau of the Census, 1998).

Rheumatoid Arthritis

Rheumatoid arthritis (RA) is thought to be one of the autoimmune disorders that involve both environmental and genetic factors (Davis, 1995). It may occur at any age, but it tends to become more frequent in individu-

---

Table 19-3

Nursing Interventions in Osteoarthritis

PAIN MANAGEMENT

Behavioral-cognitive pain control (imagery, relaxation, distraction)
Analgesic medications
Localized applications of heat

EXERCISE

Range of motion initially, progressing to aerobic exercise as tolerated/prescribed
Exercise alternated with rest
Avoiding prolonged rest periods

DIET

Weight loss if obese
Balanced, nutritious diet

JOINT PROTECTION

Avoiding high-impact activities in affected joints
Good body mechanics
Assistive devices: canes, commode extenders, Velcro-fastened clothing

PSYCHOSOCIAL PARAMETERS

Assess coping strategies, self-efficacy beliefs, social support

EDUCATION

Nature of osteoarthritis disease process
Purpose of prescribed interventions

From Kee C et al: Perspectives on the nursing management of osteoarthritis, *Geriatr Nurs* 19(1):19-27, 1998.

---

als, particularly women, after age 60. In contrast to OA, wherein the synovial covering of a joint is worn away, in RA the affected synovium becomes massively hypertrophic and edematous with projections of synovial tissue protruding into the joint cavity (Davis, 1995). This is thought to be possibly due to a smoldering infection stimulated by an unknown antigen. Generally, it begins with bilateral swelling and inflammation of the synovial membrane of small, peripheral joints, particularly of the wrist, knee, ankle, and hand, although it affects large joints as well. It is unpredictable in its course and may have periods of remission and exacerbation that seem influenced by psychosocial factors, as well as changes in synovia. Significant joint damage can occur during the first 2 years of disease onset. The course usually continues downward in spite of periods of remission. Ten years after onset, 50% of afflicted individuals are unable to work and have other limitations in function, and life expectancy may be shortened (Marino, McDonald, 1991). Symptoms in late life tend to be acutely uncomfortable and spread throughout the joints of the body. Sometimes the disorder affects systems other than joints.

Assessment

Early diagnosis is important because irreversible destruction of affected joints may occur within 1 to 2 years after onset (Paget, 1995). Unfortunately, over half of the individuals with symptoms have not been diagnosed, and of those who have, half do not know what type of arthritis they have (Arthritis Foundation, 1999). Early signs include generalized fatigue, malaise, stiffness with swelling, erythema, and warmth over affected joints. Weight loss is common. Usually joint involvement is symmetric rather than asymmetric as in osteoarthritis. An elevated rheumatoid arthritis factor (RF) and an elevated erythrocyte sedimentation rate (ESR) are most suggestive of RA.

Interventions

Prostaglandins play a primary role in both the onset and relief of the inflammation of arthritis, and the balancing of prostaglandins is the key to controlling inflammation (Dalton, 1995). Excess prostaglandins and other metabolic by-products can be inactivated and flushed from the body by increased dietary fiber and sufficient fluid intake; lacking these, arthritis may be either induced or aggravated. Certain dietary substances such as the "nightshades" (tomatoes, peppers, potatoes, and eggplant) may exacerbate symp-

Table 19-4

Highlights From Selected References Regarding Management of Osteoarthritis

	Investigators	Year	Topic	Findings	Nursing significance
General overview	Jones and Doherty	1995	General overview of osteoarthritis	N/A	Good review of the osteoarthritis process, types, and treatment strategies
	Puett and Griffin	1994	Review of osteoarthritis treatments other than surgery and drugs	Overall, the literature is deficient in addressing alternative osteoarthritis treatments	Research deficits in identifying effective treatment strategies other than surgery and drugs mean that alternative treatments should be verified on an individual basis
Pain management	Burckhardt	1990	Chronic pain	N/A	Overview provided of pain mechanisms, assessment, and a variety of management strategies
	Dekker et al	1992	Pain and disability in osteoarthritis	Pain and disability associated with muscle weakness, bone degeneration, and psychologic effects	Pain control is critical so patients will not avoid exercising; lack of exercise has both physically and psychologically harmful effects
	Duncan and O'Koon	1995	Laypersons' guide to drugs used to treat common arthritic conditions	N/A	Useful as a quick reference for arthritis drugs (NSAIDs and analgesics); provides possible side effects and contraindications
	Keefe et al	1987	Pain-coping strategies	Pain control and rational thinking are important to pain management	Pain-coping strategies need careful assessment; training in coping skills may be helpful
Exercise	Bunning and Materson	1991	Overview of exercise and osteoarthritis	N/A	Review article that provides definitions for exercise types, exercise myths, and practical strategies
	McKeag	1992	Relationship of exercise and osteoarthritis	N/A	Provides overview of physiology of osteoarthritis; discusses exercise as cause and treatment for osteoarthritis

From Kee C et al: Perspectives on the nursing management of osteoarthritis, *Geriatr Nurs* 19(1):19-27, 1998.
N/A, Not applicable; *NSAIDs*, nonsteroidal antiinflammatory drugs.

Continued

Table 19-4—cont'd

Highlights From Selected References Regarding Management of Osteoarthritis

	Investigators	Year	Topic	Findings	Nursing significance
Diet	Felson et al	1992	Weight loss and osteoarthritis	Decreases in weight decrease chances of developing osteoarthritis	Emphasizes attention to weight maintenance within recommended standards
Psychosocial variables	Burke and Flaherty	1993	Coping strategies in women with osteoarthritis	Self-control is used most often	Important to assess coping strategies and their effectiveness
	Downe-Wamboldt	1991	Stress, emotions, and coping in osteoarthritis	Osteoarthritis has physical, psychologic, and social consequences	Must be aware that osteoarthritis has daily impact on work and leisure activities
	Weinberger et al	1990	Social support, stress, and functional status	Social support directly impacts functional status	Assesses all aspects of social support for possible deficits: self-esteem, appraisal, belonging, and tangible support
Education	Bill-Harvey et al	1989	Osteoarthritis education for patients with low literacy skills	Teaching about osteoarthritis by use of indigenous instructors was an effective method	Planning osteoarthritis community health education programs with the target audience and community residents helps ensure appropriateness and success
	Goeppinger et al	1989	Compared home and small group osteoarthritis study programs	Small group intervention improved pain and depression; home study intervention improved perceived helplessness	Individual assessment important in selecting educational program type
	Lorig et al	1987	Extensive review of patient education	Patient education has been effective in symptom management	Education for pain control is of primary importance; interactive educational modes work best

toms and, if so, should be eliminated from the diet (Dalton, 1995).

The client needs psychologic support, rest, analgesics, and antiinflammatory medications (both NSAIDs and corticosteroids). Flexion contractures of the involved joints are common, resulting in limitation of movement and pain. Pain in all stages of arthritis is

a serious consideration. See Chapter 17 for suggestions regarding pain management.

Most recent philosophy tends toward vigorous treatment of RA with disease-modifying antirheumatic drugs (DMARDs) and use of NSAIDs as adjunctive rather than primary modes of pain management. Nurses must advocate for clients because they may not be aware of the importance of rapid and aggressive treatment. The Arthritis, Rheumatism, and Aging Medical Information System (ARAMIS) data banks have clearly shown the following: (1) RA is not a benign, self-limiting disease but one that increases morbidity and mortality; (2) NSAIDs are not benign but create serious gastrointestinal disorders and hemorrhage, and although they may relieve pain, they have no effect on the progression of the disease; and (3) even though DMARDs are more toxic than NSAIDs, the disability and pain are significantly reduced (Fries, 1995). For further discussion of drugs see Chapter 15.

Because of the unknown causes and unpredictable but persistent nature of arthritis, people often fall prey to worthless cure tactics. However, some may be effective because they act as placebos. Self-help and support groups are useful, but the individual often must simply learn to live with a certain degree of constant discomfort. It seems that feelings of self-efficacy, induced by increased knowledge and feelings of control, may have more positive outcomes even in the presence of increasing debilitation.

Management of arthritis through classes in specially designed exercises, relaxation, and pain management techniques has been useful. Box 19-4 lists management goals.

Participants in these classes are also given general information about their disease and taught to use medication wisely. These classes have shown that patients with arthritis can take control of their situation and increase functional independence with a minimal amount of discomfort. Based on the success of this effort, the National Arthritis Foundation is now offering similar courses throughout the United States. Many medical centers and senior care centers now have arthritis clinics, and these should be sought for a thorough evaluation and individualized treatment program. At present, arthritis cannot be prevented or cured.

Gout

Gout is an acutely painful and recurrent arthritic inflammation of the peripheral joints. The joint of the great toe is the most typical site of an attack. Sometimes the ankle, knee, wrist, or elbow is involved. There is often a low-grade temperature, although this is less usual in the elderly. The disorder is similar to rheumatoid arthritis in symptomatology. The cause is hyperuricemia that creates deposits of urate crystals in

---

Box 19-4   GOALS OF NURSING MANAGEMENT AND INTERVENTIONS IN ARTHRITIS

Goals

Pain management and promotion of comfort
Exercise and rest interspersed
Psychologic support
Reduction of swelling and inflammation
Prevention of deformity
Promotion of optimal life-style

Suggested Interventions

Provide realistic information.
Teach client self-care to promote comfort.
Assist client in modifying life-style appropriately.
Prescribe exercises for muscle maintenance.
Promote participation in weight reduction program if necessary.
Have client balance rest and activity.
Teach relaxation and stress reduction.
Teach client to avoid bending painful joints and to splint when joints are inflamed.
Teach client to maintain body alignment when standing, sitting, and lying down.

Data from Heckheimer EF: *Health promotion of the elderly in the community,* Philadelphia, 1989, Saunders.

---

soft tissue. In acute gouty arthritis, synovial fluid shows inflammatory changes and an elevated white blood cell (WBC) count, as well as visible urate crystals in the fluid when seen under a polarized light microscope. Gout may be exacerbated by drugs commonly taken by the elderly, particularly thiazide diuretics and salicylates (even in small dosages). Effective treatment of gouty arthritis involves NSAIDs, avoidance of drugs or foods that increase uric acid, and sometimes injection of long-lasting steroids into the synovial fluid cavity (Ettinger, 1995).

Geriatric Shoulder Pain

Shoulder pain in the geriatric patient is commonly seen by primary physicians. Often it is dismissed as rather inconsequential, because it does not inhibit general mobility, tends to persist for long periods, and is difficult to assess properly (Glockner, 1995). Proper evaluation requires an understanding of patient anatomy, a thorough physical examination, and a knowledge of common shoulder disorders that occur in the aged population (Vecchio et al, 1995). Because it is seldom seen as serious by the client or the physician, the nurse may be the one to observe the limitations imposed by a shoulder disorder.

The most demonstrable effects of a shoulder disorder are impairment of personal care, inability to accomplish some household tasks, and pain on movement (Vecchio et al, 1995). Often the pain interferes with sleep, and the client has difficulty moving the arm to eat if the pain is in the dominant side. One man suffered intense pain for a period of 6 months, but because the physicians attending him paid little attention, he thought he was doomed to have the pain for the remainder of his life. Medications did not seem to help, and most of the activities he enjoyed required the use of his right arm, which he could not extend or rotate externally. He held his arm as if he were hemiplegic. With aggressive examination and diagnosis it was determined that he had a rotator cuff tear. Intensive therapy, prescribed exercises, and medication finally alleviated the problem.

Shoulder pain may be a result of inflammatory disorders, degenerative problems, fractures or contusions, shoulder separation involving the clavicle, impingement syndrome involving the rotator cuff, biceps tendinitis, or referred pain from other areas (Glockner, 1995).

Assessment

The shoulder comprises four separate articulations: the glenohumeral, acromioclavicular, sternoclavicular, and scapulothoracic. The combined motion of these joints provides the wide range of motion possible in the shoulder. The shoulder has a more extensive range of motion than any other joint. To effectively use this wide range of motion, the soft tissues of the shoulder must provide the necessary stability.

During assessment, the onset, nature, location, and duration of pain and its relationship to daily activities should be determined. Pain patterns can provide important diagnostic clues. Pain that increases with activity suggests tendon impingement or degenerative arthritis. Pain with numbness and tingling may indicate cervical radiculopathy. Pain that occurs most severely at night is often seen with rotator cuff tears.

Chronic rotator cuff tears are most commonly seen in elderly patients. They represent the cumulative ef-

fects of many years of wear as the rotator cuff tendons glide under the acromion. Repetitive overhead motion impinges on the undersurface of the acromion (Zuckerman, Shapiro, 1987). Range of motion of the shoulder should be tested with the patient sitting, and roentgenographic examination should include two views taken at 90 degrees to each other. When these are not done, the assessment will be incomplete. The drop-arm test may be helpful in diagnosing a rotator cuff tear. While sitting, the patient is asked to slowly lower the arm. Inability to do so indicates a rotator cuff tear. However, depending on the location and extent of the tear, there may be limitations in lifting and lowering objects.

Interventions

Antiinflammatory medications and injected steroids may provide relief. When pain persists for more than 2 months, surgical treatment may be indicated. Shoulder replacement has been shown to provide excellent pain relief in 90% to 95% of persons undergoing the surgical procedure, but shoulder replacement has been reserved for patients in severe pain unalleviated by other methods. The nursing role in dealing with persons who have intractable shoulder pain is to encourage them to emphasize to the physician the need for a thorough examination and to keep an extensive log of the patterns of pain, its intensity, its frequency, and specific positions that cause the most pain. A complete discussion of pain management can be found in Chapter 17. Often the nurse must act as patient advocate to encourage surgery if pain resolution has not occurred within 6 to 8 weeks (Glockner, 1995). Surgical intervention for older patients is not to be discouraged. Hattrup (1995) reports that in those over 65 years of age, 77% had excellent results.

COMPLEMENTARY AND ALTERNATIVE MEDICINE

Chronic diseases are particularly responsive to complementary therapies of various kinds. Complementary and alternative medicine (CAM) has been used extensively and effectively for centuries, particularly in the Orient. Although there is an office of Complementary and Alternative Medicine in the U.S. Department of Health and Human Services, we prefer to consider these holistic alternative therapies more than a branch of medicine. These therapies are particularly effective approaches in the management of chronic conditions such as osteoarthritis and rheumatoid arthritis. Just as the triggers for disease flare-ups are poorly understood, so are the reasons why the alternative, nonmedical interventions are often very helpful. Some of the complementary therapies now are included in Medicaid and Medicare health coverage. The nurse is advised to caution the suffering individual to thoroughly investigate the credentials and durability of the providers of complementary therapies. Many methods of self-directed care are costly and may be ineffectual or actually hazardous. As in all forms of therapy, the consumer is urged to proceed slowly and moderately and to try only one approach at a time to determine effects. Above all, one should listen to one's body signals. See Resources at the end of this chapter for guidance.

Chiropractic

Chiropractic is the most widely used of all complementary therapies and is sought chiefly for musculoskeletal pain. Originally, chiropractic therapy involved manipulation of the spine and its effects on the nervous system, but chiropractic has now expanded into a more holistic approach that involves "disease prevention and health promotion through structural integrity and harmony with the environment" (Haldeman, 1992).

Homeopathy

Homeopathy was established as an alternative medical practice by Samuel Hahnemann, a German physician and pharmacist, over 200 years ago. In the late nineteenth century it was a very popular medical model involving the "law of similars." Homeopathy uses minute doses of substances with properties that resemble the symptoms of the patient and that correctly administered will stimulate the individual's immune reactive system toward self-healing potential. The present model of homeopathic medicine is best seen in immunizations. Breedveld's studies (1995) seem to have originated in homeopathic principles. We still have much to learn about how homeopathy may be effective in chronic and autoimmune disorders.

Acupuncture and Acupressure

Acupuncture and acupressure have been used in China since 2500 BC. These therapies are thought to be effective because the techniques balance body, mind, and spirit through manipulation of the universal life-sustaining energy *(chi)*. Acupressure exerts pressure at

various spots along the 12 meridians, or pathways, through which *chi* flows to nourish the body. Acupuncture uses fine-needle twirling at these points. When these points are stimulated, the nervous system releases endorphins and cortisol. Usually 10 to 12 visits with an accredited or certified acupuncturist are sufficient (Lorenzi, 1999). Again, individuals must be cautioned to determine the credentials of alternative care providers (see Resources at the end of this chapter).

Reflexology

Reflexology most often involves pressure on certain zones of the feet or hands that are thought to access the major organs. The thumb or finger is applied with deep pressure to the reflex point on the hand or foot. The goal is similar to that of acupressure in that it is intended to restore the *chi* balance and improve the circulation of blood and lymph. Elders with lower extremity circulatory problems should not use this therapy.

Other Therapies

The therapeutic value of massage, aromatherapy, crystal therapy, and magnet therapy is not documented as well as or as consistently as that of some of the other alternative therapies, but all of these therapies are based on some idea of energy exchange, redirection, or enhanced circulation, and all have been found to be effective by some individuals in dealing with bone, joint, and arthritic disorders.

• • •

We encourage nurses to ask individuals what self-initiated practices they use to manage their chronic disorders more effectively and which therapies have not been helpful. Not only is this often a very interesting and illuminating discussion, but it opens the topic of alternative therapies for discussion and consideration.

▶ KEY CONCEPTS

- As many as 90% of people over 70 years of age have osteoarthritis (the "wear and tear" syndrome) with accompanying discomfort of muscles and joints.
- Osteoporosis is a crippling problem for many elders, especially women. It can usually be prevented by early interventions: exercise, weight bearing, and calcium intake. Some medications are helpful, but

genetics is an important contributor to the development of osteoporosis.

- Rheumatoid arthritis may occur at any age, but the incidence increases in the later years. It is thought to be one of the immune disorders. It produces swelling, inflammation, intense pain, and distortion of the joints.

- Gout is a disorder of metabolism, and although it was thought to be a result of "high living," this has proved to be untrue, although certain amino by-products form extremely painful crystals in the joints, particularly of the great toe. Dietary changes may be helpful, but usually medication is needed.

- Certain types of complementary and alternative medicine have proved very helpful to individuals with joint disorders and chronic discomfort. The buyer must beware because there are many hucksters selling to the distressed.

- Because of the chronic and painful nature of bone and joint disorders in the later years, many individuals seeking solutions to their discomfort are vulnerable to faddish, unproven remedies.

▶ Activities and Discussion Questions

1. What are the most effective ways of preventing osteoporosis?
2. What life-style issues would you discuss with an individual with advanced osteoporosis?

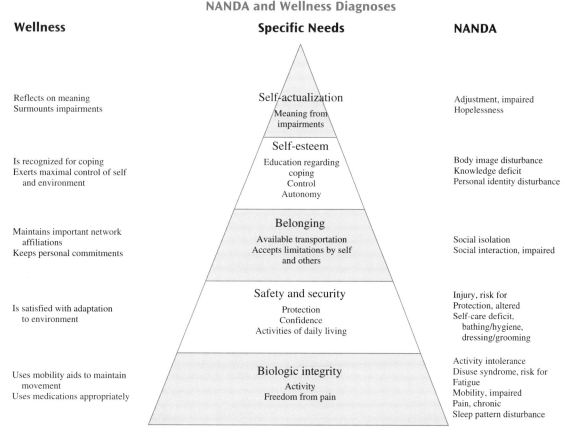

NANDA and Wellness Diagnoses

Wellness	Specific Needs	NANDA
	Self-actualization	
Reflects on meaning	Meaning from	Adjustment, impaired
Surmounts impairments	impairments	Hopelessness
	Self-esteem	
Is recognized for coping	Education regarding	Body image disturbance
Exerts maximal control of self	coping	Knowledge deficit
and environment	Control	Personal identity disturbance
	Autonomy	
	Belonging	
Maintains important network	Available transportation	Social isolation
affiliations	Accepts limitations by self	Social interaction, impaired
Keeps personal commitments	and others	
	Safety and security	
Is satisfied with adaptation	Protection	Injury, risk for
to environment	Confidence	Protection, altered
	Activities of daily living	Self-care deficit, bathing/hygiene, dressing/grooming
	Biologic integrity	Activity intolerance
Uses mobility aids to maintain	Activity	Disuse syndrome, risk for
movement	Freedom from pain	Fatigue
Uses medications appropriately		Mobility, impaired
		Pain, chronic
		Sleep pattern disturbance

These are not all of the possible wellness or NANDA diagnoses that may be identified. The above are frequent examples of nursing diagnoses that should be considered when planning care for the older adult in whatever setting.

3. What are the differences in appearance of osteoarthritis and rheumatoid arthritis?
4. What advice would you give someone who is experiencing joint pain and mobility limitations?
5. Explain what could be done for an elder complaining of shoulder pain.
6. Discuss your thoughts and experiences relating to alternative methods of dealing with chronic pain.
7. Which of your favorite activities would be difficult if you were afflicted with osteoarthritis?

RESOURCES

American Holistic Nurses' Association
    PO Box 2130
    2733 Lakin Drive, Suite 2
    Flagstaff, AZ 86003-2130
    (800) 278-AHNA
American Massage Therapy Association
    820 Davis Street, Suite 100
    Evanston, IL 60201
    (847) 864-0123
    www.amtamassage.org
Institute of Classical Homeopathy
    1336-D Oak Avenue
    St. Helena, CA 94574
    (415) 248-1632
    www.classical homeopathy.org
National Certification for Acupuncture and Oriental Medicine
    (703) 548-9004
    www.nccaom.org
National Certification Board for Therapeutic Massage and Body-work
    8201 Greensboro Drive, Suite 300
    McLean, VA 22102
    (800) 296-0664
    www.ncbtmb.com
National Institute of Health
    Office of Alternative Medicine
    www.altmed.od.nih.gov

REFERENCES

Ali N, Twibell R: Barriers to osteoporosis prevention in perimenopausal and elderly women, *Geriatr Nurs* 15(4):201, 1994.

Arthritis Foundation: *Arthritis Foundation launches "edit RA"— a national consumer education campaign on rheumatoid arthritis,* Press release, Atlanta, Aug 30, 1999.

Bauer DC: Factors associated with appendicular bone mass in older women, *Ann Intern Med* 118:657, 1993.

The best ways to relieve osteoarthritis of the hand, *Johns Hopkins Med Lett* 5(8):3, 1993.

Bill-Harvey D et al: Outcome of an osteoarthritis education program for low-literacy patients taught by indigenous instructors, *Patient Educ Couns* 13:133-142, 1989.

Breedveld F et al: Therapeutic regulation of T cells in rheumatoid arthritis, *Immunol Rev* 144:5, 1995.

Bunning RD, Materson RS: A rational program of exercise for patients with osteoarthritis, *Semin Arthritis Rheum* 21(3 Suppl 2):33-43, 1991.

Burckhardt CS: Chronic pain, *Nurs Clin North Am* 25:863-870, 1990.

Burke M, Flaherty MJ: Coping strategies and health status of elderly arthritic women, *J Adv Nurs* 18:7-13, 1993.

Copstead LC: *Perspectives on pathophysiology,* Philadelphia, 1995, Saunders.

Cowan K, Galanos AN: Fitness walking for osteoarthritis of the knee, *Geriatr Med Curr* 13(2):7, 1992.

Cummings SR: Raloxifene hydrochloride lessens risk of invasive breast cancer, *JAMA* 281:2189-2196, 1999.

Dalton C: Complementary therapies in arthritis treatment, *Adv Nurse Pract* 3(11):33, 1995.

Davis J: Disease mechanisms and therapeutic options. In *Diagnosis and treatment of rheumatoid arthritis: a special report for primary care physicians,* The Institute for Medical Studies, Inc, Laguna Niguel, Calif, 1995, HP Publishing.

Dekker J et al: Pain and disability in osteoarthritis: a review of biobehavioral mechanisms, *J Behav Med* 15:189-214, 1992.

Downe-Wamboldt B: Stress, emotions, and coping: a study of elderly women with osteoarthritis, *Health Care for Women International* 12:85-98, 1991.

Duncan MA, O'Koon M: The drug guide, *Arthritis Today* May: 1-14, 1995.

Ettinger WH: Bone, joint and rheumatic disorders. In Abrams WB, Beers MH, Berkow R, editors: *The Merck manual of geriatrics,* ed 2, Whitehouse Station, NJ, 1995, Merck Research Laboratories

Ezzati TM, Massey JT, Waksberg J: Plan and operation of the Third National Health and Nutrition Examination Survey, 1988-1995, National Center for Health Statistics, *Vital Health Stat* 1(32):48825, 1994.

Felson D: The course of osteoarthritis and factors that affect it, *Rheum Dis Clin North Am* 19(3):607, 1993.

Felson D et al: Alcohol intake and bone mineral density in elderly men and women: the Framingham study, *Am J Epidemiol* 145(5):495, 1995.

Felson DT et al: Weight loss reduces the risk for symptomatic knee osteoarthritis in women: the Framingham study, *Ann Intern Med* 116:535-539, 1992.

Fries J: A new treatment approach: DMARD-based sequential therapy. In *Diagnosis and treatment of rheumatoid arthritis: a special report for primary care physicians,* The Institute for Medical Studies, Laguna Niguel, Calif, 1995, HP Publishing.

Galanos AN: Effect of obesity on symptomatic knee osteoarthritis, *Geriatr Med Curr* 13(2):6, 1992.

Galsworthy TD, Wilson PL: Osteoporosis: it steals more than bone, *Am J Nurs* 96(6):27, 1996.

Gertz BJ et al: Monitoring bone resorption in early postmenopausal women by an immunoassay for cross-linked collagen peptides in urine, *J Bone Miner Res* 9(2):135, 1994.

Ginsburg M: Weights strengthen older women's bones, *San Francisco Examiner* 171:A1, 1994.

Glockner SM: Shoulder pain: a diagnostic dilemma, *Am Fam Physician* 51(7):1677, 1995.

Goeppinger J et al: A reexamination of the effectiveness of self-care education for persons with arthritis, *Arthr Rheum* 32:706-716, 1989.

Guralnik JM et al: *The Women's Health and Aging Study: health and social characteristics of older women with disability,* NIH Pub No 95-4009, Bethesda, Md, 1995, National Institute on Aging.

Haldeman S: *Principles and practice of chiropractic,* ed 2, Norwalk, Conn, 1992, Appleton & Lange.

Hattrup SJ: Rotator cuff repair: relevance of patient age, *J Shoulder Elbow Surg* (2):95-100, 1995.

Hazzard WR et al: *Principles of geriatric medicine and gerontology,* ed 4, New York, 1999, McGraw-Hill.

Helmes E et al: A questionnaire to evaluate disability in osteoporotic patients with vertebral compression fractures, *J Gerontol* 50A(2):M91, 1995.

Hochberg M et al: Guidelines for the medical management of osteoarthritis, *Arthritis Rheum* 38(11):1535, 1995.

Jones A, Doherty M: Osteoarthritis (ABC of rheumatology), *Br Med J* 310:457-460, 1995.

Kee CC et al: Perspectives on the nursing management of osteoarthritis, *Geriatr Nurs* 19(1):19-27, 1998.

Keefe FJ et al: Pain-coping strategies in osteoarthritis patients, *J Consult Clin Psychol* 55:208-212, 1987.

Kessenich C: Osteoporosis in aged men, *Geriatr Nurs* 17(4): 171, 1996.

Lindsay R: The burden of osteoporosis: cost, *Am J Med* 98:9S, 1995.

Looker AC et al: Prevalence of low femoral bone density in older US women from NHANES III, *J Bone Miner Res* 10:796, 1995.

Lorenzi EA: Complementary/alternative therapies: so many choices, *Geriatr Nurs* 20(3):125-133, 1999.

Lorig K et al: Outcomes of self-help education for patients with arthritis, *Arthritis Rheum* 28:680, 1985.

Lorig K, Konkol L, Gonzalez V: Arthritis patient education: a review of the literature, *Patient Education and Counseling* 10:207-252, 1987.

Mann D: *New blood test quickly assesses bone health,* Medical Tribune News Service, Oct 24, 1996.

Marino C, McDonald E: Differential diagnosis of rheumatoid arthritis, *Arthritis* 90:237, 1991.

Mastrangelo R: The silent disease: diagnosing and treating osteoporosis, *Adv Nurse Pract* 2(4):23, 1994.

Mayo Foundation for Medical Education and Research: Neck pain, *Mayo Clin Health Lett* 12(10):4, 1994.

McKeag DB: The relationship of osteoarthritis and exercise, *Clin Sports Med* 11:471-487, 1992.

National Osteoporosis Foundation: *Osteoporosis facts,* Legislation Issue Brief, Washington, DC, Feb 1996, The Foundation.

Osteoporosis research, education and health promotion, part I, Bethesda, Md, 1990, US Department of Health and Human Services, Public Health Service, National Institutes of Health.

Paget S: Diagnostic guidelines. In *Diagnosis and treatment of rheumatoid arthritis: a special report for primary care physicians,* The Institute for Medical Studies, Laguna Niguel, Calif, 1995, HP Publishing.

Pak CY et al: Treatment of postmenopausal osteoporosis with slow-release sodium fluoride, *Ann Intern Med* 123(6):401, 1995.

Prestwood KM et al: The short-term effects of conjugated estrogen on bone turnover in older women, *J Clin Endocrinol Metab* 79(2):366, 1994.

Puett DW, Griffin MR: Published trials on nonmedicinal and noninvasive therapies for hip and knee osteoarthritis, *Ann Intern Med* 121:133-140, 1994.

Sanofi Pharmaceuticals: *Hyalgan (sodium hyaluronate),* Press release, New York, 1998.

Sogaard CH, Mosekilde L, Richards A: Loss of trabecular bone strength and bone quality after 5 years of fluoride therapy for osteoporosis, *Ugeskr Laeger* 157(14):2004, 1995.

Toufexis A: Why the bones break, *Time* 143:97, Jan 31, 1994.

US Bureau of the Census: *Statistical abstract of the United States: 1998,* ed 118, Washington, DC, 1998, US Government Printing Office.

US Department of Health and Human Services, National Institutes of Health, Institute of Arthritis and Musculoskeletal and Skin Diseases (NIAMS): *Research news,* News release, Bethesda, Md, 1995.

Vecchio PC et al: Community survey of shoulder disorders in the elderly to assess the natural history and effects of treatment, *Ann Rheum Dis* 54(2):152, 1995.

Watts N: Prevention of osteoporosis: the role of primary physicians, *J Fam Pract* 32(3):119, 1991.

Weinberger M et al: Social support, stress, and functional status in patients with osteoarthritis, *Soc Sci Med* 30:503-508, 1990.

Zuckerman J Shapiro I: Geriatric shoulder pain: common causes and their management, *Geriatrics* 42(9):43, 1987.

chapter

20

Coping With Cardiac and Respiratory Disorders

▶LEARNING OBJECTIVES

Upon completion of this chapter, the reader will be able to:

- Explain the two types of congestive heart failure (CHF) and the associated symptoms in the older adult.
- Discuss assessment of and intervention for the elder with CHF.
- State the most common respiratory disorders affecting the older adult.
- Discuss the interventions necessary to meet therapy goals for an older adult with chronic obstructive pulmonary disease (COPD).
- Explain the significance of pneumonia and tuberculosis in the older population and discuss means of prevention of each of these diseases.
- Develop a nursing care plan for the elder with CHF; COPD.

▶GLOSSARY

Anergy An immunodeficient condition characterized by lack of or diminished reaction to an antigen or group of antigens.

Co-morbidity More than one disease or health condition existing at the same time.

Congestive heart failure (CHF) The abnormal condition that reflects impaired cardiac pumping action secondary to temporary or permanent heart damage.

MET A unit of measure of heat produced by the body.

Nosocomial Pertaining to the hospital as the source (as in nosocomial infection).

▶THE LIVED EXPERIENCE

When I first had that heart attack, I was so frightened it seemed I would die just from the fear. It was the first time I realized how comforting calm and efficient nurses could be. Then there was the one who came into the room a few days later and talked to me about the cardiac rehab program and that I could continue doing the things I had always done, except for changes in diet and more exercise. Even sex! I would never have asked that young thing, but she just told me it was OK.

Jerry, age 63

When Dad had that heart attack, it really scared us all, and I know we were afraid we would say or do something that would bring on another. I think he was also afraid of everything. I'm so grateful for the cardiac rehab program at the hospital. They seem to give him lots of attention and information about the things he needs to know. He seems quite relaxed with himself now.

Ruth, Jerry's youngest daughter

424

*N*ormal age changes of the cardiovascular and respiratory systems precipitate or exacerbate several similar symptoms. One is interference with adequate oxygenation, another is depletion of energy or fatigue, and another is limited reserve capacity on which to draw when there is system disequilibrium.

The interrelationship or dependency of one system on another indicates that when the nurse is addressing a cardiovascular problem, such as congestive heart failure, the respiratory system must also be seriously considered in the nursing interventions. Conversely, in the elder with serious respiratory problems such as pneumonia or emphysema, the cardiac status must be a part of nursing care. Nursing interventions, then, frequently overlap. One carefully planned action can address several systems at the same time and achieve goals of homeostasis and energy conservation.

CARDIAC DISORDERS

Congestive Heart Failure

Cardiac diseases at some point will precipitate or exacerbate a complex of symptoms known as *congestive heart failure (CHF)*. CHF occurs when there is myocardial involvement and overall cardiac dysfunction. The severity of malfunctioning is dependent on either mechanical or functional abnormality of the structure. Heart failure is best characterized by its related diseases, which are well documented in medical and nursing texts. The most common are coronary artery disease, by far the greatest single cause of heart failure, valvular disease, and hypertension. The commonality among these conditions and CHF is the substantive and irreversible damage to the heart muscle. People do not recover from heart failure; once the heart muscle is damaged, it does not regenerate, nor can it be repaired, short of heart transplantation, which is not readily available for the number of individuals suffering from severe heart failure. Damage is insidious over time because of poor control of hypertension and atherosclerosis, which initiates a chain of adverse events leading to coronary artery disease, heart failure, and end-stage heart disease. Fever, hypoxia, myocardial ischemia, anemia, and infection are some of the acute conditions that can lead to heart failure. Chronic conditions such as valvular disease (aortic stenosis), ventricular hypertrophy, metabolic disease (hyper-hypothyroid), and hypertension are also considered as contributors to heart failure (Wei, 1995) (Box 20-1). Such factors as bad diet, smoking, and lack of exercise and the normal age-

related changes in the cardiovascular system (see Chapter 7) aggravate the development of heart disease, especially for those who happen to have a family history of heart disease and the genetic makeup for heart disease.

Clinical heart failure is categorized as left-sided, right-sided, or biventricular heart failure. Others describe heart failure as systolic or diastolic dysfunction (Marek et al, 1999). Left-sided failure is the most common form and is the most common type in the elderly. In turn, it is responsible for eventual right-sided failure (Braunwald, 1992). A formal functional classification for heart failure was established by the New York Heart Association (Box 20-2). This classification does not speak to the pathogenesis of heart failure, its progres-

---

Box 20-1   CAUSES OF HEART FAILURE

Impeded Forward Ejection
Systemic arterial hypertension or elevated systemic vascular resistance
Aortic valve stenosis
Coarctation of aorta
Subaortic stenosis
Obstructive hypertropic cardiomyopathy
Pulmonary hypertension

Impaired Cardiac Filling
Ventricular hypertrophy
Prolonged myocardial relaxation time (diastolic dysfunction)
Pericardial constriction or tamponade
Restrictive endocarditis or myocardial heart disease
Ventricular aneurysm

Volume Overload
Valvular regurgitation
Increased intravascular volume
Metabolic demands: thyrotoxicosis; anemia
Arteriovenous shunts/fistulas

Myocardial Failure
Loss of muscle function (myocardial infarction; ischemia)
Cardiomyopathy
Myocarditis
Drug induced
Systemic disease (hypothyroid)
Chronic overload

sion, or treatment; it provides assessment guidelines for establishment of severity (Ebersole, Hess, 1998; Gross, 1999).

Assessment

As with any assessment, obtaining a pertinent history of the events leading up to and including the presentation of heart failure is essential whether the history is from the elder patient or the caregiver. Monitoring of vital signs; assessment of the cardiac and respiratory systems by inspection, palpation, percussion, and auscultation; and obtaining a mental status level, as well as kidney function (output), are essential. These and other assessment guidelines are listed in Box 20-3. In addition, the nurse should be on the alert for the clinical presentation of heart failure. Classic presentations can be the "wet profile," which is a result of fluid overload, or the "dry profile," which is due to low cardiac output (Gross, 1999). The wet profile includes dyspnea on exertion, paroxysmal nocturnal dyspnea, orthopnea, cough that is usually worse at night, edema and weight gain, nocturia, nausea and vomiting, and right quadrant pain. The dry profile presents with fatigue, malaise,

weight loss, cachexia, and sleep disorders. Both the wet and dry presentations of heart failure reflect a decrease in activity tolerance and a decreased appetite, or anorexia.

Elders do not always reflect the classic presentation of CHF; instead, an abnormal presentation of acute CHF might include delirium or confusion as an early sign that CHF is beginning to manifest itself. The elder may also complain of dizziness or may have syncopal episodes. Subtle symptoms of CHF may be observed with a perceptible decline from the elder's baseline in functional ability in activities of daily living (ADLs) or in instrumental activities of daily living (IADLs) (Marek et al, 1999). The nurse should be alert to these signs and symptoms in the elderly.

One of the major ways that cardiac conditions and subsequent CHF differ from other chronic problems is that most exacerbations require acute hospitalization and intensive treatment, whereas many other chronic disorders are essentially managed at home the majority of the time. With changing medical care, elders with CHF may be initially admitted to the hospital for stabilization and then either returned home for care or placed in a skilled care facility temporarily or permanently.

Interventions

The goals of therapy are to provide relief of symptoms, improve the quality of life, reduce mortality and mor-

---

Box 20-2   CLASSIFICATION OF HEART FAILURE

Class I: Basically Asymptomatic
Cardiac disease without resulting limitations of physical activity

Class II: Mild Heart Failure
Slight limitation of physical activity
Comfortable at rest
An increase in activity may cause fatigue, palpitations, dyspnea, or anginal pain

Class III: Moderate Heart Failure
Marked limitation in physical activity
Comfortable at rest
Ordinary walking or climbing of stairs can quickly bring on symptoms of fatigue, palpitations, dyspnea, or anginal pain
Substantial periods of bed rest required

Class IV: Severe Heart Failure
Almost permanently confined to bed
Inability to carry out any physical activity without discomfort or severe symptoms
Some symptoms occur at rest
Chronic shortness of breath is common

Box 20-3   ASSESSMENT FOR HEART FAILURE

Brief history of onset and course of condition
Vital signs
Cardiac and respiratory inspection and auscultation of heart and breath sounds
Mental status check
Activity capabilities
Life-style
Genitourinary: nocturia; oliguria
Weight change
Client's perception of condition, reaction to diagnosis, and treatment
General laboratory values: electrolytes, hemoglobin, hematocrit, coagulation

Data from Saunders SA: Atherosclerotic heart disease: heart failure. In Rogers-Seidl FF, editor: *Geriatric nursing care plans,* St Louis, 1991, Mosby; and Havens LL, Weaver JW: Cardiovascular system. In Hogstel MO: *Clinical manual of gerontological nursing,* St Louis, 1992, Mosby.

bidity, and slow or stop progression of left ventricular dysfunction through the use of aggressive drug therapy (Gross, 1999). Concurrent and supportive therapies include diet modification by decreasing fat, cholesterol, and sodium intake; exercise such as walking 30 minutes a day or several times a week; education; and family and social supports (Living With Heart Disease, 1994; Schultz, 1998; Johnson, 1999). The ultimate goal for elders with chronic heart failure is quality, not prolongation of survival (Brown et al, 1999).

Nursing interventions assist in the accomplishment of these goals. What specific interventions are used will depend on the severity of the CHF. Nursing actions range from teaching the older adult about life-style changes in diet, activity, and rest to acute measures such as the administration of oxygen and other emergent procedures in acute situations. In general, interventions about which the nurse should be knowledgeable include the following:

- Activity tolerance
- Prescribed exercise
- Medication administration and the evaluation of medication effects
- Monitoring for signs and symptoms of CHF
- Monitoring intake and output
- Monitoring weight (either daily, biweekly, or weekly)
- Checking for jugular distention
- Auscultating heart and lung sounds
- Noting laboratory values
- Education: low-sodium, low-fat, and low-cholesterol diet; medication regimen; signs and symptoms to report to the physician, such as a 2- to 3-pound weight gain within a few days, increased nocturia, increasing shortness of breath, persistent cough, and ankle and leg swelling

Vitally important for older adults, as well as for younger adults, is cardiac rehabilitation. Coronary problems are likely to produce a "cardiac cripple" when the individual believes that any exertion overtaxes the heart and may potentiate a heart attack or death. In reality, few elders develop activity-induced ischemia. Complicating illnesses, such as infections and bleeding episodes, are more likely to trigger an attack. A decline or lack of activity actually makes individuals with cardiac problems more vulnerable to decompensation (Heart Failure, 1994; Schultz, 1998). Because of this, cardiac exercise rehabilitation programs must be encouraged for the physical, as well as mental, health of the individual. Exercise training of elderly coronary patients has been found to increase work capacity and va-

gal tone and decrease resting heart rate, body weight, and the percentage of body fat (Wenger, 1990; Stanley, 1999). Typical programs are prescribed by the physician and begin with light activity and progress to moderate activity under the supervision of a nurse or physical therapist.

The level of activity is often expressed in metabolic equivalents (METs). For example, light to moderate housework is equivalent to 2 to 4 METs; heavy housework or yard work is equivalent to 5 to 6 METs. A person, old or young, would be tested for a baseline ability of 4 to 5 METs. The results of testing provide a guide for a prescriptive activity program at home or in a structured rehabilitation program center (Itoh, 1995), which takes into account the need for building in longer periods for the exercise heart rate to return to its resting level and low-level activity between components of exercise training.

Postexercise orthostatic hypotension is more likely to occur with the older adult as a result of decreased baroreceptor responsiveness. Because thermoregulation is impaired, exercise intensity must be reduced in hot, humid climates. Specific cardiac rehabilitation programs for elders should emphasize activities that build endurance, increase fitness, reduce the risk of new cardiac problems, and promote self-reliance to facilitate self-care and improve the quality of life (Rhodes et al, 1992; Schultz, 1998). For more impaired elders, it is necessary to identify energy-conserving measures applicable to their daily tasks.

Risk reduction programs should be instituted with a clear understanding of the difficulties involved in attempts to alter harmful life-style practices such as smoking, overeating, habitual anger or irritation, and sedentary life-style. These practices are often deeply embedded in the personality structure of the individual and are not easily eliminated by "education." The nurse's role in these instances is to discuss these practices in a nonjudgmental manner, providing acceptance, encouragement, resources, knowledge, and affirmation of the elder's right to choose.

Gender is a factor in cardiac rehabilitation outcomes. Schuster et al (1995) found that women knew less about their heart disease and supportive treatment than men and were the poorest adherents to exercise regardless of whether the cardiac rehabilitation program was at home or in a rehabilitation center.

Peripheral Vascular Disease

Most common vascular disorders of the older adult are venous insufficiency or arterial insufficiency, which results in venous stasis ulcers or arterial complications (gangrene). A discussion of vascular and arterial insufficiency and venous stasis ulcers is provided in Chapter 13.

RESPIRATORY DISORDERS

Diseases of the respiratory system are acute or chronic and involve the upper or lower respiratory tract. Further definition suggests classifying disorders as *obstructive*—preventing airflow out as a result of obstruction or narrowing of the respiratory structures (such as chronic obstructive pulmonary disease [emphysema]); or *restrictive*—causing a decrease in total lung capacity as a result of limited expansion (Lewis, Haggerty, 1999).

Chronic Obstructive Pulmonary Disease

Chronic obstructive pulmonary disease (COPD) is a nonspecific term used to "characterize persistent slowing of airflow during forceful expiration" (American Thoracic Society, 1995) and is a major concern in old age. As a category that includes chronic bronchitis, asthma, and emphysema, it is responsible for 7 deaths per 1000 individuals 65 years of age and over (US Bureau of the Census, 1995). COPD is the fifth leading cause of death in elders, second only to heart disease (Kennedy-Malone et al, 2000). Most frequently, COPD is a result of the cumulative and residual effects of long-term cigarette smoking (80% to 90% of cases), occupational and community pollutants, exposure to secondhand smoke, and, to a lesser extent, familial and genetic factors. Normal age changes in the respiratory system (see Chapter 7) are also contributors to COPD, particularly if any of the previously mentioned risk factors are or were present (Terry, 1995; Lewis, Haggerty, 1999; Kennedy-Malone et al, 2000).

The elderly population is most affected because of the natural history of the development of COPD, which has a preclinical period of damage of approximately 20 to 40 years. The progressive nature of COPD can lead to malnutrition because energy is consumed by the tremendous effort expended for breathing. Eating requires further effort and is often neglected. Individuals and their families may be so concerned with the breathing difficulties that they are hardly aware of the diminished caloric intake. Anxiety and depression are associated with the disease because of the difficulty breathing and the progressive and debilitating aspects of the condition.

Assessment

Assessment focuses on obtaining a history that explores the onset and setting of dyspnea. Usually this is insidious and occurs with exertion, particularly when climbing stairs. Lewis and Haggerty (1999) suggest a visual analog scale similar to the analog scale for pain to assess the quantity of dyspnea that the individual is having. The dyspnea scale goes from 1 (no dyspnea) to 10 (the worst dyspnea). The elder might complain of a productive cough with clear to white sputum triggered by postnasal drip, respiratory irritants, and retained secretions from impaired mucociliary action. Exploration into fears and socialization are necessary to establish reasonable functional expectation. Physical assessment or examination used for cardiac assessment is also applicable to COPD because it tends to be unclear whether symptoms such as fatigue and shortness of breath are cardiac or respiratory in nature. Observation of airway clearance, breathing patterns, and mobility; pulse oximetry; and a mental status examination facilitate a clearer picture of the current status. Pulmonary function testing is most definitive in terms of lung capacity and along with a chest x-ray examination can show the extent of respiratory damage. Box 20-4 presents a model of respiratory assessment. Additional information on respiratory assessment can be found in physical assessment texts. Assessment data are valuable in management and nursing interventions for persons with COPD.

Interventions

Management goals include stabilizing the disease, reducing the risk of exacerbations, promoting maximal functional capacity, and preventing premature disability. Aspects that should be included are smoking cessation; secretion clearance techniques; identification and management of exacerbations; breathing retraining; education; rehabilitation; psychologic support; management of depression and anxiety; nutritional support; and supplemental oxygen (O_2) therapy if and when it is necessary (Brown et al, 1999; Monahan, 1999).

Interventions should be designed to maintain or restore an acceptable quality of life for the elder with COPD and to minimize the number of hospitalizations through attention to smoking cessation, secretion clearance techniques, identification and management of exacerbations, breathing retraining, education, rehabilitation, management of depression and anxiety, nutritional support, supplemental O_2 therapy if and when it is needed, and the proper use and administration of medications.

Box 20-4   COPD ASSESSMENT

History
Respiratory diseases
Smoking history
Symptoms

Physical Examination
Inspection*
    Posture
    Chest symmetry, shape, expansion
    Respirations
    Skin color
    Capillary fill
    Sputum (color, amount, consistency)
Palpation
    Tenderness
Percussion
    Areas of hyperinflation, consolidation
Auscultation*
    Breath sounds

Functional Activity Mobility
Levels of activity before dyspneic
Interferences from sensory impairments

Knowledge
Educational attainment
Understanding of disease processes in COPD

COPD, Chronic obstructive pulmonary disease.
*Most important of the four assessment techniques.

Education. Education should be considered in every aspect of pulmonary care. The older adult should be taught to recognize the signs and symptoms of respiratory infection, how to maintain adequate nutrition, how to use an inhaler/nebulizer, how to clean it, the use of oxygen and oxygen safety, the type of exercise that is beneficial, how to pace activities, coping strategies, and other issues such as sexual function. Each of these areas requires teaching and has specific interventions that will be helpful to older adults and their families or their appointed caregivers.

Diet education should address the reason for monitoring weight and the signs of malnutrition. Weight loss can occur rapidly because of the energy expenditure needed to breathe. Dyspnea interferes with eating. In addition, satiation results from the intake of small amounts of food because of congestion in the abdomen by a flattened diaphragm. Anorexia or decreased appetite occurs as a result of sputum production and gas-tric irritation from the use of bronchodilators and steroids. The interventions that might lessen these problems appear in Box 20-5.

Exercise tolerance should be assessed by the physician and activities prescribed to increase endurance and improve respiratory status. Exercise may be done with or without oxygen as a supplement to control symptoms so that the older adult can spend enough time in exercise to gain benefit from it.

Medications are used to control dyspnea, cough, and sputum production (Terry, 1995). Older adults generally do better with inhalers/nebulizers than with oral medication because of the more rapid onset, local efficiency of reaching the target organ, and fewer side effects. The older adult should learn about the medication he or she is taking, its side effects, and what to do if side effects occur. Instruction on the use of the inhaler is also very important, since less than 30% use the inhaler correctly (Lewis, Haggerty, 1999). Inhalers may be troublesome for some older adults because of the coordination of inspiration with the inhaler or impaired manual dexterity, such as in patients with arthritis. Metered-dose or spacer devices may help elders use inhalers better and facilitate maximal drug delivery. They are also useful for those who have some visual impairment. Lewis and Haggerty (1999) advise instructing the elder to take a "drag" on the inhaler as if smoking a cigarette to learn the technique. This seems reasonable, since most persons with COPD were once smokers. Fig. 20-1 illustrates the use of the inhaler.

The client should be informed that sex is still possible and be provided with education and counseling information, either by the nurse or the professional counselor.

An older adult with COPD would be considered a candidate for pulmonary *rehabilitation* as long as he or she does not have severe COPD without pulmonary reserve, unstable heart disease, or psychiatric illness (Terry, 1995). Rehabilitation programs for the older adult with COPD consist of drug therapy, reconditioning exercises, and counseling. A multidisciplinary team of health professionals work collectively to help the aged adult achieve the following goals:

- Increase the level of independence.
- Maintain individuality and autonomy.
- Improve function in his or her environment.
- Decrease the number of hospitalizations and need for hospitalization.
- Increase exercise tolerance.
- Increase self-esteem.
- Improve the quality of life.

Box 20-5   INTERVENTIONS FOR CHRONIC OBSTRUCTIVE PULMONARY DISEASE

Nutrition

Eat small, frequent, nutrient-intense meals.
Eat foods with high protein and caloric content.
Serve meals on small plates (servings will not look overwhelming).
Select foods that do not require a lot of chewing.
Have food cut in bite-size pieces to conserve energy.
Establish a plan for fluid intake; drink 2 to 3 L of fluid daily (pineapple juice helps cut secretions; keep a liter of water in the refrigerator or on the kitchen counter to be consumed each day in addition to other fluids).
Weigh at least twice a week.

Exercise

(Based on an established plan suggested by physician or rehabilitation team)
Walk daily all year round (in good weather, outdoors; in bad weather, go to the mall and walk indoors).
    Walk up and down stairs in home (if present).
Use a stationary bicycle.
When buying shoes for activity and everyday wear, avoid shoes that require bending over to tie; instead, get a slip-on type and use a long-handled shoehorn to assist the heel into the shoe.

Activity Pacing

Avoid high levels of exertion in the early morning.
Arrange rest periods throughout the day.
Allow plenty of time to complete activities; do not hurry.
Schedule activities in advance to reduce pressure and anxiety.
Obtain and follow prescribed exercise program for maintenance of heart/lung capacity.

Activities of Daily Living (ADLs)

Allow ample time for bathing and dressing. Have a chair in the bathroom for bathing.
Arrange toiletries in easy reach.
Wear shoes that slip on or have Velcro closures, not ties.
Select clothing with elasticized waistbands; avoid constrictive clothing; use suspenders rather than belts.
Select and wear clothing that is easy to put on and remove.

Safety

Attempt to keep a dust-free environment.
Minimize or eliminate use of aerosol sprays, fumes, contaminants, dander.
Place plastic covers over mattresses; use hypoallergenic pillows and blankets.
Avoid carpet and rug floor coverings.

Emotional Support

Accept/encourage expression of emotions.
Be an active listener.
Be cognizant of conversational dyspnea; do not interrupt or cut off conversations.

Education

Teach breathing techniques:
    Pursed-lip breathing
    Diaphragmatic breathing
    Cascade coughing (series)
Teach postural drainage.
Teach medications:
    What, why, frequency, amount, side effects, and what to do if side effects occur
    Use and care of inhalers
Teach signs and symptoms of respiratory infection.
Teach about sexual activity:
    Sexual function improves with rest.
    Schedule sex around best-breathing time of day.
    Use prescribed bronchodilators 20 to 30 minutes before sex.
    Use a position that does not require pressure on the chest or support of the arms.
Avoid the use of alcohol or eating large quantities of food.

General Instructions

Listen to weather reports.
    Avoid going out in inclement weather.
    Wear a scarf over the nose and mouth in cold and windy weather; wear a hat.
    Avoid going out when air pollution is high.
Use an air conditioner to filter air and make it drier.
Avoid situations where you may encounter individuals with influenza or upper respiratory tract infections.
Obtain an annual flu shot if not allergic.
Obtain one-time multivalent pneumococcal immunization.
Notify physician of any temperature above 99° F (37.2° C).
Examine sputum; recognize and report changes to physician.
Do not use over-the-counter drugs unless physician approves.

COPD, Chronic obstructive pulmonary disease.

1. Remove the cap, and hold the inhaler upright.
2. Shake the inhaler.
3. Tilt your head back slightly, and breathe out.
4. Use the inhaler in any one of these ways. (A and B are the best ways. B is recommended for young children, older adults, and those taking inhaled steroids. C is okay if you are having trouble with A or B.)
   A. Open mouth with inhaler 1 to 2 inches away.
   B. Use spacer (ask for the handout on spacers).
   C. Put inhaler in mouth, and seal lips around the mouthpiece.

5. Press down on the inhaler to release the medicine as you start to breathe in slowly.
6. Breathe in *slowly* for 3 to 5 seconds.
7. *Hold* your breath for 10 seconds to allow the medicine to reach deeply into your lungs.
8. Repeat puffs as prescribed. Waiting 1 minute between puffs may permit the second puff to go deeper into the lungs.

NOTE: Dry powder capsules are used differently. To use a dry powder inhaler, close your mouth tightly around the mouthpiece and inhale very fast.

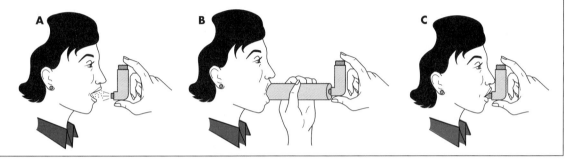

Fig. 20-1   Using a metered-dose inhaler. (Redrawn from Nurses' Asthma Education Working Group: *Nurses: partners in asthma care,* NIH Pub No 95-3308, 1995.)

Outcomes of interventions and rehabilitation measures do not suggest a cure and may be elusive. It may not appear that physiologic changes have been effected, but the individual may feel and function better. This, however, is dependent on coexisting conditions that the older adult may have.

Economic issues become important when there is chronicity and especially when there is COPD. The expense of oxygen therapy for elders with a limited income may interfere with the adequacy of therapy and create feelings of anxiety. The questions arise whether Medicare will reimburse the elder if the exact criteria are not met. Inhalers and certain medications may be restricted in certain health maintenance organization/preferred provider organization (HMO/PPO) formularies.

All of the efforts of professionals, family caregivers, and the older adult are directed toward creating a safe and comfortable environment that will maximize individual function and attainment of the highest level of function and wellness, with or without direct assistance.

There is the potential for caregiver burden when an elder's spouse is the chief caregiver. Usually nurses in acute care settings do not see the extent of care given by the spouse. It is important to be cognizant of the potential for depression, financial burden, and perhaps social isolation (Brown et al, 1999).

Pneumonia

Pneumonia is a lower respiratory tract infection that causes inflammation of the lung parenchyma, generally by a bacterial agent. Pneumonia is the fifth leading cause of death in the United States and the fourth leading cause of death in the elderly (Bartlett, 1995). The old-old (85 years and older) are five times more likely to die of pneumonia than young-old or old adults. Particularly susceptible are elders with coexisting morbidity such as alcoholism, asthma, COPD, or heart disease or those who have been institutionalized (Koivula et al, 1994). Other factors that affect the risk of acquiring pneumonia relate to normal age changes of the respiratory system, such as a diminished cough reflex, increased residual volume, decreased chest compliance, and reduced oxygen saturation. Pneumococcal pneumonias are the most common bacterial respiratory infection of the aged. Other, less common bacterial pneumonias are caused by *Haemophilus influenzae, Staphylococcus, Streptococcus,* or *Klebsiella* (Brown et al, 1999; Lewis, Haggerty, 1999).

Assessment

Pneumonia is classified as community acquired or nosocomial and is incurred through exposure in the hospital or nursing home. The usual signs and symptoms of pneumonia manifested in younger persons are not commonly seen in the aged. Instead, mental status changes or signs of confusion, general deterioration, weakness, anorexia, tachycardia, and tachypnea occur in the older adult. These atypical responses can easily lead to an incorrect diagnosis or a diagnosis made too late in the progression of the pneumonia (Kennedy-Malone et al, 2000).

Interventions

Where treatment is given is a critical issue. If there is a responsible caregiver who can minister to the older adult in the home environment and if the home environment is supportive, then therapy can occur in the elder's home with or without temporary home health service support. When the elder fails to improve or deteriorates, then hospitalization is essential. Any time there is failure to drink fluids or evidence of hemodynamic imbalance, the hospital setting is necessary to reestablish homeostasis. When an individual is in a long-term care setting, if at all possible the elder should be maintained in his or her familiar setting if oxygen therapy, parenteral fluids, and antibiotics can be administered by the nursing staff. Some insurance policies will cover such an arrangement; others do not and require hospitalization.

Treatment of pneumonia should include antibiotics for a specified period of time, depending on the responsible organism. Adequate nutrition is important, as well as an increase in fluid intake; daily intake should usually be 2000 ml unless fluid overload is a possibility because of co-morbidity such as cardiac or renal disease. Adequate rest is needed to preserve limited reserve capacity, and oxygen therapy is provided unless emphysema is present. Then the use of oxygen should be limited to 1 or 2 L. Pulmonary ventilation should be attended to with deep breathing and coughing, frequent position changes, and ambulation as soon as possible during the acute recovery period. Also, provision should be made to dispose of sputum. These measures are appropriate both at home and in the hospital. Because the individual may need more acute care and have exacerbated co-morbidities in the hospital setting, additional therapies may be used.

The nurse's role in caring for elders with pneumonia in the acute hospital setting is to administer and monitor the antibiotic therapy. It also includes mobilizing elders as quickly as the condition allows and referring them for physical and occupational therapy to prevent or stop functional decline. Monitoring nutrition and obtaining a nutrition consult may be necessary, as well as suggesting respiratory therapy (if it is not already in place) and ensuring that the elder is adequately hydrated while monitoring fluid volume to prevent overload in elders with cardiovascular disease and CHF. Finally, consideration should be given to elders' desire for treatment if they are terminally ill.

The care role in the extended care facility should include administration and monitoring of antibiotic therapy, mobilizing elders by position changes, getting them out of bed, and ambulating them. Mouth care is very important, since ignoring it allows the propagation of bacteria to confound an already-serious situation. Be sure that elders have an advance directive; if not, assist them in completing the document so that all know the individual's desire for treatment.

Prevention of pneumonia should be encouraged by ensuring that older adults know that every year between October and November they should be inoculated against the flu (influenza). Influenza is among the viruses that can set the stage for secondary infection by bacteria and subsequent pneumonia. Adults older than 65 years of age and those with chronic conditions should be encouraged to receive the one-time pneumococcal vaccine (Pneumovax) unless they are at high risk, in which case current recommendations are to receive the vaccine every 6 years. Because the risk of pneumonia increases with age and is compounded by age-related changes (see Chapter 7), it is a way to decrease the chance of succumbing to pneumonia-related death. Yearly dental examinations should be encouraged, since dental caries predispose to pneumonia secondary to increased oral bacteria.

Tuberculosis

Tuberculosis (TB) is a chronic pulmonary and extrapulmonary infectious disease characterized by particular symptoms, although these may be modified or not apparent in the very old. In the United States today there are 22,860 reported cases (Centers for Disease Control and Prevention, 1996). This number has steadily decreased from the 37,100 reported in 1970 (US Bureau of the Census, 1995). However, there has been an upsurge since 1985. In the population over age 65, incidence is highest among male Asians/Pacific Islanders (225 per 100,000) and lowest among white women (6 per 100,000). In all cultures reported, men had a much higher incidence than women (Kennedy-Malone et al, 2000). TB has been thought to be a malady of the Victorian Age or of those deprived by circumstances of poverty and overcrowding. It has lain dormant and quiescent for decades in previous victims who were actively treated, only to rise quietly as a phoenix from the ashes, stronger and more virulent than ever. Identified cases have increased 60% since 1985, and some individuals have a particularly strong multiple drug–resistant (MDR) type. *Mycobacterium tuberculosis* was considered to be conquered in the 1950s by the development of isoniazid (INH). Many of our present elders were treated following their acquisition of the disease during World War II. Many others contracted the disease in childhood. As they become immunocompromised as a result of chemotherapy, extreme old age, or human immunodeficiency virus (HIV) infection, the bacterium is reactivated.

Our chief concern is the management of TB in congregate living situations. Elders living in nursing homes or congregate settings are particularly at risk and have an incidence nearly four times that of the general population (Hopkins, Schoener, 1996; Kennedy-Malone et al, 2000). In long-term care facilities the percentage of TB cases reported varies tremendously depending on diligence in monitoring and numbers of long-term care residents under surveillance. Although TB is not as contagious as once believed, the tubercle bacillus that is becoming resistant to combinations of drugs (MDR) is tenacious. Therefore prevention is of high priority, especially among groups in close contact who have compromised immune systems; are malnourished; have co-morbidities such as diabetes mellitus, malignancies, and chronic renal failure; and have a body weight 10% below ideal, such as the very old in nursing homes (Brown et al, 1999; Kennedy-Malone et al, 2000). TB is becoming a public health problem of real concern to elders and health care workers who may be exposed to it.

Currently it is recommended that Mantoux skin testing (with purified protein derivative [PPD]) be conducted routinely regardless of whether the individual was vaccinated in the past with BCG (bacille Calmette-Guérin) (Centers for Disease Control and Prevention, 1996). The test should be read within 48 to 72 hours. A reaction of ≥10 mm is a positive test measure. The two-step PPD test should be performed on elders who test

---

Box 20-6   GUIDELINES FOR EXTENDED CARE MONITORING FOR TUBERCULOSIS

Screen all new residents on admission using two-step purified protein derivative (PPD).

Screen all residents every 2 years.

Perform chest x-ray examination of new residents on admission and of residents with documented positive reaction or in whom reactions turn positive or in whom suggestive symptoms are present.

Perform PPD testing on all previously negative residents immediately and again in 12 weeks if an active case of tuberculosis (TB) is documented in the facility.

Collect sputum for acid-fast bacillus (AFB) testing if a previously positive resident develops cough, bronchitis, pneumonia, or unexplained weight loss.

Notify local and state health departments as indicated.

---

negative and are suspect for TB or who may be persons with anergy.* By initiating a booster effect, a more sensitive response can be established in an institutionalized elder who may have TB without symptoms. When the test is positive but the chest x-ray finding is negative, a course of isoniazid prophylaxis should be instituted. When there is active TB, a four-drug regimen should be instituted and the patient closely monitored for 6 months to 1 year. Anyone in contact with a person diagnosed with TB should be tested and, if positive, given a course of prophylactic therapy with isoniazid. New laboratory tests make diagnosis much quicker than traditional methods. The BACTEC® system is a rapid radiometric culture technique that can detect mycobacterial growth in 5 to 8 days. Deoxyribonucleic acid (DNA) probe technology can detect mycobacteria in sputum within hours (Lewis, Haggerty, 1999).

Elders do not exhibit the usual symptoms of TB. Indications that an active process may be occurring are reflected in altered mental status, unusual behavior, fever, anorexia, and weight loss. Often co-morbidities and polypharmacy confuse the picture for the diagnosis and treatment of TB (Bergman-Evans, 1998).

Persons over 55 years of age account for 50% of new cases. The aged and others with compromised immune systems are particularly vulnerable, especially those in

---

*Anergy is a reaction less than 5 mm in the presence of tubercular infection.

collective living situations or institutions. The Centers for Disease Control and Prevention has identified residents of long-term care facilities and health care workers as being at particular risk. TB surveillance for the vulnerable old must be systematic. Recommendations are summarized in Box 20-6. Although these suggestions are specifically designed for nursing home residents, nurses working with the frail or vulnerable old in any setting would be wise to inquire regarding PPD testing and any history of TB or exposure to it and to recommend a preventive/therapeutic regimen when indicated.

▶ **KEY CONCEPTS**

- Congestive heart failure is one of the most prevalent chronic problems of the aged. Any condition that stresses the heart may precipitate heart failure.
- Pneumonia and tuberculosis in the elderly can be prevented through Pneumovax immunization and periodic screening for tuberculosis.
- The goal of therapy for cardiac and respiratory disorders is to relieve symptoms, improve the quality of life, reduce mortality, stabilize and slow the progression of the disease, reduce the risk of exacerbation, and maximize functional capacity.

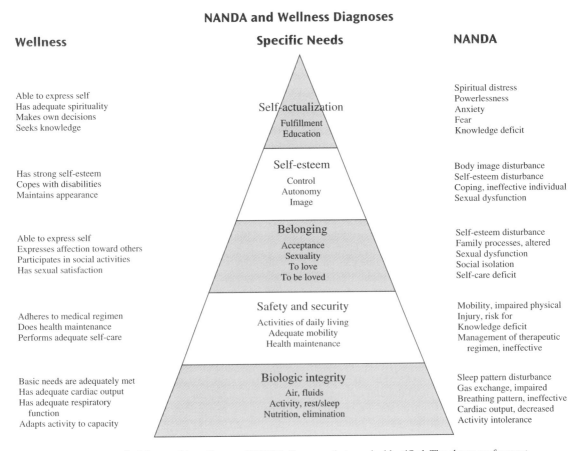

NANDA and Wellness Diagnoses

Wellness	Specific Needs	NANDA
Able to express self Has adequate spirituality Makes own decisions Seeks knowledge	**Self-actualization** Fulfillment Education	Spiritual distress Powerlessness Anxiety Fear Knowledge deficit
Has strong self-esteem Copes with disabilities Maintains appearance	**Self-esteem** Control Autonomy Image	Body image disturbance Self-esteem disturbance Coping, ineffective individual Sexual dysfunction
Able to express self Expresses affection toward others Participates in social activities Has sexual satisfaction	**Belonging** Acceptance Sexuality To love To be loved	Self-esteem disturbance Family processes, altered Sexual dysfunction Social isolation Self-care deficit
Adheres to medical regimen Does health maintenance Performs adequate self-care	**Safety and security** Activities of daily living Adequate mobility Health maintenance	Mobility, impaired physical Injury, risk for Knowledge deficit Management of therapeutic regimen, ineffective
Basic needs are adequately met Has adequate cardiac output Has adequate respiratory function Adapts activity to capacity	**Biologic integrity** Air, fluids Activity, rest/sleep Nutrition, elimination	Sleep pattern disturbance Gas exchange, impaired Breathing pattern, ineffective Cardiac output, decreased Activity intolerance

These are not all of the possible wellness or NANDA diagnoses that may be identified. The above are frequent examples of nursing diagnoses that should be considered when planning care for the older adult in whatever setting.

▶ ## Activities and Discussion Questions

1. What is congestive heart failure?
2. Discuss assessment and intervention for elders with a diagnosis of congestive heart failure, chronic obstructive pulmonary disease, and pneumonia.
3. Why are pneumonia and tuberculosis so common and a danger to the older adult?
4. What preventive measures can be instituted to prevent or lessen the severity of pneumonia and tuberculosis among the elder population?
5. Develop a nursing care plan for an elder with congestive heart failure or a respiratory condition using wellness and NANDA diagnoses.

RESOURCES

American Association of Cardiovascular and Pulmonary Rehabilitation
7611 Elmwood Avenue, Suite 201
Middletown, WI 53562
American Disabilities Association
2121 8th Avenue N., Suite 1623
Birmingham, AL 35203
American Heart Association at the local level
American Lung Association at the local level

REFERENCES

American Thoracic Society, Medical Section of the American Lung Association: Standards for the diagnosis and care of patients with chronic obstructive pulmonary disease (COPD) and asthma, *Am J Respir Crit Care Med* 152:S77-S120, 1995.

Bartlett JG: Pneumonia and tuberculosis. In Abrams WB, Beers MH, Berkow R, editors: *The Merck manual of geriatrics,* ed 2, Whitehouse Station, NJ, 1995, Merck Research Laboratories.

Bergman-Evans B: Tuberculosis in long-term care settings, *Adv Nurse Pract* 6(12):67, 1998.

Braunwald E: Pathophysiology of heart failure, *Heart Dis* 14:327, 1992.

Brown JB, Bedford NK, White SJ: *Gerontological protocols for nurse practitioners,* Philadelphia, 1999, Lippincott.

Centers for Disease Control and Prevention: *National Center for HIV/STD and TB Prevention report,* Tammy Nunnally, Office of Communications, Atlanta, Oct 9, 1996, The Centers.

Ebersole P, Hess P: Common chronic problems and their management. In *Toward healthy aging: human needs and nursing response,* ed 5, St Louis, 1998, Mosby.

Gross SB: Heart failure: a review of current treatment strategies, *Adv Nurse Pract* 7(6):27, 1999.

Heart failure sounds final; it's not, *Well Taken,* p. 2, San Francisco, 1994, San Francis Memorial Hospital.

Hopkins ML, Schoener L: Tuberculosis and the elderly living in long term care facilities, *Geriatr Nurs* 17(1):27, 1996.

Itoh M: Rehabilitation. In Abrams WB, Beers MH, Berkow R, editors: *The Merck manual of geriatrics,* ed 2, Whitehouse Station, NJ, 1995, Merck Research Laboratories.

Johnson MA: Cardiovascular conditions. In Stone JT, Wyman JF, Salisbury SA, editors: *Clinical gerontological nursing,* ed 2, Philadelphia, 1999, Saunders.

Kennedy-Malone L, Fletcher KR, Plank LM: *Management guidelines for gerontological nurse practitioners,* Philadelphia, 2000, Davis.

Koivula I, Sten M, Pirjo H: Risk factors for pneumonia in the elderly, *Am J Med* 96(4):313, 1994.

Lewis MFR, Haggerty MC: Topics in respiratory care. In Molony SL et al, editors: *Gerontological nursing: an advanced practice approach,* Stamford, Conn, 1999, Appleton-Lange.

Living with heart disease: is it heart failure? AHCPR Pub No 94-0614, Rockville, Md, June, 1994, US Department of Health and Human Services, Public Health Service, Agency for Health Care Policy and Research.

Marek MA, Wilcox JA, Cocks AE: Topics in cardiovascular care. In Molony SL, Waszynski CM, Lyder CH, editors: *Gerontological nursing: an advanced practice approach,* Stamford, Conn, 1999, Appleton-Lange.

Monahan K: A joint effort to affect lives: the COPD wellness program, *Geriatr Nurs* 20(4):200, 1999.

Rhodes R, Morrissey MJ, Ward A: Self-motivation: a driving force for elders in cardiac rehabilitation, *Geriatr Nurs* 13(2):94, 1992.

Schultz S: Living with congestive heart failure, *Focus Geriatr Care Rehabil* 12(2):1, 1998.

Schuster PM, Wright C, Tomich P: Gender differences in the outcome of participants in home programs compared to those in structured rehabilitation programs, *Rehabil Nurs* 20(2):93, 1995.

Stanley M: Congestive heart failure in the elderly, *Geriatr Nurs* 20(4):180, 1999.

Terry PB: Chronic obstructive pulmonary disease (COPD). In Abrams WB, Beers MH, Berkow R, editors: *The Merck manual of geriatrics,* ed 2, Whitehouse Station, NJ, 1995, Merck Research Laboratories.

US Bureau of the Census: *Statistical abstract of the United States: 1995,* ed 115, Washington, DC, 1995, US Government Printing Office.

Wei JY: Heart failure and cardiomyopathy. In Abrams WB, Beers MH, Berkow R, editors: *The Merck manual of geriatrics,* ed 2, Whitehouse Station, NJ, 1995, Merck Research Laboratories.

Wenger NK: Rehabilitation of the elderly coronary patient. In Frengley JD, Murray P, Wykle M, editors: *Practicing rehabilitation with geriatric clients,* New York, 1990, Springer.

21

Cognitive Impairment and Older Persons

Upon completion of this chapter, the reader will be able to:

- List several purposes of a cognitive assessment.
- Describe similarities and differences between dementia and delirium.
- Relate several ways in which cognitive impairment is measured.
- Explain the differences between hemorrhagic and ischemic stroke.
- Describe the effects of Parkinson disease.
- Develop a nursing care plan for an individual with irreversible dementia.
- Develop a nursing care plan for an individual with reversible dementia.

Aberrant Abnormal or not following the expected course.

Ataxia An impaired ability to coordinate movement, especially a staggering gait.

Catastrophic A frantic response to a situation perceived as threatening.

Contracture An abnormal fixed position of a joint secondary to lack of movement, loss of elasticity, and shortening of muscle fibers.

Degenerative Gradual deterioration and changing to a less functional form.

Dysphagia Difficulty swallowing caused by obstruction or motor disorders of the esophagus.

Emboli A quantity of air, gas, or tissue that circulates and becomes lodged in a blood vessel.

Global cognitive impairment Partial or total loss of all mental abilities.

Grandiosity Unrealistic belief in one's own abilities.

Hyperreflexia Increased reflex reactions.

Hypokinetic Diminished power of movement or motor function.

Intracerebral Within the tissue of the brain.

Mentation Any mental activity whether conscious or unconscious.

Milieu The environment or setting.

Multiinfarct dementia Deterioration of intellectual functioning caused by vascular disease that impairs circulation to the brain.

Nosocomial An infection acquired during hospitalization.

Pseudodelirium An unstable mental state caused by crises and disorientation.

Pseudodementia Affective disorder that mimics dementia, particularly, severe depression.

Rudimentary Elementary, basic; not fully developed.

Subarachnoid The space under the arachnoid membrane and above the pia mater, which may fill with blood during cerebral hemorrhage.

Thrombi A lump of platelets, fibrins, and cellular elements attached to the inner wall of an artery or vein, sometimes blocking the flow of blood.

Tomography An x-ray technique that produces a film representing a detailed cross section of tissue. Used primarily to diagnose space-occupying lesions.

I simply can't find my things. I know I had many things, a houseful, in fact. Where are they? I looked through all the drawers in my room for that picture of Joe, and I couldn't find it. I'll look again. I'm sure it is there somewhere. I wonder where my friends and family are. I don't think I have seen any of them in a long while.

Sarah, age 90

I just don't know what to do about Sarah. She keeps getting into her roommate's belongings and really gets angry when I try to stop her. Even in the middle of the night, she is pawing through drawers and closets and keeping everyone awake. Yesterday she took everything out of the linen closet and had most of it on the floor before we saw her.

Esther, Sarah's nurse

Common causes of cognitive impairment in the old are often related to degenerative processes of the central nervous system, such as those found in Alzheimer's disease, Parkinson disease, or cerebrovascular accident. These conditions are not a normal consequence of aging, although the incidence increases as one grows older. Older individuals are also more vulnerable to temporary disturbances in cognitive function. This chapter focuses on cognitive impairment, treatable and untreatable, which includes delirium, Alzheimer's disease, brain attack (stroke), and Parkinson disease.

Cognitive impairment (CI) is a term describing a range of disturbances in thinking capacity. Cognitive function includes attention span, concentration, intelligence, judgment, learning ability, memory, orientation, perception, problem solving, psychomotor ability, reaction time, and social abilities. Each individual is as unique in cognitive function as in personality. Recognizing the profile of each individual's mental strengths and deficits is extremely important in providing the care needed. If a client is misdiagnosed or poorly evaluated, the treatments provided may be inadequate, and in some treatable cases a needless permanent dementia may result. Immediate attention to indications of confusion is therefore critical. Identifying and removing the underlying causes and providing supportive and symptomatic care are essential interventions. The goal in all cases is to provide a milieu that will allow and encourage the individual to function at the highest level possible.

CONFUSION

Confusion is a much-used clinical term that conveys little specific information. It may be used to refer to an acute mental disturbance, a chronic state, or any situation in which a nurse does not comprehend the client's behavior. For example, a client was waving his arms excitedly and talking about flying. He was expecting his daughter to fly in to see him, but observers thought he was totally daft. Thus nurses report clients' behavioral manifestations within their own framework, seldom exploring the meaning to the individual. Any alteration in mentation may be loosely labeled *confusion,* and thus comparisons of delirium, dementia, and depression may be helpful in making a preliminary assessment. These can be seen in Table 21-1.

Acute Confusional States

Foreman (1996) defined *acute confusional state* as "an organic brain syndrome characterized by transient, global cognitive impairment of abrupt onset and relative brief duration, accompanied by diurnal fluctuation of simultaneous disturbances of the sleep-wake cycle, psychomotor behavior, attention, and affect." Foreman's definition of an acute confusional state and its associated clinical features describes delirium.

Delirium

Delirium is given many labels: *acute confusional state, acute brain syndrome, confusion, metabolic encephalopathy,* and *toxic psychosis.* Delirium is a brief mental disturbance with a fairly rapid onset, a course that typically fluctuates, disorganized thinking, difficulty in focusing and sustaining attention, and sensory misperceptions. The delirious individual is easily distracted. Perceptual disturbances result in misinterpretations, illusions, and hallucinations.

The causes of delirium are potentially reversible. The onset of disturbance may be rapid or gradual but is usually resolved within 7 days to the degree that it can be reversed (Foreman, 1993). Delirium occurs in

Table 21-1

Comparison of the Clinical Features of Delirium, Dementia, and Depression

Clinical feature	Delirium	Dementia	Depression
Onset	Acute/subacute, depends on cause, often at twilight or in darkness	Chronic, generally insidious, depends on cause	Coincides with major life changes, often abrupt
Course	Short, diurnal fluctuations in symptoms, worse at night, in darkness, and on awakening	Long, no diurnal effects, symptoms progressive yet relatively stable over time	Diurnal effects, typically worse in the morning, situational fluctuations, but less than with delirium
Progression	Abrupt	Slow but uneven	Variable, rapid or slow but even
Duration	Hours to less than 1 month, seldom longer	Months to years	At least 6 weeks, can be several months to years
Awareness	Reduced	Clear	Clear
Alertness	Fluctuates, lethargic or hypervigilant	Generally normal	Normal
Attention	Impaired, fluctuates	Generally normal	Minimal impairment but is easily distracted
Orientation	Generally impaired, severity varies	Generally normal	Selective disorientation
Memory	Recent and immediate impaired	Recent and remote impaired	Selective or "patchy" impairment, "islands" of intact memory
Thinking	Disorganized, distorted, fragmented, incoherent speech, either slow or accelerated	Difficulty with abstraction, thoughts impoverished, judgment impaired, words difficult to find	Intact but with themes of hopelessness, helplessness, or self-depreciation
Perception	Distorted, illusions, delusions, and hallucinations; difficulty distinguishing between reality and misperceptions	Misperceptions usually absent	Intact, delusions and hallucinations absent except in severe cases
Psychomotor behavior	Variable, hypokinetic, hyperkinetic, and mixed	Normal, may have apraxia	Variable, psychomotor retardation or agitation
Sleep/wake cycle	Disturbed, cycle reversed	Fragmented	Disturbed, usually early-morning awakening
Associated features	Variable affective changes, symptoms of autonomic hyperarousal, exaggeration of personality type, associated with acute physical illness	Affect tends to be superficial, inappropriate, and labile, attempts to conceal deficits in intellect, personality changes, aphasia, agnosia may be present, lacks insight	Affect depressed, dysphoric mood, exaggerated and detailed complaints, preoccupied with personal thoughts, insight present, verbal elaboration
Assessment	Distracted from task, numerous errors	Failings highlighted by family, frequent "near miss" answers, struggles with test, great effort to find an appropriate reply, frequent requests for feedback on performance	Failings highlighted by individual, frequently answers "don't know," little effort, frequently gives up, indifferent toward test, does not care or attempt to find answer

From Foreman MD et al: Assessing cognitive function, *Geriatr Nurs* 17(5):228, 1996.

30% to 50% of elderly medical-surgical clients. Any interruption in biologic processes is likely to produce perceptual disorganization in the elderly. Common causes can be seen in Box 21-1. Delirious states may be hypokinetic (characterized by somnolence and apathy), hyperkinetic (characterized by excitability, hallucinations, and delusions), or mixtures of these factors. Imagined odors or sensations of bugs crawling on the skin and other similar hallucinations are highly indicative of metabolic disturbances. The severity of delirium is related to the level of physiologic disturbance and degree of cerebral edema. The diagnosis of dementia cannot be made when delirium is present but must be assessed when the individual's delirious condition has stabilized.

These acute brain disorders are often accompanied by overwhelming anxiety; frightening illusions; and tactile, visual, and olfactory hallucinations. For example, an elderly woman insisted that the sprinkler spigot on the ceiling was a giant spider and the bell cord was a snake. These illusions were very frightening to her. Illusions, or frightening misinterpretations of the environment, that occur when one is under physiologic stress are common. Illusions may be the most significant signal of a toxic condition. In addition to psychologic manifestations of acute cerebral impairment, physical symptoms such as vasomotor instability; elevated pulse and respiratory rate; temperature fluctuations; tremors of the fingers, hands, lips, and facial muscles; headache; and generalized weakness are often present. An individual with acute organic brain disorder is physically ill, as well as cerebrally impaired. Delirium is a more common signal of physical illness of the very elderly than body symptoms such as fever, pain, or tachycardia (Lipowski, 1986). Elderly individuals with some degree of dementia are particularly apt to develop transient delirium in response to physical illness, drug intoxication, and psychosocial stressors. Unsurprisingly, medications are frequent offenders.

Pseudodelirium

Pseudodelirium is a delirium-like state that occurs as a result of psychosocial stressors, depression, mania, or severe anxiety. It is often mixed with the pseudodementia of depression and can appear as dementia, delirium, or manic behavior. For example, an elderly woman was restlessly pacing around her house looking for a book to take with her to the hospital while the paramedics were administering cardiopulmonary resuscitation (CPR) to her husband.

Prevention

Acute confusional states often occur during hospitalizations. Approximately 16% of all older clients admitted to hospitals exhibit some symptoms of acute confusion (Foreman, 1993). The exacerbation of delirium during hospitalization depends on the client's illness and care management while hospitalized. Preventing or minimizing these occurrences is often possible through careful use of short-term medications, especially the benzodiazapines (Marcantonio et al, 1994; Buffum, Buffum, 1997), prevention of nosocomial infection, maintenance of fluid balance, and promotion of electrolyte balance.

Nursing interventions are beneficial in reducing the discomfort of delirium. Simple interventions such as having continuity of personnel attending the person, encouraging family presence, correcting sensory deficits with glasses and hearing aids, and providing orientation and frequent reassurance that the condition is temporary can be very helpful. The continuous presence of one reliable family member or friend who will provide ongoing reassurance is ideal. Students nurses are very effective in this role.

IRREVERSIBLE DEMENTIA

In contrast to delirium, which is usually a reflection of physiologic disturbance or depression (see Chapter 25), dementia is an irreversible mental state characterized by decreased intellectual function, personality change,

---

Box 21-1	COMMON CAUSES OF CONFUSION IN THE ELDERLY*

1. Drug intoxication
2. Circulatory disturbances
3. Metabolic imbalances
4. Fluid imbalance
5. Major medical and surgical treatments
6. Neurologic disorders
7. Infectious processes
8. Nutritional deficiencies
9. Abrupt loss of significant person
10. Multiple losses in short span of time
11. Moves to radically different environments

*Shown in rank order of occurrence.

impaired judgment, and often a change in affect (expression of feelings) caused by permanently altered cerebral metabolism. Dementia is a syndrome consisting of loss of intellectual abilities of sufficient severity to interfere with social or occupational functioning. The essential feature of dementia is impairment in short- and long-term memory.

Dementia involves memory, judgment, abstract thought, reasoning, and changes in behavior and personality. The diagnosis is not made if these features are due to clouding of consciousness, as in delirium; however, delirium and dementia may coexist (American Psychiatric Association, 1994). The most common reasons for delirium in older persons with dementia are multiple medications, fluid and electrolyte imbalance, systemic disease, and malnutrition. There are, of course, numerous other disorders causing or simulating dementia that are noted in Box 21-2. The non-Alzheimer's dementias include multiinfarcts (strokes), Parkinson disease, Pick disease, Creutzfeldt-Jakob disease, human immunodeficiency virus (HIV) dementia, and several other uncommon conditions that produce irreversible dementias (Berkow et al, 1995). The percentage of persons affected increases with age. These disorders have higher mortality rates than those of Alzheimer's disease. An individual with Alzheimer's dementia may live many years if well cared for physically. It is estimated that over 70% of cases of dementia are of the Alzheimer's type (DAT) (Ott et al, 1995).

Diagnosing Dementia

Dementia is the decline of memory and other cognitive functions as compared with the client's previous level of function. Components of a dementia syndrome include the following: a history of decline in cognitive and functional performance; abnormalities in thought processes noted from clinical examination; and neuropsychologic tests indicating deficits in recall, attention, spatial perception, and psychomotor performance. The diagnosis of dementia is based on behavior and cognitive responses and cannot be determined by computerized tomography (CT), an electroencephalogram (EEG), or other laboratory measurements, although some specific causes of dementia may sometimes be identified by these means. When consciousness is impaired by delirium, drowsiness, stupor, or coma, or when other clinical abnormalities prevent adequate evaluation of mental status, a diagnosis of dementia cannot be made until these conditions are reversed to the maximum possible degree.

HIV-Related Dementia

HIV-related dementia is the neurologic impairment that is estimated to occur in up to 75% of people with acquired immunodeficiency syndrome (AIDS). HIV can infiltrate the central nervous system (CNS) directly and produce a distinctive AIDS dementia complex. AIDS dementia complex is characterized by cognitive, motor, and behavioral changes. Only rudimentary intellectual and social functioning remain intact, and psychomotor retardation (slowed and awkward movement) is evident. Overall verbal and motor slowing are prominent characteristics, as well as gait ataxia and hyperreflexia (Scharnhorst, 1992). Depression, agitation, delusions, hallucinations, grandiosity, and paranoia are common symptoms. The end result of AIDS dementia complex closely resembles Alzheimer's disease (Havarth et al, 1995). Clinicians must consider HIV infection as a possible cause of dementia in elderly persons even when they are not initially known to be in any high-risk group. Nurses must be aware that in some cases of dementia that progress more rapidly than is typical of Alzheimer's disease, the AIDS dementia complex must be considered.

The compromised immune system of an aged individual may make him or her more susceptible to AIDS than a younger person. Some of the aged have undergone massive blood transfusions (before the advent of careful monitoring of blood products) during surgeries before entering long-term care. Others have been sexually active and not taken precautions against transmission of the disease. A few elders have discussed their condition, and more will be identified as the public becomes less biased and more inclined to accept HIV testing as a routine procedure. Those persons over 60 years of age presently identified with AIDS constitute 2.9% of all cases in the United States (US Bureau of the Census, 1998).

A limited number of long-term care facilities knowingly accept AIDS clients, and among those that do, the geriatric AIDS client competes for extended care services with nongeriatric AIDS clients and non-AIDS geriatric clients. One of the major concerns is that the needs of young persons dying of AIDS may be quite different from those of the old. If these patients are indiscriminately mixed in long-term care settings, neither group is likely to have its needs well met.

Box 21-2   DISORDERS CAUSING OR SIMULATING DEMENTIA

Disorders Causing Dementia

Degenerative diseases:
  Alzheimer's disease
  Pick's disease
  Huntington's disease
  Progressive supranuclear palsy
  Parkinson's disease (not all cases)
  Cerebellar degenerations
  Amyotrophic lateral sclerosis (ALS) (not all cases)
  Parkinson-ALS-dementia complex of Guam and other island areas
  Rare genetic and metabolic diseases (Hallervorden-Spatz, Kufs', Wilson's late onset metachromatic leukodystrophy, adrenoleukodystrophy)
Vascular dementia:
  Multi-infarct dementia
  Cortical micro-infarcts
  Lacunar dementia (larger infarcts)
  Binswanger disease
  Cerebral embolic disease (fat, air, thrombus fragments)
Anoxic dementia:
  Cardiac arrest
  Cardiac failure (severe)
  Carbon monoxide
Traumatic dementia:
  Dementia pugilistica (boxer's dementia)
  Head injuries (open or closed)
Infectious dementia:
  Acquired immune deficiency syndrome (AIDS)—dementia and opportunistic infections
  Jakob-Creutzfeldt disease (subacute spongiform encephalopathy)

Progressive multifocal leukoencephalopathy
Post-encephalitic dementia
Behçet's syndrome
Herpes encephalitis
Fungal meningitis or encephalitis
Bacterial meningitis or encephalitis
Parasitic encephalitis
Brain abscess
Neurosyphilis (general paresis)
Normal pressure hydrocephalus (communicating hydrocephalus of adults)
Space-occupying lesions:
  Chronic or acute subdural hematoma
  Primary brain tumor
  Metastatic tumors (carcinoma, leukemia, lymphoma, sarcoma)
Multiple sclerosis (some cases)
Auto-immune disorders:
  Disseminated lupus erythematosus
  Vasculitis
Toxic dementia:
  Alcoholic dementia
  Metallic dementia (e.g., lead, mercury, arsenic, manganese)
  Organic poisons (e.g., solvents, some insecticides)
Other disorders:
  Epilepsy (some cases)
  Post-traumatic stress disorder (concentration camp syndrome—some cases)
  Whipple disease (some cases)
  Heat stroke

Disorders That Can Simulate Dementia

Psychiatric disorders:
  Depression
  Anxiety
  Psychosis
  Sensory deprivation
Drugs:
  Sedatives
  Hypnotics
  Anti-anxiety agents
  Anti-depressants
  Anti-arrhythmics
  Anti-hypertensives
  Anti-convulsants
  Anti-psychotics
  Digitalis and derivatives
  Drugs with anti-cholinergic side effects
  Others (mechanism unknown)
Nutritional disorders:
  Pellagra (B_6 deficiency)

Thiamine deficiency (Wernicke-Korsakoff syndrome)
Cobalamin deficiency (B_{12}) or pernicious anemia
Folate deficiency
Marchiafava-Bignami disease
Metabolic disorders (usually cause delirium, but can be difficult to differentiate from dementia):
  Hyper- and hypo-thyroidism (thyroid hormones)
  Hypercalcemia (calcium)
  Hyper- and hypo-natremia (sodium)
  Hypoglycemia (glucose)
  Hyperlipidemia (lipids)
  Hypercapnia (carbon dioxide)
  Kidney failure
  Liver failure
  Cushing syndrome
  Addison's disease
  Hypopituitarism
  Remote effect of carcinoma

From Office of Technology Assessment: *Losing a million minds: confronting the tragedy of Alzheimer's disease and other dementias,* Washington, DC, 1987, US Government Printing Office.

Alzheimer's Disease or Senile Dementia of the Alzheimer's Type

Alzheimer's disease (AD or senile dementia of the Alzheimer's type [SDAT]) was described by Alzheimer in 1906 and is a cerebral degenerative disorder of unknown origin. AD destroys proteins of nerve cells of the cerebral cortex by diffuse infiltration with nonfunctional tissue called *neurofibrillary tangles* and *plaques.* The disease is progressive and is accompanied by increasing forgetfulness, confusion, inability to concentrate, personality deterioration, and impaired judgment. The cause of the disorder is still unknown.

Because more people are living into the seventh, eighth, and ninth decades, the number of diagnosed cases of AD is estimated to increase. However, estimates of incidence vary greatly because AD is often mentioned with the generic term *dementia,* which includes both AD and other related and unrelated conditions.

Diagnosis

Presently, the only accurate method of diagnosing AD is to perform a brain biopsy or autopsy. The clinical criteria for the diagnosis of probable, possible, and definite AD are quite complex, but nursing observations of behaviors and affect are important. AD is most thoroughly diagnosed on the basis of tests ruling out other disorders that may mimic AD.

Probable AD can be clinically diagnosed if there is a typical insidious onset of dementia with progression and if there are no other systemic or brain diseases that could account for the progressive cognitive deficits. The course of this disease ranges from 1 to 15 years, with death usually occurring because of pulmonary infections, urinary tract infections, decubitus ulcers, or iatrogenic disorders.

Drug Treatment for Cognitive Aspects of Dementia

Drugs are being developed to enhance memory, stall cognitive deterioration, or stimulate remaining functional neurons to increased activity for persons with AD. One compound that has shown some promise is tacrine hydrochloride (THA, Cognex). Physostigmine, bethanechol, and lecithin have also been touted, with mixed results. All of these substances are used to stimulate the synthesis of the neurotransmitter acetylcholine, which is abnormally low in clients with AD. Drugs appear to be most effective in slowing the progression of the disease in its early stages.

Tacrine is a cholinesterase inhibitor that increases brain acetylcholine levels. Ideally, tacrine should be given an hour before meals because absorption is reduced by about 25% when it is taken with or 2 hours after meals (Kaplan, Sadock, 1996). Troublesome side effects include nausea, vomiting, diarrhea, headache, dizziness, myalgia, anorexia, and rash. The major problem with high doses of tacrine is hepatotoxicity, which is seen in about 40% to 50% of clients. If jaundice occurs, tacrine should be discontinued (Kaplan, Sadock, 1996).

Dementias, including AD, can worsen with certain antidepressants. The anticholinergic properties of tricyclic antidepressants (TCAs), such as amitriptyline (Elavil), will decrease cognitive abilities and should be avoided in clients with all types of dementia-related (vascular and nonvascular) CI.

Developmentally Disabled Elders

The number of developmentally disabled elders (DDEs) is rapidly increasing because of medical advances and healthier living conditions that keep them alive longer than in previous generations. Functional limitations in the biologic, social, and psychologic spheres may be a major cause of frailty in DDEs. These elders are particularly dependent on their environment for stimulation, and in the absence of stimulation, behaviors suggestive of dementia may emerge.

Many aspects of the aging process apparently are prematurely experienced by the developmentally disabled. Thus they may experience musculoskeletal changes, sensory decline, and certain disease states early on.

Both previously institutionalized and noninstitutionalized adults with mental retardation adapt well to group homes (Maisto, Hughes, 1995). Elderly mentally retarded persons may be kept in a more restrictive setting than necessary because no one has carefully assessed their abilities. A more humanistic and individualized model of care is necessary (Mooney et al, 1995).

Dementia of Vascular Disease Origin

Vascular brain disease results from anything that interferes with circulation to the brain. Dementia of vascular disease origin is marked by several distinguishing characteristics: remission and fluctuation, preservation of personality and insight, lability of emotion, and epileptiform attacks. The extent of damage or particular deficits in function will be seen in various incapacities, depending on the area of the brain affected. Box 21-3 lists conditions that may create cerebral anoxia or hypoxia. In addition to major brain attacks, there are transient ischemic attacks (TIAs) caused by impaired circulation. The attacks occur suddenly and are completely resolved within 24 hours (Kelly, 1995) but leave small spaces (lacunae) of nonfunctional cerebral tissue. Numerous TIAs result in multiinfarct dementia that may appear symptomatically as AD and are often prodromal to major brain attacks.

Because of the numerous ways in which circulation to cerebral cells can be impaired and the multiplicity of sites in which this may occur, vascular dementia may be initially seen with varied symptoms and may run an unpredictable course. These factors are especially threatening. An individual may feel as if he or she were living with an internal time bomb. The following may restore some sense of security to the client:

1. Install a telephone with a long cord or a portable phone and post emergency numbers on the phone.
2. Advise the client to wear antiembolic hose and avoid rising rapidly from a lying to a standing position.
3. Engage family, friends, or agencies in a daily telephone check to determine the client's status.
4. Subscribe to Lifeline through a community hospital.

Some TIAs occur gradually but may eventually trigger acute brain attack, more commonly known as *stroke.*

Box 21-3   VASCULAR BRAIN DISEASE

Vascular brain disease may result from any of the following:

- Arteriosclerotic plaques blocking circulation to cerebral cells
- Blood dyscrasias interfering with platelet and clot formation
- Cardiac decompensation resulting in insufficient perfusion to the brain
- Cerebrovascular hemorrhage (strokes) of small or large magnitude
- Diabetic deterioration of blood vessels
- Primary hypertension causing deterioration of capillary walls because of sustained pressure (Cerebral cells dependent on the deteriorated capillaries no longer function. Over time, hypertensive persons show greater decrements in cognitive performance than persons with normal blood pressure.)
- Rupture of cerebrovascular or aortic aneurysms
- Sustained severe anemia
- Systemic emboli lodging in cerebrovascular pathway
- Transient ischemic attacks (TIAs) lasting up to 24 hours, resulting from spasms of blood vessels in certain segments of the brain, which produce temporary disturbances in sensation, cognition, and motor activity and are often a warning sign of impending stroke

---

Stroke

Stroke is the leading cause of long-term disability among adults in the United States and the third leading cause of death. Diabetes, hypertension, atherosclerosis, and atrial fibrillation are primary risk factors for stroke. Strokes are cerebrovascular accidents (CVAs) that affect cerebral circulation through occlusive thrombi and emboli that cause infarction or hemorrhagic incidents occurring in the intracerebral or subarachnoid space. These variations account for differences in severity and symptomatology.

Hemorrhagic strokes are the most life threatening, but they occur much less frequently than thrombotic strokes. Intracerebral hemorrhage with interruption of an adequate supply of blood and nutrients to the brain, resulting in tissue damage, accounts for about 80% of strokes in the elderly (Caplan, 1995). Thrombotic strokes are most frequently a consequence of atrial fibrillation, which predisposes one to systemic emboli. Anticoagulant therapy is advised for conditions in which thrombotic strokes may occur (Laupacis et al, 1992) but is dangerous in hemorrhagic strokes. It is now thought that immediate treatment, within 6 hours of the CVA, may prevent some of the brain cell death. The degree of recovery from stroke is related to the severity of the accident and the immediacy of treatment. Despite the effectiveness of tissue plasminogen activator (t-PA) in reducing brain damage from infarction, few individuals are treated rapidly enough to derive its benefits (Miller, Woo, 1999). Box 21-4 lists possible stroke symp-

---

Box 21-4   SYMPTOMS SUGGESTING STROKE

- The abrupt onset of hemiparesis (one-sided weakness) or monoparesis (one-limb weakness)
- Sudden decline in level of consciousness
- Cataclysmic headache
- Acute dysphasia (language difficulties) or dysarthria (speech difficulties)
- Sudden loss of vision in one or both eyes or loss of vision in half the visual field
- Double vision
- Ataxia (clumsiness or balance loss)
- Weakness in all four extremities
- Loss of sensation in half of body

NOTE: Acute ataxia, vertigo, and vomiting—especially when associated with acute headache—may indicate stroke in the cerebellum.

From National Stroke Association: *Stroke, the first hours: emergency evaluation and treatment,* NSA consensus statement, Englewood, Colo, 1997, The Association.

toms that should alert individuals to seek treatment as soon as possible.

Difficulties and handicaps following stroke often involve communication, continence, and functional impairments. Communication problems such as aphasia are discussed in Chapter 3. The particular functional impairments will depend on the area of the brain attack. Fig. 21-1 maps the regions of the brain that will result in certain deficits. Some of the methods of testing functional disorders of the poststroke client can be seen in Box 21-5.

Rehabilitation involves timing and persistence. The expected functional improvement is based on the severity of disability 1 month after the stroke (Anderson, 1992). Most clients with stroke disabilities regain the most function possible in terms of prestroke performance of activities of daily living (ADLs) within 9 months. At 18 months following the stroke there actually tends to be a small decline, which is thought to be a result of lowered motivation or discouragement with progress. Functional improvement is delayed in those of advanced age, social isolation, and emotional distress. Up to one third of stroke victims become profoundly depressed in the year following stroke.

Assessment of needs. We know now that to maximize the benefits of interventions, a multidisciplinary team must activate a comprehensive rehabilitation plan as soon as the individual is physiologically stabilized. The assessment of needs following stroke is extremely complex and requires evaluation by neurologists, physiatrists, speech therapists, ophthalmologists, physical therapists, psychologists, and environmental planners. A multidisciplinary team is essential in the evaluation of the needs of an elder following stroke. Caretakers of the client, as well as the elder, must be included at every stage of planning to the extent possible. The nursing role involves coordinating team efforts in recognition of the client's energy levels and capacities. This involves clearly documenting all of the functional capacities that are retained and those that are impaired. The assessment must be redone routinely to adjust care plans to the client's progress and areas of need.

Stroke support groups. Nurses are becoming much more aware of the devastation a stroke produces as they study the reported experiences of elders recovering from stroke. Easton (1999) analyzed several reports and identified six stages common to stroke survivors: agonizing, fantasizing, realizing, blending, framing, and finally owning. The important idea is that the individual stroke survivor goes through many stages toward acceptance. Nurses must respect the process and realize that some never accept the assault to their sense of self.

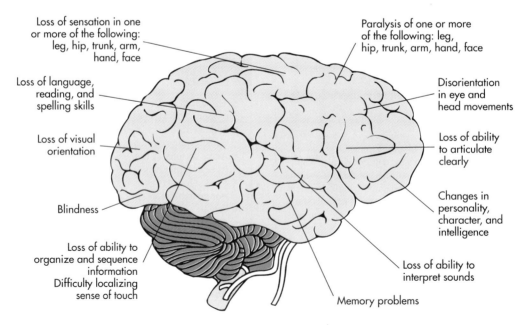

Fig. 21-1 Brain areas affected by strokes.

Small-group support is an ideal way for victims of stroke to become aware of the various stages they experience. The group ideally provides an environment for problem solving and feedback, support, acceptance, and encouragement to relearn and understand from others with similar limitations and struggles. When members have great difficulty verbalizing, it may be useful and relieve some tension to have part of each group designed toward nonverbal, nondominant brain expressions, such as art, music, or psychomotor activities. The success of a stroke group largely depends on the skill of the group facilitator. Experience with neurosurgical disorders and a background in gerontology and rehabilitation are desirable. When such specialized nurses are not available, it may be best to have co-facilitators whose combined skills most closely meet the members' biopsychosocial needs.

Use of art in stroke therapy. Adsit and Lee (1986) found art an excellent medium of expression for stroke clients. It allowed them to communicate feelings and moods when verbal articulation was impaired. In addition, it provided movement integration and a visible personal accomplishment accepted at face value without judgment. The unconscious imagery or symbolism is undoubtedly important in these artistic expressions, although the overall objective for these groups is to provide an opportunity for the client to express himself or herself emotionally and physically without the struggle for words.

The following guidelines may be useful: keep the group size under 10; tape paper to tables to prevent sliding; provide constant verbal and physical cueing to compensate for lapses in attention; and, if they are able, have clients discuss their art. Speech, music, and art therapy can each provide the client with various opportunities for self-expression.

Parkinson Disease

Parkinson disease (PD) describes a group of symptoms arising from disorders of the basal ganglia, the islands of gray matter in the cerebral hemispheres. It is a slowly progressive disease that leads to difficulty with movement. PD affects over 1 million people in the United States, is the most common of neurologic syndromes, and has an average onset at age 68. The incidence peaks at age 75 and then seems to decline in frequency. In persons over 80 years old, about 1 in 100

Box 21-5   TESTS OF SPECIFIC DISABILITIES THAT COMMONLY FOLLOW STROKE

Hemianopia (Loss of Part of Visual Field)
Sitting opposite the patient, hold up simultaneously two pens of different colors 30 cm in front of the patient and 30 cm apart; patients with hemianopia will be unable to see one of the pens or may turn the head toward the hemianopic side in an effort to see.

Proprioception (Awareness of Body in Space)
The wrist of the affected arm is held between the thumb and forefinger of the examiner; the patient's hand is raised and lowered, and the patient, with closed eyes, is asked the position of the hand; this exercise can also be done with fingers to determine even more specific loss of proprioception.

Sensation (Feeling Generated by Sensory Receptors)
With the patient's eyes closed, the examiner strokes the back of the unaffected hand and then the affected hand and in both cases asks the patient to describe the sensation. The affected side may have varying degrees of loss of sensation or total loss of feeling.

Balance (Bodily Poise)
The patient is asked to sit on the side of the bed with feet off the floor and maintain balance and sit unaided for 1 minute; it is usually readily apparent if the individual has a problem maintaining balance.

Arm Function (Range of Motion and Control)
The patient is asked to lift the affected arm to shoulder height and press against the examiner's upheld hand:
Complete paralysis = inability to move arm
Severe weakness = can move arm but not lift up or push
Moderate weakness = able to lift arm but unable to push
Slight weakness = able to do task requested but cannot push as hard as with unaffected arm
No weakness = no difference in abilities of either arm

Data from Anderson R: *The aftermath of stroke: the experience of patients and their families,* Cambridge, UK, 1992, Cambridge University Press.

will experience some degree of PD. Men are more commonly affected than women. In addition, many elders develop parkinsonian reactions (abnormal involuntary movements) in response to psychotropic drugs. This secondary PD is caused by several medications (see Chapter 15).

Although the etiology of primary parkinsonism is unknown, the death of substantia nigra cells within the basal ganglia results in a marked reduction in dopamine and is the cause of symptoms of tremor, muscular rigidity, akinesia, and loss of postural reflexes (Berkow et al, 1995; Kaszniak, 1995). Depression and anxiety are common in individuals with primary or secondary parkinsonism and may occur in 80% of these individuals.

Symptoms

Early signs are mild tremor of the hands and feet, generalized slowing of movement, rigidity, loss of motor skills and facial expression, and characteristically small handwriting. The most common initial symptom is tremor of one hand and the pill-rolling motion of the fingers. There is also a tendency toward stooped posture, shuffling gait, and keeping the arms slightly flexed and fixed at the side when walking (Parkinson's Disease Foundation, 1996). Some individuals with PD have a festinating gait in which steps become smaller and smaller and faster and faster.

Invisible symptoms, including erosion of recent memory, depression, hallucinations, low backache secondary to poor posture, mild vision loss, cramps, and burning sensations of the thighs and legs, become very troublesome. Although tremor, rigidity, and slowness of movement are the characteristic triad of symptoms, other problems that occur quite frequently include freezing (sudden difficulty in walking or turning around), dementia, excessive perspiration, oily skin, and feeling hot or cold. Box 21-6 lists symptoms of PD. There is uncertainty about the cause and predictability of symptoms. Risk factors are not clear, but preliminary investigation suggests that environmental toxins may be a factor.

Essential Tremor

Essential tremor (sometimes called *familial tremor*) is somewhat similar in appearance to PD and is said to be the most prevalent movement disorder, peaking in the sixth decade of life. It primarily affects the hands and the head and may significantly impair communication and activities requiring fine motor

control, as well as impact psychosocial adjustment. The disorder may become apparent in young adulthood and will grow progressively worse as one ages (Lundervold, Poppen, 1995). Etiology and management are poorly understood, although tremorlytic

---

Box 21-6 | PRIMARY SYMPTOMS OF PARKINSON DISEASE

Resting Tremor
- Occurs in approximately 50% to 75% of all PD patients and is often the initial symptom
- Affects mainly hands and feet but may also involve the head, neck, face, lips, tongue, or jaw
- Appears regular and rhythmic; approximately four to six beats per second

Rigidity
- Sustained muscle contraction; often mistaken for common stiffness or achiness
- Walking with arms held stiffly at the sides (rather than swinging naturally)
- Most common types include:
  - Cogwheeling: muscles move in a series of short jerks
  - Lead-pipe: muscles move smoothly, yet stiffly
- May affect breathing, eating, swallowing, and speech

Bradykinesia Slow *(brady)* movement *(kinesia)*
- Slowing of ordinary movements, such as walking, sitting down, and getting dressed
- Reduction in semiautomatic gestures, such as crossing the legs or scratching
- Reduction of spontaneous facial movements, resulting in mask-like stare
- Handwriting begins large and becomes smaller as patient fatigues
- Voice may become soft and trail off

Postural Instability
- Difficulty maintaining balance when walking or standing
- Leans forward in an effort to maintain center of gravity
- May result in injuries from frequent falls

From The American Parkinson Disease Association, Inc., 60 Bay Street, Staten Island, NY 10301.
PD, Parkinson disease.

medications and alcohol are helpful in reducing tremor in most cases.

Management

Typically, individuals are maintained on a combination of carbidopa and levodopa (Atamet, Sinemet), which often loses effectiveness as the amino acid levodopa competes with other amino acids for absorption at both the intestinal wall and the blood-brain barrier. Restricting dietary protein is sometimes effective. In many clients with PD the medication regimen may create illusions or hallucinations. Meco et al (1990) found that these were more common in individuals with CI. The Parkinson's Disease Foundation (1996) warns that clients with PD must be maintained on their medication even during acute illness because some persons deprived of their antiparkinsonian medication have died.

Because of the slow progression of the disease and the disability that accompanies it, individuals experience a change in role, activities, and social participation. Tremors may produce embarrassing moments. The expressionless face, slowed movement, and soft, monotone speech may give the impression of apathy, depression, and disinterest. Others, observing these symptoms, may react with disinterest. A sensitive nurse is aware that the visible symptoms produce an undesired facade that may hide an alert and responsive individual who wishes to interact and generate interest. Persons with PD experience great functional problems in mobility, communication, and home management (Longstreth et al, 1992). Two commonly identified problems are trouble with writing or typing and decreased sexual activity. Another problem, studied by Madeley et al (1990), was that of marked impairment in driving skills in severe cases of PD. A problem of lesser frequency but very distressing is dystonic cramps, particularly those that result in curling and twisting of the toes and the feet. Surgery does not correct this problem. A neurologic consultation is advised.

Topp (1987) suggests the following ways of coping with some of the symptoms that disturb the client with PD:

1. Movement of the limbs decreases the tremors; when walking, one should swing the arms.
2. Holding an object helps control the tremors; individuals should hold something in their hands when sitting quietly.
3. Contractures and deformities are avoided if the individual walks as much as possible and avoids remaining still for long periods; range of motion and balancing exercises need to be prescribed by a physical therapist and practiced faithfully.
4. Skin must be kept dry and clean, and oil-free lotion applied every few hours to avoid seborrhea and skin breakdown; air mattresses and sheepskins are advisable for beds.
5. Constipation may be avoided by high fluid intake and a high-residue diet.
6. Speaking and reading aloud should be encouraged to enhance communication; sometimes speech therapy is warranted.
7. Depression and low self-esteem may be partially countered by direct discussion of feelings about changes in self-image, sexuality, and functional ability.
8. Support system encouragement and information about the disease are essential if the family is to cope with the slow responses, clumsiness, and poor communication of the afflicted individual.
9. Self-help groups are often useful, because the members solve their problems collectively.

Parkinson Dementia

There is a correlation between increased incidence of dementia and PD in late life (Marder, 1992). It remains controversial whether the dementia that occurs in about 25% of clients with PD is related to the pathologic findings of the disease or whether it is a disorder quite distinct from PD without dementia (Hazzard et al, 1994). However, the *Diagnostic and Statistical Manual of Mental Disorders (DSM-IV)* (American Psychiatric Association, 1994) states that dementia is a direct result of pathophysiologic changes that occur in the presence of PD. Early signs of dementia are subtle and are somewhat related to age and age of onset, although specific cognitive changes commonly occur early in the course of PD (Levin, Katzen, 1995). The incidence of dementia in PD is associated with depression, institutionalization, older age at onset of PD, and atypical neurologic features (Aarsland et al, 1996).

Nurses may be instrumental in assessing and dealing with the mood disorders that often accompany PD. Depression and mania may mimic dementia and must be relieved to the greatest extent possible to increase client comfort and determine the actual amount of impairment from dementia. Medications and individualized treatment plans are critical to the care of the person with PD. The challenge to client, family, and nurse is to maintain the highest possible level of hope. At times the deterioration is rapid, but most clients remain functional for many years (Berkow et al, 1995).

ASSESSMENT OF COGNITIVE IMPAIRMENT

Foremost in assessment of CI is a thorough medical workup to rule out factors that may be clouding consciousness. Following that, an evaluation for depression is necessary because the effects of severe depression are a significant problem and frequently are severe enough to mimic dementia. Nurses' recognition and primary assessment of CI are most likely to be accurate if appropriate instruments are employed. Nurses are the only professionals who see the client throughout the course of the day and night and are able to observe mentation and behavior in many circumstances, as well as the diurnal variations.

Self-appraisal is also important, and the nurse should discuss abilities and problems with the client and family. However, it is known that individuals with dementia may overestimate their capacities, whereas those with depression are inclined to underestimate them (McDougall, 1996). In addition, families typically underestimate the performance of their elders.

Memory

Memory testing may be used primarily for establishing the presence of dementia and assessment of other cognitive functions for determining the severity of CI. Although it is extremely common in individuals over 75 years of age, CI is rarely assessed by primary care providers, even for those with moderate to severe impairment (Callahan et al, 1995). Loss of short-term memory is the first indication of some CI. There are many tests that establish short- and long-term memory deficits. Some of these are discussed in Chapter 14.

Orientation

Many nurse clinicians use the client's orientation to time, place, and person as a quick evaluator of cognitive function; however, orientation items are inaccurate indicators of the degree and severity of CI. Orientation screening is unacceptable and insensitive as a means of establishling cognitive function.

Perception

Perception is one criterion used to assess a person's level of CI. Investigations reveal a relationship between the quality of the sensory apparatus and cognitive functioning. Auditory status and cognitive functional decline may be associated. Hearing impairment not only interferes with comprehension but significantly reduces stimulation needed to maximize cerebral function.

Psychomotor Ability

Psychomotor behaviors are the motor effects of cerebral or psychic activity. These do not necessarily lead to purposeful behaviors in clients with CI. An example of this is seen in sundowner's syndrome (SS). SS was first identified by Cameron in 1941 and was called "nocturnal neurosis and wandering." It resembles delirium, and nurses often see the agitation, restlessness, confusion, and wandering behavior of older adults when the sun goes down. Evans (1987) identified risk factors for SS in institutionalized elderly persons. Physiologic factors were dehydration, mental impairment, frequent night awakening, and odor of urine. Psychosocial factors included being in a room less than 1 month, recent admission to a facility, and fluctuating levels of orientation.

Functional Ability

The Functional Dementia Scale (FDS) is designed to objectively monitor the course of dementia and to evaluate treatment. The items of the FDS were selected to assess the major problems associated with dementia, such as emotional lability, wandering, agitation, incontinence, memory loss, and need for supervision. The FDS is a brief scale capable of distinguishing varying degrees of functional limitation and is useful in establishing the level of impairment and assessing the impact of interventions over time. This scale may be useful to clinicians and families caring for demented clients and is easily administered by nursing home personnel or families (Moore et al, 1983) (see Chapter 14).

A mini-mental status examination is the mostly commonly used instrument to detect problems with orientation, immediate and recent memory, attention, calculation, and language and motor skills. The mini-mental status examination is unique because it allows assessment of fluid (nondominant; right brain) and crystallized (dominant; left brain) intelligence. Symptoms in AD usually progress in five stages: (1)

loss in memory, (2) loss in powers of reasoning, (3) loss in comprehension, (4) deterioration in personality, and (5) a terminal vegetative state (McDougall, 1990). This and other tools to measure CI are included in Chapter 14.

Affectual Disturbance

Affect (expression of feelings and emotions) is often unstable, heightened, or flattened in dementia; in some, particularly stroke victims, emotional incontinence is characteristic. Emotional incontinence simply means that the person will laugh or cry uncontrollably without any triggering event or thought. In the later, severe stages of dementia, affect seems totally lacking.

Social Intactness

Inappropriate behaviors, particularly abusive and violent behaviors that may be present in CI, are signals that a client may not understand or be unable to conform to the routines and rules of the environment and should have a need-driven assessment (discussed later in this chapter).

CARING FOR THE PERSON WITH DEMENTIA

Much of dementia care takes place in the home and is provided by an aging spouse or middle-age child (see Chapter 23) or in a nursing home, where it is provided by aides. Therefore nurses will be most effective when they assist the direct caregivers, in whatever setting, in understanding the nature of dementia and the interventions likely to be most effective. Interventions must match expectations with capabilities; incorporate earlier life skills and interests; and provide a calm, caring, and structured environment.

Identifying the strengths of the dementia-afflicted older person requires staff commitment and patience. Too often the obvious deficits create an unwarranted assumption that the individual has nothing left of the personality that is valuable. In an atmosphere of acceptance, individuals will show maximal potential. Staff can reinforce areas of capability and prevent shame by helping the client only with things he or she has tried and is unable to accomplish. This requires patience and hope, as well as assistance only at the necessary level.

Environmental Alterations

The present trend to have special care units designed for the needs of persons with CI is meant to ensure maximal function and safety for impaired individuals. Good lighting, soothing colors and pictures, clearly visible signs indicating space functions, individual photos on the doors of clients' rooms, noise control, large areas for wandering, and protection from dangerous objects and places all contribute to a functionally supportive environment. Music may be soothing if it is used appropriately and if it is of a type that the individual enjoys. Families are encouraged to provide information about the individual's previous habits, pleasures, and preferences and to bring significant items to the client's room. Mildly confused people find clocks, calendars, and an indoor sign showing the name of the institution helpful.

Reality Orientation

Reality orientation is a term much used and abused. Approximately 30 years ago a specific program of reality orientation (called *RO*) was begun in Tuscaloosa, Alabama, to stimulate staff members' interest and hope for the profoundly disoriented clients in their care. This program was useful because it provided caregivers with a specific program and structure that resulted in increased interaction with clients and some hopeful interventions. In the intervening years it has been found that some of the expectations were unrealistic, but the interest in communicating with the individual resident has been sustained. At present, the thrust of programs is toward identifying elements of the individual's past and helping the individual and staff to appreciate the connections and the feelings. It remains important to retain the following concepts that evolved out of the RO programs:

1. A calm, caring atmosphere
2. Dependable routines and structured expectations
3. Clear communication in simple words; brief and consistent instructions
4. Consistent caregivers
5. An RO board containing information about the date and place that is consistently maintained to give residents an opportunity to remain oriented to dates, times, and important events
6. Connecting present situations with past similar experiences to emphasize strengths and remote memories to assist in dealing with the present

Rather than insistently reminding an apparently confused individual of the present time and place, it may be far more revealing and therapeutic to join the individual in his or her time and place. Validating his or her inner orientation as expressive of a particular need or feeling can restore self-esteem and give staff members a deeper understanding of the individual. Thoughtfully consider repetitious or unusual behaviors and link behavior to previous life activities. This may provide reassurance and increase staff understanding.

Nutrition

Chapter 10 deals with the nutritional needs of elders. Individuals with dementia, PD, or CVA exhibit numerous behaviors that interfere with adequate nutritional intake. Many conditions may contribute to swallowing disorders. Assessment must be done by a certified speech therapist. The nurse must be alert to signs and symptoms of swallowing disorders (Box 21-7). The nursing challenge is to increase functional behaviors during the process of eating or being fed (Van Ort, Phillips, 1992). Common problems encountered in the feeding process include the following:
- Refusal to open the mouth without extra stimulation (such as coaxing it open with a spoon)

Box 21-7	**SIGNS AND SYMPTOMS OF DYSPHAGIA**

Person (or family) complaints that swallowing is difficult

Inability to control food or saliva in the mouth (e.g., drooling or leakage of food from mouth)

Facial droop

Coughing before, during, or after swallowing food or liquids

Choking while eating or drinking

Increased congestion or secretions after a meal

Change in voice quality (e.g., a wet, gurgling, or hoarse voice)

Recurrent upper respiratory infections and/or pneumonia

Refusal of food or reluctance to have food placed in mouth

Retention of food in mouth or pharynx

Resistance to being fed quickly (i.e., turning head to the side to avoid having food placed in mouth or attempting to push nurse away)

Refusal to open mouth and/or to accept a large bite of food

Unexplained weight loss

From Kayser-Jones J: Dysphagia among nursing home residents, *Geriatr Nurs* 20(2):77-82, 1999.

- Closing the mouth inappropriately; extrusion and disturbed tongue movements; hoarding food in the mouth
- Inability to swallow
- Coughing when swallowing
- Spitting out food

Van Ort and Phillips (1992) suggest that general interventions should include leaning toward the person, addressing the person by name, touching the person, explaining the content of each bite, offering sips of fluid between bites, holding the spoon ready while talking to and touching the resident, and hugging the resident when he or she successfully takes and swallows a bite.

Dysphagia

Dysphagia is a common problem and requires nursing time, skill, and compassion to ensure that the resident will maintain sufficient nutrition (Kayser-Jones, 1999). Kayser-Jones (Box 21-8) provides guidelines to facilitate safety when feeding the dysphagic person. For each resident there are particular behaviors of the nurse that will facilitate the process of eating. The caregiver with sensitivity to the individual's eating patterns, preferences, life history, and present symptoms can respond more effectively to the client's eating abilities and preferences. Food is often one of the few pleasures remaining for a cognitively impaired person.

Wandering

Wandering is one of the most difficult management problems encountered in institutional settings. Each year some residents wander away from a facility and are later found injured or dead. Media attention and litigation may suggest that staff has been lax in allowing this to happen, even though an elder determined to leave will usually find a way.

Ambulation, in and of itself, is necessary, and providing sufficient opportunities to ambulate in areas that are not hazardous is necessary in institutional settings. Individuals whose life-style has included great amounts of ambulation are particularly in need of opportunities to continue this behavior. The rate or amount of ambulation may seem excessive, but if it is not inherently dangerous, it should be allowed without interference. The pattern and route of ambulation and the point at which it terminates are significant. There are many possible patterns and causes for wandering behavior. Some of the most predominant include the following:
- Akathisia-induced ambulation, which is usually a result of long-term use of neuroleptics and is associ-

ated with other signs of akathisia, such as inability to sit still, repetitive movements, and other extrapyramidal symptoms. Antiparkinsonian medication may reduce motor restlessness. Usually these persons will not do anything dangerous if they are made aware of the hazards.

- Self-stimulatory behavior that takes the form of ambulation. This is often seen in advanced dementia and is associated with other stereotyped actions, such as furniture rubbing, hand clapping, and repetitive vocalizations. Little has been done to deal effectively with stereotypy—the persistent, inappropriate mechanical repetition of actions or verbalizations. These may be a form of self-stimulation in the absence of stimulation that is more meaningful. Providing other forms of stimulation such as paper, cloth, or stuffed toys to manipulate may reduce the meaningless repetitive behavior. Continuous self-stimulation may indicate a lack of external sensory stimulation in the environment.

- Modeling, which occurs when a severely demented client shadows an ambulator and will follow him or her everywhere. Engagement in other activities has proved useful to deter the shadowing.

- Exit-seeking behavior, which is most often exhibited in recently admitted patients on locked wards. The behavior is accompanied by statements reflecting a desire to go home. Distracting activities may be temporarily useful. Exit-seeking behavior is highly motivated and may persist until the individual finds some gratifications in the present environment that reduce the desire to leave. It may be useful to bring some significant items from the home to help the individual feel more comfortable in the unfamiliar setting. It is important for the nurse to determine how actively the individual was involved in the decision to move to the institution and whether there was adequate orientation to the move.

The first two behaviors listed are secondary forms of wandering that are not motivated by the primary desire to move about and are in fact evidence of neurologic or cognitive disorders. The interruption of these behaviors may cause more distress for the client and is usually not necessary. When any behavior is negated or discouraged, it is important to provide something to take its place. It is most productive to modify the environment so that the wandering is not likely to be hazardous. As an example, in one facility it was noted that a client always tended to walk out of his room and turn right, toward the exit. By recognizing this pattern and changing his room so that a right turn led him to the lounge area, staff members were able to abate his tendency to wander outside. Past patterns undoubtedly had something to do with his penchant to make a right turn whenever leaving his room. We might assume that in his home the kitchen was to the right of his bedroom.

The stimulus for wandering arises from many internal and external sources. Agenda behaviors were identified and studied by Rader et al (1985). They found that many wanderers had a specific pattern that gave clues to their needs. When the need was met, the wandering abated. For example, one individual frequently went toward a window with a view of a lake. A large

---

Box 21-8   INTERVENTIONS TO FACILITATE EATING SAFELY

Use an interdisciplinary team approach (RN, speech pathologist, physician, dietitian, and dentist) for the assessment and management of dysphagia.

Provide a pleasant, quiet environment free from distractions.

Place residents in an upright, comfortable, well-supported position.

Feed residents only when they are wide awake and alert.

Keep residents in upright position for 1 hour after meals.

Offer small bites of food (that the resident will enjoy) slowly.

Do not force residents to eat quickly.

Make sure residents have swallowed one bite before giving them another by watching movement of larynx.

Thicken thin liquids if recommended by the speech pathologist.

Alter food consistency as recommended by the speech pathologist.

Focus on the resident when feeding, not on television set or others.

Observe and report any change in resident's respiratory rate, voice quality, or other changes in general condition that may indicate that aspiration has occurred.

Provide oral hygiene and examine resident's mouth after the meal to make certain food that could be aspirated does not remain in the mouth.

Observe for any change in resident's swallowing ability that may indicate need for reassessment of swallowing and report change to speech pathologist immediately.

Provide frequent (every 3 to 4 months) in-service staff education by a speech pathologist.

From Kayser-Jones J: Dysphagia among nursing home residents, *Geriatr Nurs* 20(2):77-82, 1999.

mural of a lake scene posted in her room seemed to decrease the wandering.

Three psychosocial factors are correlated with types of wandering: previous work roles, lifelong patterns of coping with stress, and the search for security. Attention to the wanderer's nonverbal behavior, past coping strategies, and present mood is essential. Before attempting to manage wandering behavior, you need answers to the following questions:

- What is being sought?
- When does the behavior most frequently occur?
- What would be done if the person were 20 years old instead of 80?
- Is the present setting too restrictive?
- How dangerous is the wandering?
- What psychologic need or energy process causes the wandering?

Discussion of these questions with caregivers and the wanderer may help arrive at interventions that will diminish the need to search. The following interventions may be helpful:

- Care plans that include past coping styles and work orientation
- Memory-training group sessions for wanderers
- Assistance to residents in building cognitive maps
- Interesting activity programs to meet varied needs
- Interpersonal contact with significant people
- Availability of items to meet basic needs (e.g., food, drinks, blanket)
- Activities that dissipate energy
- Continuity of personnel
- Group relationships and meetings to establish feelings of connection
- Established territory and cognitive maps
- Music, exercise groups, and dances to provide opportunities to move in an integrated manner
- Massage to reduce generalized tension
- Imagery exercises to take mental trips to places one enjoyed
- Nature walks outside the facility to provide relief from the institutional setting
- Visits to places of importance such as work sites and homes

Most important, on admission the patient and family should discuss the hazards of wandering versus the hazards of confinement and make a deliberate decision about when and if an individual should be restricted or restrained. Electronic ankle bracelets embedded in plastic, for comfort and ease of bathing, can be put on individuals who have been identified as "wanderers." These will activate alarms that are installed at exits. A lighted panel alerts staff to the exit the resident has crossed. This system allows others to enter and leave the facility at will and eliminates the need for locked exits. There are other electronic tracking devices that are being used to follow the wanderings of some individuals to determine patterns.

A particularly appealing method of dealing with the wandering patient is to form a buddy system with an individual who is willing and able to provide companionship for varying periods and can account for the patient's presence. This might increase the socialization of each, protect the wanderer, and enhance the ego of the "buddy." The "buddy" must not be coerced into such an arrangement. Sometimes these arrangements form spontaneously.

We have found no better guidelines than those proposed by Rader et al (1985) to manage an individual who is trying to leave a protected setting. Following this plan reinforces the nurse's interest in the patient's feelings and needs and may relieve distress. It seems that tone of voice and eye contact may provide sufficient focus, somewhat like a radar beam, that keeps an individual on course. Perhaps the personal attention fills the empty restlessness that activated the wanderer.

A wanderer's lounge was developed in a nursing home in Long Beach, California, to provide beneficial activities for confused residents and respite for staff and the more alert residents who were annoyed by the intrusions of the wanderers. The lounge was made safe, and everything in it could be touched by the residents. Each day just before 3 PM, the time when these residents seemed to become the most confused and agitated, a small group of 15 to 20 residents was taken to the designated area. The group members were introduced to each other daily and involved in simple exercises and activities. Refreshments were served. The program employed music, exercise, sensory stimulation, nourishment, and dancing each day. Activities varied from day to day and included entertainers, poetry readings, sing-alongs, cosmetic sessions, and reminiscing. The program lasted for about $1\frac{1}{2}$ hours (McGrowder-Lin, Bhatt, 1988).

Holmberg (1997) reported the success of an "evening walkers'" group in reducing aimless wandering in a group of persons who had various degrees of dementia but were physically quite active. Conducted in the early evening by volunteers, 8 to 10 individuals would be assembled each evening just after dinner for a planned walk. The volunteers were given information about past interests of individual group members and used this knowledge to keep a conversation going during the walk. Those who participated in the walks seemed calmer afterward and tended to sleep well.

It has been suggested that regular outdoor walking programs be instituted as a standard intervention for all nursing home residents who are ambulatory, even if canes and walkers are necessary. In urban settings where traffic and crime may present special problems, internal courtyards may be created or special routes selected for elements of safety. It might also be possible to transport groups to more pleasant settings for walking. Staff accompaniment is usually necessary for the walking group, but in certain cases individuals may be encouraged to walk in pairs or small groups without staff accompaniment. Visitors can also be encouraged to take residents for walks outside a facility.

Dealing With Agitation

Agitation is pervasive among individuals suffering from CI. They become agitated easily and frequently, and caregivers often have great difficulty knowing the cause or how to intervene. Frequent causes of agitation include hypoxia, delirium, urinary tract infection, fatigue, or pain. Agitation may result from unexpected reactions to medications, anxiety related to an overload of adaptational stresses for which the elder does not have the psychic reserve or available supports, and disturbances in biologic rhythmicity. It is quite possible that the aged individual is less integrated biorhythmically when stressed. Minor environmental changes and psychologic stress must be considered. Providing a routine, structured environment that is clearly understood and is designed according to the individual's life-style patterns may reduce agitation. Too often the agitation is considered just another demonstration of dementia.

Norris (1986) states that restlessness that seems random is really an indication of the individual's coping efforts and, even though ineffective, signals the potential for coping when appropriate assistance is provided. A systematic and individualized approach is necessary because agitation is a multidimensional problem. It is often demonstrated in aggressive behaviors, motor restlessness, aberrant vocalizations, and resistance to care (Gerdner, Buckwalter, 1994).

Most difficult behaviors usually occur at bath time (Bergener et al, 1992). It is quite easy to understand how being undressed, being suspended in a Hoyer lift, and lowered into a tub of water would be upsetting to anyone and much more so when dementia clouds the

understanding of what is happening. Kovach and Meyer-Arnold (1997) provide tips for decreasing agitation during bath time (Box 21-9).

Preventing Catastrophic Reactions

Goldstein (1952) coined the term *catastrophic reaction* to describe the overreaction toward minor stresses that occurs in demented clients. It is precipitated by fatigue, overstimulation, inability to meet expectations, and misinterpretations. Interventions to avert or minimize this reaction include those proposed by Wolanin and Phillips (1981) in their classic work on confusion (Box 21-10).

Coping With Problem Behaviors

Behavioral problems frequently encountered include physically aggressive behavior such as biting, spitting, hitting, and throwing objects; verbally aggressive behavior such as cursing and shouting; and nonaggressive behaviors such as pacing, dressing or disrobing inappropriately, incontinence, wandering, and repetitive vocalizations. Nursing responsibilities include the following:

1. Carefully observe and record mood, behavior, and patterns; where and with whom the problems occur.
2. Manage behaviors with the use of as few psychotropic medications as possible. They tend to increase the client's difficulty negotiating the environment.
3. Avoid changing routines; make surroundings as predictable as possible.
4. Groom the client carefully; encourage independence in this area, but if he or she is unable to provide self-care in this area, do not leave him or her untidy.
5. Provide occupational therapy geared to the client's abilities. Boredom may instigate problem behaviors.
6. Provide the client with consistent orientation to activities and expectations.
7. Avoid using physical or chemical restraints.
8. Provide a mildly stimulating environment.
9. Interact in a caring and supportive manner.
10. Make every effort toward consistency of caregivers.

Chapter 3 discussed the communication problems likely to be encountered with impaired individuals. The inability to communicate one's needs is often at the root of behavioral problems. It is worth mentioning again that although verbal communication may be quite

Box 21-9	TIPS FOR DECREASING ENVIRONMENTAL STRESS AND AGITATION DURING BATH TIME

- Keep room and water temperatures comfortable. Install an extra heater in the tub room so the air and water temperatures are not as disparate.
- Avoid background noises and conversations. Hang beach towels in the bathing room if there is a lot of "echo" from sounds.
- Install a shampoo sink on your unit. Shampoo hair on a separate day for residents who cannot tolerate both a bath and shampoo or for residents who become agitated when water sprays on their head or face.
- Give the person a tub bath, shower, or bed bath depending on preference of the resident. Assess the best time of day for the person's bath—usually when the resident is the most calm and does not have other activities or appointments challenging their stress threshold.
- If the person is very resistive, consider postponing the bath. Avoid getting into long explanations and cajoling about why a bath is needed. Offer an incentive for getting the bath done, such as "After your bath we can go to the coffee shop together." Another suggestion along the lines of incentive is to make an appointment for the bathing experience. Showing the fearful person the tub room frequently decreases the fear of that unknown room.
- Transfer residents with sufficient staff, proper techniques, and proper equipment. Do not use a shower chair to transfer the person to the bathing room. Replace tubs with hydraulic chair lifts with ones that use an easy-access side panel.
- Undress the person in the bathing room. As the person is undressed, cover each unclothed area with a bath blanket. If comforting, put the person in the tub with bath blankets or towels that cover the person and are raised only in the area needed to allow a hand and washcloth to do the washing. Use blankets and towels that have been warmed in a dryer to pamper the person.
- Run the water into the tub before the person enters the bathing room. Running water before bringing the person to the tub room not only keeps the tub room warm, it also controls unwanted noise and distraction. It also allows the caregiver and person to engage in conversation. Some people can tolerate one inch of water and some aren't bothered by five inches. Keep this and other likes and dislikes in the care plan.
- Have all equipment, linens, and clothing ready and organized before the person enters the bathing room to facilitate an organized and consistent bathing process.
- Allow the resident to feel the water before getting into the tub. Use reassuring phrases such as "This is nice" or "This feels good."
- Try some aromatherapy. Give the resident a choice between two. For example, allow the resident to smell the bath oils and ask, "Do you like the rose or herb scent?"
- Use a calm unhurried approach. Have one consistent caregiver give the bath, explaining what will be done and asking the person if he or she is comfortable. Use reassuring words, especially when the person seems confused or fearful. Acknowledging the different or conflicting agendas may give the person being bathed more control of the experience.
- Keep stimulation as singular and focused as possible. For example, two people should not bathe different parts of the body. If water is running, decrease or stop tactile stimulation.
- Encourage the resident to participate in the bath when possible. If the person has difficulty, try putting your hand over the person's hand while washing.
- Give the person a washcloth or shampoo bottle to hold during the bath. This keeps hands busy, decreases striking out, and allows you to thank the person for helping.
- Placing a sock or pillowcase over the shower head decreases the force of the spray. Use only a hand-held shower to provide focused and controlled spraying.
- Use music to redirect and relax. Songs with which the caregiver and person can sing along can be helpful in giving the person control of the bath.
- Decorate the tub room in a homelike fashion. The tub room should look like a bathroom, not a laboratory. Encourage the staff to bring their personalities into the bathing routine. Pictures of children and pets, familiar landscapes and objects are helpful for supporting engaging behaviors.
- "Seize the moment." If an accidental food spill soils the clothes, it may be the perfect time to change clothes in the tub room and suggest a bath. "As long as we're changing your clothes let's freshen up, wash your face and hands, and soak your feet a while."

From Kovach CR, Meyer-Arnold EA: Preventing agitated behaviors during bath time, *Geriatr Nurs* 18(3):107-111, 1997.

meaningless, a quiet, calm tone of voice, smooth cadence, and gentle actions will have more influence than the words.

Recognize that the feelings of distress may linger in a client after he or she has forgotten the precipitant. Relief should be available to the caregiver who becomes angry or irritated. It is important for nurses to express their annoyance or impatience to another staff member. We believe it is futile to talk of being caring, patient, and gentle with clients without providing opportunities

| Box 21-10 | WHAT TO DO FOR CATASTROPHIC BEHAVIOR |

The patient with Alzheimer's may exhibit a sudden temporary worsening in behavior related to buildup of stress, fatigue, and/or physical discomforts. Thinking deteriorates (cognitive inaccessibility) and the patient becomes unable to communicate (social inaccessibility). The patient experiencing a catastrophic episode is generally frightened or panicked, unsafe, and exhibits strong potential for injuring himself or others.

How to prepare for it: A person's catastrophic episodes are usually the same each time. Ask the caregiver how the patient usually acts when tired or overwhelmed: Does he become fearful? Agitated? Wander? Act more confused? Become combative? Ask what the caregiver does to calm the patient.

Immediate measures: Place the patient in a quiet room, eliminating all extraneous stimuli, including people. Regard the patient as frightened. Focus your interventions on returning his sense of mastery or control over his environment.

- Assess for and eliminate all potential stressors, such as full bladder, restraints, catheters, pain.
- Provide a "time out" of at least one-half to one hour. If possible, ask the caregiver to sit quietly with the patient. (No TV or talking except quiet, gentle reassurance.)
- If the patient's combative behavior poses an immediate hazard to himself or others, provide physical or chemical restraints in the least restrictive manner possible. *However,* if the patient is not combative unless approached, simply supervise while maintaining a safe distance, using the "time-out" to defuse the situation.
- Remain calm: this is a time-limited event. Talk in low, calm, reassuring tones to help the patient feel safe and secure. Do not attempt to argue with the patient's belief. ("They are not constructing that building in your yard, you are in the hospital!") Usually the patient will not believe such a comment; instead, it will heighten his anxiety.
- Chart the symptoms of the event, time of onset, duration, and successful interventions.
- Prevent further episodes by simplifying the daily schedule, increasing rest periods, evaluating environmental stressors, limiting visitors, controlling pain, and using other interventions described in this article.

From Hall GR: The hospital patient has Alzheimer's, *Am J Nurs* 91(10):45-50, 1991.

for caregivers to express their frustration and anger at appropriate times.

In a demonstration project at the Blumenthal Jewish Home in Clemmons, North Carolina, residents with AD were removed from the setting for 2 hours in the afternoon four times a week and placed in another protected environment in which a structured program of activity, music, exercise, memory recall, sensory stimulation, and nourishment was provided. This allowed the staff respite from the difficulty of managing the residents' behaviors, and (more important) the participating residents rapidly became more manageable; had fewer episodes of rummaging, combativeness, and incontinence; and demonstrated more acceptable social behavior. For some, wandering decreased slightly, and they were able to sleep uninterrupted through the night (Sawyer, Mendlovitz, 1982).

Cohen (1996) focuses attention on the treatment of AD in the absence of cure and prevention strategies. The growing attention to considerate pharmacologic, behavioral, and psychosocial approaches to care of both the family and the individual is promising. For example, the catastrophic reaction of certain clients responds quite readily to distraction. The infectious nature of agitated behaviors often results in overreactions of caregivers as well. Slow, calm, deliberate action is much more likely to be effective.

Need-Driven Dementia Behaviors

Even the most bizarre misinterpretations and actions carry a message of need that can be addressed appropriately if the individual's past history and habits, physiologic status, and physical and social environment are carefully evaluated (Kolanowski, 1999). This implies that all behavior has meaning and is driven by need. This does not mean that we reinforce the client's action or misinformation but that we respond to the underlying problem and meet or alter the need that underlies the disruptive action. This perspective moves the burden off the client and encourages problem resolution by assessing the need of the client. There is much to learn about this approach, but we have made a beginning effort based on Maslow's framework of human needs (Fig. 21-2).

• • •

Care must be individualized to preserve dignity. In spite of cognitive deficits and behavioral abnormalities, these clients are sensitive to attitudes and seem to know instinctively whom they can trust. Body language of the caregivers sets an emotional climate: facial expression, eye contact, gestures, and fluidity of movement convey

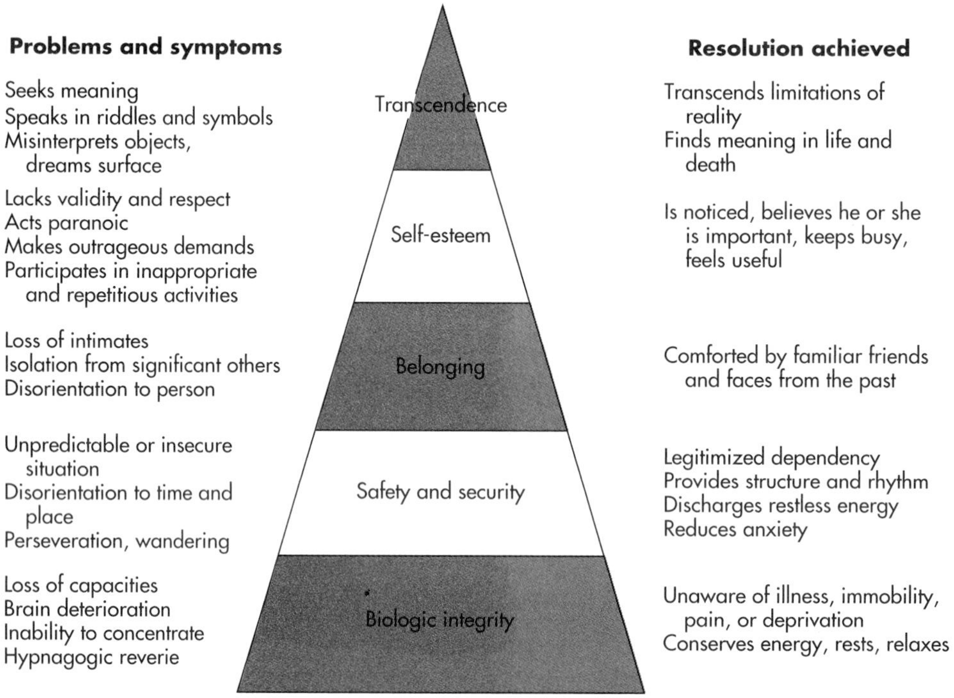
Problems and symptoms
Seeks meaning
Speaks in riddles and symbols
Misinterprets objects, dreams surface
Lacks validity and respect
Acts paranoic
Makes outrageous demands
Participates in inappropriate and repetitious activities
Loss of intimates
Isolation from significant others
Disorientation to person
Unpredictable or insecure situation
Disorientation to time and place
Perseveration, wandering
Loss of capacities
Brain deterioration
Inability to concentrate
Hypnagogic reverie
Transcendence
Self-esteem
Belonging
Safety and security
Biologic integrity
Resolution achieved
Transcends limitations of reality
Finds meaning in life and death
Is noticed, believes he or she is important, keeps busy, feels useful
Comforted by familiar friends and faces from the past
Legitimized dependency
Provides structure and rhythm
Discharges restless energy
Reduces anxiety
Unaware of illness, immobility, pain, or deprivation
Conserves energy, rests, relaxes

Fig. 21-2 Needs met through confusional states. (Developed by Priscilla Ebersole.)

messages of acceptance or disinterest (Bartol, 1979). Moments of pleasure and joy must not be overlooked as sources of brief satisfaction, distraction, and respite from the underlying anxiety. Affection, appreciation, and touch may provide some moments of meaning. Bergener et al (1992) found that the most significant calming effect was achieved by a relaxed, smiling caregiver.

Even grossly demented persons, often seen as helpless and hopeless, may briefly respond with warmth and pleasure when stimulated. For those persons the goal is not orientation but, rather, human contact. Care should be directed toward fostering good general health and maintaining locomotor skills and functional preservation to the extent possible in all areas of behavior. Listening with respectful attention to any attempts to communicate is most important. There are currently no known cures for dementia, an overabundance of descriptive data, and few medical treatments; thus the meaning of the individual's last years lies with nursing personnel. The quality of life provided the client depends directly on the skill and interest of care providers.

KEY CONCEPTS

- Cognitive impairment that is significant is a disease process and must be regarded as such. Some of the dementias are treatable, and some are not. Nurses need to advocate for thorough assessment of any elder who appears to be experiencing genuine cognitive decline and inability to function in important aspects of life.
- Delirium, sometimes referred to as *acute confusional state,* is a result of physiologic imbalances and may be caused by a variety of biologic disturbances. Delirium is characterized by fluctuating levels of consciousness, sometimes in a diurnal pattern, and frequent misperceptions and illusions.
- Medications are frequently the cause of delirious states in the aged.
- Irreversible dementias follow a pattern of inevitable decline accompanied by decreased intellectual function, personality changes, and impaired judgment. The most common of these is Alzheimer's disease.
- Alzheimer's disease has been the subject of enormous amounts of research in attempts to understand the causes. Genes, latent viruses, enzyme and neurotrans-

NANDA and Wellness Diagnoses

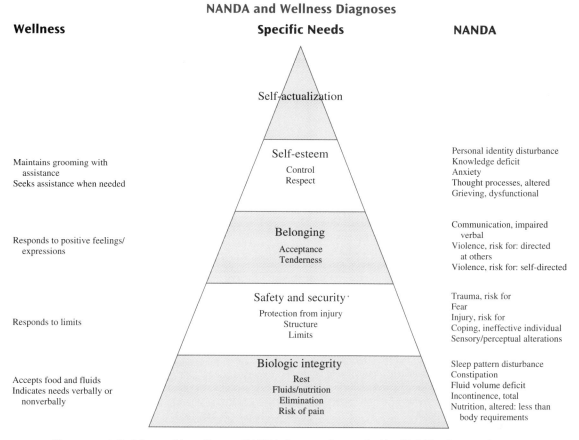

Wellness	Specific Needs	NANDA
	Self-actualization	
Maintains grooming with assistance Seeks assistance when needed	Self-esteem Control Respect	Personal identity disturbance Knowledge deficit Anxiety Thought processes, altered Grieving, dysfunctional
Responds to positive feelings/expressions	Belonging Acceptance Tenderness	Communication, impaired verbal Violence, risk for: directed at others Violence, risk for: self-directed
Responds to limits	Safety and security Protection from injury Structure Limits	Trauma, risk for Fear Injury, risk for Coping, ineffective individual Sensory/perceptual alterations
Accepts food and fluids Indicates needs verbally or nonverbally	Biologic integrity Rest Fluids/nutrition Elimination Risk of pain	Sleep pattern disturbance Constipation Fluid volume deficit Incontinence, total Nutrition, altered: less than body requirements

These are not all of the possible wellness or NANDA diagnoses that may be identified. The above are frequent examples of nursing diagnoses that should be considered when planning care for the older adult in whatever setting.

mitter deficiencies, environmental toxins, and psychosocial stressors have all been implicated to some degree. Research is continuing in attempts to discover ways to protect against or halt the progression of the disease. At this time there is no known cure, although some medications being developed seem to slow the progression of the dementia for a time.

- HIV-related dementia is often overlooked in the aged; there is an ageist assumption implicit in this neglect.
- Vascular brain disorders (brain attacks) are caused by interruption of the blood supply to the brain because of clots, hemorrhages, and vascular spasm or occlusion. Many of these situations can be remedied and serious brain damage prevented if treatment is immediate.
- Developmentally disabled elders are a rather new phenomenon because in the past these individuals

usually died long before they reached old age. Those who have survived have special needs related to the levels of development they may or may not have achieved. These individuals should not be treated as if demented but given opportunities carefully matched to the level of their abilities.

- Assessment of cognitive impairment is complex. Nurses may do a cursory assessment with any number of brief mental status examinations and need to request more thorough assessment when there is an indication of dementia.
- Individuals who are mentally impaired respond best to calmness, few demands, clear communication, and predictable routines. They are hypersensitive to chaotic situations and may develop catastrophic reactions when demands exceed their ability.

► Activities and Discussion Questions

1. Discuss methods for assessing cognitive status and the problems encountered in doing so.
2. Explain reasons why nurses may provide the most accurate assessment of cognitive status.
3. How might you recognize delirium in a cognitively impaired individual?
4. Discuss the most useful way to provide information for a delirious person.
5. What are some of the strategies that are helpful to a person with dementia?
6. Describe how you would design a special care unit for individuals with Alzheimer's disease.
7. What would you suggest to an elder with a developmentally disabled 50-year-old son?
8. What would you say to an individual who has experienced a stroke and is fearful of another one?
9. Describe the appearance of an individual with Parkinson disease.

RESOURCES

Diagnostic and Statistical Manual of Mental Disorders (DSM-IV), 4th edition (1994, American Psychiatric Association). For those interested in studying specific diagnostic criteria.

Alzheimer's Disease and Related Disorders Association, Inc.
919 N. Michigan Avenue, Suite 1000
Chicago, IL 60611-1676
(312) 335-8700; (312) 335-1110 (fax)

American Parkinson Disease Association
60 Bay Street
Staten Island, New York 10301
(800) 223-2732 or (805) 934-2216

National Stroke Association
96 Inverness Drive E., Suite 1
Englewood, CO 80112-5311
(800) STROKES or (303) 649-9299

REFERENCES

Aarsland D et al: Frequency of dementia in Parkinson's disease, *Arch Neurol* 53(6):538, 1996.

Adsit J, Lee R: Art for stroke therapy, *Rehabil Nurs* 11(3):120, 1986.

American Psychiatric Association: *Diagnostic and statistical manual of mental disorders (DSM-IV),* ed 4, Washington, DC, 1994, The Association.

Anderson R: *The aftermath of stroke: the experience of clients and their families,* Cambridge, UK, 1992, Cambridge University Press.

Bartol M: Dialogue with dementia: nonverbal communication in clients with Alzheimer's disease, *J Gerontol Nurs* 5:21, 1979.

Bergener SC et al: Caregiver and environmental variables related to difficult behaviors in institutionalized, demented elderly persons, *J Gerontol* 47(4):P242, 1992.

Berkow R, Butler RN, Sunderland J: Cognitive failure: delirium and dementia. In Abrams WB, Beers MH, Berkow R, editors: *The Merck manual of geriatrics,* ed 2, Whitehouse Station, NJ, 1995, Merck Research Laboratories.

Buffum M, Buffum J: Medication usage in the elderly, *Geriatr Nurs* 17(3), 1997.

Callahan CM, Hendrie HC, Tierney WM: Documentation and evaluation of cognitive impairment in elderly primary care clients, *Ann Intern Med* 122(6):422, 1995.

Caplan LR: Cerebrovascular disease. In Abrams WB, Beers MH, Berkow R, editors: *Merck manual of geriatrics,* ed 2, Whitehouse Station, NJ, 1995, Merck Research Laboratories.

Cohen G: Treatment of Alzheimer's disease in the absence of cure and prevention, *High Notes Newsletter,* spring 1996.

Easton KL: The poststroke journey: from agonizing to owning, *Geriatr Nurs* 20(2):70-75, 1999.

Evans LK: Sundown syndrome in institutionalized elderly, *J Am Geriatr Soc* 35(2):101, 1987.

Foreman MD: Acute confusion in the elderly, *Ann Rev Nurs Res* 11:3, 1993.

Foreman MD et al: Assessing cognitive function, *Geriatr Nurs* 17(5):228, 1996.

Gerdner LA, Buckwalter KC: A nursing challenge: assessment and management of agitation in Alzheimer's clients, *J Gerontol Nurs* 20(4):11, 1994.

Goldstein K: The effect of brain damage on the personality, *Psychiatry* 15:245, 1952.

Havarth TA et al: Dementia-related behaviors in Alzheimer's disease and AIDS, *J Psychosoc Nurs Ment Health Serv* 33(1):35, 1995.

Hazzard W et al, editors: *Principles of geriatric medicine and gerontology,* ed 3, New York, 1994, McGraw-Hill.

Holmberg S: A walking program for wanderers: volunteer training and development of an evening walker's group, *Geriatr Nurs* 18(3):120, 1997.

Kaplan HI, Sadock BJ: *Synopsis of psychiatry,* ed 8, Baltimore, 1996, Williams & Wilkins.

Kaszniak AW: Parkinson's disease. In Maddox GL, editor: *The encyclopedia of aging,* ed 2, New York, 1995, Springer.

Kayser-Jones J: Dysphagia among nursing home residents, *Geriatr Nurs* 20(2):77-82, 1999.

Kelly M: Transient ischemic attack, *Am J Nurs* 95(9):42, 1995.

Kolanowski AM: An overview of the Need-Driven Dementia-Compromised Behavior Model, *J Gerontol Nurs* 25(9):7-9, 1999.

Kovach CR, Meyer-Arnold EA: Preventing agitated behaviors during bath time, *Geriatr Nurs* 18(3):107-111, 1997.

Laupacis A et al: Antithrombotic therapy in atrial fibrillation, *Chest* 102(Oct suppl):4265, 1992.

Levin BE, Katzen HL: *Arch Neurol* 65:85, 1995.

Lipowski Z: A comprehensive view of delirium in the elderly, *Geriatr Consult* 7:26, 1986.

Longstreth WT et al: Utility of the sickness impact profile in Parkinson's disease, *J Geriatr Psychiatry Neurol* 5:142, 1992.

Lundervold D, Poppen R: Biobehavioral rehabilitation for older adults with essential tremor, *Gerontologist* 35(4):556, 1995.

Madeley P et al: Parkinson's disease and driving ability, *J Neurosurg Psychiatry* 53:580, 1990.

Maisto AA, Hughes E: Adaptation to group home living for adults with mental retardation as a function of previous residential placement, *J Intellect Disabil Res* 39(1):15, 1995.

Marcantonio ER et al: A clinical prediction rule for delirium after elective noncardiac surgery, *JAMA* 27:134, 1994.

Marder K: Epidemiology of PD in Northern Manhattan, *Parkinson's Disease Foundation Newsletter,* summer 1992.

McDougall GJ: A review of screening instruments for assessing cognition and mental status in older adults, *Nurse Pract* 15:11, 1990.

McDougall GJ: Predictors of memory improvement strategy use in older adults, *Rehabil Nurs* 21(4):202-209, 1996.

McGrowder-Lin R, Bhatt A: A wanderer's lounge program for nursing home residents with Alzheimer's disease, *Gerontologist* 28(5):607, 1988.

Meco G et al: Hallucinations in Parkinson disease: neuropsychological study, *Ital J Neurol Sci* 11:373, 1990.

Miller RM, Woo D: Stroke: current concepts of care, *Geriatr Nurs* 20(2):66-69, 1999.

Mooney RP, Mooney DR, Cohernour KL: Applied humanism: a model for managing inappropriate behavior among mentally retarded elders, *J Gerontol Nurs* 21(8):45, 1995.

Moore JT et al: A functional dementia scale, *J Fam Pract* 16:499, 1983.

Norris C: Restlessness: a disturbance in rhythmicity, *Geriatr Nurs* 7(6):302, 1986.

Ott A, Breteler MM, van Harskamp F: Prevalence of Alzheimer's disease and vascular dementia: association with education, *BMJ* 310(6985):970, 1995.

Parkinson's Disease Foundation: About Parkinson's disease, *Parkinson's Disease Foundation Newsletter,* summer 1996.

Rader J, Doan J, Schwab M: How to decrease wandering, a form of agenda behavior, *Geriatr Nurs* 6:196, 1985.

Sawyer JC, Mendlovitz AA: *A management program for ambulatory institutionalized clients with Alzheimer's disease and related disorders.* Paper presented at the meeting of the Gerontological Society of America, Boston, Nov 21, 1982.

Scharnhorst S: AIDS dementia complex in the elderly, *Nurse Pract* 17(8):37, 1992.

Topp B: Toward a better understanding of Parkinson's disease, *Geriatr Nurs* 8(4):180, 1987.

US Bureau of the Census: *Statistical abstract of the United States: 1998,* ed 118, Washington, DC, 1998, US Government Printing Office.

Van Ort S, Phillips L: Feeding nursing home residents with Alzheimer's disease, *Geriatr Nurs* 13(6):249-253, 1992.

Wolanin MO, Phillips LR: *Confusion: prevention and care,* St Louis, 1981, Mosby.

BIBLIOGRAPHY

Beffer U, Poirier J: Apolipoprotein E, plaques, tangles and cholinergic dysfunction in Alzheimer's disease, *Ann NY Acad Sci* 777:166, 1996.

Christensen D: *Hardening of the arteries linked to Alzheimer's disease,* Medical Tribune News Service, Jan 16, 1997.

Matteson MA, Linton AD, Barnes SJ: Cognitive developmental approach to dementia, *Image J Nurs Sch* 28(3):233, 1996.

Royston MC, Mann D, Pickering-Brown S: Apo E2 allele, Down's syndrome and dementia, *Ann NY Acad Sci* 777:255, 1996.

Smith MA et al: Radical aging in Alzheimer's disease, *Trends Neurosci* 18(4):172, 1995.

Ying W: Deleterious network hypothesis of Alzheimer's disease, *Med Hypotheses* 46(5):421, 1996.

chapter 22

Maintaining Mobility and Environmental Safety

chapter 22

▶LEARNING OBJECTIVES

Upon completion of this chapter, the reader will be able to:

- Discuss the effects of impaired mobility on general function and quality of life.
- Specify risk factors for impaired mobility.
- Be familiar with factors that increase vulnerability to falls.
- List several measures to prevent falls, and identify those at high risk.
- Describe assessment measures to determine gait and walking stability.
- Name several assistive devices that facilitate mobility for elders.
- Develop a nursing care plan appropriate to an elder at risk of falling.
- Understand the effects of restraints and alternative measures of protection.
- Recognize hazards in the home and environment that threaten the safety of elders.
- Identify numerous factors in the environment that contribute to the safety and security of the aged.
- Relate strategies for protecting the aged person from injury and accidents in the home and in the community.

▶GLOSSARY

Extrapyramidal Pertaining to structures outside the pyramidal tracts of the brain that are associated with body movement.

Hemiplegia Paralysis of one side of the body.

Hypoxia Inadequate oxygen for cellular metabolism.

Ischemia A decreased supply of oxygenated blood to a body part or organ.

Micturition Urination.

Paresthesia A subjective sensation experienced as numbness, tingling, or "pins and needles."

Proprioception Sensations from within the body regarding spatial position and muscular activity.

Syncope A brief lapse in consciousness caused by transient cerebral hypoxia.

Vertebrobasilar Pertaining to the vertebral and basilar artery junction at the base of the skull.

Vestibular In this chapter it is associated with the sense of equilibrium.

▶THE LIVED EXPERIENCE

After that fall last year when I slipped on the urine in the bathroom, I feel so insecure. I find myself taking small, shuffling steps to avoid falling again, but it makes me feel awkward and clumsy. When I was younger, I never worried about falling, but now I'm so afraid I will break a bone or something.

Betty, age 75

It really bugs me sometimes; Betty is so slow and shuffles so, it seems as if she is 100 years old rather than barely past 70.

Marie, Betty's caregiver

MOBILITY, SAFETY, AND SATISFACTION

Mobility is the capacity one has for movement within the personally available environment. In infancy, moving about is the major mode of learning and interacting with the environment. In old age, one moves more slowly and purposefully, sometimes with more forethought and caution. Throughout life, movement remains a significant means of personal contact, sensation, exploration, pleasure, and control. Movement is integral to the attainment of all levels of need as conceived by Maslow. Needs met by maintaining mobility include basic biologic function, activity, security, social contacts, pride, and dignity. Thus maintaining mobility is an exceedingly important issue.

This chapter focuses on maintaining maximal mobility in health and in the presence of various disorders, the assessment of gait and mobility status, the effects of restraints and immobility, risk factors related to falls and preventive actions that nurses may take to reduce the risks, and aids and interventions that are useful when mobility is impaired. Specific information will be provided to promote a safe environment.

Mobility and Agility

Mobility and comparative degrees of agility are based on muscle strength, flexibility, postural stability, vibratory sensation, cognition, and perceptions of stability. Aging produces changes in muscles and joints, particularly of the back and legs. Strength and flexibility of muscles decrease markedly, and endurance decreases to a somewhat lesser extent. Movements and range of motion become more limited. Normal wear and tear reduce the smooth coverings (synovial membrane and cartilage) of joints. Movement is less fluid as one ages and joints change as regeneration of tissue slows and muscle wasting occurs. Some normal gait changes in late life include a narrower standing base, wider swaying when walking, the appearance of a "waddle," bowing of the legs, and less muscular control of the lower extremities. Steps are shorter and with a decreased stepping motion. These changes are less pronounced in those who remain active and at a desirable weight.

Inappropriate clothing may hinder mobility. Fitted, back-closing, and knee-length clothing is not comfortable for persons confined to wheelchairs, those with limited range of motion, or those who require catheters or prosthetic devices. Elders living alone have no one to help them button or zip the back of clothing. This can make dressing and undressing a time-consuming and frustrating experience. Adaptive fashions have been designed to facilitate ease of independent dressing and include features such as back and side openings, Velcro front openings, raglan sleeves, and cape-style clothing. Slacks with front flaps or extra room in the back, or longer skirts are helpful. The fabric should be chosen for comfort, durability, attractiveness, and ease of laundering. Other items to facilitate moving about include wheelchair bags, catheter bags, and carefully chosen footwear (discussed in Chapter 13).

Maintaining mobility may mean the difference between an independent, active community life and maintenance of self-respect versus institutionalization and a sedentary life-style. Mobility may be limited by paresthesias; hemiplegia; neuromotor disturbances; fractures; foot, knee, and hip problems; and illnesses that deplete one's energy. Diabetes, cardiac disease, arthritis, gout, hypertension, and peripheral vascular disease all affect mobility. These conditions are likely to occur more frequently and have more devastating effects as one ages. More than one third of those over 65 years of age and more than half at age 75 have some of these afflictions, with women significantly outnumbering men in this respect (US Bureau of Census, 1998). Therefore an individual's complete medical history must be known if one is to prevent various degrees of immobility.

A gross assessment of ambulatory mobility involves the individual's ability to rise from a chair, maintain balance, initiate and maintain a steady gait, turn, and return to a sitting position in the chair. The ability to climb stairs and walk for 5 minutes indicates that the individual is functionally mobile (Ettinger, 1995).

Gait and Balance Disorders

Gait involves a complex set of simultaneous movements. Gait disorders make one vulnerable to tripping and falling. In addition, they impede activity and increase anxiety in the elder who is aware of instability in gait. Elders with Parkinson disease, discussed in Chapter 21, are acutely aware of problems with gait. Routine examination of the elderly should include descriptions of gait and posture. Normal gait involves the vestibular system (equilibrium), balance, proprioception (sensitivity to the body in motion), neurophysiologic integrity, and vision. Arthritis of the hip, knee, or foot is the most common cause of instability. Arthritis of the knee may result in ligamentous weakness and instability, causing the legs to adduct at the knee, give way, or collapse. Muscle weakness (sarcopenia) may be a result of hyperthyroidism or hypothyroidism, hypokalemia, hyperparathyroidism, osteomalacia, or hypophosphatemia and in some cases is brought on by various drug therapies.

Diabetes, alcoholism, and vitamin B deficiencies may cause neurologic damage and resultant gait problems. Vestibular dysfunction causes unsteadiness in walking and listing to one side or the other when eyes are closed. The individual cannot focus well on a fixed target while moving or on a moving object while standing still. Elderly persons with diabetes and individuals taking certain medications may experience dizziness, unsteadiness, and light-headedness. Postural instability increases and is exacerbated by some medications. Extrapyramidal symptoms produce a shuffling gait in some individuals taking psychotropic medications (see Chapter 15) and in those who have Parkinson disease. Postural reflex impairment occurs with aging, and postural sway, forward and backward, can be observed when an individual stands still. A cane or supportive device may be essential to provide a sense of security.

Assessment

A thorough physical and medication review is needed to identify, describe, and assess causes of gait and balance disorders. The physical examination must include vision, blood pressure, range of motion, muscle strength, balance, posture, podiatric examination, and neurologic and cognitive assessment. Neurologic damage is best determined by a positive Romberg sign and impaired vibratory sense in the legs (Catanasos, Israel, 1991). Gait speed and agility have been found to correlate well with functional level (Potter et al, 1995). Gait disorders may be a prelude to increasing loss of mobility. Some senile balance and gait disorder is thought to be an aspect of advanced age, but marked gait disorders are not normally a consequence of aging and are more likely indicative of an underlying pathologic condition.

The nurse is responsible for initial assessment of gait disturbance and for obtaining appropriate professional evaluation for gait training or a prosthesis. A guide that nurses can use for gait and balance assessment is provided in Box 22-1. A complete analysis of gait patterns and characteristics requires special equipment and expertise, but simple gait observation by nurses can yield valuable descriptive information. Rehabilitative teams are usually responsible for assessment and for teaching patients corrective measures, but nurses must understand concepts and specific methods because they will assist the patient in carrying out correct procedures on a daily basis.

Box 22-1   GAIT DESCRIPTION AND ASSESSMENT

Pain in back and lower limbs	Antalgic gait; short steps flexed toward affected side
Contracture or ankylosis	Short-leg gait; wide outward swing of affected side; unaffected knee flexed and body bent forward
Foot deformities	Loss of spring and rhythm in step; toes inward or outward bilaterally or unilaterally
Footdrop	Foot slap heard as a result of knee raised higher than usual
Gluteus medius weakness	Waddle gait; drop and lag in swing phase of unaffected side; seen in osteomalacia and senile gait in women
Stroke	Wide, open, flinging foot on affected side; uncoordinated
Cerebroarteriosclerosis	Bilateral involvement manifested by extremely short steps
Parkinsonism	Festinating gait; short, hurried, often on tiptoe, or rigid, tremorous, slow; tends toward retropulsion, mincing
Etat lacunaire	Similar to parkinsonian gait; irregular footsteps
Dementia	Slow, shuffling, apraxic, short steps
Peripheral neuropathy	Difficulty lifting feet; stumbles easily
Subdural hematoma	Ataxic; prominent feature is gait disturbance
Cerebellar ataxia	Staggering, unsteady, irregular, wide-based gait; inappropriate foot placement
Vitamin B_{12} deficiency	Paresthesias, unsteadiness, foot dragging
Endocrine disorders	Gait ataxia, particularly with hypothyroidism
Medications	Ataxia, parkinsonian gait, imbalance

Interventions

In most gait disturbances, nervousness or anxiety aggravates the condition. Nurses may assist by gently holding the arm on the unaffected side and supporting the client's efforts. Often, well-fitting shoes, canes, leg braces, pain relief, handrails, or walkers may improve the client's mobility status.

Exercise. Exercise often produces improvements in gait and balance. Lord et al (1996) found that older persons actively engaged in exercise develop strength in lower limbs, faster walking pace, longer strides, and improved ankle dorsiflexion strength. Exercise can also benefit individuals with arthritis, increase bone density in osteopenia, and enhance cognitive function. Specific gait-training exercises as individually prescribed by a physical therapist were found to be effective in reducing falls in individuals who were prone to falls (Galindo-Ciocon et al, 1995).

The interventional problem is not only to "educate" the individual but also to identify ways to motivate the elderly person to routinely exercise in a manner designed to facilitate health. Exercises to improve flexibility and muscle tone while lying, sitting, standing, and walking are included in Chapter 12. We must remember that the very problems exercise may impact are the ones that may cause the individual to avoid participation: lack of strength, fear of falling, and lethargy. Creating security and confidence in movement includes encouraging the elder to employ the following strategies:
- Participating in home exercise programs
- Wearing carefully fitted, low-heeled, and rubber-soled shoes
- Walking with a companion on smooth ground as a form of exercise and muscle strengthening
- Asking bystanders for help in navigating high curbs or other hazards to walking
- Participating in gait training
- Practicing good posture
- Evaluating and modifying home hazards
- Keeping a weekly log of functional gains made through following an exercise program

Care of the feet. Care of the feet is an important aspect of comfort, stable gait, and mobility and one that is often neglected. Some aged persons in the hospital have been unable to walk comfortably, or at all, because of neglect of corns, bunions, and overgrown nails. Other causes of problems may be traced to loss of fat cushioning and foot resilience with aging, ill-fitting shoes, poor arch support, excessively repetitious weight-bearing activities, obesity, and uneven distribution of weight on the foot (Mayo Foundation for Medical Education and Research, 1996). As many as 35% of persons living at home may have significant foot disability that goes untended. The following are common disorders:
- Arthritic foot disorders resulting from rheumatoid arthritis, osteoarthritis, or gout

- Atrophy of the plantar pad that leads to loss of shock absorption and metatarsalgia with increased difficulty in walking
- Onychogryphosis, or overgrown, clawlike toenails that cause walking pain, immobility, and falls
- Corns that cause pain and may reduce mobility
- Hallux valgus (the great toe angles away from the midline and rides over the other toes), which may cause little difficulty unless ulceration or bursitis sets in
- Foot surgery, which may give rise to severe walking difficulty for several months (Cunha, 1988)

Therefore a careful examination of the feet may be the initial action of the nurse concerned with gait disorders. Podiatric examination and care may have been long neglected and can be a first-line intervention to improve gait. Appropriate care of the feet is discussed in Chapter 13.

FALLS: CAUSES AND CONSEQUENCES

Falling is one of the most serious and frequent problems associated with the aging process. Falls are a symptom of a problem, although the consequences of a fall incur many problems. Disease processes, psychologic factors, and environmental hazards all contribute to a greater vulnerability to falls as one ages. Box 22-2 lists fall risk factors for elders in an institution and in the community.

Factors Contributing to Falls

Falls may indicate neurologic, sensory, cognitive, medication, or musculoskeletal problems. It is important for nurses to evaluate each elder's biopsychosocial vulnerability to falling (Table 22-1). Specific precipitants to falls include the following:
- Transient ischemic attacks with vertigo, syncope, or stroke
- Muscle weakness
- Interference with the sense of balance
- Poor eyesight and faulty evaluation of spatial relationships
- Urinary frequency and urgency leading to unsafe maneuvering at toileting
- Unsteady gait because of pain, fatigue, arthritic changes, or osteoporosis
- Improper footwear or podiatric difficulties
- Improper clothing, such as long nightclothes or robes
- Improper use of wheelchairs and walkers, especially on transfer

Box 22-2   FALL RISK FACTORS FOR ELDERS

Conditions

Female or single (incidence increases with age)
Sedative and alcohol use, psychoactive medications
Previous falls, unsteadiness, dizziness
Acute and recent illness
Pathologic conditions, drop attacks
Cognitive impairment, disorientation
Disability of lower extremities
Abnormalities of balance and gait
Foot problems
Depression, anxiety
Decreased vision or hearing
Fear of falling
Terminal drop (dies in following year to 2 years)
Skeletal and neuromuscular changes that predispose to
    weakness and postural imbalance
Acute and severe chronic illness, debilitation
Functional limitations in self-care activities
Women (75 years and older)
Multiple disorders and medications
Wheelchair bound
Sensory deficits
Impaired locomotion
Predisposing physiologic and psychologic conditions
Preoccupation with stressors
Anxiety related to previous falls
Confusion, dementia

Situations

Urinary urgency, particularly nocturia
Environmental hazards
Recent relocation
Assistive devices needed for walking
Inadequate or missing safety rails, particularly in bathroom
Poorly designed or unstable furniture
Low stools
High chairs and beds
Uneven floor surfaces
Glossy, highly waxed floors
Wet, greasy, icy surfaces
Inadequate lighting
General clutter
Pets that inadvertently trip an individual
Electrical cords
Loose or uneven stair treads

Data from Tinetti M, Speechley J, Ginter S: Risk factors for falls among elderly persons living in the community, *N Engl J Med* 319(26):1701, 1988; Craven R, Bruno P: Teach the elderly to prevent falls, *J Gerontol Nurs* 12(8):27, 1986; Kaufmann M: *Falls and the consequences,* Lecture, Francis Payne Bolton School of Nursing, Cleveland, Nov 9, 1988, Case Western Reserve University; Barbieri EB: Patient falls are not patient accidents, *J Gerontol Nurs* 9(3):171, 1983; and Fife D, Solomon P, Stanton M: A risk/falls program: code orange for success, *Nurs Manage* 15(11):50, 1984.

• Mental confusion and faulty judgment
• Incontinence and dribbling of urine

Acute Illness

Acute illness is associated with an increased risk of falling. Confusion, multiple medical problems, generalized weakness, postural instability, and an unfamiliar environment are major contributors to falling when a person is hospitalized. Diminished proprioception in the legs resulting from bed rest and disuse may also be a factor. There is an increased vulnerability if the individual has a history of falls, is receiving intravenous therapy, has impaired mental status, or needs assistive devices to walk.

Visual Problems

Sudden unexpected visual problems become major fall risks; changes in vision may be transient, a symptom of other problems such as hypotension, cardiac dysrhythmia, temporal arteritis, or vertebrobasilar artery insufficiency. In addition, new eyeglasses or recent cataract surgery may be impediments. The more gradual and progressive visual changes become serious fall risks when they interfere with depth vision.

Balance Problems

Vertigo and dizziness are a result of dysfunction in balance control systems and vestibular apparatus. Disequilibrium may arise from many diseases, including Parkinson disease, Alzheimer's disease, peripheral neuropathy caused by pernicious anemia, alcoholism, or diabetes. These patients experience unsteadiness and a tendency to fall and often need an assistive device for walking (Tideiksaar, 1990). Contributing factors are summarized in Box 22-3.

Table 22-1

Fall Factors

Psychogenic	Physiologic	Environmental

Dementia
  Alterations in gait and
    vitamin B_{12} level;
    poor evaluation
    of ability and
    environment
Depression
  Disinterest in
    surroundings, no
    concern for safety,
    subliminal suicide
Fear/anxiety
  Distraction, scattered
    perceptions
	Neurologic
	  Dementias
	  Somnolence
	  Normal-pressure hydrocephalus
	  Neurosensory and visual deficits: loss of
	    proprioception; peripheral neuropathy;
	    vestibular dysfunction; dizziness; vertigo;
	    syncope; seizures, brain tumors, or le-
	    sions; Parkinson disease; cervical
	    spondylosis
	Cardiovascular disorders
	  Cerebrovascular insufficiency, strokes and
	    TIAs, carotid sinus syncope, vertebral
	    artery insufficiency
	  Dyshythmias: Stokes-Adams
	  Valvulopathies
	  Congestive heart failure
	  Hypotension: postural hypotension, postpran-
	    dial drop in blood pressure, medication in-
	    duced, male micturition when urethral ob-
	    struction present, hypovolemia
	    (dehydration, hemorrhage), impaired ve-
	    nous return (venous pooling, Valsalva), im-
	    paired vasoconstriction (autonomic disor-
	    ders, vasovagal)
	Metabolic disorders: anemia, hypoxia, hypo-
	  glycemia, hyperventilation
	Debilitating disease: cancer, pulmonary dis-
	  ease, immunosuppressant disorder
		Slippery floor: urine or fluid on
		  floor, loose throw rugs
		Uneven and obstructed walking
		  surfaces; electrical cords, fur-
		  niture, pets, children, uneven
		  door steps or stair risers,
		  loose boards, cracked side-
		  walks
		Inadequate visual supports:
		  glare; low-wattage bulbs; lack
		  of night-lights for bathroom,
		  stairs, and halls; poor mark-
		  ing of steps and other hazards
		Inadequate construction: ab-
		  sence of railing, lack of grab
		  bars on shower or tub, poorly
		  designed stairs and walkways

TIAs, Transient ischemia attacks.

Interruption of Cerebral Oxygenation

Sufficient oxygen circulating to the brain may be interrupted by brief cerebral arterial spasms (transient ischemic attacks) or by syncope associated with such causes as hypotension, medications, emotional trauma, or cardiac or vagal nerve disorders. These are brief, unpredictable events that often result in falls and injury. Certain preventive actions may be helpful in those who are subject to these occurrences.

Transient ischemic attacks. Transient ischemic attacks (TIAs) affect the perfusion of the brain and cause intermittent dizziness. It is estimated that up to 25% of falls are due to drop attacks (a feeling of the legs giving way) associated with TIAs. The individual may not lose consciousness. Patients subject to these attacks should wear cervical collars to prevent backward flexion of the head.

Syncope. Syncope, or a brief loss of consciousness secondary to cerebral ischemia, has many causes. Baroreflex responses mediate both hypertension and hypotension, and in old age the efficiency of this function progressively declines; thus the aged are more vulnerable to episodes of cerebral ischemia with rapid changes of posture. Orthostatic syncope occurs with rapid rising to a standing position when depletion of body fluids or medications interfere with a rapid venous return. Occasionally, postprandial reductions in blood pressure may be sufficient to produce syncope. Hypoglycemia is usually syncopal in a diabetic person 3 to 5 hours after a meal.

Box 22-3 ASSESSMENT OF FALL RISK

Obtain history of previous falls and precipitants.

Evaluate for orthostatic hypotension (increases with age).

Evaluate visual acuity: peripheral, depth, and color vision.

Determine presence of dysrhythmias.

Massage carotid bulb for carotid sinus sensitivity.

Rotate neck to assess vertebrobasilar artery involvement.

Observe movements and evaluate muscle strength and balance:

Test of functional reach

Rising from chair

Performing deep knee bend

Walking 10 feet in a straight line, turning full circle

Climbing and descending stairs

Romberg test for increased sway

Standing on tiptoes and reaching upward

Bending down to pick up object from floor

Raising feet while walking; tandem walking

Check feet for abnormalities that affect gait.

Evaluate mental status and medication regimen; particularly note psychoactive drugs.

Observe ease of routine daily mobility maneuvers.

All of these evaluations must be carried out with sufficient support and encouragement to avoid activities threatening to the individual's sense of security or that are potentially dangerous.

Data from Tideiksaar R: Falls in the elderly: etiology and prevention. In Bosker G et al, editors: *Geriatric emergency medicine,* St Louis, 1990, Mosby; and Tinetti M, Speechley M, Ginter S: Risk factors for falls among elderly persons living in the community, *N Engl J Med* 319(26):1701, 1988.

Vasodepressor (vasovagal) syncope typically occurs during emotional upset, injury, excessive fatigue, or prolonged standing in a warm environment.

Carotid sinus syncope occurs frequently in older people who have sinus node disease. This hypersensitivity to pressure or mechanical obstruction makes the individual vulnerable to syncope when pressure is applied to the carotid in shaving, turning the head sharply to one side, or wearing tight collars. Drugs such as propranolol and digitalis may produce carotid hypersensitivity (Tideiksaar, 1990).

Micturition syncope is unusual and rarely mentioned. It occurs immediately following voiding in some elderly men with bladder outlet obstruction (often prostatic hypertrophy). The loss of consciousness is due to vagal bradycardia. These individuals should sit during urination.

Cardiac dysrhythmias are a common cause of syncope, particularly supraventricular tachycardias. Heart monitoring for 24 to 48 hours is often necessary to reveal these bradyarrhythmias or tachyarrhythmias.

Fatigue Factors

Poor posture contributes to the incidence of falls. Fatigue, osteoarthritis, muscle weakness, and lifelong habits may contribute to poor posture. Postural training can have benefits for some individuals. Physiotherapists should be engaged to teach nurses and clients correct postural habits.

Fear of Falling

Fear of falling can result in avoidance phobias that gradually restrict an individual's life space (area in which an individual carries on activities). Anxiety, depression, and slowed walking pace may result from the fear of falling. Older persons may be at risk of falling when reaching into cabinets or closets, taking a bath or shower, walking about in unfamiliar places, and getting in and out of bed. Individuals tend to stiffen their posture when they are afraid of falling, and this actually increases falls.

Drop Attacks

Falls that occur in an older person "just because my leg went out from under me," are called *drop attacks.* These falls cause hip trochanter cracks or femur fractures or both and are often due to extensive osteoporotic bone erosion. When osteoporosis of this magnitude occurs, the bone can no longer bear the weight of the individual in walking. It is sometimes difficult to determine whether the fall creates the fracture or the fracture creates the fall. Numerous conditions may precipitate a drop attack. A fractured hip will result in some degree of immobility and the physical ailments that tend to follow immobility, especially in the very old and in frail elders.

Fractures

Osteoporosis of the hip increases with each decade of women's lives, particularly after menopause. Decreased bone mass density puts one at high risk for future hip fractures. This is an important cause of hip fractures in older women (Wolinsky, Fitzgerald, 1994). Prevention of hip fractures can be accomplished in many cases by wearing padded undergarments that protect the hips. Several types of these are under investigation and have proved effective in reducing hip fractures in those prone to falls (University of California, San Francisco, 1995; Chipman, 1996).

Age and preoperative health status affect postfracture ambulation. A younger person has the most possibility of returning to prior function. Those over 70 years of age with previous disabilities are most likely to experience increased disability following a fracture. The expectation of complete recovery includes the ability to maintain (1) balance, (2) motor coordination, (3) stamina, and (4) walking and activities of daily living (ADLs) within 2 weeks after surgery.

Maximal recovery for the client entails intensive and consistent physical therapy, including muscle building, range-of-motion exercises, and regaining strength. The client needs to participate in decisions regarding care, maintain social contacts and feelings of self-worth, and tolerate some dependency during the recovery period. The prefracture level of activity provides a baseline for the formation of appropriate goals. When progress is slow, small signs of progress must be discussed with the individual and frequent encouragement given. Emphasis on the activities the individual desires and is capable of achieving is essential.

Fall Assessment

A thorough physical examination, including attention to the conditions and situations noted above, and nursing observations of function are essential to establishing an accurate diagnosis. The nurse is most likely to have had extended opportunities to observe the elder's function whether in the community or in an institution. Families' observations also provide important data. Chipman (1990) recommends that any patient with an unexplained fall should have postural pulses and blood pressures taken, a rectal examination for stool guaiac testing, and evaluation of hematocrit level.

Interventions and Prevention of Falls

Prevention of falls requires education of the individual in all aspects of environmental hazards and the awareness that falling may be an indication of other underlying problems. Box 22-4 lists actions that help prevent falls. In addition, each facility needs a well-developed fall prevention protocol tailored to their patients, staff, and environment.

Environmental factors (extrinsic) may need modification for safety. Any interventions that enhance sen-sory function and spatial awareness will reduce fall risk. All older persons should be cautioned against sudden rising from a sitting or supine position, particularly after eating. As a general principle, any action that increases the individual's confidence and ability to relax is likely to decrease the tendency toward falls.

Actions to increase patient safety include the following:

- Individualize care planning in terms of the patient's level of orientation.
- Reduce anxiety and uncertainty in new residents. Fear and agitation create clumsiness.
- Review medications, especially psychotropic medications and antihypertensives.
- Modify the environment to meet clients' special needs.
- Teach the safe use of wheelchairs and walkers.
- Observe for signs of weakness or fatigue and assist as necessary.
- Initiate a program of accident prevention.

Box 22-4	ACTIONS TO PREVENT FALLS

Have regular testing for vision and hearing; use aids if needed; keep glasses clean and ears free of cerumen and infection.

Seek evaluation and modification of medications (e.g., diuretics, nitrates, hypnotics, antidepressants, antianxiety agents, antihypertensives, and hypoglycemics) that affect balance, coordination, and cardiovascular sufficiency.

Limit alcohol intake.

Rise slowly from bed or chair to avoid sudden drop in blood pressure; avoid sudden changes in position.

When outdoors watch for wet or slippery surfaces; use extra care getting into and out of vehicles, negotiating curbs and crowds.

Ask for assistance when needed.

Reduce hazards in home.

Stay physically and socially active; increase activities gradually.

Wear appropriate footwear; avoid high heels and slippery soles.

Use assistive devices for ambulation.

Consult with physician if feeling unsteady or ill.

Data from Tideiksaar R: Falls in the elderly: etiology and prevention. In Bosker G et al, editors: *Geriatric emergency medicine,* St Louis, 1990, Mosby; and Tinetti M, Richman D, Powell L: Falls efficacy as a measure of fear of falling, *J Gerontol* 45(6):239, 1990.

- Encourage the elder to use a cane or walker to help maintain balance.
- Purchase beds that are as low to the floor as possible; possibly invent beds that are safe.
- Increase muscle strength through carefully designed exercise programs.
- Teach walking exercises in which the client learns to lift the feet rather than shuffling.
- Provide appropriate shoes and slippers that have non-skid soles and broad heels of a height comfortable to the individual.

A fall prevention program must include a thorough assessment of persons who have fallen, including a detailed history and physical examination and assessment of the risk of falling.

MOBILITY AIDS

Four-and-one-half million persons over 65 years of age use some mobility device, the most common being canes and walkers (US Bureau of the Census, 1998). Numerous mobility aids are available of various designs that can be fitted to the needs and preference of any individual. Medical supply houses often have consultants available to advise regarding the best device based on individual need.

Assistive Devices

In Victorian times a walking stick was essential to a gentleman's attire. Even now, many older persons carry elaborate walking sticks even though canes and walkers are primarily designed to augment security and independence.

Arthritic hips and knees may cause considerable pain. To relieve the pressure, the use of a cane on the uninvolved side is helpful. When both sides are involved, a walker may relieve the pressure equilaterally. Many devices are available that are designed for very specific benefits (Fig. 22-1).

When helping someone select a walking assistance device, begin with correct shoes. If you think your client could benefit by using an assistive device, consult specialists and/or rehabilitation therapists. Assist your client in obtaining a written prescription from the appropriate therapist, because Medicare may cover up to 80% of the cost of the device if this is done; other insurance coverage is variable.

When the correct device is obtained, the client will need assistance in learning to use it. This, again, should be taught by specialists in physical therapy. In general, the following principles should be observed:
- Move the assistive device first, then the weaker leg, and finally the stronger leg.
- Always wear low-heeled, nonskid shoes.

A **B** **C** **D**

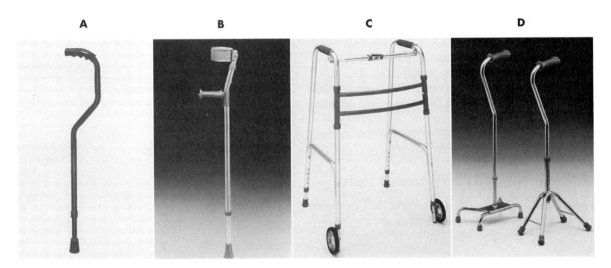

Fig. 22-1 Assistive devices. **A,** Standard ortho cane with swan neck. **B,** Forearm crutch stabilizes the elbow as the person walks. **C,** Walker with front wheels allows constant contact with the ground. **D,** Quad cane offers more support than a single-stem walker. (Courtesy Lumex, Inc., New York.)

- When using a cane on stairs, step up with the stronger leg and down with the weaker leg. Use the cane as support when lifting the weaker leg. Bring the cane up to the step just reached before climbing another step. When descending, place the cane on the next step down and move the disabled leg down, followed by the good leg.
- When using a walker, stand upright and lift the walker with both hands.
- Place all of the walker's legs down at a comfortable distance. Step toward it with the weaker leg, and then bring the stronger leg forward. Do not climb stairs with a walker.
- Every assistive device must be adjusted to individual height; the top of the cane should align with the crease of the wrist.
- Choose a size and shape of cane handle that fits comfortably in the palm; like a tight shoe, it will be a constant irritant if it is not properly fitted.
- Cane tips are most secure when they are flat at the bottom and have a series of rings. Replace tips frequently, because a worn tip is not reliable.

Wheelchairs

Wheelchairs are a necessary adjunct at some level of immobility. Medicare coverage is available for wheelchairs when needed. Ideally, a physical therapist or medical supply specialist will assist in the selection of a wheelchair that is appropriate to the size of the individual and is comfortable. There are various types of motorized chairs that can be handled with ease. These are more expensive than hand-propelled chairs but are sometimes available secondhand through advertisements, senior center bulletin boards, or congregate care settings.

ENVIRONMENTAL SAFETY

A safe environment is one in which one is capable, with reasonable caution, of carrying out the activities of daily living (ADLs) and the instrumental activities of daily living (IADLs), as well as the activities that enrich one's life, without fear of attack, accident, or imposed interference. It is the job of nurses and other health team members to ensure, to the greatest extent possible, a safe environment for individuals within their care in the institution or in the home.

Accidents and Injury

Accidental death rates for those over 65 years of age is 87 per 100,000, with the rate for men being 105 per 100,000 and the rate for women being 74 per 100,000. Individuals over age 75 are particularly subject to falls, suffocation, and motor vehicle accidents. Falls create the most accidental fatalities, and the majority of these occur in the home. The second highest cause of accidental deaths of individuals over 80 years of age is motor vehicle accidents. The incidence of these deaths has gradually increased since 1980, whereas in all other age categories the incidence of vehicular accident deaths has decreased significantly (US Bureau of the Census, 1998).

Environmental Hazards

The aged are more susceptible than younger people to the impact of environmental variations, including pollutants, pesticides, impure water supplies, toxic substances, and climatic and altitudinal environmental extremes. Rice (1999) provides an extensive list of potential toxins in the home. Many of these may also be found in institutions. These are included in Appendix 22-A, and methods for reducing environmental toxins are explained in Appendix 22-B.

High Altitude

When elders briefly visit areas of high altitude, they may become hypotensive or develop cardiac symptoms. Older persons may experience dizziness, shortness of breath, and headache at high altitudes. They should be advised to rise to a standing position slowly and to reduce their activity level to a point of comfort. They may need additional rest periods. High altitudes and air travel may precipitate aural discomfort or disequilibrium as a result of changes in atmospheric pressure. It is helpful to let people know that any major environmental change is likely to be physically stressful, but specific discomforts should not be ignored. When an older person experiences a specific, intermittent uncomfortable reaction or one sustained over several hours, he or she should seek medical attention. Too often, a real problem is dismissed as just a symptom of old age.

Hyperthermia

Hyperthermia is a temperature-related illness and is classified as a medical emergency. There are numerous deaths among elders annually from temperature extremes, and these could be almost entirely prevented with education and caution. Although most of these problems occur in the home among individuals who do not have air conditioning or sufficient heat during temperature extremes, older adults with multiple physical problems residing in institutions may be especially vulnerable to temperature changes. Elders with cardiovascular disease, diabetes, or peripheral vascular disease, and those taking certain medications (anticholinergics, antihistamines, diuretics, beta-blockers, antidepressants, and antiparkinsonian drugs) are at risk. Interventions to prevent hyperthermia when ambient Fahrenheit temperature exceeds 90 degrees include the following:

• Drink 2 to 3 L of cool fluid daily.
• Minimize exertion, especially during the heat of the day.
• Stay in air-conditioned places or use fans when possible.
• Wear hats and loose clothing of natural fibers when outside; remove most clothing when indoors.
• Take tepid tub baths or showers.
• Apply cold wet towel compresses or immerse the hands and feet in cool water.
• Avoid heavy, hot foods.
• Evaluate medications for risk of hyperthermia.
• Avoid alcohol.

Hyperthermia in institutionalized individuals is seldom a problem, but certain pyschotropic medications may induce a hyperthermic crisis (see discussion of neuroleptic malignant syndrome in Chapter 15).

Hypothermia

Hypothermia and the prevalence of deaths from exposure and cold have paralleled the increase in energy costs, indicating that many older persons may not be able to afford sufficient heat in their homes. Unfortunately, a dulling of awareness accompanies hypothermia, and persons experiencing it rarely recognize the problem or seek assistance. For the very old and frail, environmental temperatures below 65° F (18° C) may cause a serious drop in core body temperature to 95° F (35° C) or less. The median oral temperature of elderly persons is 96.8° F (36° C). Factors that increase the risk of hypothermia are numerous, as shown in Box 22-5.

Nurses are responsible for keeping frail elders warm for comfort and prevention of problems. Recognition of the clinical signs and the severity of hypothermia is the first nursing responsibility, because it frequently goes unrecognized (Table 22-2). Specific interventions to prevent hypothermic reactions are shown in Box 22-6.

Because much of nursing care has moved into the home, it is imperative to assess the available warmth

---

Box 22-5   FACTORS THAT INCREASE THE RISK OF HYPOTHERMIA IN THE ELDERLY

Thermoregulatory Impairment

Failure to vasoconstrict promptly or strongly on exposure to cold
Failure to sense cold
Failure to respond behaviorally to protect oneself against cold
Diminished or absent shivering to generate heat
Failure of metabolic rate to rise in response to cold

Conditions That Decrease Heat Production

Hypothyroidism, hypopituitarism, hypoglycemia, anemia, malnutrition, starvation
Immobility/decreased activity (e.g., stroke, paralysis, parkinsonism, dementia, arthritis, fractured hip, coma)
Diabetic ketoacidosis

Conditions That Increase Heat Loss

Open wounds, generalized inflammatory skin conditions, burns

Conditions That Impair Central or Peripheral Control of Thermoregulation

Stroke, brain tumor, Wernicke's encephalopathy, subarachnoid hemorrhage
Uremia, neuropathy (e.g., diabetes, alcoholism)
Acute illnesses (e.g., pneumonia, sepsis, MI, CHF, pulmonary embolism, pancreatitis)

Drugs That Interfere With Thermoregulation

Tranquilizers (e.g., phenothiazines)
Sedative/hypnotics (e.g., barbiturates, benzodiazepines)
Antidepressants (e.g., tricyclics)
Vasoactive drugs (e.g., vasodilators)
Alcohol (causes superficial vasodilation; may interfere with carbohydrate metabolism and judgment)
Other: methyldopa, lithium, morphine

From Worfolk JB: Keep frail elders warm, *Geriatr Nurs* 18(1):7, 1997.
MI, Myocardial infarction; *CHF,* congestive heart failure.

Table 22-2

Clinical Presentation of Hypothermia: Stages and Assessment Findings

Mild (89.6°-95° F)	Moderate (82.4°-89.6° F)	Severe (82.4° F and below)
Cold skin; pallor	Very cold skin; increasing pallor	Extremely cold skin; extreme pallor, blue blotches, cyanosis
May not complain of cold	Puffy face; generalized edema	Deathlike appearance
Slurred speech	Speech difficult	Comatose; unresponsive to stimuli
Intense shivering (elderly may not shiver)	Shivering stops; muscle rigidity develops	Muscle rigidity; may become flaccid below 80° F
Incoordination; slow gait; may stumble and fall	Slowed reflexes; poorly reactive pupils	Areflexia; pupils fixed and dilated
Confusion, disorientation	Stupor; semicomatose	
Apathy or irritability, may be combative (elderly may sit immobile in a chair)		
Increased BP, HR	Bradycardia, hypopnea	Apnea
	Atrial and ventricular arrhythmias (atrial common in the elderly)	No detectable pulse; ventricular fibrillation
	Polyuria or oliguria	
	Dehydration; signs of shock	

From Worfolk JB: Keep frail elders warm, *Geriatr Nurs* 18(1):7, 1997.
BP, Blood pressure; *HR,* heart rate.

Box 22-6   **NURSING INTERVENTIONS TO PREVENT COLD DISCOMFORT AND THE DEVELOPMENT OF ACCIDENTAL HYPOTHERMIA IN FRAIL ELDERS**

Desired outcomes: Hands and limbs warm; body relaxed, not curled; body temperature >97° F; no shivering; no complaints of cold.

Interventions

Maintain a comfortably warm ambient temperature no lower than 65° F. Many frail elders will require much higher temperatures.

Provide generous quantities of clothing and bedcovers. Layer clothing and bedcovers for best insulation. Be careful *not* to judge your patient's needs by how *you* feel working in a warm environment.

Limit time patients sit by cold windows to short periods in which they are warmly dressed.

Provide a headcovering whenever possible—in bed, out of bed, and particularly out-of-doors.

Cover patients well during bathing. The standard—a light bath blanket over a naked body—is not enough protection for frail elders.

Cover naked patients with heavy blankets for transfer to and from showers; dry quickly and thoroughly before leaving shower room; cover head with a dry towel or hood while wet.

Dry wet hair quickly with warm air from an electric dryer. *Never* allow the hair of frail elders to air dry.

Use absorbent pads for incontinent patients rather than allow urine to wet large areas of clothing, sheets, and bedcovers. Avoid skin problems by changing pads frequently, washing the skin well, and applying a protective cream.

Provide as much exercise as possible to generate heat from muscle activity.

Provide hot, high protein meals and bedtime snacks to add heat and sustain heat production throughout the day and as far into the night as possible.

From Worfolk JB: Keep frail elders warm, *Geriatr Nurs* 18(1):7, 1997.

in the environment, demonstrate how to prevent heat loss and maintain core body temperature, and give clients information about the energy assistance that is available in most communities for those on limited incomes.

Generally, older persons in hospitals and long-term care settings are in comfortable ambient temperatures. The major considerations are to prevent wandering out of doors (see Chapter 21) in extreme temperatures and to be aware that certain illnesses and medications, as noted in Box 22-5, tend to alter the body's hypothalamic thermoregulatory processes.

Injury Prevention in the Environment

In general, the most dangerous rooms for elders are the bedroom and the bathroom. Injuries, other than falls, include burns, suffocation, poisoning, scalding, electrical shock, and drowning. The kitchen is the source of many nonfatal injuries such as cuts, burns, and falls. Many of the problems can be avoided with good home maintenance. Environmental assessment and appropriate modification may prevent many problems. A home assessment checklist is provided in Chapter 14 (see Box 14-12).

Restraints

Restraints have been used historically for the "protection" of the client and for the security of the client and

Table 22-3

Common Reasons That Patients Are Restrained

Reason	Chronic	Acute
Facilitate treatment	3%	50%
Prevent falls	80%	75%
Altered mental status	50%	88%
Other's safety	33%	25%
Prevent patient from harming self	57%	70%
Wandering	13%	38%
Noncompliance	7%	13%
Agitation	40%	63%
Other	7%	5%

From Bryant H, Fernald L: Nursing knowledge and use of restraint alternatives: acute and chronic care, *Geriatr Nurs* 18(2):57, 1997.

staff. Some common reasons for restraining patients are enumerated in Table 22-3 (Bryant, Fernald, 1997).

Physical Restraints

Physical restraints are devices, material, and equipment that prevent free bodily movement to a position of choice (standing, walking, lying, turning, sitting) and cannot be controlled or easily removed by the patient. The most frequently used restraints are seat belts, "geri-chairs," and jacket vests (Bryant, Fernald, 1997). Temporary immobilization of a part of the body for the purpose of treatment, such as casts, splints, and arm boards, is not included in this definition. Factors that increase the likelihood of restraint application are cognitive impairment, severe limitation in ADLs, depression, wandering (Burton et al, 1992), and dementia. Paradoxically, although they are often used for protection, mechanical restraints have caused serious injuries and deaths.

The prevalent use of physical restraints for the "protection" of the institutionalized elder was first brought to the forefront of nursing attention by Doris Schwartz. Through the research efforts of Evans and Strumpf, the use of restraints has been drastically reduced (Evans, Strumpf, 1989; Strumpf, Evans, 1988; Strumf et al, 1992).

Within the last decade and in compliance with the Omnibus Budget Reconciliation Act (OBRA) of 1987 requirements, there has been a concerted effort to reduce the use of restraints in long-term care settings. OBRA requires, within residents' rights, that restraints, physical or chemical, be used only to ensure the resident's safety or the safety of other residents and only on the written order of a physician that specifies the duration and circumstances under which restraints are to be used. They may not be imposed for purposes of discipline or convenience (OBRA, 1991, Section 1819). Mion and colleagues (1994) have developed a nursing standard-of-practice protocol for the use of mechanical restraints (Box 22-7).

Whereas physical restraints were the first consideration in preventing falls, they have now been largely replaced by methods of reducing the agitation that precipitates falls and interference with treatments (Bryant, Fernald, 1996). Fear of litigation was often the impetus for restraints. Now, family members and the client are engaged in discussions regarding legalities and problem solving to avoid the use of restraints. In acute care settings more than 90% of nurses are not aware of OBRA requirements and tend to use restraints to prevent the patient from detaching invasive devices (Bryant, Fernald, 1997).

Electronic devices are available to alert nurses when an individual is attempting to get out of bed; these are being used much more frequently as human rights are more rigidly enforced. However, nursing skills are often needed far more than restraints or electronic devices. Communication and creative planning can reduce anxiety and agitation in the client (Werner et al, 1994). Questions the nurse needs to address include the following: What is frightening the patient? Is there anything in the environment that is familiar to provide security for the client? Is the client cognitively impaired? Is the client isolated, or can contact with the environment be more constant? Information given in measured quantities and frequent brief interactions may reduce the anxiety and agitation to manageable levels. Some alternatives to restraint use are enumerated in Table 22-4. The methods are limited only by the creativity of the nurse. When the safety and agitation of the client cannot be managed by any known methods, it is the nurse's obligation to insist that the family or facility engage a sitter or companion for the individual.

Historically, side rails have been used to prevent falling from the bed, but this practice is being replaced by careful evaluation of the need and benefits of side rails. Capezuti et al (1998) have developed interventions to resolve some of the problems that have typically resulted in restraint or side rail use (Box 22-8).

Reducing environmental hazards, keeping an individual moving about to increase endurance and function, and identifying persons most at risk of falling are methods that may be used to avoid accidents and falls and maintain mobility. Thoughtful and clear communication, creative planning, and nursing skills can reduce the need for restraints.

Transportation

Even though one is physically able to move about, there may be many hindrances to full use of public space. Available transportation is a critical link in the ability of the elderly to remain independent and functional. The lack of accessible transportation may contribute to other problems, such as social withdrawal, poor nutri-

---

Box 22-7	**NURSING STANDARD-OF-PRACTICE PROTOCOL: USE OF MECHANICAL RESTRAINTS WITH ELDERLY PATIENTS**

I. Background
  A. Physical restraint is the use of any manual method of physical/mechanical device that the patient cannot remove, that restricts the patient's physical activity or normal access to his/her body, and that:
    • Is not a usual and customary part of a medical, diagnostic, or treatment procedure indicated by the patient's medical condition or symptoms
    • Does not serve to promote the patient's independent functioning
  B. The standard of care for hospitalized elderly patients is nonuse of mechanical restraints, except under exceptional circumstances, after all reasonable alternatives have been tried.
  C. Risk factors for use of mechanical restraints in the acute care setting include:
    • Fall risk
    • Tubes or IVs that need stability
    • Severe cognitive or physical impairments
    • Diagnosis or presence of a psychiatric condition
    • Surgery

  D. Morbidity and mortality risks associated with mechanical restraint use include:
    • Nerve injury
    • New-onset pressure ulcers
    • Pneumonia
    • Incontinence
    • Increased confusion
    • Inappropriate drug use
    • Strangulation/asphyxiation
  E. Appropriate alternatives exist to the use of mechanical restraints.
II. Assessment parameters
  A. Request information about the use of mechanical restraints from pre-hospital settings.
  B. On admission, identify as "at risk for restraint use" any elderly patient who is agitated, at risk of falling, or disrupting therapy.
  C. Use 1:1 observation or behavior monitor logs to identify and document specific risks. For example, for fall risk, assess impaired cognition, poor balance, impaired gait, orthostatic hypotension, impaired vision and hearing, and the use of sedative and hypnotic agents.

From Mion LC, Strumpf N, NICHE faculty: Use of restraints in the hospital setting: implications for nursing, *Geriatr Nurs* 15(3):127-132, 1994.

Table 22-4

Alternatives to Restraint Use

Type of method used	Chronic	Acute
Pain relief	34%	54%
Other comfort measures, i.e., repositioning	69%	71%
Reality orientation	62%	86%
Pet therapy	3%	0%
Music therapy	36%	14%
Therapeutic touch	31%	11%
Reminiscence	24%	3%
Behavior modification	66%	26%
Companionship	55%	60%
Crafts	21%	6%
Active listening	34%	26%
Clear pathways	31%	11%
Increased lighting	21%	43%
Placement of patient near nursing station	86%	80%
Beds lower to floor	21%	43%
Accessible call light	66%	29%
Regular routine	52%	31%
Defusing agitated behavior	66%	29%
Diversional activities	62%	46%
1:1 supervision	69%	69%
Other	14%	0%

From Bryant H, Fernald L: Nursing knowledge and use of restraint alternatives: acute and chronic care, *Geriatr Nurs* 18(2):57, 1997.

tion, or neglect of health care. Even when a municipal transportation service is available, elders may not use it. Urban buses and subways are not only physically hazardous, they are often dangerous. A "crisis in mobility" exists for many aged people because of the lack of an automobile, an inability to drive, limited access to public transportation, health factors, geographic location, or economic considerations.

Older persons may desire increased contact with friends and relatives; however, even more crucial is the need to reach medical services, shopping areas, and service agencies. The emphasis on a "barrier-free" (structurally revised) transportation system and reduced fares has been helpful to many aged, but some cannot avail themselves of public transportation because of physical disability or residence in a high-crime area. County, state, or federally subsidized transportation is being provided in certain areas to assist aged people in reaching social services, nutrition sites, health services, emergency care, medical care, recreational centers, mental health services, day care programs, physical and vocational rehabilitation, continuing education, and library services.

Some effective local transportation programs include the following services:
- Reduced fares
- Informal, volunteer drivers
- Demand-response transit vehicles
- Specially constructed vehicles for the handicapped
- Door-to-door minibuses requiring advance reservations
- Use of subsidized taxicab services
- Radio-equipped response vehicles
- Demand-response vehicles with a large pool of volunteer drivers (many of them aged)
- Dial-a-ride
- Charter bus trips to special events

The greatest problems in transportation exist among the rural aged, who may be unable to drive and have limited, if any, public transportation.

PROVIDING A SAFE ENVIRONMENT

A common assumption is that the environment is generally hazardous to older persons. We must keep in mind that most older people are very capable, have considerable experience negotiating their environment, and have survived many dangerous situations. They are usually more aware of potential dangers and exert more caution than younger people.

Nurses most often work with elders who are in an unfamiliar environment that increases the potential for accidents. It is incumbent on us to reduce hazards. It is wise to involve family or significant others in making an environmental assessment of the home before an individual's discharge from institutional care. When that is not possible, the first home health follow-up visit should include a survey of the environment and its hazards. Poor lighting, slippery tubs and showers, and loose rugs and cords are the most common offenders.

• • •

In summary, the capacity to move about on two legs, horses, and wheeled vehicles has been portrayed from the earliest recorded time. The nurse can be significant in facilitating this most fundamental human need and assist our clients in moving as far as their reach extends and as far as our imagination will allow.

Box 22-8   RESIDENTIAL PROBLEMS AND INTERVENTIONS

Problems With Mobility

Inability to move in bed without assistance

- Install trapeze.
- Place uni/bilateral transfer enabler, such as bed handle, bed grab bar, transfer pole, quarter or half side rail.
- Refer to occupational therapist for upper extremity strengthening exercises.
- Install easily accessible call bell or bulb (pressure sensitive).

Inability to transfer safely without assistance

- Refer to physical/occupational therapist for transferring training.
- Refer to physical/occupational therapist for evaluation and instruction in balance and in strengthening for exercises of hip extensor-abductor and ankle plantar-flexor muscles.
- Encourage recreational activities to complement rehabilitation therapies (e.g., dancing and Tai Chi).
- Place uni/bilateral transfer enabler, such as bed handle, bed grab bar, transfer pole with handrail that rotates 360 degrees, quarter or half side rail.
- Place folding bed board under mattress.
- Lock or remove wheels of bed.
- Adjust bed height specific to resident's lower leg length: low beds or very low adjustable-height beds.
- Use nonskid rubber-backed rugs at bedside.
- Use nonslip bath mats or wet floor safety matting.
- Install easily accessible call bell or bulb (pressure sensitive).
- Use "nursery" or "baby" monitor.
- Place signs at strategic locations to alert staff of fall risk.
- Use weight-change sensor alarms for bed.
- Install movement sensor alarm (usually placed on thigh).

Inability to safely transfer as a result of dizziness and/or postural hypotension

- Refer to physician/nurse practitioner for evaluation, including medication review.
- Teach resident to rise slowly from lying and sitting positions.
- Refer to physical/occupational therapist re transferring training: lying to sitting to standing, standing to commode, sitting on toilet/commode to standing.
- Teach correct method of sitting on toilet: do not sit until legs are against the seat, then place hands on handrails, finally sit down slowly.
- Teach prevention of Valsalva maneuver related to excessive straining when defecating or straining to urinate in residents with BPH.

Inability to safely ambulate as a result of specific lower extremity problems: pain, weakness, limited ROM, or contractures

- Refer to physician/nurse practitioner for evaluation, including medication review and prescription of scheduled analgesic agents.
- Refer to physical/occupational therapist for evaluation, including need for specific rehabilitation therapies.
- Use hot packs.
- Consider joint mobilization.
- Incorporate conditioning, strengthening, and ROM exercises.
- Obtain assistive ambulatory devices, such as a walker "sled."
- Explore gait training.
- Encourage slow, prolonged stretching preceded by heat or ultrasound.
- Use leg length discrepancy pads.
- Use extra-wide walker.
- Use hemi-ambulator walker.
- Use slide walker or walker "sled" plus walker skis.
- Install hand grips for walker.
- Provide unit-based ROM and walking program.

Inability to navigate well because of foot problems

- Place antiskid acrylic wax on floors.
- Use nonskid rubber-backed rugs at bedside.
- Apply skid-proof strips near bed.
- Teach resident the importance of wearing footwear when walking to bathroom.
- Refer to podiatrist for evaluation.
- Obtain podiatry prescription for appropriate shoe gear and orthotics (e.g., shoes to correct leg length discrepancy and fit over deformities).

Inability to negotiate environment in low light

- Install night-lights with bulb wattage specific to resident's need.
- Keep light in bathroom on at night.
- Install pull cord for light within resident's reach in bed.
- Use motion sensor light.
- Place cordless press-on light at bedside.
- Use low buff on waxed floors.
- Install bulb (pressure sensitive) call bell.
- Ensure eyeglasses are easily accessible from bed.

Inability to negotiate path between bed and bathroom

- Rearrange furniture/objects to provide an obstacle-free path and compensate for specific problems (e.g., macular degeneration).

Modified from Capezuti E et al: Individualized assessment and intervention in bilateral siderail use, *Geriatr Nurs* 19(6):322-330, 1998.
BPH, Benign prostatic hypertrophy; *ROM,* range of motion.   *Continued*

Box 22-8   RESIDENTIAL PROBLEMS AND INTERVENTIONS—cont'd

- Use side rail on one side (resident's weaker side) to encourage one path to bathroom.
- Outline path to bathroom with fluorescent tape in contrasting color to floor or wall, such as red or orange.
- Rearrange bed closer to bathroom or provide a rest stop (e.g., chair placed midway between bed and bathroom).
- Use bedside commode (without wheels) placed on resident's stronger side, specific to resident's size.
- Provide illustration of toilet on bathroom door.
- Avoid slippery floor surface.
- Attach stop sign or material/vinyl strip across doorways not to enter.
- Use knob locks, such as "knob knots."

Difficulty transferring on and off toilet

- Refer to occupational therapist to evaluate need for toilet to be fitted with a secured raised seat and grab rails on each side, adjustable toilet seat, or adjustable toilet seat and rails.
- Apply skid-proof strips near toilet.
- Use accessible, glare-free light.
- Place cordless press-on light near commode.
- Refer to physical/occupational therapist re transfer training: standing to toilet/commode, sitting on toilet/commode to standing.
- Teach transferring techniques, including sitting on a commode: wait until legs are against the seat, then place hands on handrails, finally sit down slowly.
- Teach prevention of Valsalva maneuver related to excessive straining when defecating or straining to urinate in residents with BPH.
- Refer to physical/occupational therapist to teach exercises to increase strength of hip extensor-abductor and ankle plantar-flexor muscles.
- Use easily removable night clothing.
- Place alarm cord near toilet in bathroom.

Potential for Injury
Potential for fall-related injury from bed

- Use full body pillows or long immobilization bags.
- Use bed bolsters or pillows or rolled blanket under mattress edges.
- Use very low bed or very low adjustable-height beds.
- Adjust bed height specific to resident's lower leg length: low or very low adjustable-height beds.
- Place bed mattress on floor.
- Place nonskid rubber-backed rugs at bedside.
- Place egg-crate mattress on floor near bed if unable to walk.
- Use mat (4 × 6 to 8 feet) with nonslip surface.
- Apply hip pads.

- Use weight-change sensor alarm for bed.
- Use movement sensor alarm (usually placed on thigh).
- Apply call bell cord to clothing (alarm when disconnected) or alarm attached to clothing or adapt "mugger stopper."
- Place motion sensor light close to bed.
- Use "nursery" or "baby" monitor.
- Install video monitor.
- Place signs at strategic locations to alert staff of fall risk.

Potential for injury (skin tears) related to involuntary movements during sleep

- Position resident in center of bed (on back and both sides).
- Use body-length pillows bilaterally.
- Use full body-molded foam cushion.
- Use bed bolsters.
- Apply pillows/cushions for positioning of joints.
- Apply leg separator pads.
- Use very low beds: 5-, 8-, 11-inch deck heights or very low adjustable-height beds.
- Place bumper wedge on side rail.
- Attach sheepskin side rail pad.
- Attach side rail pad/bumper; bumper with see-through window.
- Use side rail pads for small-stature residents or sheepskin side rail pad.

Nocturia/Incontinence
Nocturia

- Conduct elimination rounds (individual-specific frequency).
- Place urinal or bedpan near bedside.
- Place bedside commode (without wheels) on resident's strongest side, specific to resident's size, drop arm commode.
- Use nonskid rubber-backed rugs at bedside that can absorb urine.
- Apply nonskid raised-tread socks.
- Place nonslip bath mats or wet floor safety matting near bed and bathroom.
- Refer to physician/nurse practitioner for evaluation if urination frequency changes.

Incontinence

- Refer to continence specialist, physician, nurse practitioner for evaluation.
- Conduct eliminations rounds (individual-specific frequency).
- Use extra-absorbent incontinence pads.
- Use bed pads.

Continued

Box 22-8   RESIDENTIAL PROBLEMS AND INTERVENTIONS—cont'd

- Apply incontinence covers for cushions.
- Install incontinence sensor with alarm.
- Apply raised-tread socks.

Sleep
Lack of comfort or inability to relax

- Refer for evaluation by physician or nurse practitioner for anxiety, depression, restless leg syndrome, paroxysmal nocturnal dyspnea, and sleep apnea.
- Refer for medication review by physician/nurse practitioner.
- Evaluate sleep hygiene: excessive daytime napping, lack of regular exercise, and exposure to daylight and overuse of caffeine.

- Install noise conditioner or "white noise."
- Turn radio/television on or off; play soothing music based on previous life-style preferences.
- Use body-length pillow.
- Install firm mattress or folding bed board under mattress.
- Use egg-crate mattress.
- Use air mattress.
- Apply sheepskin mattress pads.
- Use specific position (i.e., elevated, bent knees for back pain).
- Use pillows/cushions for positioning.
- Apply leg separator pads.
- Apply heel pads, bed cradle, and foot support.
- Install foot board.

► KEY CONCEPTS

- Mobility provides opportunities for exercise, exploration, and pleasure and is the crux of maintaining independence.
- Ease of mobility is thought to be the most visible measure of one's overall health and survival capacity.
- Changes in bones, muscles, and ligaments with aging affect one's balance and gait and increase instability.
- Muscle weakness (sarcopenia) must be investigated because it is often a result of reversible problems such as endocrine imbalances (particularly, hypothyroidism) or medication reactions.
- Gait disorders are often an obvious index of systemic problems and should be investigated thoroughly.
- A thorough nursing assessment must include descriptions of gait and mobility patterns.
- Prevention of falls is one of the most important proactive considerations to preserve health and function for the elderly.
- Each institutionalized individual should be assessed for fall risk factors to which he or she is exposed or inclined.
- Paradoxically, fear of falling and extreme caution actually increase falling propensity in the elderly.
- Physical restraints are to be used only under very specific conditions, with a physician's order, and for

a very limited time until a better solution can be found. They are not appropriate for "safety" and are not allowed under OBRA guidelines except in very specific situations.
- Transportation for the elderly is critical to their physical, psychologic, and social health.

► Activities and Discussion Questions

1. Put your shoes on the wrong feet, and then ask another student to analyze your gait.
2. Borrow a pair of bifocals from someone, and then attempt to go up and down stairs.
3. Evaluate the safety of your living quarters using Box 14-12 as a guide.
4. Discuss your activities that increase your fall vulnerability.
5. Discuss falls you have had and their consequences. Consider how it might have been different if you were 75 years old.
6. Obtain a wheelchair, and sit in it for 20 minutes with a restraining belt around your waist. Discuss your feelings with a partner. Reverse the process with your partner.
7. Discuss the various reasons why you might want to use restraints for an individual and identify several alternatives that might be satisfactory.

NANDA and Wellness Diagnoses

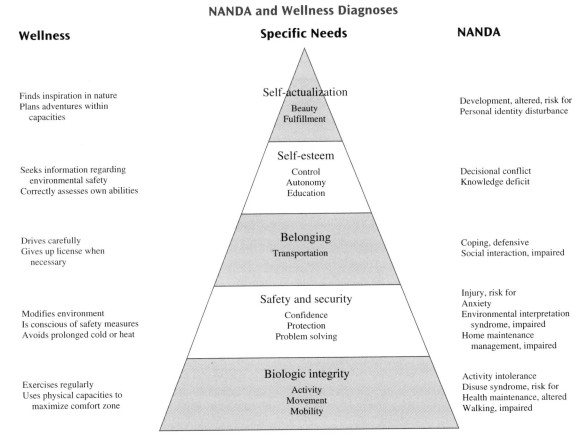

Wellness

Finds inspiration in nature
Plans adventures within
  capacities

Seeks information regarding
  environmental safety
Correctly assesses own abilities

Drives carefully
Gives up license when
  necessary

Modifies environment
Is conscious of safety measures
Avoids prolonged cold or heat

Exercises regularly
Uses physical capacities to
  maximize comfort zone

Specific Needs

Self-actualization
  Beauty
  Fulfillment

Self-esteem
  Control
  Autonomy
  Education

Belonging
  Transportation

Safety and security
  Confidence
  Protection
  Problem solving

Biologic integrity
  Activity
  Movement
  Mobility

NANDA

Development, altered, risk for
Personal identity disturbance

Decisional conflict
Knowledge deficit

Coping, defensive
Social interaction, impaired

Injury, risk for
Anxiety
Environmental interpretation
  syndrome, impaired
Home maintenance
  management, impaired

Activity intolerance
Disuse syndrome, risk for
Health maintenance, altered
Walking, impaired

These are not all of the possible wellness or NANDA diagnoses that may be identified. The above are frequent examples of nursing diagnoses that should be considered when planning care for the older adult in whatever setting.

RESOURCES

Making Your Community Livable: Programs That Work. Booklet available free from the Public Policy Institute, American Association of Retired Persons (AARP), 601 E Street NW, Washington, DC 20049. Describes programs in crime prevention, home repair and modification, and transportation that have proved effective in helping older people live independently in their homes.

Restraint and Seclusion Standards for Ambulatory Care, Hospital and Behavioral Health Care. Available from the Joint Commission on Accreditation of Healthcare Organizations (JCAHO), 1 Renaissance Boulevard, Oakbrook Terrace, IL 60181; (630) 792-5000; www.jcaho.org.

Selection Guide for Restraint-Free Resident Positioning and Safety Aids. Available from Akil-Care Corporation; 167 Saw Mill River Road; Yonkers, New York 10701; (800) 431-2972.

REFERENCES

Bryant H, Fernald L: Nursing knowledge and use of restraint alternatives: acute and chronic care, *Geriatr Nurs* 18(2):57, 1997.

Burton L et al: Mental illness and the use of restraints in nursing homes, *Gerontologist* 32(2):164, 1992.

Capezuti E et al: Individualized assessment and intervention in bilateral siderail use, *Geriatr Nurs* 19(6):322-330, 1998.

Catanasos G, Israel R: Gait disorders in the elderly, *Hosp Pract* 26(12):67, 1991.

Chipman A: Airbag for hip protects elderly, *San Francisco Examiner,* p B1, April 8, 1996.

Chipman C: Evaluation of falls and their traumatic consequences. In Bosker G et al, editors: *Geriatric emergency medicine,* St Louis, 1990, Mosby.

Cunha U: Differential diagnosis of gait disorders in the elderly, *Geriatrics* 43(8):33, 1988.

Ettinger HW: Joint and soft tissue disorders. In Abrams WB, Beers MH, Berkow R, editors: *The Merck manual of geriatrics,* ed 2, Whitehouse Station, NJ, 1995, Merck Research Laboratories.

Evans L, Strumpf N: Tying down the elderly: a review of literature on physical restraint, *J Am Geriatr Soc* 37:65, 1989.

Galindo-Ciocon D, Ciocon J, Galindo D: Gait training and falls in the elderly, *J Gerontol Nurs* 21(6):10, 1995.

Lord S et al: The effect of exercise on gait patterns in older women: a randomized controlled trial, *J Gerontol* 51A(2):M64, 1996.

Mayo Foundation for Medical Education and Research: Heel pain, *Mayo Clin Health Lett* 14(7):1, 1996.

Mion LC, Strumpf N, NICHE faculty: Use of restraints in the hospital setting: implications for nursing, *Geriatr Nurs* 15(3):127-132, 1994.

Omnibus Budget Reconciliation Act of 1987 (OBRA): Amendment to the Social Security Act, Public Law 100-203, Nursing Home Reform Law, US Department of Health and Human Services.

Potter J, Evans A, Duncan G: Gait speed and activities of daily living function in geriatric patients, *Arch Phys Med Rehabil* 76(11):997, 1995.

Rice R: Environmental threats in the home: home care nursing perspectives, *Geriatr Nurs* 20(6):333-334, 1999.

Strumpf NE, Evans LK: Physical restraint of the hospitalized elderly: perceptions of patients and nurses, *Nurs Res* 37(3):132, 1988.

Strumpf NE et al: Reducing physical restraints: developing an educational program, *J Gerontol Nurs* 18(11):5-11, 1992.

Tideiksaar R: Falls in the elderly: etiology and prevention. In Bosker G et al, editors: *Geriatric emergency medicine,* St Louis, 1990, Mosby.

US Bureau of the Census: *Statistical abstract of the United States: 1998,* ed 118, Washington, DC, 1998, US Government Printing Office.

University of California, San Francisco: A hip pad to prevent injuries during a fall, *To Our Neighbors* 20(4):1, 1995.

Werner P et al: Individualized care alternatives used in the process of removing physical restraints in the nursing homes, *J Am Geriatr Soc* 42:321, 1994.

Wolinsky F, Fitzgerald J: The risk of hip fracture among noninstitutionalized older adults, *J Gerontol* 49(4):S165, 1994.

Appendix 22-A Sources of Potential Toxins in the Home

Moisture
Pressed wood furniture
Humidifier
Moth repellents
Dry-cleaned goods
House dust mites
Personal care products
Air freshener
Stored fuels
Car exhaust
Paint supplies
Paneling
Wood stove
Tobacco smoke
Carpets
Pressed wood subflooring

Drapes
Fireplace
Household chemicals
Asbestos floor tiles
Pressed wood cabinets
Unvented gas stove
Asbestos pipe wrap
Radon
Unvented clothes dryer
Pesticides
Stored hobby products
Lead-based paints
Cockroaches
Pets
Flowering plants
Contaminated drinking water

From Environmental Protection Agency: *The inside story: a guide to indoor air quality,* EPA Pub No 402-K-93-0013, Washington, DC, 1995, Office of Air and Radiation.

Appendix 22-B   Make Your Home Toxin Free!

Reduce Exposure to Particulates and Biologic Contaminants

Install and use exhaust fans in kitchens and bathrooms that are vented to the outdoors.

Vent clothes dryers outdoors.

Ventilate the attic and crawlspaces to prevent moisture build-up.

Thoroughly clean and dry water-damaged carpets and building materials (within 24 hours if possible) or consider removal and replacement with tile or hardwood flooring.

Keep the house clean by vacuuming and dusting weekly. If a vacuum is not available, dust and sweep daily. Dust mites, pollens, animal dander, and other allergy-causing agents can be reduced—but not eliminated—through regular cleaning.

Do not smoke, especially in the presence of children and elderly people.

If you must have pets in the home, don't sleep with them.

Consider using miniblinds in bedrooms instead of drapes.

Heat dry pillow on "high" three times a week to reduce bacteria and mold growth.

Have your well water tested for biologic contaminants.

Reduce Exposure to Volatile Organic Compounds

Take special precautions when operating fuel-burning unvented space heaters.

Install exhaust fans over gas cooking stoves and ranges; keep burners properly adjusted.

Keep woodstove emissions to a minimum; choose properly sized new stoves that are certified as meeting EPA emission standards.

Do not idle the car in the garage.

Inspect and clean central air handling systems, including furnaces, flues, and chimneys, annually (replace air filters annually); open and ventilate the home the first day the furnace or air conditioner is turned on.

To reduce exposure to household chemicals, follow label instructions carefully.

Throw away partially full containers of old or unneeded chemicals safely.

Buy limited quantities of paints, paint strippers, and kerosene for space heaters or gasoline for lawn mowers; buy only as much as you need right away.

Minimize exposure to methylene chloride and benzene, both of which are used in household products and are known carcinogens.

Keep exposure to perchlorethylene (perc) emissions from newly dry-cleaned materials to a minimum because this chemical has been shown to cause cancer in animals.

Avoid using pressed wood products in the home because they emit formaldehyde, a known carcinogenic agent.

Run water through the faucet a few minutes before using it.

Have well water tested for presence of toxic chemicals.

Reduce Exposure to Radon

Test your home for radon. Fix your home if your radon level is 4 picocuries per liter or higher and contact your state radon office.

Reduce Exposure to Pesticides

Use sparingly, according to manufacturer's instructions; consider natural and nonchemical methods of pest control when possible. Store chemicals in sealed glass jars, preferably in a shed away from home.

Wear a mask and gloves when spraying pesticides.

Allow plenty of fresh air when using these products; ventilate the area well after use.

Mix or dilute solutions outdoors.

Dispose of pesticides according to label directions or public health directives.

Take pets or plants outdoors when applying pesticides.

Store clothes with moth repellents in separately ventilated areas, if possible.

Keep indoor spaces clean, dry, and well-ventilated to avoid pest and odor problems.

Reduce Exposure to Lead

Leave lead-based paint undisturbed if it is in good condition; do not sand or burn off paint that may contain lead.

Do not bring lead dust into the home. If the workplace or hobby involves lead, change clothes and use doormats before entering the home.

Vacuum the inside of the car weekly.

Run cool water through a faucet for a few minutes before using it for eating or cooking purposes; do not use hot faucet water for cooking purposes.

Eat a balanced diet rich in calcium and iron.

From Environmental Protection Agency: *The inside story: a guide to indoor air quality,* EPA Pub No 402-K-93-0013, Washington, DC, 1995, Office of Air and Radiation.
EPA, Environmental Protection Agency.

►LEARNING OBJECTIVES

Upon completion of this chapter, the reader will be able to:

- Identify several dynamics of family relationships and their significance.
- Relate several functions of grandparenting and the contributions elders make to family life.
- Specify factors that make caregiving of the aged particularly difficult.
- Describe the nursing role in supportive networks serving elders.
- Relate essential aspects of conservatorships and guardianships and nursing responsibilities in relation to these.
- Explain several of the dynamics of elder abuse.
- Describe several situations that may trigger elder abuse.
- Discuss the nurse's responsibility in regard to assessing, intervening, and reporting in cases of suspected elder abuse.

►GLOSSARY

Competent Having the ability to meet the necessary requirements in a given situation.

Idiosyncrasy Pertaining to personal peculiarities or mannerisms.

Maligned Treated in a way that is injurious physically or emotionally.

Passivity Behavior and attitudes that allow others to override an individual's personal needs and desires.

Psychopathologic Behavioral manifestations of mental disorders.

Scapegoat An individual who is blamed for problems and thus allows others to avoid any responsibility for them.

Skewed Ideas, statistics, or facts that are incorrect because certain important factors have not been considered.

►THE LIVED EXPERIENCE

I just can't stand watching as my father becomes weaker and is unable to do the things he always did so naturally and well. Yesterday he got lost on his way to the market. He was always my guide and protector. I knew I could count on him no matter what. It makes me feel sort of alone in the world.

Madge, an adult offspring

It is so irritating when Madge tries to help me do things. After all, I have lived 85 years and have done very well. I think she wants to put me away somewhere. I wish she would just leave me alone. I'm sure I could manage if she just wouldn't interfere.

John, the aged father

We wish to thank Mary Joy Quinn, Director of Probate Court Services, San Francisco Superior Court, City and County of San Francisco, who has contributed substantially to the accuracy and content of this chapter and whose contribution is essential to the substantive aspects of the chapter.

FAMILIES

Ideally, families are the primary source of material and emotional support of members. The greatest emphasis on families of the aged has been on describing the burden of caring for them. This approach neglects to examine the reciprocal nature of family relationships. There can be no accurate estimates of how much material and financial support flows from the older generation to the younger ones, but a considerable amount is given to educate and launch the younger generations. In addition, there is usually a massive transfer of goods, assets, and titled and nontitled properties on the death of an elder. The younger generations provide a sense of meaning and purpose to the elders, who wish to bequeath knowledge, history, and wisdom. Functional and physical assistance also flow from the young to the frail old, and the burden of caring may become quite overwhelming.

It is thought that more than 8 million elders need, and get, some form of assistance from family and friends that allows them to live at home. As the population shifts toward increasing numbers of frail aged with multiple problems, these numbers will increase markedly. Older family members, themselves impaired, will often find it necessary to take care of very old parents. The quality, meaning, and reliability of relationships with family members are significant factors in maintaining morale and experiencing life satisfaction in one's final years.

This chapter deals with the nature of family dynamics and relationships, aspects of caregiving, the abuse of elders, and legal protection for frail elders.

Family History

A potent force, often overlooked in families with aged members, is the influence of the family history. Gender and sibling position in a family profoundly influence relationships with parents and other siblings. Motivation, socialization, affiliation, and aggression are rooted to some degree in family configuration. Early sibling relationships, parental expectations, and parental favoritism remain influential in reactions to aged parents. These early beginnings are never totally dismissed and many years later have significant effects. In caregiving situations each sibling may have a specific role in meeting the parents' needs. Nurses may be helpful in pointing out to each family member how their contributions sustain and enrich the lives of their parents in their own unique way. Nurses also may ask family members what aspects of their lives they attribute to parental influence.

Parents in their old age may depend on the eldest child to care for them, just as they depended on that child to care for younger siblings decades before, or each parent may have a different "favorite" child. Sometimes a "rejected" child may attempt to gain love and recognition by attending the aged parent or may unconsciously punish the parent for injustices experienced in the distant past. Nurses may help all family members understand the present situation as reflecting many conflicts from the past.

Rivalry among family members for the approval of aged parents is common when there is awareness of a potential inheritance. Many people are reluctant to admit to themselves that such thoughts enter their minds. It is helpful to recognize the reality of such considerations and that it may be just as natural to entertain such feelings as it was to attempt to gain more than one's share of the parental love in the early stages of childhood. Most close relationships are fraught with ambivalence. Helping family members to recognize and accept these feelings will ease feelings of guilt or shame.

If the family has never been close and supportive, it will not magically become so when the parents are old. Resentments long buried may crop up and produce friction or psychologic pain. One of the tasks of middle-age adults centers on their ability to work through youthful feelings and attitudes toward parents. The mature adult begins to see parents as individuals rather than extensions of one's own needs. However, long-submerged conflicts and feelings often return to surprise adult children (Townsend, Franks, 1995).

Mature acceptance of aged parents, with all their foibles and personal idiosyncrasies, is an ongoing task. Nurses may help family members accept their own and others' idiosyncrasies as meaningful and valid, even though the relationships are always complex, clouded with ambivalence, and influenced by the past. Some families can be encouraged to express their feelings more openly, although if they have never done so, it may be difficult to break long-standing habits within the family relationships. Most important, each family member needs to be accepted and understood as significant to the family system.

Deference

Old people may play games with their children, perhaps ones they have always played or ones invented to avert fear and loneliness. Some manipulate, dwell on infirmities, belittle themselves, or use their money to wield power. Children may rightfully feel used and angry.

Among health care providers it is common to believe that the old are maligned and neglected by families. Rarely are situations as simple as they appear on the surface. Nurses can help people see their situation more clearly and recognize the reality of their situation and also that one need not put up with games or avoid confrontation in deference to old age.

Scapegoating

We are aware of the detrimental effects of consistently being the scapegoat for others, although most people are given this role occasionally or cast it on others at times. Aged parents are often scapegoats. The focus of energy usually flows toward the younger generations as the bearers of unfulfilled dreams, whereas the elders are the carriers of disappointment and worn traditions. They may personify all of the facets of life that we are conditioned to avoid: death, illness, depression, and uselessness. It is easy to displace responsibility and project feelings onto an aged parent who may in fact have already internalized the social rejection of the generalized aged.

As nurses, perhaps the most useful approach to families who seem to scapegoat the aged members would be to explore the individual's fears and concerns related to his or her own aging. For example, the nurse might say, "Having your parent in your home must stimulate a lot of thoughts about your own aging process." It is recognized that when a family crisis occurs, the elderly member is likely to be identified as the source of the problem and removed from the family group in attempts to restore order. If the older person has sapped the family energy system, the move may temporarily restore family balance, even though solution of the real problem will only be deferred. Losing a younger member from a family system is a major crisis, particularly if it is by death or an abrupt and traumatic separation. It is then that one is likely to hear, "Why couldn't it have been Grandma; she has had a full life. It is so unfair."

Family Caregiving

According to the National Alliance for Caregiving (1997; see Resources at the end of this chapter), nearly one in four Americans over age 50 feels responsibility for an elder needing long-term care. About 43% of noninstitutionalized elders over the age of 85 need assistance with basic activities of daily living. Relatives provide 84% of all care to men and 79% of all care to women. More than 1 in 3 elderly men needing assistance is cared for by a wife, but only 1 in 10 disabled elderly women is cared for by a husband (American Association of Homes and Services for the Aging, 1996).

If an aged parent is beginning to need help, the following suggestions to family members may be useful:
1. Involve the parent in all decisions that affect care.
2. Assist the elderly parent in remaining as independent as possible and provide assistance only for those things that are especially stressful or depleting.
3. Seek resources that provide options between independent living and a nursing home.
4. If the parent insists on promises to never be put in a nursing home, the family may promise that they will do everything possible to prevent it.

Before inviting an elder to move into the family's home, consideration should be given to items in Box 23-1.

At present, families provide 80% to 90% of the long-term care of elders in the community (Family Caregiver Alliance, 1996). Numerically, about 3 million adult children provide "hands-on care" for disabled elders; far more spouses than adult children provide care, and it is assumed that they will do so when a spouse exists.

Historically, family support and care for older members have always been voluntary or tolerated because there were no other alternatives. In the past, unmarried women were particularly vulnerable to the assumption that they would take care of aged parents (Brody et al, 1994). Now, we are much more likely to expect the government to help and to develop programs to assist families with various social needs, including the burden of caregiving. This has occurred as changes in societal demands and expectations of family members make it more difficult, if not impossible, for any one adult child to be available around the clock. Even when a caregiver is available, the burden may be onerous. Elderly spouses often find themselves available but not physically capable of the demands of constant caregiving.

Recently there have been questions about the real extent of the "sandwich" generation—that generation wedged between obligations to children and those to elderly parents. On average there are 5 years, between the ages of 50 and 55, when one is likely to have the care of both a parent and a minor child. The percentage of the population group in this situation fluctuates. Being caught in the middle is far from a typical experience (Rosenthal et al, 1996), but when it does occur, the pressures and conflicts are so tremendous that they can be absolutely overwhelming.

Box 23-1   PLANNING TO ADD AN AGED MEMBER TO THE HOUSEHOLD

Questions you need to ask:
- What are the needs of the new member and of the family?
- Where will space be allotted for the new member?
- How will this new member be included in existing family patterns?
- How will responsibilities be shared?
- What resources in the community will assist in the adjustment phase?
- Is the environment safe for this new member?
- How will family life change with the added member, and how does the family feel about it?
- What are the differences in socialization and sleeping patterns?
- What are the aged person's strong needs and expectations?
- What are the aged person's skills and talents?

Modifications you need to make:
- Arrange semiprivate living quarters if possible.
- Consider a "granny flat" (see Chapter 27).
- Regularly schedule visits to other relatives to give each family times of respite and privacy.
- Arrange day care and senior activities for the older person to help keep contact with members of his or her own generation.

Discuss potential areas of conflict:
- *Space:* especially if someone has given up his or her space to the aged relative.
- *Possessions:* old person may want to move possessions into house; others may not find them attractive or may insist on replacing them with new things.

- *Entertaining:* times when old and young feel the need or desire to exclude the other from social events.
- *Responsibilities and chores:* old may feel useless if they do nothing and in the way if they do something; young may feel that their position is usurped or may be angry if they wait on parent.
- *Expenses:* increased cost of home maintenance, food, clothing, and recreation may not be shared appropriately.
- *Vacations:* whether to go together or alone; the young may feel uneasy not taking older person but resentful if they must.
- *Child rearing:* disagreement over child-rearing policies.
- *Child care:* grandparental babysitting may be welcomed by family and resented by older person, or if not allowed, older person may feel lack of trust in capability.

Decrease areas of conflict by:
- Respecting privacy
- Discussing space allocations
- Discussing elderly person's furnishings before move
- Making it clear ahead of time when social events include everyone or exclude someone
- Clearing decisions about household tasks—all should have responsibility geared to ability
- Paying a share of expenses and maintaining a separate phone reduce strain and increase feelings of independence

Caregiving as a Women's Issue

It is estimated that 72% of care is given by women (Family Caregiver Alliance, 1996). One in four women becomes a caregiver at some time between ages 35 and 44, and one in three between ages 55 and 64. Only 45% of the oldest cohort studied (born 1905 to 1917) were ever caregivers of elderly relatives, compared with 64% of the present cohort (born between 1927 and 1934) (Moen et al, 1994). To a large extent, this is a result of the great increases in elderly women living to advanced old age, and this trend is on the upswing. Because of increasing numbers of frail elderly and strong trends toward their management in the home, nurses must support policies to provide supports for the female caregiver in the home. The Older Women's League has made remarkable progress in this respect.

The Older Women's League. The Older Women's League (OWL) was one of the first groups established specifically for the purpose of assisting older women in

their caregiving roles. They have established a functional grass roots organization to respond directly to the concerns of caregivers in their own communities. Some volunteer groups, such as those reported by Sheehan (1989), have been developed to assist caregivers. "Natural" volunteer helpers from churches within a metropolitan area were recruited for a training program in aging and caregiver support. From these efforts several programs were developed in various churches to reach out to community caretakers with assistance in problem solving and respite.

The needs of caregivers largely fall into a few categories: (1) support groups or allies, (2) knowledge of aging, (3) knowledge of resources, (4) respite, (5) financial assistance, and (6) recognition. George and Gwyther (1983, 1986) have designed a tool to assist the elderly and family in determining need for formal and informal supports (Fig. 23-1). This is a simple questionnaire and the most practical that we have found.

Support for Caregivers

"Now I'd like to ask you about some of the ways your family and friends may help you out—either how they help you personally or the way they help you to care for your confused relative. For each question below, please check one column to indicate how often your family or friends give you that kind of help. Then please tell us the relationship of the person who gives you the most help of that type (for example, sister, friend, daughter-in-law)."

| Type of Help | How often do you receive this help? | | | | | Relationship |
Do your family or friends:	Never	Rarely	Only if I ask	Now and then	Regularly	of helper
1. Help you out when you are sick?						
2. Shop or run errands for you?						
3. Help you out with money or bills?						
4. Fix things around your house?						
5. Keep house for you or do household chores?						
6. Give you advice on business or finances?						
7. Provide companionship for you?						
8. Give you advice on dealing with problems?						
9. Provide transportation for you or your confused relative?						
10. Prepare or provide meals?						
11. Stay with your confused relative while you are away?						
12. Provide personal grooming services for your confused relative?						

13. Do you wish that your family and friends would give you more help with these kinds of things?
    1. No
    2. Yes

Fig. 23-1   Informal support. (From George LK, Gwyther LP: *Duke University caregiver well-being survey,* Durham, NC, 1983, Duke University Center for the Study of Aging and Human Development; and George LK, Gwyther LP: Caregiver well-being: a multidimensional examination of family caregivers of demented adults, *Gerontologist* 26:253, 1986.)

Caregivers of Elders With Dementia

Caregivers of demented elders are thought to have the most difficult job; yet in one study 96% agreed that it was a "labor of love" (Hoffman, 1996). Eighty-one percent of these caregivers were women, 51% lived in the same household, and 30% were the sole caregiver. A "labor of love" may or may not mean that the care is lovingly given, as the phrase seems to imply. "Labor of love" is often used to describe any labor that is unpaid. On the other hand, it may be an indication of the caregiver's sense of duty or obligation, or simply having no other available alternative. Fig. 23-2 provides a hierar-

Motivations	Needs	Examples of modes

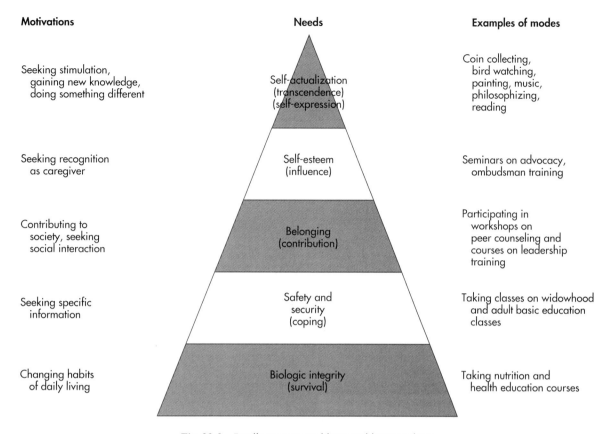

Fig. 23-2   Family support problems and interventions.

chy of needs and supports for those in these difficult situations.

A daughter caring for her elderly mother afflicted with Alzheimers disease said she had previously thought it was important to focus on reality. On one occasion, after trying unsuccessfully to convince her mother that the month was May and not April, she went to get a calendar to show her. By the time she returned, her mother had forgotten all about it. "It was then I realized that reality doesn't matter. That was the biggest breakthrough. If she thought it was April, what did it matter? I found that when I stopped correcting her and went along with her, it saved us both a lot of heartache. The content of the conversation did not matter as much as the feeling" (Hoffman, 1996).

Elderly spouses caring for disabled partners have special needs. Often the spouse has significant health problems that are neglected in deference to the greater needs of the incapacitated partner. Life satisfaction tends to be limited when illness, low income, multiple demands, and the loss of intimacy and companionship

converge on a conscientious mate. It is most difficult when the partner is aphasic or incontinent. Availability of children, relatives, and friends is significant in easing the load and increasing satisfaction. Respite from continuous care is essential (Feinberg, Kelly, 1995).

Women who care for a demented spouse seem to fare better if the relationship before illness was close and remains so. From a practical standpoint, nurses may encourage caregiving spouses to be alert to subtle signs of responsiveness. Periods when the patient is calm and content should be documented and a log kept to help identify the times when the caregiver may feel gratified. These methods restore a sense of control and increase awareness of the positive aspects of caregiving. Small gains are significant in maintaining the morale of a caregiving spouse.

Four sets of risk factors seem significant to the durability and acceptability of a caregiving relationship with a demented elder: the caregiving relationship, family life stressors outside of caregiving, individual and family coping styles, and the caregiver's perception

of the situation (Rankin et al, 1992). The caretaker who fares best is one who has the following characteristics:
- Can accept the psychologic changes occurring in the patient
- Can facilitate effective communication while understanding the patient's inability to comprehend reality
- Can use the relationship to strengthen the patient's sense of self
- Is compassionate
- Is willing to try unusual solutions to problems
- Maintains a sense of humor
- Talks without expecting an answer
- Interacts with the individual even if he or she does not respond

Five coping strategies were significant in reducing the perceived burden of care: (1) confidence in problem-solving ability, (2) ability to perceive the problems in alternative ways, (3) passivity in reference to things that could not be changed, (4) spiritual supports, and (5) an extended family (Pratt et al, 1985).

Caregiving: A Cultural Perspective

It is often thought that various cultures have stronger bonds, are more effective in caring for their elders, and in general have formed tighter communities. These attributes are often not really culturally based but are simply measures to cope with fewer resources, limited opportunities, and lack of appropriate assistance from the community at large. Some argue that culturally competent care is dependent on immersion in a given culture, whereas others believe that genuine caring goes beyond culture and is universally recognized. Language arises from the framework of a world view, and the subtleties may not be understood simply by a working knowledge of a second language. In working with culturally diverse families, the basic issues are respect for their traditional approaches (regardless of our understanding) and recognition of the efforts of the family to maintain its solidarity. However, regardless of the cultural or ethnic orientation, each situation must be approached as unique.

For general information about cultural orientations see Chapter 4. We would advise students to review these when considering the needs and strengths inherent within a particular cultural framework. Avoiding stereotypes is very important.

Caring for Developmentally Disabled Adults

Although we tend to think of caregivers as middle-age adults caring for elders, an unknown number of elders are caring for their middle-age children who are physically and mentally disabled. Earlier in the century these

developmentally disabled children usually died before reaching adulthood; now, with improved care they are surviving. Often this has been a burden carried by parents for their entire adult life and will end only with the death of the parent or the adult child. In a study of 115 older mothers (ages 58 to 96 years) caring for mentally retarded offspring, religion and prayer emerged as critical aspects of their coping, although they often questioned why God was letting them suffer so (Tobin et al, 1994). At present, little is being done about this situation, but the Society of Friends is giving serious attention to it as an issue of aging that has been neglected (Schwartz, Kelly, 1996).

Caregiving in the Nontraditional Family

There are 11 million blended families in the United States (Vinick et al, 1996) and numerous nonconventional family configurations. This trend is expected to continue and increase in the future. The long-range implications for elders in nontraditional families is stirring interest among gerontologists. The generational reciprocity that is so fundamental to our present system of survival of young and old may develop in entirely different ways or simply break down. Prenuptial agreements regarding asset inheritance are common in later marriages, but agreements regarding inheritance of caregiving responsibilities are notorious by their absence.

In countries that are seriously limiting population growth, such as China, filial responsibility will necessarily be problematic, since one child when grown may have the responsibility of parents and several grandparents. In addition, as more and more youth are dying of acquired immunodeficiency syndrome (AIDS) in their prime years, more elders will be left with one or no children to carry on. Costs of caregiving, emotionally and economically, are a worldwide problem that will continue to tax the ingenuity of world populations as longevity increases.

Assessment

Assessing the family's needs, strengths, and stresses, as well as its support system and family dynamics, will assist the nurse in gaining a holistic picture of the interventions that may strengthen the family unit (Fig. 23-3 and Box 23-2). A mutually constructed, written assessment of a family's needs and coping capacities can be comprehensive and specific and becomes a document of their strengths in times of stress. Foci to be included are sources of stress, particular coping methods, resources that are used or can be used, and the rewards and problems of caregiving.

Problems	Collective need	Interventions

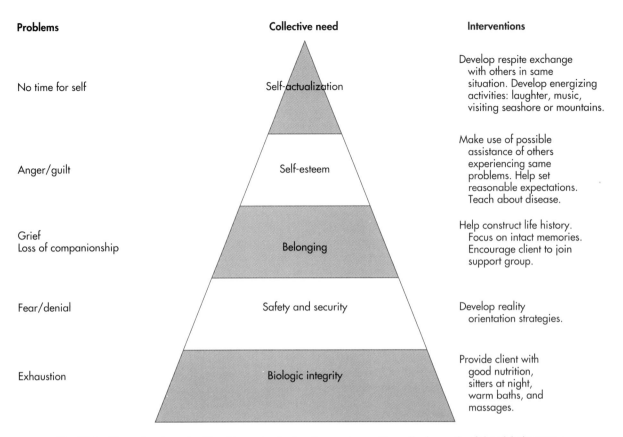

No time for self	Self-actualization	Develop respite exchange with others in same situation. Develop energizing activities: laughter, music, visiting seashore or mountains.
Anger/guilt	Self-esteem	Make use of possible assistance of others experiencing same problems. Help set reasonable expectations. Teach about disease.
Grief / Loss of companionship	Belonging	Help construct life history. Focus on intact memories. Encourage client to join support group.
Fear/denial	Safety and security	Develop reality orientation strategies.
Exhaustion	Biologic integrity	Provide client with good nutrition, sitters at night, warm baths, and massages.

Fig. 23-3 Hierarchy of needs of families caring for family members with senile dementia of the Alzheimer type (SDAT).

Box 23-2   FAMILY SUPPORT SYSTEM ASSESSMENT

Size	Number in extended family who are accessible	Functions	Contributions to aged member
	Number of daughters who are accessible		Money
			Chores
	Number of sons who are accessible		Transportation
	Number of grandchildren, nephews, nieces, confidants, siblings		Listening/psychologic support
			Functional assistance
		Deterrents	Other demands
Ability	Economic status of each		Work
	Poverty		Travel
	Lower middle		Adolescent children
	Middle	Recent stresses	Poor health
	Upper middle		Job change
	Wealthy		Moves
Willingness	Frequency of involvement		Deaths
	Monthly		
	Weekly		
	Daily		
	Constant		

Although staff develop written care plans and evaluate patient progress, these are seldom discussed with or given to the family. Inclusion in the development of a nursing care plan and periodic evaluation may help family members assess their effectiveness even in the face of patient decline. Factors that are indexes of coping in the caretaking role include perceived well-being, perceived social support, promotion of functional ability of the care receiver, and a positive relationship with the care receiver (Georgemiller et al, 1987).

Interventions

Interventions with caregivers must always take into account the great variability in family structures, resources, traditions, and history. The range of adaptations is enormous, and the goal is always to restore the balance of the system to the greatest extent possible while avoiding scapegoating and harmful practices. The family can be visualized as a mobile with many parts, and when one is touched, each part shifts to regain the balance. The intrusion of professionals into a family system will temporarily unbalance the system and may provide an opportunity to restore the balance in a healthier manner, sometimes by adding an element or increasing the weight of one or decreasing the weight of another.

Respite

Respite is, perhaps, the most significant intervention with families when elder members require considerable assistance. Stephens (1996) found that day care respite can be effective for some caregivers if it allows sufficient relief, creates no additional stress, is at least partially subsidized, and provides information about other resources that may be helpful. Transportation of the elder is frequently a problem, since programs do not necessarily fit their hours to a working family's needs.

Audiotapes and videotapes that provide mild stimulation or entertainment for elders and respite for their caregivers have been developed and show some promise of being used effectively (Camberg et al, 1996). Fortunately or unfortunately, depending on the situation, many elders and their families use television programming as a source of respite.

Employee Assistance Programs

Middle-age working women must often carry on the demands of caregiving in addition to work and other responsibilities (Boaz, 1996). The age-group most involved with elder care is between 40 and 49 years of age; many also have children for whom they are still responsible. Many companies provide employee respite time, "flex time," and/or unpaid personal leaves to assist the employee in caring for elders. Some employee assistance programs (EAPs) have hot lines and community resource booklets for the support of working caregivers.

Community experts with local knowledge may be of assistance to employers developing EAP programs. Features of comprehensive programs include the following:

- Personalized consultation
- Information about the range of service options in the area
- Individualized referrals currently available
- Consumer education
- Guidance through the process of decision making
- Follow-up to determine whether needs were met
- Readily available emergency leaves when necessary

The corporate nurse working with the family and the aged person is in a unique position to maximize all of these supports. Family needs can be identified, and through empowering the support network, encouraging reciprocity within it, and linking the client system with the service system, goals can be accomplished.

Long-Distance Caring

Long-distance caregiving is most challenging for concerned families. The usual impulse is to move the elder to an accessible location for the family, but this may not be best for an elder who has lived a long time in one community and has many supports there. Plans and alternatives should be discussed before emergency events and will prevent the need for hasty decisions. Conferring with a case manager in advance of any evidence of problems may forestall the need to move the parent into the adult child's home. Issues that need to be considered include identifying the person who will be available quickly in emergency situations; identifying reliable individuals or services that will provide daily monitoring; identifying acceptable facilities for assisted living if that becomes necessary; determining which family member is most likely to be free to travel to the elder if needed; and being sure that legalities regarding advance directives, a will, and a possible power of attorney have been established.

A network of services has emerged to assist the geographically distant family member to ensure that an elderly relative will be taken care of. City and county referral services or case managers through private agencies may assist family members in solving difficult problems in caring for a distant elderly parent. Often they know of resources that can allow the elder to remain independent and yet assure the family that safety and other needs are being met. Case management services can be particularly useful to families who are geographically remote. Some nurses and social workers have developed this type of service. At present these services are available only to those who are able to pay, since they are not covered by private insurance or public agencies of any kind.

Institutionalization

Families may feel defeated when a parent must be institutionalized. The efforts they have expended are rewarded with decline. It is imperative that nurses reinforce the family's adequacy and importance to the aged member. Family support groups may be helpful in dealing with the ambivalence and distress of institutionalizing an elder. Goals of these groups can be seen in Box 23-3.

Caregiving issues are likely to remain in the forefront of discussions of public policy and concerns about family life. There is a continuing need for investigations that identify potentially modifiable features of caregivers' situations and that contribute to the development and evaluation of interventions to assist families (Zarit, 1991).

Counseling Families

Nurses involved in counseling families are advised to encourage all involved family members to participate. Including young and aged family members is most likely to produce satisfactory results. Too often, plans are made for the aged rather than with them. It is important to anticipate needs and options and form contingency plans before crises occur that result in emergency actions, poorly thought through (Wolanin, 1979).

Families may not know where to turn for support and guidance when needed. Nurses in contact with middle-age people might ask about aged family members and their plans and expectations for the future and explore their awareness of possible resources or agencies to contact during times of crisis. Area Agency on Aging offices are located throughout the United States, and these are able to direct people to community services and agencies.

Health care workers consulting with middle-age people might routinely ask, "What is happening with your aging relatives?" Discuss functional state, quality of relationships, and tentative plans that have been considered.

Box 23-3   GOALS OF FAMILY SUPPORT GROUPS
Learn to accept the elder as he or she is now; let go of the past.
Learn the balance between protectiveness and smothering.
Recognize one's own needs as fundamental to caring for others.
Learn to share and cope with disappointment.
Discuss resurgence of feelings of loss during holidays and anniversaries.
Share knowledge of how to deal with family and community.
Develop a caring and sharing network within the group.
Deal with feelings of guilt, helplessness, and hopelessness.
Identify realistic ways to assist in the care of the elder.

Modified from Richards M: Family support groups, *Generations* 10(4):68, summer 1986.

Sometimes people just need an opportunity to share the difficulties they are experiencing. Having an attentive listener without any emotional commitment may allow ventilation, release of stored-up feelings, and a restoration of energy to continue in a difficult situation. Some problems are not totally resolvable but may be borne if a supportive network is available, such as help from immediate and extended family and friends. Recognizing this, nurses may see their most important function as sustaining the intimate network of supports.

Rice (1996) points out that families have the option of refusing to provide care if they feel incapable or not so inclined. However, many families do not know this and are reluctant to refuse. As well, there are elders who do not wish to be cared for by family. Family relations that have never been warm or supportive will likely be less so with the dependencies of aging. It is the nurse's responsibility to accept and support the decisions of the aged and their family members in this regard and to alleviate any sense of guilt that may accompany these decisions.

Sibling Supports in Old Age

The late-life sibling support system is poorly understood and neglected by professionals. There are many possible sibling relationships in old age: intimate, congenial, loyal, apathetic, distant, friendly, hostile, advisory, competitive, and envious. For some elders, the significance of siblings grows as one grows old. Siblings share a unique history—a similar biologic and cultural heritage—albeit with numerous variable personal interpretations.

It is common in large families for siblings to have formed childhood alliances that last throughout life. Elder female siblings often have mothering relationships with the youngest siblings, or there may be little, if any, relationship when the chronologic distance is great. Siblings very close in age may have a leader/follower alliance that can be either comforting or irritating to the follower. There are numerous configurations and loyalties. It is interesting for nurses to ask about siblings, particularly ones who are emotionally close and geographically available.

The significance of these long-term parallel surviving relationships cannot be denied. They become particularly important when they are part of the support system, especially among single or widowed elders living alone. Sometimes they band together for economic or psychologic reasons and share living space. Elders seldom rely on siblings for financial help or care during illness but (especially those from larger families) believe the siblings are a backup support that can be called on for moral support and help in emergencies. As one would expect, unmarried and/or widowed siblings were found to be more likely to go to each other for assistance and support. They harbor strong feelings of reciprocity in the relationships. Freedman (1996) found that having even one sibling significantly reduced the likelihood of institutionalization.

The loss of siblings has a profound effect in terms of awareness of one's own mortality, particularly when those of the same gender die. When an elder reaches the age of the sibling who died, the reaction can be quite disruptive. Not only is grieving activated, but rehearsal for one's own death may occur. In cases where an elder sibling survives younger ones, there may be not only a deep grief but also some pangs of guilt: "Why them and not me?"

Grandparenting

Traditionally, expected behavior from grandparents included providing gifts, money, and access to travel for grandchildren; knowledge of family heritage, rituals, news, and folklore; respite for parents; aid in raising the grandchildren; and emotional comfort. In recent years more grandparents have become, by default, the primary caregivers of grandchildren because the parents are incapable of providing the care needed. Major antecedents to this situation are child abuse, imprisonment, joblessness, drug and alcohol addictions, illness, and social problems of the parents (Kelly, 1993). These grandparents have been called the "silent saviors" (Jendrek, 1994). Most say they never intended to parent children again, but when the parents proved unable or unfit to do so, the grandparents stepped into the role. Grandparents are fast becoming a crucial resource on which society and the younger generation increasingly rely. Interestingly, the children raised solely by grandparents seem to maintain health and make good school adjustments (Solomon, Marx, 1995).

Grandparents frequently report financial and health problems related to the additional burden of caring for grandchildren. Nearly half report increased stress, illness, anxiety, and depression (Burton, 1992). In spite of all that, grandmothers tend to report that the grandchildren provide purpose that keeps them going. As this situation becomes more prevalent, organizations are developing to provide resources and assistance for grandparents (see Resources at the end of this chapter).

Jendrek (1994) found three major categories of grandparents assisting in the raising of children: the custodial grandparent, in which case the child lives with the grandparents because of severe problems in the nuclear family; the live-in, in which case the grandparent lives in the home of the grandchild and provides variable amounts of assistance to the family and the grandchild; and the day care provider, in which case the grandparent cares for the child while parents work.

Grandparental functions may include any of the following:

Surrogate parent
Provider of support in times of crisis
Babysitter
Homemaker
Housesitter
Income provider/financial resource
Teacher
Confidant/wise counselor
Keeper of the family heritage

Grandparenting is not a static state but a developmental stage. The grandparent role can be a mutually significant one, with the burden for making it so lying within the realm of the role (Kivett, 1991). Several strategies that are helpful are suggested in Box 23-4. These provide young adult grandchildren with advice, affirmation, and a sense of roots and continuity. The

Respect the rights and desires of parents.

Ask parents before overriding rules of their home.

Interfere in parenting only if the child is in danger of abuse.

When possible, give parents time away from their children.

Share interesting and entertaining anecdotes of parents' childhood.

Share tales of your own childhood.

Write memoirs for grandchildren.

Develop rituals and traditions for special occasions but be flexible.

Spend time with each grandchild individually.

Write, phone, and send amusing cards when child is distant.

Make pages of scrapbook on special childhood occasions.

Develop photo albums of relatives for child to enjoy.

Be aware that grandparents occupy varied roles in a child's life, depending on age and situation.

Remember your own grandparenting, and incorporate the best of it.

young often gain an understanding of aging and mortality through sharing with grandparents. It is a loss to everyone when grandparents are incorporated into family life only as they become feeble and ill. The child will then have a skewed view of what aging means, and it will be a source of dread and avoidance.

Grandparents' memories are stories and can be a special treasure for children. One woman in middle age wished that her grandparents had identified relatives in old snapshots, passed along their favorite recipes, told more about their school days, explained where they had obtained the land they owned, and kept a family tree. These suggestions may be helpful in talking to elders about something useful they might do for their grandchildren. Nurses may find it interesting and useful to discuss the meaning and satisfaction older people find in the grandparenting role. Those who are not grandparents may wish to discuss their feelings about that. If they feel cheated, there are surrogate grandparent roles they may wish to assume, such as those in foster grandparent programs. Grandparents are no longer just the "fun seekers." The diversity of family life-styles and cultural differences have resulted in numerous types of grandparenting. Grandparents' Day is observed the first

Sunday after Labor Day. It is observed nationally, particularly in nursing home settings.

Friendships in Old Age

The significance of friendships in old age has been largely ignored in research. Friendships across the life span can be sustained in the face of overwhelming disasters. They often provide the critical elements of satisfactory living that family may not, providing commitment and affection without judgment, personality characteristics that are compatible because they are chosen, availability without demands, and caring without obligation. Friends may share a long-life perspective or may bring a totally new intergenerational viewpoint into one's life. Late-life friendships often develop out of changing situations such as shared tenancies, widowhood, moves, and involvements in volunteer pursuits (O'Connor, 1993). As desires and pursuits change, some friendships evolve that the persons never would have considered in their youth.

Friends function in many ways: (1) to provide surrogate kin, (2) to ease the loneliness of widowhood or widowerhood, (3) to replace lost siblings, and (4) to validate one's generational viewpoint. Considering the obvious importance of friendship, it seems to be a neglected area of exploration and a seldom-considered resource by professionals assisting the aged.

Relationships may at times be one-sided in terms of benefits, but that seems of little consequence among real friends (Sherman, Antonucci, 1996). The critical issue for women seems to be the opportunity for intimate disclosure within the relationship. This is less significant for men.

Among older men, Akiyama et al (1996) found a distinct shift from same-sex alliances toward the development of more and closer relationships with women, possibly because there are more women in the older men's network as they move out of work relationships and as male life expectancy diminishes. If married, they become more involved in their wives' activities; possibly because of frailty and dependency, they are more comfortable with women.

Nurses may help older people to maintain and revive old friendships by assisting them in letter writing, taking care to deliver phone messages, and discussing the nature of friendships. When considering an elder's needs, nurses should assess the size, composition, and structure of the person's friendship network, the nature of the needed task, and the person's feelings about receiving certain types of help from friends. New friendships are facilitated by the opportunity for both closeness and distance. The impact of loss of a close friend seems dependent to some extent on the number of other close friends who remain in the network, particularly if the friend was mutual and the remaining friends share the loss. Friends are an excellent reservoir of strength, support, and help when needed. Finally, the importance of intergenerational friendships should be mentioned. These often sustain the old and illuminate the young.

Contributions of the Old to Family Life

Although the focus of this chapter primarily relates to the needs of the old in relation to their families, the flow of help from adult child to parent is not unidirectional. The aged provide a family history perspective, models for growing old, assistance with grandchildren, a sense of continuity, and a philosophy of aging. In many cases the old continue to contribute money, gifts, status, and services to their adult children. Soldo and Hill (1993) contend that it is far more likely that elderly parents will give financial help to children and grandchildren than it is that they will receive it.

In addition, if one moves beyond the moment, it is apparent that the old have contributed their time and energy across the adult life span to provide opportunities for their children. Perhaps even more important, they appreciate the success of their children and convey their approval and pride. Although adults are motivated in the process of maturation more by personal motivation than by external motivation, there is still pleasure in knowing that one's parents are pleased with various accomplishments. Just as Scott-Maxwell (1968) noted the tendency to always remain a parent concerned about the development of one's child, so the adult child benefits from the interest of the parent.

Not only mature adults but also their children benefit from the influence of a vital old person. They provide anticipatory socialization into old age. Elders often serve as "kin-keepers." *Kin-keeper* is a term used to denote a family member who arranges get-togethers, develops the family history and rituals, and in other ways promotes solidarity and unity among the kin (Rosenthal, 1985).

Consider the example of Grandma Daisy, who always merited a special visit from any of the kin in her vast Northwestern network. A pioneer settler in her small community, she knew the names, ages, and whereabouts of the children and spouses and the grand-

children and spouses of all of her eight children. They seldom saw each other but always felt a connecting link through Grandma Daisy. When she died at age 94, a great portion of the family history and sense of solidarity died with her. She was a true kin-keeper.

ABUSE AND NEGLECT OF THE AGED

The terms *abuse* and *neglect of the elderly* are used to describe situations in which individuals over the age of 65 experience battering, verbal abuse, exploitation, denial of rights, forced confinement, neglected medical needs, or other types of personal harm, usually at the hands of someone responsible for assisting them in their activities of daily living (ADLs) (Fulmer, O'Malley, 1987).

In a society becoming increasingly more violent, it is reasonable to assume that abuse of elders and other vulnerable persons will continue to increase. Estimates are that from 1.5 to 2 million adults experience abuse or neglect each year in the United States (Aravanis et al, 1993). The National Center on Elder Abuse (1996) estimated the number to be between 1 million and 2 million. It is impossible to get an accurate estimate because there is no place where elders are routinely exposed to scrutiny, as in the case of children in school.

Although we often think of physical abuse as the most likely form, one study found that 46% of substantiated charges were of financial exploitation (Shiferaw et al, 1994). Many situations of abuse arise around family conflicts. Verbal abuse and neglect have been found to be significantly related to long-standing problems in the relationship and occur long before caregiving is necessary. Often the abuse is precipitated or augmented by alcohol abuse. The caregivers may willingly talk about their difficulties, but the elders rarely do so. Neglect by self and other is by far the most frequent type of mistreatment (Fig. 23-4). Nurses must remember that elders are often embarrassed or afraid to admit that they are being abused or neglected.

Increasing awareness of neglect and abuse of elders has led the American Medical Association (AMA) (1992) to issue guidelines for the identification and treatment of abuse. The AMA has identified five classifications of elder abuse: (1) physical or sexual abuse, (2) psychologic abuse, (3) exploitation (misuse of assets), (4) medical abuse (withholding necessary treatment or aids for ADLs), and (5) neglect.

There are many reasons for abuse beyond the typically identified frustration and exhaustion of a caregiver.

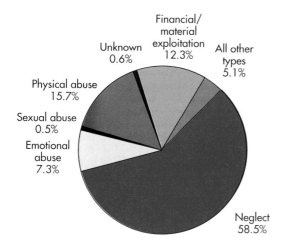

Fig. 23-4   Types of domestic elder abuse. (From Tatara T, Blumerman LM: *Elder abuse in domestic settings,* Elder Abuse Informational Series, No 3, Washington, DC, 1996, National Center on Elder Abuse.)

Some of the others include psychopathology of the abuser (often also includes alcoholism), extreme dependency of the elder, turbulent life-styles, and lack of resources (financial, emotional, family, community). The AMA guidelines suggest that practitioners ask direct questions to determine the presence and nature of abuse. However, elders often refuse to divulge information because of loyalty or fear of reprisal. The National Center on Elder Abuse has provided clear definitions and signs of the various types of abuse that provide guidelines for health professionals (see Appendix 23-A).

Dynamics of Abuse

The abuser is most usually thought to be an adult child, but the abusers are more often spouses. Elder abuse may be spouse abuse grown old and reversed. Wives who are caregivers may abuse their frail husbands, possibly in retaliation for past abuse. On the other hand, it must be acknowledged that the abuse or neglect could have commenced with old age and that elderly men are much more likely to be living with a spouse than are elderly women.

There are undoubtedly numerous cultural differences in identification and definitions of abuse. Given our diverse society, this must be taken under consideration. Moon and Williams (1993) obtained responses from black, white, and Korean-American elderly women regarding their perceptions of abusive situa-

tions. The Korean-Americans were much less likely than the others to perceive a given situation as abusive. Additional studies in this respect would be enlightening and particularly important in identification and intervention. There is no universal acceptance of actions that constitute abuse.

Frail elders are most often cared for in the home, and the demands of such care on the family are thought to increase the incidence of abuse. Alzheimer's disease and other dementias are particularly intolerable. Caretakers sometimes admit that they have pinched, kicked, bit, struck, or shoved the elder in their care.

Abuse predictive factors to consider include socialization to abusive actions, pathologic or authoritarian personality characteristics that increase tolerance for abuse infliction, decreased tolerance for stress, inability to provide satisfactory care, intolerance for the intimacy of caregiving, and vulnerability of the victim. There is speculation that some abusive persons are abused in retaliation as they become old and frail.

One dynamic of abuse that has not been seriously explored is that of the son who must care for an incontinent mother. The deep societal abhorrence of incest and particularly the taboo against a sexualized mother/son relationship may produce an irrationally strong response to the necessity of exposing a mother's perineum when giving care. Nurses may provide some anticipatory guidance and understanding when dealing with such cases. Reassurance that the nurse understands how difficult this can be may reduce the revulsion and anxiety the caregiving son feels. Vulnerability factors have been summarized by Frost and Willette (1994) (Table 23-1).

Studies provide profiles of abusive situations, family dysfunction, and abusive persons, but none could be found that address macro issues such as climatic conditions, seasons, culture, geographic differences, disaster situations, excessive political pressures, and stressors. For instance, are farm or urban/suburban families more inclined toward abuse and neglect, in the South or North, in summer or winter, following floods or preceding tax deadlines? Will tax relief for the expense of caring for an elder change the prevalence of abuse? When a family depends on the elder's Social Security or Supplemental Security Income, does that have an effect on how abusive they may be? These and many other questions that might shed light on the general topic of abuse seem not to have been asked or given serious consideration. We know only that the incidence is rising rapidly throughout society and toward all vulnerable persons.

Table 23-1

Assessment of Elderly Vulnerability

General assessment	Specifics
Physiologic	Diminished endurance/weakness
	Decreased mobility/ambulation/range of motion, unstable ambulation
	Bruises easily, often evidence of ecchymosis
	Decreased cardiac output
	Ineffective airway
	Shortness of breath interferes with activities of daily living (ADLs)
	Unstable blood glucose
	Inability to speak
	Altered vision
	Poor nutritional or fluid intake
	Incontinence
	Fragile skin integrity (breaks in skin or potential for)
	Potential infection
	Unable to see wound
	Numbness
	Dizziness
	Dysphagia
Environmental	Factors that create safety concerns in and outside the home
	Potential for falls
	Injuries from various sources in and outside the home
Cognitive	Knowledge deficit
	Signs of brain dysfunction/poor memory
	Confusion
Psychosocial	Lacks confidence in self-care abilities
	Absence of social supports
	Loneliness
	Overwhelmed by treatment
	Anxiety about caregiver's health
	Depression
Caregiver	Dependence on caregiver with limited physical abilities
	Dependence on caregiver with limited mental abilities
	Need for caregiver respite
	Nonacceptance of caregiver
Other	Need for physical assistance
	Self-care deficits
	Inability to adhere to medication or treatment regimens

Modified from Frost MH, Willette K: Risk for abuse/neglect: documentation of assessment data and diagnosis, *J Gerontol Nurs* 20(8):37, 1994.

Abuse and Neglect in Home Care

Most abuse of elders occurs within the home by family, but it also occurs with appalling frequency by hired caregivers in the home. Reports of problems include the following: inadequate supervision of patient care, poor coordination of services, inadequate staff training, theft and fraud, drug and alcohol abuse by staff, tardiness and absenteeism, unprofessional and criminal conduct, and inadequate record keeping. Theft of belongings seems to be the most common problem, and the aged who have complained are often dismissed as "confused" or "paranoid." More frequently than we know, undue influence is exerted on the elder, and a companion or home care provider will manage to convince the elder to transfer assets and even the deed to the home. These situations are being examined more carefully in the courts, and some states are activating legal protections against undue influence (Quinn, Tomita, 1997; Quinn, 1999).

The number and diversity of providers, both licensed and unlicensed, make monitoring of care extremely difficult. In a personal conversation, a director of one home care agency said, "Yes, we know it happens, even though all our people are bonded. We really can't do much as we don't witness the abuse and we do not inventory homes, so what can we prove?"

It is clear that even though it may be costly, more care must be exerted in investigating the background of workers who are sent into the home to care for the dependent aged, and their work must be monitored more closely.

Assessment

Risk factors include a history of mental illness, alcohol/drug abuse, a family history of violence, isolation of the victim, a limited social network, minority status, a stressful life-style for the victim and/or abuser, the presence of dementia, behavioral problems, incontinence, and the need to be fed. Dimensions of maltreatment include deprivation; verbal, physical, psychologic, material, and sexual abuse; violation of rights; passive and active neglect; and financial exploitation. To make an adequate assessment, it is necessary to observe the living arrangements and evaluate the financial status, social supports, interactions of family members, and emotional stressors in the present situation (Lachs et al, 1994; Paris et al, 1995).

Elder abuse tends to be episodic and recurrent rather than an isolated event (Lett, 1995). Thus, it is also important to review past records of accidents and emergency room visits that may create a "high index of suspicion" when taken in total (Kingston, Penhale, 1995). Assessment of mistreatment involves several components as noted in Box 23-5.

Interventions

The goals of intervention are to stop exploitation of elders, protect the victim and society from inappropriate

---

Box 23-5   EVALUATIVE COMPONENTS OF MISTREATMENT

- Safety of elder: Is the elder in immediate danger?
- What can be done immediately to increase safety?
- Are there barriers to reaching the elder (cognitive, family interference, emotional)?
- Are adequate physical, social, and financial resources available to properly care for the elder?
- What medical problems may make the elderly particularly vulnerable to abuse and neglect?
- What type of mistreatment has occurred, how frequently, and of what severity?

---

and illegal acts, hold perpetrators of mistreatment accountable, rehabilitate the offender, and order restitution of property and payment for expenses incurred as a result of the perpetrator's conduct. The rules of the court dictate the procedures to accomplish these goals. Both civil and criminal laws require that the accused be given notice of what they have allegedly done (Heisler, Quinn, 1993). This may create additional problems for the victim unless immediate removal from the abusive setting can be accomplished. Few states have legal alternatives that can quickly be brought to play to immediately remove the elder to a protected situation.

There are three basic dynamics of abuse: the psychopathologic, the learned, and situational stress causation. The design of appropriate interventions depends on understanding the dynamic, since each requires different strategies of intervention.

The *psychopathologic dynamic* presents the greatest challenge and generally requires removal of the offender or the elder from the situation, perhaps by legal intervention.

Learned abuse, theoretically, can be unlearned and may respond to a close working relationship with a mentoring professional who can demonstrate positive problem solving and new ways of managing difficult situations.

Most frequent are the *stress-related situations.* These are responsive to almost anything that eases the burden: removal of the stressor (often this is the elder), support groups for ventilation of frustrations and peer support, respite, crisis hot lines, professional consultation, victim support groups, victim volunteer companions, and, above all, thoughtful and compassionate care for the victim and the perpetrator (Wolf, Pillemer, 1994; Reis, Nahmiash, 1995; Quinn, Tomita, 1997).

Preventive interventions include the following (Patwell, 1988):

- Make professionals aware of potentially abusive situations.
- Educate the public about normal aging processes.
- Help families develop and nurture informal support systems.
- Link families with support groups.
- Teach families stress management techniques.
- Arrange comprehensive care resources.
- Provide counseling for troubled families.
- Encourage the use of respite care and day care.
- Obtain necessary home health care services.
- Inform families of resources for meals and transportation.
- Encourage caregivers to pursue their individual interests.

Reis and Nahmiash (1995) have developed a process protocol for the identification and subsequent actions to be taken in cases of elder abuse (Box 23-6). The essential elements are the availability of advice teams that can design health, financial, and legal supports for victims and an available "buddy" to provide personal attention, assistance, companionship, and advocacy. In addition, the "buddy" would quite obviously provide respite for the usual caregiver.

Mandatory Reporting

Most states now have mandatory laws requiring the reporting of elder mistreatment. Nurses must be aware of the definitions and reporting policies within their area of practice. Even though the intent of mandatory reporting laws is protection of the abused person, at times it can create more abuse unless immediate action for removal is taken.

The procedure for reporting suspected elder abuse is explained by DeLong (1995) and may entail any of the following actions:

- If you work in an agency or hospital, call the social worker or social service department to report the problem and manage the case.
- Call the elder abuse hot line listed in the front of the telephone book for advice and assistance; often counseling for the abused and abusers is also available.
- If there is immediate danger to the victim, it is best to call the police.
- Contact adult protective services to alert them to investigate.
- A written report, including the name, sex, race, and address of the abused and the type of abuse that occurred, must be filed promptly. Careful documentation is important. Some say to identify the suspected abuser, but we believe that great caution must be exerted in this respect lest someone be accused inaccurately.

Box 23-6	IDENTIFICATION AND SUBSEQUENT ACTION FOR ELDER ABUSE

Team

- BASE: *Brief Abuse Screen for the Elderly*—screens abuse: specifies types, sources of abuse, urgency for treatment.
- Abuse Checklist
- The Intervention Teams *Home Care Team:* Trained Basic Intervention unit: screens using the Tool Package, intervenes.
- *Multidisciplinary Team:* about three to five home care team members: confirm/disconfirm abuse (using the BASE); brainstorm, plan, monitor, and evaluate intervention strategies.
- *Empowerment Support Group:* Victims discuss problems, strengths, solutions, resources, appropriate responses.
- *The Community Senior Abuse Committee:* An independent group of volunteers: arrange programs and publications to educate/sensitize the community to abuse; advocacy functions; liaison with home care team members.

Interventions

1. Abuse cases are tagged. The initial intervention strategies are planned and implemented. Screens abuse; specifies caregiver/care receiver indicators for intervention focus.
2. Home care team members make initial home visits to further assess and make written plans. They brainstorm the case with the multidisciplinary team and consult with the expert consultant team for specialized advice and help. They enlist specialized advice and additional assistance as needed (e.g., buddies, empowerment group). They improve and continue the planned intervention strategies.
3. Empowerment group works to improve self-esteem, active responding; increase personal control and empowerment of victims.
4. Committee refers clients, volunteers to the intervention; provides community involvement in combating abuse.

Modified from Reis M, Nahmiash D: When seniors are abused; an intervention model, *Gerontologist* 35(5):667, 1995.

LEGAL PROTECTIONS FOR THE VULNERABLE AGED

Nurses have rarely had sufficient exposure to the legalities of the court system to make decisions regarding the protection of the vulnerable aged, especially in cases where there may be some mistreatment. For the most part, these situations occur when the elder is either not strong enough or competent enough to exert measures to protect his or her own interests. A review of state statutes on conservatorship and guardianship will clarify specifics. It may be necessary to contact a geriatric legal counselor in your area. These can be found through your county's legal services to the elderly and are listed in the phone book.

Conservatorships

Many aged persons are judged incapable of managing their finances or their basic needs and are given adult protective services under the laws of conservatorship, which vary from state to state. *Conservatorship* generally means that a court-appointed conservator (who may be a family member) makes decisions about where an individual lives and how his or her needs are met. Conservatorship hearings are presented in court at periodic intervals to determine necessity for continuation. Limits are set according to the degree of protection needed. *Total dependency* means the person cannot meet basic needs for survival and is unable to manage the environment in any self-sustaining way. *Some dependency* means the person may be able to manage certain challenges of life; health or judgment may interfere with management of other needs. Conservatorships (termed *guardianships* in some states) are the most legally restricting way that an individual's person and property can be handled short of imprisonment or commitment to a locked mental health facility.

A conservator of person may be appointed for a person who is unable to properly provide for his or her personal needs for physical health, food, clothing, or shelter. A conservator of the estate may be appointed for a person who is substantially unable to manage his or her own financial resources or resist fraud or undue influence. Substantial inability may not be proved solely by isolated incidents of negligence or improvidence.

Guardianships

The reliance on legal guardianships is increasing as a result of the numbers of vulnerable elders who are surviving and the effect on families and communities.

However, even with the best of intentions, these can lead to further decline in the elders' capacities as they relinquish decision-making power. It has usually been assumed that guardianships have been instituted for the protection of an elder who needs help. Now, reforms are being instituted because it is increasingly realized that sometimes persons seeking guardianship of an elder are acting in their own interests and may take advantage of the elder (Heisler, Quinn, 1993).

Adult Protective Services

The term *adult protective services* refers to a wide range of services—medical, social, and legal—that are delivered to the frail, endangered elderly. Many referrals for adult protective services involve reports from persons concerned that an elder is unable to care for self (self-neglect) (Lachs et al, 1996).

Programs vary from one community to another. There are many gaps in services. The frail, vulnerable old usually need several services at one time. Coordination among the various service providers (i.e., community health nurses, social workers, physicians, clinic nurses, discharge planners, lawyers, clergy members, family, and friends) is necessary lest the elder feel invaded. Team coordination and case management are essential and are apparent in good health maintenance organizations (HMOs). When intervening with the frail, vulnerable elderly, the following fundamentals must guide decisions:
1. The vulnerable adult client is the primary person the nurse is serving.
2. When interests compete, the aged adult client is in charge of decision making until he or she delegates responsibility voluntarily to another or until the court grants responsibility to another.
3. Freedom is more important than safety; that is, the person can choose to live in harm or even self-destructively provided that he or she is capable of choosing, does not harm others, and commits no crimes.
4. Protection of vulnerable adults strives to achieve the following (in order of importance): freedom, safety, least disruption of life-style, and least restrictive care (Quinn, 1989).

Power of Attorney

Power of attorney is a legal device that affords some assistance in handling legal affairs. It can be valid only if the person granting the power of attorney is capable of doing so. There are three types, one of which, the durable power of attorney, is valid even after mental impairment has set in. There is no bonding involved as there is with conservatorships, so there is less protection for the frail person. Nevertheless, it is helpful and appropriate for some people.

Assessment

When older people are in need of adult protective services, they are upset and often deny the need. Family and friends are usually equally distressed. Perhaps they are exhausted from trying to help the impaired person over a long period of time. Maybe the elder is demanding, even hostile. People in need of help may be confused, frightened, dependent, and unwilling or unable to make decisions for themselves. Often, there is pressure on the worker to "do something—now." But help and services, except in emergencies, cannot be adequate without thoughtful, interdisciplinary conferences with family and client. Generally, assessment goes forward at the pace the client can tolerate, although some services may need to be put in place as the assessment proceeds. Priorities must be developed.

Interventions

Nurses would do well to familiarize themselves with the laws that specifically affect older adults in their state. This can be done by speaking with an attorney or selecting continuing education programs to update knowledge in the field of client legal protections.

Once informed of the laws affecting frail elders, nurses are in a position to assist elders and family members in seeking legal representation when necessary. For instance, knowing conservatorship and guardianship law would enable the nurse to guide family members and elders to appropriate individuals for assistance in the process of filing for conservatorship or guardianship when necessary.

Nurses can also help conservators and guardians fulfill their roles through careful documentation of clients' status and family interactions. Families may need considerable encouragement and assistance to assume increased responsibility for the affairs of aged members.

Advocacy

Because so many older frail people cannot speak for themselves, nurses often find themselves in the position of having to do the "talking"—being an advocate. An advocate is one who maintains or promotes a cause; defends, pleads, or acts on behalf of a cause for another;

fights for someone who cannot fight; and often gets involved in getting someone to do something he or she would not otherwise do.

Many frail elders' situations seem globally desperate to middle-class workers not used to extreme hardships in life. In these situations the danger exists that workers will "overadvocate" and bring in services the client really does not want and cannot use. An advocate needs to be clear at all times just whose position and needs are being met. The client is the focus.

Topics for advocacy can include protection of specific rights, such as promoting the least restrictive alternative for a client, finding the best nursing home, or telling court personnel one's opinion of a proposed conservator. Other areas include the rights of medical patients, the right to have in-home supportive services, and maintenance of government benefits such as veterans' benefits, Medicare, Social Security (SS) and Supplemental Security Income (SSI), and food stamps.

Advocates function in various arenas: with their own and other disciplines within their own agencies, with other agencies, with physicians, with families, with neighbors and community representatives, with legislators, and with courts when conservatorships are at issue.

STRENGTHENING THE PRIMARY SUPPORT SYSTEMS

In this era of diverse life-styles and family patterns, it is becoming increasingly important to preserve the integrity of the primary support systems. There is a prevalent feeling in the United States that too little is being done to help families maintain their elders. The aged, when needing assistance, must rely on the good will and intentions of those closest to them, whether nuclear or extended family, alternative family systems, friends, or neighbors. Support networks, families, and others are made up of ordinary people with needs, frailties, and frustrations. Each participant sometimes functions well and sometimes barely. At times it becomes necessary to bring legal action into situations that become destructive or dysfunctional. Considerable effort is needed to preserve the integrity of primary support systems in some situations, yet without these systems life loses meaning. Making resources available that decrease stress and increase effectiveness may restore the balance of the system. A particularly important nursing function is to make individuals fully aware of the bonds that connect them and the special qualities each person appreciates of the other.

▶ **KEY CONCEPTS**

- The aged and each of their family members carry a long history. Current family dynamics must be understood within the context of family history.
- Sibling relationships may increase in importance during old age as individuals cope with various losses.
- Grandparenting is a significant role among elders. Frequently grandparents are the primary provider for young children and function as parents.
- Caregiving of elderly parents is one of the major social issues of our times. Adult children most often will spend some time caring for aged parents.
- "Parenting" one's parents is a commonly used misnomer. Parents, no matter how vulnerable, do not become children. The life they have lived must be considered regardless of the present situation.
- Women most often provide the "hands-on" care, whereas men are more frequently involved in the economic and practical aspects of caregiving.
- Frail elders are generally considered to be those who are in tenuous physiologic, mental, or emotional balance and maintain their integrity within a small margin.
- Vulnerable elders are those who are placed under the legal protections of another who may or may not advocate or make decisions to their best advantage.
- Vulnerable elders are also those who live in situations that are potentially neglectful or outright abusive.

NANDA and Wellness Diagnoses

Wellness	Specific Needs	NANDA
	Self-actualization	
Seeks stimulating interests Explores new ventures of family Deals ethically with different decisions	Ethics Fulfillment	Parenting, altered Role performance, altered
	Self-esteem	
Carries out appropriate role responsibly Recognizes each member's contributions Expresses appreciation	Recognition Respect Control Appreciation	Social isolation Caregiver role strain Decisional conflict Role performance, altered
	Belonging	
Accepts limitations of each member Avoids scapegoating Expresses tenderness Is sexually appropriate	Acceptance Belonging Tenderness Sexuality	Caregiver role strain Coping, ineffective family, disabling Family processes, altered
	Safety and security	
Discusses problems and solutions Checks perceptions with others Is assured of protection	Problem solving Reality perception Protection	Violence, risk for: directed at others Protection, altered Caregiver role strain Coping, ineffective family: compromised Family processes, altered
	Biologic integrity	
Gives consideration to family, individual biologic needs Receives regular physical care Monitors health problems	Rest/sleep Health maintenance	Caregiver role strain Health maintenance, altered Sleep deprivation

These are not all of the possible wellness or NANDA diagnoses that may be identified. The above are frequent examples of nursing diagnoses that should be considered when planning care for the older adult in whatever setting.

- Abuse may be physical, financial, psychologic, or extreme neglect, either intentional or unintentional.
- Adult protective services are usually public agencies who oversee the care of the vulnerable aged. There are some privately founded and funded adult protective services, and at times these have been found to take financial advantage of those under their protection.
- Nursing responsibilities are to be alert to signs of abuse and neglect of an elder and to report known cases to the appropriate state agency, as required by law.
- Abusive situations can emerge from overburdened caregivers who have little assistance, great frustration, and little respite.
- Abusive situations also often arise as a result of substance abuse by willing or unwilling caregivers.
- Elders rarely report family members who abuse them because they are uncertain whether an alternative situation would be an improvement.
- Nursing responsibilities include assisting caregivers in finding resources to alleviate or partially relieve a stressful situation.

▶ Activities and Discussion Questions

1. Discuss your position in the family and how that has affected your relationship with siblings and parents.
2. What do you suppose your role will be when your parent or parents need help?
3. Write a brief essay discussing the ways in which your grandparents have affected your life.
4. What would you find most difficult in regard to assisting your aged parent?
5. In what ways are nurses involved in protection of the rights of elders?
6. Discuss with a group the situations you have encountered in which you felt an elder was vulnerable or had been mistreated. What were the factors that influenced your feelings about this situation?

RESOURCES

National Alliance for Caregiving
4720 Montgomery Lane, Suite 642
Bethesda, MD 20814
(301) 718-8444; (301) 652-7711 (fax)

National Center on Elder Abuse
c/o American Public Welfare Association
810 First Street NE, Suite 500
Washington, DC 20002-4267
AARP Grandparent Information Center
American Association of Retired Persons
601 E Street NW
Washington, DC 20049

REFERENCES

Akiyama H, Elliott K, Antonucci TC: Same-sex and cross-sex relationships, *J Gerontol* 51B(6):P374, 1996.

American Association of Homes and Services for the Aging: Burden weighs heavy on caregivers: study, *Currents* 11(4):2, 1996.

American Medical Association: *AMA issues guidelines for physicians to treat abused, neglected elderly,* News release, Chicago, Nov 23, 1992, The Association.

Aravanis SC et al: Diagnostic and treatment guidelines on elder abuse and neglect, *Arch Fam Med* 2(4):371, 1993.

Boaz RF: *Full-time employment and informal caregiving in the 1980s,* Paper presented at the meeting of the Gerontological Society of America, Washington, DC, Nov 19, 1996.

Brody EM et al: Marital status of daughters and patterns of care, *J Gerontol* 49(2):S95, 1994.

Burton LM: Black grandparents rearing children of drug addicted parents: stressors, outcomes and social service needs, *Gerontologist* 32(6):744, 1992.

Camberg L et al: *Methods to evaluate an audiotape intervention for Alzheimer's patients,* Paper presented at the meeting of the Gerontological Society of America, Washington, DC, Nov 19, 1996.

DeLong MF: Part I: Elder abuse, *NurseWeek* 8(4):11, 1995.

Family Caregiver Alliance: Selected caregiver statistics, *Family Caregiver Alliance Newsletter* V IV(2):2, 1996.

Feinberg LF, Kelly KA: A well-deserved break: respite programs offered by California's statewide system of caregiver resource centers, *Gerontologist* 35(5):701, 1995.

Freedman VA: Family structure and the risk of nursing home admission, *J Gerontol* 51B(2):S61, 1996.

Frost MH, Willette K: Risk for abuse/neglect: documentation of assessment data and diagnoses, *J Gerontol Nurs* 20(8):37, 1994.

Fulmer T, O'Malley T: *Inadequate care of the elderly: a health care perspective on abuse and neglect,* New York, 1987, Springer.

George LK, Gwyther LP: *Duke University caregiver well-being survey,* Durham, NC, 1983, Duke University Center for the Study of Aging and Human Development.

George LK, Gwyther LP: Caregiver well-being: a multidimensional examination of family caregivers of demented adults, *Gerontologist* 26:253, 1986.

Georgemiller R, Iacono G, Browne E: Factors related to coping in caretakers of cognitively impaired elderly, *Proceedings of the*

Third Congress of the International Psychogeriatric Association 3:36, 1987. Summary of presentations. (abstract) Rochester, Minn, Mayo Foundation for Medical Education and Research.

Heisler CJ, Quinn MJ: A legal perspective. In Johnson TF, editor: *Elder mistreatment: ethical issues, dilemmas, and decisions,* New York, 1993, Haworth.

Hoffman D: Complaints of a dutiful daughter, *Alzheimer's Caregiver* 9(1):1, 1996.

Jendrek MP: Grandparents who parent their grandchildren: circumstances and decisions, *Gerontologist* 34(2):206, 1994.

Kelly SJ: Caregiver stress in grandparents raising grandchildren, *Image J Nurs Sch* 25(4):331, 1993.

Kingston P, Penhale B: Elder abuse and neglect: issues in the accident and emergency department, *Accid Emerg Nurs* 3(3):122, 1995.

Kivett VR: The grandparent-grandchild connection, *Marriage Fam Rev* 16(3/4):267, 1991.

Lachs MS et al: A prospective community-based pilot study of risk factors for the investigation of elder mistreatment, *J Am Geriatr Soc* 42(2):169, 1994.

Lachs MS et al: Older adults: an 11-year longitudinal study of adult protective service use, *Arch Intern Med* 156(4):449, 1996.

Lett JE: Abuse of the elderly, *J Fla Med Assoc* 82(10):675, 1995.

Moen P, Robison J, Fields V: Women's work and caregiving roles: a life course approach, *J Gerontol* 49(4):S176, 1994.

Moon A, Williams O: Perceptions of elder abuse and help-seeking patterns among African-American, Caucasian-American, and Korean-American elderly women, *Gerontologist* 33(3):386, 1993.

National Alliance for Caregiving: *Family caregiver fact sheet,* Bethesda, Md, 1997, The Alliance.

National Center on Elder Abuse: *Elder abuse in domestic settings,* Elder abuse informational series, No 3, Washington, DC, 1996, The Center.

O'Connor P: Same-gender and cross-gender friendships among the frail elderly, *Gerontologist* 33(1):24, 1993.

Older Women's League (OWL): *Administration on aging awards support for national caregiving information project,* OWL press release, Washington, DC, 1992, The League.

Paris BE et al: Elder abuse and neglect: how to recognize the warning signs and intervene, *Geriatrics* 50(4):47, 1995.

Patwell T: Familial abuse of the elderly: a look at caregiver potential and prevention, *Home Healthc Nurse* 4(2):10, 1988.

Pratt C et al: Burden and coping strategies of caregivers to Alzheimer's patients, *Fam Relations* 34(1):27, 1985.

Quinn M, Director, San Francisco City and County Probate Court: Personal communication, June, 1999.

Quinn M: Probate conservatorships and guardianships: assessment and curative aspects, *J Elder Abuse Neglect* 1(1):91, 1989.

Quinn M, Tomita S: *Elder abuse and neglect: causes, diagnosis, and intervention strategies,* ed 2, New York, 1997, Springer.

Rankin ED, Haut MW, Keefover RW: Clinical assessment of family caregivers of dementia, *Gerontologist* 32(6):813, 1992.

Reis M, Nahmiash D: When seniors are abused: an intervention model, *Gerontologist* 35(5):666, 1995.

Rice R: *Home health nursing practice: concepts and application,* ed 2, St Louis, 1996, Mosby.

Rosenthal CJ: Kinkeeping in the familial division of labor, *J Marriage Fam* 47:965, 1985.

Rosenthal CJ, Martin-Matthews A, Matthews SH: Caught in the middle? Occupancy in multiple roles and help to parents in a national probability sample of Canadian adults, *J Gerontol* 51B(6):S274, 1996.

Schwartz D, Kelly C: Personal communication, Sept 16, 1996, Gwynedd, Pa.

Scott-Maxwell E: *The measure of my days,* New York, 1968, Knopf.

Sheehan NW: The caregiver information project: a mechanism to assist religious leaders to help family caregivers, *Gerontologist* 29(5):703, 1989.

Sherman A, Antonucci T: *Reciprocity in best friend relationships,* Paper presented at the meeting of the Gerontological Society of America, Washington, DC, Nov 18, 1996.

Shiferaw B et al: The investigation and outcome of reported cases of elder abuse: the Forsyth county aging study, *Gerontologist* 34(1):123, 1994.

Soldo BJ, Hill MS: Intergeneration transfers: economic, demographic and social perspectives. In Maddox GL, Lawton MP, editors: *Annual review of gerontology and geriatrics,* vol 13, New York, 1993, Springer.

Solomon JC, Marx J: To grandmother's house we go: health and school adjustment of children raised solely by grandparents, *Gerontologist* 35(3):386, 1995.

Stephens MAP: *Day care and family strain: testing the effects of interventions.* Paper presented at the meeting of the Gerontological Society of America, Washington, DC, Nov 19, 1996.

Tobin S, Fulimer E, Smith GC: Coping with a developmentally disabled offspring. In Thomas E, Eisenhandler S, editors: *Aging and the religious dimension,* Westport, Conn, 1994, Auburn House.

Townsend AL, Franks MM: Binding ties: closeness and conflict in adult children's caregiving relationships, *Psychol Aging* 10(3):343, 1995.

Vinick BH, Lanspery S, Hoy E: *Stepfamilies in later life: a neglected area of research.* Paper presented at the meeting of the Gerontological Society of America, Washington, DC, Nov 20, 1996.

Wolanin M: Personal communication, 1979, San Francisco.

Wolf RS, Pillemer K: What's new in elder abuse programming? Four bright ideas, *Gerontologist* 34(1):126, 1994.

Zarit SH: Methodological considerations in caregiver intervention and outcome research. In Lebowitz BD, Light E, Niederche G, editors: *Alzheimer's disease and family stress,* Rockville, Md, 1991, National Institute of Mental Health.

Zusman RM: Oldest old. In Maddox GL, editor: *The encyclopedia of aging: a comprehensive resource in gerontology and geriatrics,* New York, 1995, Springer.

Appendix 23-A *The National Elder Abuse Incidence Study*

DEFINITIONS OF DOMESTIC ELDER ABUSE, EXPLOITATION, AND NEGLECT

The following definitions of domestic elder abuse, exploitation, and neglect pertain to elders living in domestic settings. The perpetrator of this abuse may or may not be the caregiver of an elderly person or a member of the elderly person's family. Furthermore, some signs and symptoms are characteristic of several kinds of maltreatment and should be regarded as indicators of possible maltreatment. The most important of these are:
- an elder's frequent unexplained crying; and
- an elder's unexplained fear of or suspicion of a particular person(s) in the home.

Physical abuse is defined as the use of physical force that *may* result in bodily injury, physical pain, or impairment. Physical abuse may include but is not limited to such acts of violence as striking (with or without an object), hitting, beating, pushing, shoving, shaking, slapping, kicking, pinching, and burning. In addition, the inappropriate use of drugs and physical restraints, force-feeding, and physical punishment of any kind also are examples of physical abuse.

Signs and symptoms of physical abuse include but are not limited to:
- bruises, black eyes, welts, lacerations, and rope marks;
- bone fractures, broken bones, and skull fractures;
- open wounds, cuts, punctures, untreated injuries, and injuries in various stages of healing;
- sprains, dislocations, and internal injuries/bleeding;
- broken eyeglasses/frames, physical signs of being subjected to punishment, and signs of being restrained;
- laboratory findings of medication overdose or underutilization of prescribed drugs;
- an elder's report of being hit, slapped, kicked, or mistreated;
- an elder's sudden change in behavior; and
- the caregiver's refusal to allow visitors to see an elder alone.

Sexual abuse is defined as nonconsensual sexual contact of any kind with an elderly person. Sexual contact with any person incapable of giving consent also is considered sexual abuse. It includes but is not limited to unwanted touching, all types of sexual assault or battery such as rape, sodomy, coerced nudity, and sexually explicit photographing.

Signs and symptoms of sexual abuse include but are not limited to:
- bruises around the breasts or genital area;
- unexplained venereal disease or genital infections;
- unexplained vaginal or anal bleeding;
- torn, stained, or bloody underclothing; and
- an elder's report of being sexually assaulted or raped.

Emotional or psychological abuse is defined as the infliction of anguish, pain, or distress through verbal or nonverbal acts. Emotional/psychological abuse includes but is not limited to verbal assaults, insults, threats, intimidation, humiliation, and harassment. In addition, treating an older person like an infant; isolating an elderly person from his/her family, friends, or regular activities; giving an older person a "silent treatment"; and enforced social isolation also are examples of emotional/psychological abuse.

Signs and symptoms of emotional/psychological abuse may manifest themselves in such behaviors of an elderly person as:
- being emotionally upset or agitated;
- being extremely withdrawn and noncommunicative or nonresponsive;
- unusual behavior usually attributed to dementia (e.g., sucking, biting, rocking); and
- an elder's report of being verbally or emotionally mistreated.

Neglect is defined as the refusal or failure to fulfill any part of a person's obligations or duties to an elder. Neglect may also include a person who has fiduciary responsibilities to provide care for an elder (e.g., pay for necessary home care services, or the failure on the part of an in-home service provider to provide necessary care). Neglect typically means the refusal or failure to provide an elderly person with such life necessities as food, water, clothing, shelter, personal hygiene, medicine, comfort, personal safety, and other essentials included in the responsibility or agreement to an elder.

Signs and symptoms of neglect include but are not limited to:
- dehydration, malnutrition, untreated bedsores, and poor personal hygiene;

From National Center on Elder Abuse: Elder abuse informational series No 3, Washington, DC, 1996, National Center on Elder Abuse.

- unattended or untreated health problems;
- hazardous or unsafe living conditions/arrangements (e.g., improper wiring, no heat or no running water);
- unsanitary and unclean living conditions (e.g., dirt, fleas, lice on person, soiled bedding, fecal/urine smell, inadequate clothing); and
- an elder's report of being mistreated.

Abandonment is defined as the desertion of an elderly person by an individual who has assumed responsibility for providing care for an elder, or by a person with physical custody of an elder.

Signs and symptoms of abandonment include but are not limited to:
- the desertion of an elder at a hospital, a nursing facility, or other similar institution;
- the desertion of an elder at a shopping center or other public location; and
- an elder's own report of being abandoned.

Financial or material exploitation is defined as the illegal or improper use of an elder's funds, property, or assets. Examples would include but are not limited to: cashing an elderly person's checks without authorization/permission; forging an older person's signature; misusing or stealing an older person's money or possessions; coercing or deceiving an older person into signing any document (e.g., contracts, a will); and the improper use of conservatorship, guardianship, or power of attorney.

Signs and symptoms of financial or material exploitation include but are not limited to:
- sudden changes in bank account or banking practice, including an unexplained withdrawal of large sums of money by a person accompanying the elder;
- the inclusion of additional names on an elder's bank signature care;
- unauthorized withdrawal of the elder's funds using the elder's ATM card;
- abrupt changes in a will or other financial documents;
- unexplained disappearance of funds or valuable possessions;
- substandard care being provided or bills unpaid despite the availability of adequate financial resources;
- discovery of an elder's signature being forged for financial transactions and for the titles of his/her possessions;
- sudden appearance of previously uninvolved relatives claiming their rights to an elder's affairs and possessions;
- unexplained sudden transfer of assets to a family member or someone outside the family;
- the provision of services that are not necessary; and
- an elder's report of financial exploitation.

Self-neglect is characterized as the behaviors of an elderly person that threaten his/her own health or safety. Self-neglect generally manifests itself in an older person's refusal or failure to provide himself/herself with adequate food, water, clothing, shelter, personal hygiene, medication (when indicated), and safety precautions. The definition of self-neglect *excludes* a situation in which a cognitive/mentally competent older person (who understands the consequences of his/her decisions) makes a conscious and voluntary decision to engage in acts that threaten his/her health or safety as a matter of personal preference.

Signs and symptoms of self-neglect include but are not limited to:
- dehydration, malnutrition, untreated or improperly attended medical conditions, and poor personal hygiene;
- hazardous or unsafe living conditions/arrangements (e.g., improper wiring, no indoor plumbing, no heat or no running water);
- unsanitary or unclean living quarters (e.g., animal/insect infestation, no functioning toilet, fecal/urine smell);
- inappropriate and/or inadequate clothing, lack of the necessary medical aids (e.g., eyeglasses, hearing aid, dentures); and
- grossly inadequate housing or homelessness.

NATIONAL CENTER ON ELDER ABUSE (NCEA)

Consortium Organizations

American Public Welfare Association (APWA)
810 First Street NE
Suite 500
Washington, DC 20002-4267

National Association of State Units on Aging (NASUA)
1225 I Street NW
Suite 725
Washington, DC 20005

University of Delaware
College of Human Resources
Department of Textiles, Design, and Consumer Economics
Newark, Delaware 19716

National Committee for the Prevention of Elder Abuse (NCPEA)
c/o Institute on Aging
The Medical Center of Central Massachusetts
119 Belmont Street
Worcester, Massachusetts 01605

24

Health Care in a Changing System

▶LEARNING OBJECTIVES

Upon completion of this chapter, the reader will be able to:

- Specify nursing roles as case managers.
- Become familiar with the mechanisms of and controls in our present health care delivery system.
- Explain fundamentals of Medicare and Medicaid sufficiently to assist elders in obtaining more specific information.
- Assist elders in finding information they need to make decisions about health care systems.
- Describe the role of the nurse-advocate in relation to health and consumer protections.

▶GLOSSARY

Fiduciary Accounts held in trust for another's use.

Health Care Financing Administration (HCFA) The federal agency under the Department of Health and Human Services that is responsible for the administration of Medicare and Medicaid.

Minimum Data Set (MDS) A standardized comprehensive assessment tool devised by the HCFA and legalized by the Omnibus Budget Reconciliation Act (OBRA) that must be completed and updated periodically for each individual in a long-term care setting.

Omnibus Budget Reconciliation Act (OBRA) Federal requirements dictating certain minimum requirements of care for individuals in long-term care that must be met to qualify for reimbursement of services. These were established in 1983 and have been updated periodically since that time.

Plethora A superabundance, as in "a plethora of advice and a paucity of assistance."

Title XVIII of the Social Security Act The federal legislation providing for Medicare to all individuals over age 65 and the disabled.

Title XIX of the Social Security Act The federal legislation providing for Medicaid to qualified individuals over age 65, the disabled, and economically qualified individuals.

Title XX of the Social Security Act The federal legislation providing for the establishment of senior centers throughout the United States.

▶THE LIVED EXPERIENCE

I'm so grateful to be able to stay here in my apartment, but it seems like every hour someone else arrives to do something for me or to me. Those dressings twice daily take so much time and seem always to interrupt my afternoon nap. I guess it's because I have been alone so long I just can't get used to people coming and going all day long. I wonder if there is some way I can get some quiet time just for resting and thinking.

John, age 84

It seems as if John doesn't really like me. I have been coming here twice daily now for a month, and yet he hardly seems to notice me and never really talks to me. I'll bet if someone else came next week, he wouldn't even know the difference. Nursing is so much more gratifying when I feel appreciated.

Al, home nursing provider

This chapter is designed to inform and update students and practitioners on the health policies that one must comprehend to provide appropriate guidance and resource information to elders within nursing care or jurisdiction. Because of the many changes in the health care system, individuals must, more than ever before, have knowledge of the options available to them and the resources and advocates they can trust. The movement in general is toward increasing client and family responsibility for their own welfare, developing numerous methods to provide care outside of institutions, and moving away from the private provider model. The Balanced Budget Act of 1997 allows greater flexibility for states in the administration of Medicaid programs and greater choices for elders in the selection of Medicare health provider plans. However, this has produced a plethora of options and has created confusion for the consumer.

The federal government has played a central role in the organization, financing, and delivery of health care to elders in the United States since Medicare was implemented in 1965. Presently most care of the aged is subsidized in one way or another by state and federal funds. We are relentlessly moving toward nationally controlled health care but without the availability of national health care. Over 44 million people (6.3% of the total population) in the United States have no health coverage of any kind. Of all subpopulations, the aged are best served by the present system. However, there is no consistent or comprehensive plan for financing and delivery of services over time but, rather, a continuously shifting plan in reaction to problems that occur within the system.

Nurses are increasingly in the front lines as primary care providers, case managers, and gatekeepers to care. Advanced practice nurses are being given more responsibility in triage and management of elders within the health care system.

MULTIDISCIPLINARY CARE PLANNING

In our complex, sophisticated health care delivery system, collaboration is essential. The special knowledge and skills of a dozen or more professionals are often required in a single case. To reduce redundancy, fragmentation, and waste, we must consciously and routinely organize multidisciplinary planning sessions and use the skills of expert case managers.

The major players in the multidisciplinary approach to care management are physicians, nurses, and social workers. Brickner et al (1997) suggest that physicians must learn to work effectively with nonphysician members of the team, nurses must have more education in administration and management, and social workers must be capable of developing long-term plans for the use of resources.

The basic case management team for the care of an individual and family involves a physician, nurse, and social worker. Until recently, physicians have not necessarily needed to collaborate with nurses and social workers and may find this new role difficult. Nurses, although best qualified to see the whole picture of patients' needs and constraints, have seldom taken an equal position in team planning. Social workers are still carving out their role and specialty with the aged and therefore require consistent inclusion and recognition in team planning.

To coordinate plans and involve appropriate professionals, a comprehensive documentation program must be in place and periodically reviewed with team input. The Minimum Data Set (MDS) is believed to be the instrument most likely to include a multidisciplinary appraisal and follow the patient through various levels of long-term care. Because this is not used in acute care settings, we suggest that the Nursing Needs Assessment Instrument, developed by Holland and colleagues (1998), be initiated immediately on patient admission to acute care and that this assessment follow the patient on discharge. This tool is based on the Uniform Needs Assessment Instrument (UNAI) (Health Care Financing Administration [HCFA], 1992) and can be blended into the MDS. It is ideal for case-managed care. Documentation is covered extensively in Chapter 6.

HEALTH MAINTENANCE ORGANIZATIONS AND MANAGED CARE

Health maintenance organizations (HMOs) and *managed care* are terms that are used interchangeably to indicate health care systems that provide various services for a set monthly fee. These fees may be paid by an employer, agency, individual subscriber, or any combination of these. These organizations have a vested interest in maintaining the health of their subscribers and keeping costs of care as low as possible. There are some excellent plans and some that are notoriously poor. The National Policy and Resource Center on Women and Aging (1995) provided the checklist seen in Box 24-1 of suggestions for selecting the appropriate managed care plan.

Box 24-1	**MANAGED CARE CHECKLIST**

If you now have a doctor, is he or she affiliated with a plan you can join?

Can you easily switch doctors in the plan if you are dissatisfied?

What is the quality of care rating (see Resources at the end of this chapter)?

Can you switch plans without undue difficulty if you are dissatisfied?

Are the various services conveniently located?

Are advice and care readily available on evenings and weekends?

How accessible are mental health services within the plan?

Does the plan supply information in your primary language?

Where and how can you obtain health services if you are traveling?

Does the plan cover alternative therapies such as acupuncture, chiropractic, and homeopathy?

Data from National Policy and Resource Center on Women and Aging: What do you know about managed care? *Women Aging Lett* 1(1):1, 1995.

Box 24-2	**THE SEVEN *C*'s OF MANAGED CARE: THE CORE CONCEPTS BEHIND MANAGED CARE SYSTEMS**

Common Features:

Managed care systems aim to be:
1. CONSOLIDATED in auspice and funding, so there is one-stop shopping
2. COMPREHENSIVE, offering services across the continuum
3. CONTINUOUS, following people from acute to long-term care
4. COORDINATED, with more integration of services and information
5. CONTROLLED, with authority over providers, services, and costs
6. COST-CONSCIOUS, and aim to be cost-competitive or capitated
7. COMMUNITY-BASED, emphasizing noninstitutional approaches

These systems are also becoming more and more CONSUMER-ORIENTED.

Differences Between Various Types of Managed Care Systems:

Managed Care Systems differ from one another in:
1. The RANGE OF SERVICES they provide (acute vs. long-term care; medical vs. health vs. social support services; whether or not housing is included)
2. The POPULATION targeted for recruitment, or eligible for enrollment
3. The extent to which they assume COMPLETE and LONG-TERM RESPONSIBILITY for their enrollees
4. The TYPES OF FUNDING used to support services
5. The MODEL used to bring together services and providers
6. The MECHANISMS used FOR CONTROLLING COSTS
7. The SOPHISTICATION OF their systems for INFORMATION MANAGEMENT and SERVICE COORDINATION

The above differences result in a CONTINUUM OF MANAGED CARE SYSTEMS
        basic health——augmented health——chronic care——long-term care

Courtesy Laura Reif, RN, PhD, School of Nursing, University of California, San Francisco, 1994.

The premise of Medicare managed care is that better outcomes will result from systems of care that integrate professionals in responsive teams, maximize the use of subacute care, and provide incentives to reduce the reliance on institutional acute care (Rosenfeld, 1996). Managed care systems are most effective for in-dividuals enrolled over a long period of time who use ongoing primary care and preventive strategies to maintain health and avoid high-cost emergency services and intensive treatment (Twentieth Century Fund, 1995). All managed care systems are based on a daily, monthly, or annual per capita amount designated to sustain individuals in as healthy a manner as possible. In other words, the care of every person enrolled in managed care generates a certain amount of money, often allotted through Medicare or Medicaid, to pay for the health care of that individual. Core concepts behind managed care systems can be seen in Box 24-2. The American Association of Managed Care Nurses was established in 1994 in response to an identified need to educate nurses regarding managed health care (see Resources at the end of this chapter).

CASE-MANAGED CARE

The terms *case manager* and *care manager* have slightly different connotations. In the strictest sense, a case manager works within a system with the primary intent of saving money, whereas a care manager is working for the client to provide the best service at the least cost. In real practice the roles are seldom that clear, and there is much overlap. Community-based case/care management as a method of controlling costs and avoiding premature institutionalization has increased immensely in the last 15 years. To provide more comprehensive, individualized, and economic care, case management and managed care have emerged as solutions to the cost and fragmentation experienced by elders. In some cases as many as 20 contract services are needed to adequately serve one case (Box 24-3).

Managed care simply means care that is guided by economic concerns, and *case management* implies an individual provider who functions as a primary care agent concerned about both cost and quality of services. Many variations of these mechanisms exist throughout acute and long-term care. Elders often need an advocate or individual who can provide answers based on a comprehensive view of their situation. There are many components to a successful case management program. Some of the most important include the following: convenient consumer access; a broad range of referral sources and service providers; evaluation of the effectiveness of providers; and cooperative relationships with involved departments, agencies, and businesses (Aging Consult, 1994).

In response to the emergence of case management, the Case Management Society of America (CMSA), an international, nonprofit organization, was founded in 1990 (see Resources at the end of this chapter). The CMSA developed the Standards of Practice for Case Management and the Standards of Practice and Ethics Statement. Education, research, and networking to cre-

---

Box 24-3	CONTRACT SERVICES

Adult day care	Advocacy
Chore service	Companionship
Counseling	Diagnosis and evaluation
Home-delivered meals	Homemaker
Homemaker/home health	Hospice services
aide	Medical equipment and
Housing assistance	supplies
Medically oriented day	Nutritional education
services	Skilled nursing
Respite care	Transportation/taxi
Transportation/	
specialized	

From Shoaf KG: The paper trail. In Pelham AO, Clark WF, editors: *Managing home care for the elderly: lessons from community based agencies,* New York, 1986, Springer.

ate professionalism and accountability are top priorities of the organization.

Roles of Case Managers

A few of the roles required of effective case managers include the following: broker, leader, manager, counselor, negotiator, administrator, communicator, and advocate. Case managers need to follow the client through the entire continuum of care. Peters (1986) has outlined ten commandments of care that should be observed by case managers when clients are hospitalized in acute care (Box 24-4). They must be experts regarding community resources and understand how these can best be used to meet the client's needs. They are expected to make appropriate referrals with consideration of the client's expectations and the system's limits and to monitor any nondirect brokered services. Browdie and Turwoski (1986) note that in the broker role the case manager wheels and deals for the client and his or her family. This overlaps with the advocate role, which is that of being prepared and willing to address any and all involved agencies on behalf of the client's needs. The case worker is a resource person whom the client can seek for advice and counsel, brokering the flow of services and acting as gatekeeper.

MEDICARE AND MEDICAID

In 1965 the Social Security Act was amended to provide Medicare (Title XVIII) and Medicaid (Title XIX).

Box 24-4   TEN COMMANDMENTS OF CASE MANAGEMENT DURING HOSPITALIZATION

1. Be visible in the acute care setting; the case manager must follow the client through any level of care.
2. Communicate routinely with the hospital discharge planner (HDP); when the client is hospitalized, immediately call the HDP to alert him or her to your involvement.
3. Provide support for the hospitalized client. Ideally, visit daily and keep the client informed of discharge plans.
4. Provide for necessary monitoring of the home while the client is absent, such as pet care.
5. Monitor the client's hospital progress and make staff aware of previous functional needs and abilities.
6. Recommend appropriate levels of discharge to the HDP; when meeting resistance, negotiate for a trial period in the least restrictive level of care.
7. Maximize benefits of hospitalization by initiating assessment and care of conditions that the client may have been neglecting before hospitalization.
8. Encourage early discharge; hospitalization is dangerous to elders.
9. Begin discharge planning on the day of hospital admission. Discuss with the HDP a package of potential services needed on discharge.
10. Make placement recommendations based on experience with the quality of care or special facilities in specific institutions; seek the least restrictive alternative. At times you must educate the physician or acute care staff regarding the differences in levels of long-term institutional care.

Modified from Peters B: The ten commandments of case management during hospitalization: a practice perspective. In Pelham AO, Clark WF, editors: *Managing home care for the elderly: lessons from community based agencies,* New York, 1986, Springer.

Medicare was meant to provide medical care to the elderly regardless of their financial situation. Medicaid was designed to defray expenses for those who could not meet the cost of Medicare contributions or who exhausted their Medicare benefits. Medicaid, however, is left to the individual state's discretion; therefore it varies in coverage nationwide. Almost all aged persons receive either Medicare or Medicaid benefits.

Medicare

Medicare was instituted as a federally administered universal health insurance program for people over 65 years of age and some disabled people under 65 years of age. Medicare has two parts: Part A is designed as hospital insurance, and Part B covers physician and certain outpatient service fees. Hospital insurance (Part A) is financed through a dedicated payroll tax on current workers and partially financed by current beneficiaries. Most people do not pay directly for Parts A and B, because premiums are deducted from the monthly Social Security check. If one is covered by both Parts A and B, there are still many exceptions. Claims are handled through specific major insurance companies, called *carriers,* in each state. Some of these carriers have recently opted out in favor of managed care programs.

Each year, all Social Security recipients receive a booklet explaining the many exclusions and complexities in the Medicare reimbursement system (see Appendix 24-A). Out-of-pocket costs may be considerable because of exclusions, co-payments, and deductibles. These are burdensome to the elderly poor. Medicare Part C is a recent addition, not fully activated, that gives more choices and less federal control. This will add to the confusion regarding health care choices for many elders. Even the HCFA is uncertain about the outcomes of this third component of Medicare.

At present, Medicare recipients have two choices: they may participate in the original Medicare plan as outlined above, or they may select a Medicare managed care plan (HMO). In the managed care plans the consumer is restricted to certain physicians and hospitals. There are fewer out-of-pocket costs unless an individual decides to see a physician or seek a service outside the system to which he or she has subscribed.

Medicare contracts with HMOs to provide comprehensive services for the elderly, financed by Medicare premiums. The best of these are complete health care systems with highly trained physicians and nurses working out of a single, completely equipped medical center. HMOs differ from other medical services in that they emphasize preventive medicine, comprehensive care, periodic physical examinations, and immunizations, and they cover more services than are ordinarily covered under Medicare. There is a minimum monthly charge to the participant or the participant's former employer and a service fee for each visit and for each prescription.

The plans are capitated by Medicare, which means that the HMO is paid a certain fixed amount each day for each enrollee regardless of the amount of care

- Better monitoring by the Health Care Financing Administration (HCFA) of the impact of Medicare risk programs is needed.
- Consumers need more and better information about the quality of various plans.
- Medicare beneficiaries need to understand limitations of access to providers outside the plan.
- Providers need to make the range of services and limitations clear to the participants.

given. This has created abuses and horror stories in which elders were denied needed treatments to save money for the corporate providers. Now patient protection laws are in place that allow consumers to lodge complaints and initiate legal action against these abuses. The Center for Patient Advocacy supported a much-needed bill that became law in October 1999, which allows appeals when an HMO denies care, guarantees access to specialists when needed, ensures that health-related decisions are made by physicians rather than bureaucrats, and holds HMOs legally accountable for medical decisions that cause harm. See Resources at the end of this chapter for further information regarding complaints.

HMOs that have been granted Medicare per capita waivers cannot refuse applicants based on preexisting health conditions, and the supplemental services offered may save the participant a considerable amount in medications, assistive devices, and professional consultation charges. The negative aspects of HMOs/managed care are the access barriers to specialists and high-tech procedures and treatments. Some HMOs provide extensive health education services, support groups, and telephone support services to the homebound. Information and improvements that are needed in the system are summarized in Box 24-5.

Several variations of HMOs are available to Medicare beneficiaries:

- *Medicare risk HMOs.* These are the most popular and least expensive for the breadth of health care services. These plans are required by the HCFA to provide all of the services ordinarily available through Medicare with the exception of hospice services. Access to physicians and hospitals is limited to the HMO provider network unless a feature called *point of service (POS)* is included. In those cases benefi-

ciaries may see a physician of their choice but usually will pay more for that option. The word *risk* refers to the financial risk assumed by the provider when costs exceed per capita reimbursement.

- *Medicare cost HMOs.* These are more costly to beneficiaries and companies than risk HMOs because the retrospective reimbursement through the HCFA is for actual Medicare-approved costs of care. These HMOs are less frequently available through employee health plans because they are more costly than capitated plans.
- *Medicare-eligible preferred provider organizations (PPOs).* These include a network of physicians and other providers for beneficiaries to choose from and also offer, for additional cost, the choice of physicians outside the plan. Many physicians are now forming their own small PPOs to allow themselves more freedom of practice than in the large managed care organizations.

Fundamentals of Medicare that every nurse and elder should be aware of are found in Box 24-6. The greatest inadequacies in Medicare are for the most common needs of the aged: hearing aids, eyeglasses, medications, and long-term care. However, as seniors increasingly subscribe to capitated HMOs, some of these items are provided at very low cost to the consumer.

Details about Medicare coverage can be obtained by requesting the Medicare Handbook from the HCFA (see Resources at the end of this chapter) or from the local Social Security office.

Medicaid

Medicaid provides health care insurance to more than 36 million low-income Americans, more than half of whom are poor children (US Bureau of the Census, 1998). In contrast to Medicare, Medicaid provides an array of preventive services, as well as medical services: eye care, dental care, prescription drugs, physical therapy, hospice care, and rehabilitation services with no out-of-pocket fees, premiums, co-payments, exclusions, or deductibles. Long-term care and social services programs are administered locally. Therefore the scope of services; extent of funding by county, state, and federal governments; and eligibility requirements differ from community to community. The result is a maze of services that may be duplicative, of variable quality, and of uncertain durability. Medicare was designed to ensure a basic hospital benefits package, which was well defined.

Box 24-6   FUNDAMENTALS OF MEDICARE

Medicare Part A

Medicare Part A is designed primarily to partially cover the costs of inpatient hospital care and other specialized care as listed below:

- Acute hospitalization coverage includes costs of semiprivate rooms, meals, nursing services, operating and recovery room, intensive care, drugs, laboratory and radiology fees, blood products, and other necessary medical services and supplies. Certain deductibles must be paid by the patient. These vary each year and increase incrementally as patients are hospitalized beyond 60 days. Most individuals meet these expenses through Medigap policies or health maintenance organization (HMO) membership. Further discussion of these is found later in the chapter in relation to managed care and its development.
- Skilled nursing facility care is covered by Medicare for a maximum of 100 days and then only if the individual has been hospitalized in acute care for a minimum of 3 days within the prior 30 days and only if deemed medically necessary. With the emergence of subacute care in skilled nursing facilities, these rules are likely to change, particularly the requirement for 3-day hospitalization before nursing home admission. The patients pay a deductible for each day after 20 days.
- Home health care may be covered by Medicare on an intermittent and/or part-time basis for skilled nursing care, physical therapy, and rehabilitative services; however, chronic disorders requiring custodial care, such as Alzheimer's disease, must be paid out-of-pocket by the

patient or caregiver. Cost of care is covered as long as individuals meet Medicare requirements; Medicare pays 80% of the approved amount for durable equipment.

- Hospice care is provided for terminally ill persons expected to live less than 6 months who elect to forgo traditional medical treatment for the terminal illness. Medicare pays for all but limited costs for outpatient drugs and inpatient respite care (Health Care Financing Administration [HCFA], 1996).
- Psychiatric care is limited to 190 days of care in a lifetime; partial payment and other limitations apply.

Medicare Part B

Medicare Part B is designed to pick up where Part A leaves off. It pays partially for a wide range of medical services and supplies:

- Physician's services, supplies and diagnostic tests, physical and speech therapy, durable medical equipment, and other services are included for unlimited periods; deductibles are applied.
- Clinical laboratory services are fully covered if deemed medically necessary.
- Outpatient hospital treatment, blood, and ambulatory surgical services have deductibles of $100 each and patient payment of 20% of charges (HCFA, 1996).

Booklets explaining the details of Medicare are provided annually to all beneficiaries.

At present most Medicaid beneficiaries are enrolled in managed care programs. Medicaid is the health care financing program that complements Medicare and at present provides assistance to more than 1 in 10 Americans age 65 and older; the great majority of these are in long-term care situations. Two thirds of all Americans in nursing homes receive assistance from Medicaid. An elderly Medicaid-eligible recipient residing in a nursing home costs an average of $42,000 annually.

Medicare was designed to ensure a basic hospital benefits package, which was well defined. There has been no similar national consensus for a defined package of long-term care and social services. These have been developed at state discretion under the federal guidelines of Title XIX (Medicaid) of the Social Security Act. Medicaid eligibility requirements are complicated and cumbersome (Box 24-7) and do not address the needs of the near-poor, who cannot qualify for aid

but cannot afford basic health care, even with the partial aid of Medicare.

Dual Eligibles

Some individuals who have income not exceeding 100% of the federal poverty level and whose resources do not exceed twice the limit for Supplemental Security Insurance (SSI) may qualify for Medicare with deductibles, co-insurance, and out-of-pocket costs covered by Medicaid. These are considered *dual eligibles*.

LONG-TERM CARE

Medicaid and the Veterans Administration are the chief fiduciary agents of long-term institutional care. Medicare reimbursement for nursing home care applies only to a few patients, and then it is of very short dura-

Box 24-7   VERIFICATION DOCUMENTS FOR MEDICAID ELIGIBILITY

To determine eligibility, an applicant is generally required to provide the following information when meeting with case workers.

1. Social Security cards for all household members
2. Multiple pay stubs or earnings statement from employer
3. Proof of income from rental property
4. Verification letters from Social Security, Supplemental Security Income, Department of Veterans Affairs, unemployment compensation, or workers compensation
5. Proof of support or alimony payments
6. Bank statements, checking accounts, savings accounts, credit union records, stocks, and bonds
7. Rent or mortgage payment receipts
8. Utility receipts
9. Proof of citizenship or alien status
10. Verification of age of children
11. Proof of the absence or disability of a parent
12. Verification of address
13. Collateral verification of family composition and address
14. Tag receipt of title of all motor vehicles
15. Tax notice on real estate
16. All life and health insurance policy and insurance identification cards
17. Written statement of child care expenses
18. Written statements from anyone making a contribution (cash or vendor payments)
19. If pregnant, written statement verifying pregnancy

Data from Shuptrine S: Reforming Medicaid eligibility rules, *The Safety Net,* p 5, summer 1991.

tion. The rapid discharge from acute care, originally an outcome of diagnosis-related groups (DRGs) and the strict limitations in reimbursement, has resulted in the placement in nursing homes of many patients requiring postacute care. Placement is often difficult, since some facilities are unable to provide the services required for subacute care certification. Medicaid remains the primary payer for long-term care.

Problems that confront patients and their families include the imposition of additional fees for specific services such as care for incontinence and various private-payment contractual arrangements they must agree to before a facility will accept a patient receiving Medicaid. Facilities tend to seek patients requiring the most skilled care at the most attractive subacute reimbursement rates or those who can pay for their own care.

Subacute Care

As the acute care hospital has become the site of surgical, emergency, and intensive care, the nursing home has been transformed into a center for the coordination of the continuum of care. Long-term care now includes subacute care; hospice care; home health care; social, medical, and rehabilitative day care; and assisted living and congregate care. These changes have instigated many attitudinal, administrative, and personnel shifts, as well as retraining opportunities. Nurses have always borne the major responsibility for planning and implementing the long-term care of the aged. Geriatric nurse practitioners are increasingly involved in diagnosing, directing, and monitoring the care of the aged in nursing homes.

The development of subacute care units has become a massive move by the larger nursing home chains and hospitals to meet the needs of the aged who are discharged "quick and sick." The American Health Care Association (AHCA) and the Joint Commission on Accreditation of Healthcare Organizations (JCAHO) provide the following definition of subacute care:

> Subacute care is comprehensive inpatient care designed for someone who has an acute illness, injury, or exacerbation of a disease process. It is goal-oriented treatment rendered immediately after, or instead of, acute hospitalization to treat one or more specific active complex medical conditions or to administer one or more technically complex treatments in the context of a person's underlying long-term conditions and overall situation.

The definition goes on to explain in more detail all of these factors. Copies are available from the JCAHO.

As hospitals eject patients with ever-greater rapidity, nursing homes are increasingly taking on the form and functions of the traditional medical unit in a general hospital under the category of providing subacute care. Subacute care is more intensive than traditional nursing facility care and several times more costly, but it is far less costly than similar care in an acute care hospital.

Guidelines have been established for these subacute care units for accreditation standards and physician responsibilities. These are, in large part, in response to the necessary upgrading of many long-term care facilities in which staffing, equipment, and structures were not adapted to the level of care needed by some of the patients admitted directly from acute care hospitals.

The American Medical Association (AMA) established guidelines in 1995 that are especially important in ensuring prompt and adequate care, because typically long-term care has been the stepchild of physicians. Now, physicians are required to be responsible for patient care 24 hours a day, 7 days a week. The patient is to remain under the primary coordinating care of the admitting physician rather than being transferred to a house physician. Other features of the guidelines include assurance that education and skills of staff are sufficient to provide the necessary care, that peer evaluation will monitor quality of care, that a comprehensive patient assessment and plan of care will be in place within 24 hours of admission, and that there will be a minimum of once-weekly visits and progress notes for each visit (American Medical Association, 1995).

A present concern in the long-term care provider industry is the need to institute staff development programs that include skills and procedures traditionally limited to the acute care setting. Nurses who have devoted their careers to providing the real "nursing home" care so essential to long-term residents fear that it will be lost as the industry gears up to provide hospital care.

Long-Term Care Insurance

Long-term care insurance (LTCI) to defray the cost of nursing home care and, in some policies, also home care is becoming more affordable and reliable. The triggers for benefit payments are more likely to be functional losses than medical conditions. With the shift in venue and health care delivery methods, traditional LTCI designed around a flat-fee daily reimbursement rate for nursing home care and home care is responding with reimbursement for a richer set of alternatives, particularly noninstitutional options. In August 1996 Congress passed S.1658 (the Health Insurance Reform Act of 1996), which has a number of features related to insurance portability. It also provides incentives for individuals to finance their own LTCI.

Many plans are being marketed at present. Even the American Nurses Association (ANA) has a plan available to ANA members that is underwritten by American Express. The purchaser of LTCI must be especially prudent and consider all of the exclusions most thoughtfully before enrolling. There are particular concerns related to Alzheimer's disease because many policies exclude these individuals from home benefits and include very limited institutional benefits. Guidelines for policy selection are provided in Box 24-8. It is important to review all of the benefits and restrictions before

> **Box 24-8   BENEFITS INCLUDED IN A GOOD LONG-TERM CARE POLICY**
>
> - Daily benefit of $100
> - Waiting period of not over 20 days
> - Maximum benefit for one stay of at least 4 years
> - Unlimited maximum benefit for all stays
> - Payment for skilled nursing facility (SNF), intermediate care facility (ICF), or custodial care
> - Partial payment for subacute care not covered by Medicare
> - Coverage should begin within 20 days of a hospital stay of 3 days
> - Home care benefits should be paid without requiring a hospital stay or previous nursing home care
> - Waiver of premium when hospitalized
> - Guaranteed renewability for life
> - Specific coverage of Alzheimer's disease
> - Constant premium level for life

advising consumers to purchase a policy. The best LTCI packages are those negotiated by a large employer or state organization or association.

It is advisable to check consumer reports of the particular insurance company and its reliability before recommending or applying for a policy. Congress is considering bills that would encourage individuals to purchase LTCI through tax incentives for doing so (CalPERS, 1996).

VETERANS HEALTH CARE SYSTEM

Nearly 7 million World War II veterans and 3 million Korean War veterans are now over 65 years old. Medical program expenses for the veterans of our wars have become a major fiscal responsibility, totaling $16.9 billion in 1997. The Veterans Health Administration (VA) system has long held a leadership position in geriatric research, medical care, and extended care. In fact, a great deal of the research that has guided gerontologists in earlier years was generated through the VA system, as were innovations in care. In addition, the vast majority of geriatric fellowships have been provided through the Department of Veterans Affairs (VA) hospitals. The VA system has been a forerunner of the various continua of care providers in place at present. Early on, they provided VA-run nursing homes, home care and community-based programs, respite care, blindness rehabilitation, mental health, and numerous other services in addition to acute medical/surgical provisions.

HOME CARE

Because of costs and humane concerns there is a considerable effort to keep individuals in their homes and communities and to avoid institutionalization. Home care is often thought to be less costly, but that is not necessarily true. Equipment and supplies have become outrageously expensive, and efforts to curb these home care expenses are constant. An array of public and privately financed services has developed across the United States to support the desire of impaired elders to live out their lives in the comfort and independence of their own homes. Ideally, the services provide a combination of health care, day care supervision, housekeeping, counseling, meal deliveries, transportation, visits from friendly companions, home repairs, and other services as needed. All states have received federal waivers allowing them to pay for home and community care for elderly Medicaid beneficiaries who otherwise would end up in nursing homes.

A wide range of services is available to those who can afford them out-of-pocket, but persons may be unaware of what is needed or where it can be obtained. In these situations, case managers may help individuals identify specific needs and find the appropriate services. Case managers may be found through city and county referral services or private agencies that provide case management on a fee-for-service basis.

Community services and home health care may be funded through a combination of Medicare and Medicaid (Title XVIII and XIX of the Social Security Act), the Social Services Amendment (Title XX of the Social Security Act), Title III of the Older Americans Act, and the Department of Veterans Affairs. Provision of community services focuses on the individual and may not support the family in its efforts to care for the functionally dependent older person in the home. The net effect restricts the provider's capacity to develop or manage a comprehensive treatment plan. Home care can be a desirable alternative to institutional care if caregivers, nurses, family, social workers, physicians, homemakers, and home health aides are available when needed. However, these ideal conditions may not exist, and if these services are available, there are strict Medicare limits. Some aged people manage to remain in their homes with few services and minimal assistance. Conditions may be less than desirable from professional standards, but by the standards of the individuals they are much more acceptable than institutionalization.

Supermarkets of home care supplies and medical equipment designed to provide individual and personalized service directly to consumers are appearing nationwide and drawing crowds of careful shoppers (Chriss, 1996). These retailers often have professionals available to advise, instruct, and answer questions. In one such outlet most of the employees are registered nurses or licensed vocational nurses and have special training in the use of medical equipment. In some situations follow-up home assessments are made to ensure client satisfaction and proper usage. This is reassuring evidence of the growing trend for clients to take charge of their own care. Nurses are case managers and primary care coordinators in the home, and at present, home health care is the most important issue at stake in the care of the aged. We expect that nurses will continue to occupy a pivotal role in home care as client advocates and to carefully evaluate care plans, quality outcomes, and costs.

TELECOMMUNICATION AND MONITORING

Telecommunication by phone, Internet, or television is becoming more and more popular in health care. Telephones, electronic media, and medical devices readily provide health advice, monitoring, education, and interaction and are especially accessible to elders who may be largely homebound. Rice (2000) notes that the telephone can be especially important in supplementing home visits and monitoring progress. She cautions that cellular phones do not afford privacy and that telephone management should only be supplementary to in-person interactions. Bondmass et al (2000) found that physiologic home monitoring by telephone, followed by periodic follow-up phone calls, provided immediate information to the health center, reassurance to the patient, better medication compliance, and decreased hospitalizations. Telecommunication is only one aspect of comprehensive case management and must be used judiciously and interspersed with personal contact. In the future we expect these strategies to become more prevalent as cost savers and a means of more frequently accessing homebound individuals and those in remote areas. It is extremely important to carefully document telecommunication contact, as in any other form of health care intervention.

QUALITY MANAGEMENT IN THE CONTINUUM OF CARE

Quality management must become an integral part of an organization's daily functioning, based on the agency's mission and goal. The agency or institution must have a clear idea of what is to be done, how, for whom, and for what purpose (Weber et al, 1997). The values and hopes must be conveyed to each staff member on every level to gain appropriate commitment and enthusiasm. Funding, licensing, and accreditation all depend on meeting certain requirements, but real quality depends on personal commitment to the defined vision for the future (Weber et al, 1997).

Variance among states and private accrediting organizations results in great differences from one state and agency to another. Many agencies meet only basic state requirements. However, with the institution of Omnibus Budget Reconciliation Act (OBRA) regulations in long-term care, quality concerns have shifted to the patient's rights, satisfaction, and opportunity to be an active participant in care planning.

Traditional quality assurance is of three types: (1) assessment of the adequacy of organizational and facility structure, appropriate personnel, supplies, and equipment; (2) process assessments of what is done to and for clients; and (3) outcome assessments of the effects on clients' biopsychosocial status.

Recently there has been a strong move toward outcome assessments involving efficacy, effectiveness, and efficiency. *Efficacy* is based on the expected value of an intervention in ideal circumstances; *effectiveness* is the result obtained under usual circumstances, and *efficiency* considers the benefit of the service in relation to the cost. In 1994 the Outcome-Based Quality Improvement (OBQI) system was established to measure all aspects of quality, including providers, discharge and ongoing planning, and efficacy of supports. The broad case management approach to quality care emphasizes consumer rights, client involvement, and satisfaction. Many of these elements are subjective, and clients' perspectives may be shaped by the events of the day on which they are assessed rather than by their ongoing quality of life. However, the general move toward more assessment of clients' perspectives rather than structural adequacy seems to be an important consideration.

THE SHIFTING SYSTEM

It has become clear as we face the burgeoning population of very old survivors and the entry of the "baby boomers" into the ranks of older persons that many aspects of the health care system must be modified. Because nurses are pivotal players within the system and occupy diverse roles, there are abundant opportunities for professional growth and gratification in working with the aged in our ever-shifting health care system.

▶ KEY CONCEPTS

- Most Medicare beneficiaries are now subscribers to a health maintenance organization (HMO) or managed care provider. The healthier aged are quite satisfied with the system; however, the ill aged often believe that they are not getting the expert attention they need or sufficient time with providers to properly address their complex problems.
- Nursing home care consumes the largest share of the Medicaid budget, and the provision of long-term care insurance is an ongoing concern of both young and old.
- A major nursing responsibility is to advocate for the aged who lack family or understanding to represent their own best interests.
- Good case management is a mode of care management that considers cost, quality, and coordination of services for the benefit of the client.
- Home care is thought to be the ideal for elders, but unless it is carefully supervised, it may be inadequate and very costly.
- Telemonitoring, computers, and electronic monitoring have made distance health care management a growing trend.
- Subacute care, sometimes referred to as *postacute care,* is becoming increasingly available as a specialized service in long-term care institutions.

NANDA and Wellness Diagnoses

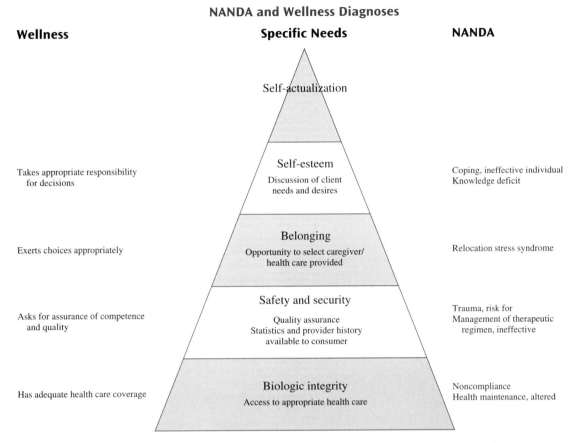

Wellness	Specific Needs	NANDA

These are not all of the possible wellness or NANDA diagnoses that may be identified. The above are frequent examples of nursing diagnoses that should be considered when planning care for the older adult in whatever setting.

▶ **Activities and Discussion Questions**

1. Interview a nurse case manager, and ask about the components of the position that are gratifying and those that are the most difficult.
2. Discuss your thoughts about specific activities that are different for case managers and care managers.
3. Describe the role of the nurse-advocate in relation to health and consumer protections.
4. Explain the fundamentals of Medicare and Medicaid sufficiently to assist elders in obtaining more specific information.
5. Interview an elder in a rehabilitation center, and ask about his or her experiences with acute hospitalization, long-term care, and Medicare.
6. Discuss with this elder his or her thoughts about Medicare and how it does or does not meet his or her needs. Write a brief summary, and present it to the class.

RESOURCES

American Association of Managed Care Nurses
4435 Waterfront Drive, Suite 101
PO Box 4975
Glen Allen, VA 23058
(804) 747-9698
Case Management Society of America
1101 17th Street NW, Suite 1200
Washington, DC 20036

Consumers' Guide to Health Plans. Publication that has rated health care maintenance organizations (HMOs) across the nation as excellent, very good, good, fair, or poor. This guide also gives information on keeping costs down and getting the best care when enrolled in a plan. Contact Health Plan Guide, 733 15th Street NW, Suite 821, Washington, DC 20005. (Cost: $12, including postage.)

Consumers' Guide to Health Plans. Similar publication; available from the Center for the Study of Services; call (202) 347-7283, (510) 397-8305, or (800) 475-7283.

1996 Accreditation Manual for Home Care. Available from the Joint Commission on Accreditation of Healthcare Organizations (JCAHO), 1 Renaissance Boulevard, Oakbrook Terrace, IL 60181; (708) 916-5800.

Self-Help for Public Benefits. Brochure prepared by the Legal Counsel for the Elderly/AARP, PO Box 96474, Washington, DC 20090-6474.

Social Security Retirement and Survivors Benefits. Booklet available from all Social Security offices listed in the telephone book or by calling (800) 772-1213.

Your Medicare Handbook. Available from the Health Care Financing Administration, U.S. Government Printing Office, U.S. Department of Health and Human Services, 7500 Security Boulevard, Baltimore, MD 21244-1850. The handbook is updated and issued each year to Medicare eligibles and may also be requested by other interested persons.

Complaints against health care service plans in California can be filed with the Department of Corporations (DOC), (800) 400-0815. This should be done only after contacting the health plan's grievance representative and attempting a resolution.

To obtain the free Status List of the National Committee for Quality Assurance, call (202) 955-3515.

REFERENCES

Aging Consult: *Keys to a successful case management program,* Creve Coeur, MO, 1994, Aging Consult.

American Medical Association: *AMA guidelines for physician responsibilities in subacute care,* Washington, DC, 1995, AMA Board of Trustees.

Bondmass M et al: The effect of physiologic home monitoring and telemanagement on chronic heart failure outcomes, *Geriatr Nurs* 21, 2000 (in press).

Brickner PW et al: Learning and training in long term home health care: physicians, nurses and social workers. In Brickner PW et al: *Geriatric home health care: the collaboration of physicians, nurses and social workers,* New York, 1997, Springer.

Browdie RM, Turwoski A: The problems of providing services to the elderly in their own homes. In Pelham AO, Clark WF, editors: *Managing home care for the elderly: lessons from community based agencies,* New York, 1986, Springer.

CalPERS: Making your health plan decision, *Perspective,* p 1, fall 1996 (California Public Employees' Retirement System newsletter).

Chriss L: Retailers cash in on home health market, *NurseWeek* 9(17):1, 1996.

Health Care Financing Administration: *Health care financing review,* Washington, DC, summer 1996, US Government Printing Office.

Health Care Financing Administration: *Report to Congress: report of the secretary's advisory panel on the development of the UNAI,* Washington, DC, 1992, US Government Printing Office.

Holland DE et al: Continuity of care: a nursing needs assessment instrument, *Geriatr Nurs* 19(6):331-334, 1998.

National Policy and Resource Center on Women and Aging: What do you know about managed care? *Women Aging Lett* 1(1):1, 1995.

Peters B: The ten commandments of case management during hospitalization: a practice perspective. In Pelham AO, Clark WF, editors: *Managing home care for the elderly: lessons from community based agencies,* New York, 1986, Springer.

Rice R: Telecaring in home care: making a telephone visit, *Geriatr Nurs* 21(1):48, 2000.

Rosenfeld A: Managed care for the elderly: what's the problem, where's the problem? *Public Policy Aging Rep* 7(2):1, 1996.

Shoaf KG: The paper trail. In Pelham AO, Clark WF, editors: *Managing home care for the elderly: lessons from community based agencies,* New York, 1986, Springer.

Twentieth Century Fund: *Medicaid reform: a Twentieth Century Fund guide to the issues,* New York, 1995, Twentieth Century Fund Press.

US Bureau of the Census: *Statistical abstract of the United States: 1998,* ed 118, Washington, DC, 1998, US Government Printing Office.

Weber C M et al: Quality management in home health care. In Brickner PW et al: *Geriatric home health care: the collaboration of physicians, nurses and social workers,* New York, 1997, Springer.

Appendix 24-A   *Your Medicare Benefits*

Medicare Part A (Hospital Insurance)
Covers:

Hospital Stays: Semiprivate room, meals, general nursing and other hospital services and supplies. This does not include private duty nursing, a television or telephone in your room, or a private room, unless medically necessary. Inpatient mental health care coverage in a psychiatric facility is limited to 190 days in a lifetime.

Skilled Nursing Facility (SNF) Care:
Semi-private room, meals, skilled nursing and rehabilitative services, and other services and supplies (after a 3-day hospital stay).

Home Health Care: Part-time skilled nursing care, physical therapy, speech-language therapy, home health aide services, durable medical equipment (such as wheelchairs, hospital beds, oxygen, and walkers) and supplies, and other services.

Hospice Care: Medical and support services from a Medicare-approved hospice, drugs for symptom control and pain relief, short-term respite care, care in a hospice facility, hospital, or nursing home when necessary, and other services not otherwise covered by Medicare. Home care is also covered.

Blood: Given at a hospital or skilled nursing facility during a covered stay.

Medicare Part B (Medical Insurance)
Covers:

Medical and Other Services: Doctors' services (except for routine physical exams), outpatient medical and surgical services and supplies, diagnostic tests, ambulatory surgery center facility fees for approved procedures, and durable medical equipment (such as wheelchairs, hospital beds, oxygen, and walkers).

Also covers outpatient physical and occupational therapy including speech-language therapy, and mental health services.

What You Pay in 2000* in the Original Medicare Plan

For each benefit period you pay:
- A total of $776 for a hospital stay of 1-60 days.
- $194 per day for days 61-90 of a hospital stay.
- $388 per day for days 91-150 of a hospital stay.
- All costs for each day beyond 150 days.

For each benefit period you pay:
- Nothing for the first 20 days.
- Up to $97 per day for days 21-100.
- All costs beyond the 100th day in the benefit period.

If you have questions about SNF care and conditions of coverage, call your Fiscal Intermediary. This is the company that pays Medicare Part A bills.

You pay:
- Nothing for home health care services.
- 20% of approved amount for durable medical equipment.

If you have questions about home health care and conditions of coverage, call your Regional Home Health Intermediary.

You pay:
- A copayment of up to $5 for outpatient prescription drugs and a $5 per day copayment for inpatient respite care (short-term care given to a hospice patient by another caregiver, so that the usual caregiver can rest). The copayment can change depending on where you live.

If you have questions about hospice care and conditions of coverage, call your Regional Home Health Intermediary.

You pay:
- For the first 3 pints of blood.

What You Pay in 2000* in the Original Medicare Plan

You pay:
- $100 deductible (pay once per calendar year).
- 20% of approved amount after the deductible, except in the outpatient setting.
- 20% of $1,500 for all outpatient physical and speech therapy services and 20% of $1,500 for all outpatient occupational therapy services. You pay all charges above $1,500. **(Hospital outpatient therapy services do not count towards the $1,500 limits.)**
- 50% for most outpatient mental health.

Extracted from Medicare & You, 2000, Health Care Financing Administration (HCFA), USDHHS, Baltimore, Md.

Clinical Laboratory Service: Blood tests, urinalysis, and more.

You pay:
• Nothing for services.

Home Health Care: Part-time skilled care, home health aide services, durable medical equipment when supplied by a home health agency while getting Medicare covered home health care, and other supplies and services.

You pay:
• Nothing for services.
• 20% of approved amount for durable medical equipment.

Outpatient Hospital Services: Services for the diagnosis or treatment of an illness or injury.

You pay:
• 20% of the charged amount (after the deductible). During the year 2000, this will change to a set copayment amount.

Blood: Pints of blood needed as an outpatient, or as part of a Part B covered service.

You pay:
• For the first 3 pints of blood, then 20% of the approved amount for additional pints of blood (after the deductible).

Part B also helps pay for:
• Ambulance services (limited coverage).
• Artificial limbs and eyes.
• Braces—arm, leg, back, and neck.
• Chiropractic services (limited).
• Emergency care.
• Eyeglasses—one pair after cataract surgery with an intraocular lens.
• Kidney dialysis and kidney transplants.
• Medical supplies—item such as ostomy bags, surgical dressings, splints, casts, and some diabetic supplies.
• Outpatient prescription drugs (very limited).
• Preventive services.
• Prosthetic devices, including breast prosthesis after mastectomy.
• Services of practitioners such as clinical psychologists, social workers, and nurse practitioners.
• Transplants—heart, lung, and liver (under certain conditions).
• X-rays and some other diagnostic tests.

Medicare Part B Covered Preventive Services

Bone Mass Measurements:
Varies with your health status.
Colorectal Cancer Screening:
• Fecal Occult Blood Test—Once every year.
• Flexible Sigmoidoscopy—Once every four years.
• Colonoscopy—Once every two years if you are high risk for cancer of the colon.
• Barium Enema—Doctor can substitute for sigmoidoscopy or colonoscopy.
Diabetes Monitoring:
Includes coverage for glucose monitors, test strips, lancets, and self-management training.
Mammogram Screening:
Once every year.
Pap Smear and Pelvic Examination:
(Includes a clinical breast exam)
Once every three years. Once every year if you are high risk for cervical or vaginal cancer, or if you are of childbearing age and have had an abnormal Pap smear in the preceding three years.
Prostate Cancer Screening:
Starting January 1, 2000
• Digital Rectal Examination—Once every year.
• Prostate Specific Antigen (PSA) Test—Once every year.

Vaccinations:
• Flu Shot—Once every year.
• Pneumonia Shot—One may be all you ever need, ask your doctor.
• Hepatitis B Shot—If you are at medium to high risk for hepatitis.

What is not paid for by Medicare Part A and Part B in the Original Medicare Plan?

The original Medicare Plan does not cover everything. Your out-of-pocket costs for health care will include but are not limited to:
• Your monthly Part B premium ($45.50 in 2000*).
• Deductibles, coinsurance or copayments when you get health care services.
• Outpatient prescription drugs (with only a few exceptions).
• Routine or yearly physical exams.
• Vaccinations except as listed.
• Orthopedic shoes.
• Custodial care (help with bathing, dressing, toileting, and eating) at home or in a nursing home.
• Most dental care and dentures.
• Routine foot care.
• Hearing aids.
• Routine eye care.
• Health care you get while traveling outside of the United States (except under limited circumstances).
• Cosmetic surgery.
Outpatient physical and occupational therapy services, including speech-language therapy except for those you get in hospital outpatient departments, have limits for each calendar year. The Original Medicare Plan does pay for some preventive care, but not all of it.
You may be able to get help to cover the costs Medicare does not cover. You may be able to join a Medicare managed care plan and get extra benefits.

chapter 25

Mental and Emotional Health in the Elderly

▶LEARNING OBJECTIVES

Upon completion of this chapter, the reader will be able to:

- Identify common emotional needs of elders.
- Relate crises and stressors that are likely to occur in the lives of the elderly in the community; list those that are likely for the institutionalized elder.
- Discuss the concept of anxiety and explain several reactions that may be used to reduce the discomfort.
- Name the three most common disturbances of the mental health of elders.
- Assess the presence of depression in an elder.
- Recognize elders at risk of suicide, and conduct a suicide assessment of an elder.
- Specify several indications of the possibility of substance abuse.
- Evaluate interventions aimed at promoting mental health in older adults.

▶GLOSSARY

Compulsion An insistent and repetitive urge to perform an act contrary to the person's ordinary desires. It is a mechanism to control anxiety, and if it is interfered with, the individual will become very anxious. The classic compulsion is repetitious hand washing.

Delusion A false belief not in keeping with the individual's experience that is not subject to logic. Attempting to convince someone that his or her delusion is false is useless.

Denial An unconscious defense mechanism to protect against realities that the individual is not able to cope with.

Dysthymia At least 2 years of depressed mood for more days than not, accompanied by additional depressive symptoms, but symptoms do not meet criteria for a major depressive episode.

Hallucination A false sensory perception in the absence of a real stimulus (e.g., hearing voices that no one else can hear).

Illusion Misinterpretation of a real experience (e.g., thinking a curled rope is a snake).

Major depression Five or more of the following symptoms are present for 2 weeks or more: (1) depressed mood, (2) diminished interest or pleasure, (3) loss or gain of more than 5% of body weight within 1 month, (4) insomnia or excessive sleeping, (5) movement agitation or retardation, (6) excessive fatigue, (7) feelings of worthlessness or inappropriate guilt, (8) inability to concentrate or make decisions, (9) recurrent thoughts of death or suicide. Detailed discussion can be

found in the *Diagnostic and Statistical Manual of Mental Disorders (DSM-IV)* (American Psychiatric Association, 1994, p. 327).

Obsession A persistent unwanted thought that cannot be eliminated by logic or reasoning; a common and benign obsession is the repetitious intrusion of a particular song into one's thoughts.

Paranoia The development of an unrealistic belief system that interprets events as persecutory. The individual may be convinced of his or her superiority or unique abilities.

Posttraumatic stress disorder Characteristic symptoms of intense psychologic distress recurring, often for years, following exposure to extremely traumatic events that have incurred horror, helplessness, and paralyzing fear.

Projection An unconscious defense mechanism in which emotions unacceptable to self are attributed to others (e.g., believing your husband is unfaithful when unconsciously you would like to have an affair).

Psychodrama A technique of group psychotherapy in which individuals dramatize their emotional problems.

Psychoneuroimmunology The investigation of how the psyche and neurologic system interact to weaken or strengthen the immune system.

Somatic displacement Physical symptoms that are caused by emotional factors and that are focused on a single organ system; commonly, back problems with no identifiable physiologic explanation.

I know my daughter is keeping something from me. I can feel it when she visits and is afraid to look me in the eye. I know she wants to sell my house and spend all the money; maybe she already has. I notice she has a lot of new clothes. She has always been greedy.

Genevieve, age 85, insecure, slightly paranoid, and newly admitted to an assisted living setting

I feel so guilty that I put Mother in this assisted living center. I wish I had talked to her about it rather than being so sneaky, but I just couldn't because I knew she would refuse to go. It is so hard to visit with her, since I'm afraid she will never trust me again.

Genevieve's daughter, Ethel, age 50

MENTAL HEALTH IN OLD AGE

Mental health of the elderly is difficult to define because the increasing life experience throughout the life span results in many variations in personality and sometimes odd adaptations in late life. Each individual becomes more uniquely himself or herself the older he or she becomes. The accumulation of life experience, as well as particular situations, emphasizes certain aspects of personality and appearance and diminishes others. Some apparently negative personality characteristics, such as being crusty, disagreeable, grouchy, or grumpy, may be adaptive. Thus an old man coping with a severe illness and stoically protecting others from awareness of his pain might be mentally healthy although extremely cantankerous.

Mental health can be defined as a satisfactory adjustment to one's life stage and situation. This chapter presents concepts of mental and emotional health and disturbances in old age and provides specific nursing strategies to maintain and promote mental health, self-esteem, and satisfaction of older individuals. Nurses caring for the aged need to consider clients' basic human needs when attempting to assess mental health and adaptation.

Assessment of mental health includes examination for cognitive function/impairment and the specific conditions of anxiety and adjustment reactions, depression, paranoia, substance abuse, and suicidal risk. Assessment of mental health must also focus on social intactness and affectual responses appropriate to the situation. Attention span, concentration, intelligence, judgment, learning ability, memory, orientation, perception, problem solving, psychomotor ability, and reaction time are assessed in relation to cognitive intactness and must be considered when making a psychologic assessment (see Chapter 14 for assessment tools). Cognitive function is considered in Chapters 8 and 21.

Obtaining assessment data from elders is best done during short sessions after some rapport has been established. Performing repeated assessments at various times of day and in different situations will give a more complete psychologic profile. It is important to be sensitive to a client's anxiety, special needs, and disabilities. The interview should be focused so that attention is given to strengths and skills, as well as deficits. It is also useful to take a psychologic inventory of the geriatric client (Box 25-1).

This chapter is designed to engage students in the process of assisting elders in keeping or rebuilding feelings of control and competence. When elderly clients may be feeling helpless, hopeless, and dependent as a result of crises, overwhelming stress, and depleting illnesses, they will need emotional "splinting" (Wolanin, Phillips, 1981)—a temporary assist to keep the structure of their lives steady. Yet, we know that anyone who has survived past 80 or so years has been inoculated numerous times by stressful events and has developed tremendous resistance. It is our task to discover the strengths and adaptive mechanisms that will assist clients in coping with stress and anxiety and to avert crises.

EMOTIONAL NEEDS

There is much that we do not yet understand about the connection between emotions and health and illness, although we know that some emotions for some people result in illness. Stress theorists are interested in understanding the process by which demands exceed the adaptive capacity of the organism and result in psychologic and biologic changes that place the person at risk

Box 25-1	INVENTORY OF THE PSYCHOGERIATRIC CLIENT: FUNCTION AND CARE PLAN

1. List client's strengths:
   - Ability to take initiative in caring for self, finances, work project
   - Ability to express feelings
   - Ability to stand up for his or her rights
   - Ability to make decisions
   - Ability to care for self (e.g., dressing, going to meals)
   - Ability to share with others or show concern for others
   - Enjoyment of music and arts
   - Active participation in organizations
   - Interest in sports
   - Enjoyment of reading
   - Imagination and creativity
   - Special aptitudes (e.g., mechanical ability, gardening)
2. Identify predominant defensive coping styles:
   - Denial
   - Projection
   - Displacement
   - Passive aggression
   - Positive identification
3. Identify highly adaptive coping styles:
   - Affiliation
   - Altruism
   - Humor
   - Self-assertion
   - Sublimation
4. Identify defensive breakdown patterns:
   - Delusional projection
   - Psychotic suspiciousness
   - Psychotic denial
   - Immobilizing fears
   - Psychotic distortions
   - Apathetic withdrawal
5. Determine client needs and problems based on:
   - Reason for seeking assistance by patient, family, and others

- Medical history and findings (physical, mental, neurologic, and psychologic examinations and tests)
- Drug use profile (use of prescribed and nonprescribed drugs)
- Laboratory and diagnostic tests
- Psychiatric history
- Social history
- Mental status
- Other background information provided by patient, family, and each staff person who has interviewed the patient
6. Develop a nursing care plan considering:
   - Patient's problems, needs, and strengths
   - Mutually identified short-term goals
   - Mutually identified long-term goals
7. State expected outcome of care in terms that can be measured. The following are examples of goals stated in measurable terms:
   - Socializes more
   - Dresses appropriately—puts on coat or jacket when going outside in cold weather
   - Improves personal hygiene—brushes teeth daily without being reminded
   - Shows improvement in problem areas
   - Improves attitude—discusses problems or concerns instead of hitting or resisting
   - Increases functional independence
   - Reduces hostility—responds when spoken to in a friendly manner
   - Improves self-esteem—goes 1 day without self-criticism
   - Reduces depression—expresses interest in one outside activity
   - States increased enjoyment of activities
   - Reduces suspiciousness—eats a meal without expressing fear of poisoning
8. Review progress periodically and revise goals as necessary and appropriate.

of disease (Cohen 1995). Many studies in psychoneuroimmunology (PNI) are being conducted to more clearly determine the connection between mind and body.

According to Maslow (1970), the author of the model we have found most useful in caring for the aged, there are certain human needs that must be fulfilled to ensure maximal function and satisfaction. In later life, when the basic physiologic systems are gradually losing efficacy over time, the need for safety and

security, a sense of belonging, and intimacy become supremely important.

Safety and Security

The external issues of safety and security are considered quite thoroughly in Chapter 22. These are relatively simple to address if there is a real desire to do so. A deep, internal sense of insecurity develops as elders discover that the body they have taken for granted most of their lives begins to betray them; organ systems work less effectively, and automatic actions and reactions require concentration. This then becomes the source of much anxiety and erodes one's security. Compensation for impairments and sensory deficits and the opportunity to continue personal rituals that provide daily structure and security will help ensure feelings of safety and reduce anxiety. Specific manifestations of anxiety and interventions are considered later in the chapter. Appropriate living situations significantly affect one's sense of security and safety. These are discussed at length in Chapter 27.

Belonging

As individuals in the support system become less readily available and the society moves forward without the elder's input or major contributions, the sense of belonging is diminished and the opportunity to be an active participant with others is steadily decreased. The family and its elder members are considered in Chapter 23. Elders without involved family or partners and geriatric orphans, especially those who are institutionalized, will need to develop surrogate family or caring groups and affiliations that meet their need for belonging.

Intimacy and Sexuality

The need for closeness and intimacy remains throughout life regardless of opportunity. Many older individuals say that they enjoy simply being cuddled and held, but others avidly seek sexual satisfaction through intercourse. The opportunity for intimacy and for sexual expression as a component of intimacy may be virtually unattainable for very old persons whose lifelong partner has died or for elders who are institutionalized. Although professionals give lip service to this need, some are surprised when actually confronted with it. Many elders consider sexual intercourse an important aspect of their lives.

In assessing the need for sexual activity, one must be wary of reticence and of inflicting one's own values. A 95-year-old man was found to be actively involved with prostitutes who would come to his low-rent high-rise apartment when he requested it. His housekeeper was upset when she discovered this, as were the nursing students involved in his health care. The housekeeper feared that the prostitutes would steal from him, and the students feared that he might contract a sexually transmitted disease (STD). These are legitimate concerns, but the first and most important issue is the confronta-

tion of health care providers' attitudes toward elders and sexual activities.

Johnson (1997) surveyed 1500 men and women over age 50 and summarized their suggestions for discussing sexuality (Box 25-2). These are helpful guidelines for nurses not sure how to approach the discussion.

The normal sexual changes of aging are considered in Chapter 7. Erectile dysfunction (impotence) is a common problem among older men and one that may be personally devastating. Erectile dysfunction in old age is frequently related to disease entities such as diabetes, medications, alcohol, depression, and long periods of abstinence. Miller (1997) provides a summary of various medical therapies for erectile dysfunction (Table 25-1), but with the advent of sildenafil citrate (Viagra), these may be less often necessary. Some men have had penile implants and find them satisfactory. The method of maintaining an erection must be effective and acceptable to the man and his partner. Nurses are responsible for identifying and addressing health-related issues that interfere with life satisfaction, and therefore it is appropriate for nurses to ask, "Are your needs for intimacy being met?" The nurse may assist the elderly in obtaining information and referrals.

Unmet Needs

Unmet needs may be submerged and appear in the form of various defense mechanisms or behavioral distortions. Deprivations result in reactions that may or may not be health enhancing. The nurse's task is to provide appropriate resources for resolving the issue to the extent possible and to listen with an "I/thou" attitude, knowing that we all are connected and will be that individual with the same need at some point. To be truly heard provides the feelings of security, belonging, and intimacy that are so necessary but often unavailable in our economically and mechanistically oriented society. When the needs are not addressed or even recognized, various manifestations will occur.

STRESS AND STRESSORS OF THE AGED

The experience of stress is an internal state accompanying threats to self. Healthy stress levels motivate one toward growth, whereas stress overload diminishes one's ability to cope effectively. Stress overload can be conceptualized as a result of poor tension management.

Ongoing stressors may create moderate anxiety and be accompanied by unconscious alterations in behavior,

---

Box 25-2   GUIDELINES FOR HEALTH CARE PROVIDERS

Health Care Providers Should Spend Time With Older Adults
- Be available to discuss the subject.
- Give us your full attention.
- Allow time to ask questions.
- Take time to answer questions.

Health Care Providers Should Use Clear and Easy-to-Understand Words
- Use plain, everyday language.
- Explain medical terms in plain English.
- Give explanations or answers to questions in simple terms.

Health Care Providers Should Help Older Adults Feel Comfortable Talking About Sex
- Help us to break the ice.
- Make us feel comfortable in asking questions.
- Offer permission to express feelings and needs.
- Don't be afraid or embarrassed to discuss sexuality problems.

Health Care Providers Should Be Open-Minded and Talk Openly
- Don't assume there are no concerns.
- Be open.
- Ask direct questions about sexual activity and attitudes.
- Discuss sexual concerns freely.
- Answer questions honestly.
- Just talk about it.
- Don't evade sexual concerns.
- Be willing to discuss sexual problems.
- Probe sexual concerns if elder wishes.

Health Care Providers Should Listen
- Be prepared to listen.
- Listen so we feel you are interested in our problems.
- Let us talk.

Health Care Providers Should Treat Older Adults With a Respectful and Nonjudgmental Attitude
- See us as individuals with sexual needs.
- Accept us for what we are: gay, straight, bisexual.
- Be nonjudgmental.
- Show genuine concern and respect.

Health Care Providers Should Encourage Discussion
- Make opportunities for one-to-one discussion.
- Provide privacy.
- Promote candid discussion.
- Provide discussion groups to ask questions.
- Develop support groups.

Health Care Providers Can Give Advice or Suggestions
- Provide information.
- Offer to find solutions and alternatives to given situations.
- Provide explicit pamphlets, explain sexual positions, lubrication.
- Discuss old taboos.
- Give suggestions of ways to help solve sexual problems.

Health Care Providers Need to Understand That "Sex Is Not Just for the Young"
- Try to eliminate the idea that sex and love are just for younger people.
- Acknowledge that sexual impulses are healthy and do not disappear as individuals age.
- Treat older adults as normal sexual beings and not as asexual elderly people.
- Recognize that sex can improve—can become even better when one is older.

From Johnson B: Older adults' suggestions for health care providers regarding discussions of sex, *Geriatr Nurs* 18(2):65-66, 1997.

---

such as repetitive actions, that discharge the anxious feelings in specific and observable symptoms. Many changes and losses compounded may result in anxiety that has no specific trigger that the elder can identify. Among the aged, stress is likely to appear as cognitive impairment (Krause, 1996).

During the course of the later years many situations and conditions occur that erode confidence in one's self and stir negative feelings. Restoration of a sense of con-

trol is basic to moving beyond the helplessness experienced during crises, stress, and illness.

No generation has faced so many changes or had its mettle so tested. This provides a beginning focus of discussion with elders feeling uncertain and incapable of making the changes necessary in their situation. It is sometimes necessary to remind an elder of all of the major events that they have survived (see Chapter 1 for discussion of these). Our task is to restore faith in one's

Table 25-1

Medical Therapies Available for Erectile Dysfunction

Medical product (examples)	Action/type of delivery
External vacuum devices (Erectaid, Catalyst, VED pump)	Airtight plastic cylinder used around penis to create a vacuum using a manual or battery-powered pump; constriction band then placed around base of penis to retain erection; cylinder then removed
Intracavernous injection therapy with alprostadil (Caverject, EDEX, Prostin VR); papaverine (Pavabid) and phentolamine (Regitine) are also widely used but not approved by the FDA for this purpose	Self-injection of medication into erectile tissue; causes vasodilation and relaxation of smooth muscles of penis
Transurethral alprostadil (MUSE)	Plastic applicator with microsuppository of a prostadil inserted into urethra, where the medication is released
Yohimbine (Yocon, Yohimex)	Traditional African aphrodisiac; approved for erectile dysfunction but has a low success rate; sometimes combined with trazodone
Testosterone replacement therapy (Andryl, Depo-Testosterone, Testoderm, Androderm)	Oral, sublingual, or transdermal hormonal therapy for small minority of men with abnorally low natural testosterone levels
Topical medications (e.g., minoxidil, nitroglyerin, aminophylline, isosorbide dinitrate, herbal combinations)	May assist in enhancing erection; not approved for this use by FDA
Sildenafil citrate (Viagra)	Assists in attaining erection—contraindicated in certain medical conditions

Modified from Miller CA: New treatments for erectile dysfunction, *Geriatr Nurs* 18(6):285-286, 1997.

adaptive capacity and self-directed action. These goals must be geared to the client's present situation and the realization that self-control, once relinquished, may be slow to return.

Stressors in the present, whether acute or chronic, require action and inner resources to avert crises. Some that are common to the aged include the following:
- Caregiving of a demented spouse
- Illness or health care system concerns
- Relocation and dispersal of significant belongings
- Loss of children, cohorts, siblings, or friends
- Incompetency proceedings
- Inheritance conflicts
- Abandonment: fear of dying alone, not being found, or painful death
- Hospitalization or institutionalization, costs, and loss of independence
- Separation from the elder's personal physician
- Sensory changes (vision and hearing)
- Housing and home maintenance
- Rent increases

- Lack of protection when frail and vulnerable
- Limited mobility and lack of transportation
- Unnamed concerns about the future
- Fears of senility
- Social losses or loss of the elder's driver's license
- Acute and chronic pain
- Medications
- Abuse and neglect
- Loss of pet
- Uncertainties about financial resources

The following are factors to consider in stress management:
- Change is stressful; therefore interventions should impose as few changes as possible.
- Continuity of personnel and having as few persons as possible to administer services leave the client more energy to deal with the problem at hand.
- Timing is important. Individuals have personal time clocks that order their peak efficiency daily, monthly, and developmentally; use the best times to introduce change.

- Another aspect of timing to consider is the recency of stresses. More energy will be needed to integrate events that have occurred within the previous 6 weeks, 6 months, or year than those occurring in the remote past.
- The aged often experience multiple, simultaneous stresses, and reduction of anxiety is necessary before options for intervention can be considered.
- Some aged are in a chronic state of grief because losses are never fully resolved before another one occurs; stress then becomes a constant state of being. Further discussion of grief can be found in Chapter 26.
- The individual needs to understand that resolution may be slower than expected if he or she has recently been bombarded with change.
- Individuals in high-stress situations should be advised to increase rest and improve nutrition, because the body chemistry changes and one is more vulnerable to illness.
- Relaxation strategies may be helpful.

Prevention and Treatment

A core set of attitudes, including optimism, self-esteem, a sense of control, connectedness, and sources of happiness and pleasure, result in the ability to deal with enormous stressors (Sobel, 1995).

Martin (1996) has developed acronyms that are reminders of important tips in stress management:

S   Collect data with a stress scale.
T   Talk about upsetting situations.
R   Relax with imagery or visualization.
E   Exercise (e.g., gardening, walking, or window shopping—these are also distracters).
S   Support groups; join those that provide affirmation and problem solving.
S   Smile.

Martin further adds the *HALT* acronym, which specifies that decisions must never be made when one is *H*ungry, *A*ngry, *L*onely, or *T*ired.

Teaching the elderly stress reduction often begins with progressive muscle relaxation (PMR). This will often reduce stress and increase awareness of muscles that are weak, tight, stressed, or inactive. The procedure for teaching progressive muscle relaxation and the sequential order of proceeding from one muscle group to another are shown in Boxes 25-3 and 25-4. There are numerous books on the market for professionals and for lay persons that provide various techniques for managing stress (Jacobson, 1938; Lusk, 1992).

Box 25-3   PROCEDURE FOR TEACHING PROGRESSIVE MUSCLE RELAXATION

1. Provide a quiet environment.
2. Arrange for a comfortable chair; a recliner is ideal.
3. Instruct the client to wear comfortable clothes and remove any contact lenses.
4. Instruct the client to focus attention on a muscle group.
5. Instruct the client to tense that muscle group and focus on feelings of tension.
6. After 5 to 7 seconds of tension, instruct the client to relax that muscle group.
7. Allow the client to relax the muscle group for 30 to 40 seconds and instruct the client to focus on feelings of relaxation.
8. Repeat the tense and relax cycle.
9. Encourage the client to practice the complete procedure twice a day for 15 to 20 minutes.

From Weinberger R: Teaching the elderly stress reduction, *J Gerontol Nurs* 17(10):23, 1991.

Box 25-4   SEQUENTIAL ORDER FOR RELAXATION OF MUSCLE GROUPS

Dominant hand and forearm
Dominant biceps
Nondominant hand and forearm
Nondominant biceps
Forehead
Upper cheeks and nose
Lower cheeks and jaws
Neck and throat
Chest, shoulders, and upper back
Abdominal region
Dominant thigh
Dominant calf
Dominant foot
Nondominant thigh
Nondominant calf
Nondominant foot

From Weinberger R: Teaching the elderly stress reduction, *J Gerontol Nurs* 17(10):23, 1991.

POSTTRAUMATIC STRESS DISORDER

Sexual and physical assault, robbery, mugging, torture, natural or man-made disasters, and life-threatening illnesses with all of the attendant medical treatments and torments are traumatic events that may leave permanent psychologic scars. These events may remain psychologically disrupting for years thereafter. The memories invoke anger, anxiety, nightmares, intrusive images and thoughts, denial, emotional numbness, and survivor's guilt.

Identifying the reactions to these deep psychologic scars as posttraumatic stress disorder (PTSD) syndrome is recent and has been largely associated with Vietnam war veterans' experiences. In World War II "shell shock" and "combat fatigue" were used to refer to the same phenomenon. Research has found that the amount and severity of combat exposure, not the soldier's personality, are related to PTSD symptom development (Buffum, Wolfe, 1995). PTSD results from exposure to overwhelmingly stressful situations, beyond the realm of the ordinary human imagination. Table 25-2 outlines the phases of PTSD. The stressors of aging and the loss of loved ones weaken the psyche's defense system, and PTSD may emerge in old age (Buffum, Wolfe, 1995).

The nurse must understand that any current loss or traumatic situation may trigger unexpected and devas-

Table 25-2

Common Posttrauma Responses, Symptoms of Denial and Intrusion, and Pathologic Intensification

Phases of PTSD	Symptoms	Pathologic intensification
Outcry: fear, sadness, anger		Overwhelmed; dazed; confused; panic; dissociative reactions; psychoses
Denial: numbing, avoidance	Daze; selective inattention; inability to appreciate significance of stimuli; amnesia; inability to visualize memories; constriction and inflexibility of thought; fantasies used to counteract reality; feeling of numbness or unreality or detachment; overcontrolled states of mind; sleep disturbances; tension-related autonomic nervous system responses, felt as fatigue or headache; frantic overactivity to crowd attention with stimuli; withdrawal from ordinary activities	Maladaptive avoidances: seclusion, drug or alcohol abuse, phobic frenzy, dissociative episodes
Intrusion experiences: unbidden thoughts and images	Hypervigilance; hypersensitivity to associated events; startle reactions; illusion, including sensation of recurrence; intrusive-repetitive thoughts or images or emotions or behaviors; overgeneralization of associations; inability to concentrate; preoccupation with event-related themes; confusion or disruption while thinking about event and themes; labile; sleep disturbances; recurrent dreams; search for lost persons or situations; bodily sensations associated with readiness for flight: tremor, nausea, diarrhea, sweating	Flooded and impulsive states; despair; impaired work and social relationships and activities; compulsive reenactments
Working through: facing reality		Anxiety and depressive reactions; physiologic disruptions
Relative completion of response: getting on with life		Inability to work, create, or feel emotions

Modified from Marmar CR, Horowitz MJ: Diagnosis and phase-oriented treatment of post-traumatic stress disorder. In Wilson JP, Harel Z, Kahana B, editors: *Human adaptation to extreme stress,* New York, 1988, Plenum.
PTSD, Posttraumatic stress disorder.

tating reactions related to those past losses and disastrous events. Long-delayed reactions may burst forth. The nurse should be available to talk about these experiences, to listen, and to respect the ones who wish to remain silent. It is useful, as in any crisis, to restore a sense of normality in the surroundings and to reassure the individual that these devastating recollections are eruptions of grief processes. Each awareness moves the person toward healing.

Benezra (1996) identified individuals who had experienced extremely traumatic events that created intense fear and helplessness. Those who coped successfully without enduring problems seemed to have secure and supportive relationships, the ability to freely express or fully suppress the experience, favorable circumstances immediately following the trauma, productive and active life-styles, strong faith/religion/hope, a sense of humor, and biologic integrity.

CRISES

Crises and stressful situations occur throughout life but are thought to occur less frequently in the later years, although with more devastating effects, when one may have less reserve adaptive capacity and fewer available supports (McLean, Link, 1994). *Stress* and *crisis* are not the same. Crisis events always create stress, but stressful situations do not necessarily precipitate crises. Any of the stressors that occur among the aged may actually be experienced as a crisis if the event occurs abruptly, is unanticipated, requires skills or resources the elder does not possess, or results in personality disorganization or psychologic immobility.

Psychologic homeostasis, comparable to and intertwined with physiologic homeostasis, fluctuates in the elderly within a reduced range of normal. The daily habits and rituals provide points of security and bolster stress immunity. When crises and cumulative stresses stretch the limits of coping capacity beyond one's individually established range, adaptive behavior temporarily deteriorates. Helplessness, lack of control, and dependency may emerge, as well as personality aberrations. It is important to remember that these are temporary conditions and will generally subside as some degree of personal power can be restored.

Crisis as referring to devastating stress was first introduced into the psychologic health care arena by Erich Lindemann in 1944. It is defined as the lack of defense or coping mechanisms to deal with sudden and unexpected intrusions into a life situation that was pre-

viously experienced as stable (Battegay, 1995). Crises common to the aged include those listed in Box 25-5.

Some individuals have developed, through a lifetime of coping with stress, a tremendous stress tolerance, whereas others will be thrown into crisis by changes in their life with which they feel unable to cope. The critical factor is personal perception of an event. The degree of personal disorganization is reflective of one's self-esteem and sense of capability more than the magnitude of the event.

Reactions to a perceived crisis include (1) anxiety, fear, a sense of unreality, and detachment; (2) restlessness, inability to sit still, searching for something to do, disorganized behavior, and repetitiously performing behaviors that are no longer effective; (3) detachment and watchful waiting; (4) ruminating thoughts of guilt, incompetence, helplessness, questioning, confusion, and paranoia; and (5) physical reactions of exhaustion, anorexia, and other symptoms of grief as explained in Chapter 26.

Recognizing characteristics of and reactions to crises will alert nurses to organize crisis intervention strategies. We have most frequently observed detachment, apathy, inability to make decisions, and disorganized behavior in elders experiencing a crisis. Crises and stressful situations may produce emotions that erode the health of the frail aged. When the events exceed a critical, but individually variable, level of de-

---

Box 25-5   CRISES COMMON TO THE AGED

- Abrupt internal and external body changes and illnesses
- Other-oriented concerns: children, grandchildren, spouse
- Loss of significant people
- Acute discomfort and pain
- Breach in significant relationships
- Fires, thefts
- Injuries, falls
- Translocation
- Aphasia, abrupt loss following stroke
- Abrupt loss of mobility or source of transportation
- Major unexpected drain on economic resources (e.g., house repair, illness)
- Abrupt changes in housing, especially without warning, to a new location, home, apartment, room, or institution
- Death of roommates in institutions

mand on the already-vulnerable physical homeostasis, illness is likely. An array of harmful neuroendocrine responses is thought to be triggered (Kopin, 1995). These neuroendocrine responses attributable to overload of the stress response system may lead to autoimmune diseases such as arthritis, heart disease, or cancer (Stratakis, Chrousos, 1995; Ulmer, 1996; Vingerhoets et al, 1996); upper respiratory tract infections (Cohen, 1995); impaired response to influenza vaccine (Kiecolt-Glaser et al, 1996); and memory loss (Krause, 1996).

The numerous unexpected natural disasters that occur each year leave many elderly displaced or homeless. Tornadoes, hurricanes, cyclones, floods, tropical storms, firestorms, and earthquakes are examples of such events. In addition, there are terrorist acts, bombings, killings, and accidents that occur suddenly and without preparation. All of these are likely to generate crises and dysfunctional coping. They may or may not resolve quickly, depending on the person, as well as the quality and immediacy of interventions. These events may trigger PTSD, as discussed earlier. Events that evoke personal bodily threat and terror are most difficult to integrate.

Crisis Intervention Strategies

Crisis intervention is designed to resolve the immediate problem and to restore the person to the level of function that existed before the crisis occurred. The immediate interventions must be geared to alleviating some of the anxiety and the problem that most disturbs the elder. Immediate actions must decrease discomfort sufficiently to gain the elder's attention and cooperation.

Dealing with older persons in crisis is different from dealing with younger persons. Increased chronic medical problems, decreased ability to manage without assistance, and living alone combine to produce a situation requiring supportive therapy. Crisis management may involve many referrals and ongoing case management. Strengthening the informal care network is important, although in some cases it may be ineffective or inappropriate and contribute to the crisis.

Some specific suggestions for crisis intervention with the aged include the following:

1. Maintain routine and usual habits as much as possible.
2. Clarify cognitive perception of the disruptive event.
3. Learn the client's characteristic behavior.
4. Encourage reminiscing to learn about self-esteem, affect, character, past coping patterns, and uniqueness and to restore a sense of control and capability.

5. Encourage expression of feelings toward tension discharge and mastery.
6. Listen to complaints; do not dismiss any as unimportant; help resolve predominant complaints.
7. Develop a readily available support system; identify and use existing systems when they are supportive.
8. Give adequate information to the client, but avoid overload; sometimes the information will need to be written and/or repeated.
9. Attend to physical comfort measures.
10. Use touch as appropriate.
11. Identify the resource person to be contacted if needed.

Crisis as Growth

Growth occurs through crisis if the process is recognized and coping efforts are supported and augmented as needed. Many of the symptoms of emotional disorder are evidence of an ineffective search for resolution of an earlier problem. Recognizing these symptoms may assist nurses in reassuring clients of their potential strength. Rather than attempting to ameliorate or ignore symptoms of crisis states, we might encourage recognition and acceptance.

Nurses may wish to pose alternative solutions long before the client has reached a state of readiness. This is not helpful. Timing is critical. Recognize stages and validate verbally (e.g., "It seems as if your thoughts are going in circles. That is a necessary step before you can move on to resolution of the problem.")

ADJUSTMENT REACTIONS

Adjustment disorders are diagnosed when one develops significant emotional or behavioral responses to an identifiable psychosocial stress or stressors (American Psychiatric Association, 1994, p. 623). Clinical significance is noted when the distress exhibited by the elder is in excess of that expected by the nature of the stressor (Box 25-6). The stressors may be single or multiple, recurrent or continuous, and some are more prominent in certain transitional periods, such as frequent moves into increasingly dependent situations experienced by elders. Typical stressors that evoke an adjustment disorder in the aged include retirement, changes in living situations, and medical diagnoses that are threatening.

Assessment of excessive emotional reactions to certain adjustments required of the aged may be difficult because personality, gender, and cultural factors must

Box 25-6	DIAGNOSTIC CRITERIA FOR ADJUSTMENT DISORDERS

A. The development of emotional or behavioral symptoms in response to an identifiable stressor(s) occurring within 3 months of the onset of the stressor(s).
B. These symptoms or behaviors are clinically significant as evidenced by either of the following:
   1. Marked distress that is in excess of what would be expected from exposure to the stressor
   2. Significant impairment in social or occupational (academic) functioning
C. The stress-related disturbance does not meet the criteria for another specific Axis I disorder and is not merely an exacerbation of a preexisting Axis I or Axis II disorder.
D. The symptoms do not represent Bereavement.
E. Once the stressor (or its consequences) has terminated, the symptoms do not persist for more than an additional 6 months.
Specify if:
   Acute: If the disturbance lasts less than 6 months
   Chronic: If the disturbance lasts for 6 months or longer

Data from American Psychiatric Association: *Diagnostic and statistical manual of mental disorders (DSM-IV)*, ed 4, Washington, DC, 1994, The Association.

be considered, as well as the availability of supportive relationships. Adjustment disorders may be exhibited by profound depression, with or without anxiety, and behavioral disturbances. Nursing interventions should include anticipatory rehearsal of the event and instigation of a reliable and ongoing support system available to the individual before and following the occurrence. In addition, options and alternatives related to the particular adjustment should be thoroughly discussed and considered. This will reduce the sense of helplessness and irreversibility.

ANXIETY REACTIONS

The *Diagnostic and Statistical Manual of Mental Disorders (DSM-IV)* (American Psychiatric Association, 1994) delineates three categories of anxiety disorder: phobic disorders, PTSDs, and anxiety states. PTSD, probably more common than has been recognized, is dealt with earlier in this chapter. Anxiety in its varied manifestations is considered extensively here.

Anxiety states are common in late life. Frequent symptoms include shakiness, trembling, inability to relax, palpitations, worry or anticipated disaster, a sense of impending doom, distractibility, poor concentration, insomnia, and excessive vigilance. In the aged, anxiety is most frequently expressed in somatic concerns (Boerner, 1995). The threat of illness is very real, as is the confrontation with mortality. Illness may precipitate loss of self-trust, changes in self-concept, alteration in interpersonal relationships, and fears of death and permanent dependency. Thus anxiety is frequently experienced as forebodings of illness.

Anxiety is a response to feelings of helplessness, isolation, alienation, and insecurity—a response to unmet needs of the human condition. Mild and moderate anxiety motivate one toward problem resolution, but intense anxiety produces a diffuse feeling of panic, dread, and lack of control that can be agonizing in the acute stages.

Extreme or prolonged personal stress is likely to bring on episodes of anxiety. Clinical levels of anxiety are seldom held for long periods because they are intolerable. They are commonly subverted into phobias or various other control mechanisms. It is thought that anxiety in the aged is likely to produce a state of hypervigilance. Following are some evidences of an anxiety state likely to be seen in the aged:

- Disorganization
- Persistent use of a single behavior (sometimes called *perseveration* [e.g., the patient may continually and repetitiously call for the nurse and then forget what was needed])
- Exaggerated emotional reactions to minor disturbances in the elder's routine
- Agitation
- Cardiac palpitation
- Disturbed memory, inability to concentrate
- Decreased problem-solving ability
- Suspiciousness
- Obsessive/compulsive actions
- Illusions, hallucinations, delusions, phobias

Some old-age strategies that might appear as maladaptive personality traits if predominant in other situations are effective in reducing anxiety in elders and should be respected (Box 25-7).

Obsessive/Compulsive Disorders

Obsessive/compulsive disorders are those recurrent thoughts or actions that significantly impair function and consume more than 1 hour each day (American Psychiatric Association, 1994, p. 417). These disor-

Box 25-7	DEFENSE MECHANISMS USED TO REDUCE ANXIETY

- *Denial* may be intrinsic to aging and necessary to maintain one's equilibrium in the face of major losses and impending demise of self.
- *Projection* is often used to give vent to inexpressible wishes and feelings; it signals high levels of internal stress.
- *Regression* may be temporarily necessary to mobilize energy and resources to cope with external stressors.
- *Displacement* may help the elder to submerge feelings of anxiety and fasten on something more concrete and controllable.
- *Somatization* is a common means of dealing with psychosocial problems and is very hard to circumvent, since it brings secondary gains if not overused.
- *Selective* memory tends to focus one on the memories that exemplify and corroborate present feelings, whatever they may be.
- *Compulsivity* allows one to keep control in a comforting way of certain aspects of life when the larger issues are overwhelming.

ders are exaggerated manifestations of a need for control and order and a way of warding off anxiety. They are common in the aged, although very often they are not sufficient to seriously disrupt function and thus are not truly considered a disorder; rather, they are a coping strategy. If they progress to the point where they disrupt the life-style, they will need clinical attention.

In the aged these disorders are often displayed as obsessions about body functions, particularly elimination and sleep. The compulsive rituals that accompany these thoughts are an effort to ward off anxiety and discharge tension. Carrying out these tension-relief behaviors must be respected if they do not interfere with important aspects of life.

Interestingly, the two most consuming compulsive disorders I (P.E.) have observed have been related to the control of time. One woman had numerous clocks with alarms set for different times of the day and night. In dealing with her, staff considered the symbolic significance of clocks and time and death from an existential perspective. The elder was gradually weaned from the clocks, one at a time, and other gratifying activities were introduced into her schedule, one at a time and on a precise timetable that the staff assured her would not vary. She was also shown her chart to show her that she

was checked each half hour at night to be sure that she was all right.

Excessive Suspicion and Paranoia

Many older people with no previous history of mental disturbance develop a suspicious or paranoid viewpoint. Various estimates of the prevalence of paranoia range from 5% to 10% of the aged population. These reactions are sometimes induced by alcoholism or medications, particularly male hormones in combination with antidepressants. The majority, however, originate in attempts to exert control in an unsatisfactory situation or to feel capable. Inability to correctly evaluate the social milieu because of isolation or cognitive disturbance is a significant factor (Blazer, 1995a). Forgetfulness may result in an elder being convinced that items are being stolen. Fear and a lack of trust originating from a reality base may become magnified, especially when one is isolated from others and does not receive reality feedback.

Men are more subject than women to those reactions. The male dilemma of expecting to be in control and to gain recognition may be a factor. Women (of the present older generation) were subject to control by others and by their body reactions throughout their young adult lives and have had more experience coping with events beyond their control.

Assessment and Treatment

Paranoia is characterized by suspiciousness and insecurity (Riley, 1990). Deafness or hearing impairment may accentuate these feelings. Delusions often incorporate significant persons rather than the global grandiose or persecutory delusions of younger persons. It is sometimes difficult to determine the reality of an apparent paranoid reaction. Many cases have been encountered in which plots against an older person were real. In the case of simple paranoid psychoses the delusions appear to serve an adaptive function. When an individual becomes incapable of obtaining life's satisfactions or of maintaining function or adequate supplies, the delusions may allow the individual to avoid depression and self-blame and maintain self-esteem by projecting blame onto others or society.

Direct confrontation is likely to increase anxiety and agitation, the sense of vulnerability, and the need for the delusion. A more useful approach is to establish a trusting relationship that is nondemanding and not too intense and to identify the client's strengths and build on them (Box 25-8). Paranoid behavior may be present

Box 25-8	GUIDELINES FOR NURSING CARE OF SUSPICIOUS PATIENTS

Remember that anger is pervasive and is not meant for the nurse per se.

Anger is a legitimate expression of feeling.

Suspicious persons will look for flaws or indications of injustice.

Attempt to accept criticism without resentment or defensiveness.

Arguing only increases the struggle for control.

The quality of nursing care may not be measurable by patient progress, particularly if the goals are unrealistic or not relevant to the patient. In other words, paranoia may lift slowly or not at all.

Nursing care should provide for the following needs:

1. Suspicious persons need to learn to trust themselves. Allow the patient to function independently in areas in which success can be achieved and identified.

2. Suspicious persons need to be able to trust others. Nurses should state what they are willing and able to do. Vague promises such as, "I'll be around whenever you need me," only increase opportunities for distrust and disappointment.

3. Suspicious persons need to test reality. When the larger reality is distorted, focus on smaller aspects of reality; for example:

   Mrs. J.: The whole world is against me.

   Nurse: What in this room gives you that feeling? Are there certain times when you feel that most strongly?

   Contact with the nurse and the nurse's accepting responses reassure the person and decrease the need for protective delusion.

4. Suspicious persons need outlets for their anger.

---

in the absence of any cognitive loss but may also be the first symptom noted in the development of dementia.

The presence of paranoid ideation is a problem only if it disturbs the patient or others in his or her environment. Paranoia may act as an effective shield against intrusion into one's vulnerable state and as such may be a useful defensive posture. When encountering suspicious elderly, the nurse's primary concern is first directed at establishing the reality of the feeling, but if the suspicions are not substantiated, the elder should not be challenged.

Nurses need to reduce the alienation and feelings of insignificance that underlie paranoid ideation. It is im-

portant that the nurse be trustworthy, that clear information be given, and that clear choices always be presented to the patient. When food, medication, treatments, or resources are being offered to the patient, relevant information should also be given. If medications must be mixed with food or liquid for ease of administration, it should be done in the elder's presence and an explanation given. When patients refuse "necessary" treatments, their decision must be respected. Focusing on decision-making power is most likely to be beneficial (e.g., "Mrs. S., it seems that you are reluctant to take these medications. I respect the fact that you are cautious about such things. I will get you more information about these drugs. Are there particular reactions you are concerned about? Let me know if you decide to take them"; or "Mrs. J., many people feel angry or afraid when they are ill. Is there anything I can do to make you more comfortable?")

Delusions

A delusional disorder is one in which conceivable ideas, without foundation in fact, persist for more than 1 month. These beliefs are not bizarre and do not originate in psychotic processes (American Psychiatric Association, 1994, p. 296). Common delusions are of being poisoned, being followed, or being deceived by a spouse or lover. Delusional disorders in the absence of psychoses usually begin between the ages of 40 and 55 when psychologic and physical stressors and major personal and social problems occur (Kaplan, Sadock, 1994). Delusions are intellectual mechanisms for maintaining a sense of control when security is threatened. They are beliefs that guide one's interpretation of events and help make sense out of disorder. The delusions may be comforting or threatening, but they always form a structure for understanding situations that otherwise might seem unmanageable. One elderly woman persistently held onto the delusion that her son was a very important attorney and was coming to force the administration to discharge her from the nursing home. Her son, a factory worker, had been dead for 10 years. The events of her day, her hopes, and her status were all organized around this belief. It is clear that without her delusion she would have felt forlorn, lost, and abandoned. I (P.E.) have encountered many delusions related to family members and their actions or intentions among the institutionalized aged.

The assessment dilemma is often one of determining the truth of the delusional belief and avoiding assumptions. It is never safe to conclude that someone is delusional unless you have thoroughly investigated his or her claims. In one case an 88-year-old man insisted that he must go and visit his mother. His thoughts seemed clear in other respects (often the case with people who are delusional), and I suspected that he had some unresolved conflicts about his dead mother or felt the need of comforting and caring. I did not argue with him about his dead mother, since arguing is never a useful approach to persons with delusions. Rather, I used the best techniques I could think of to assure him that I was interested in him as a person and recognized that he must feel very lonely sometimes. He continued to say that he must go and visit his mother. When I could delay his leaving no longer, I walked with him to the nurses' station and found that his 104-year-old mother did indeed live in another wing of the institution and that he visited her every day.

Hallucinations

Hallucinations are best described as sensory perceptions of nonexistent external stimuli and may be spurred by the internal stimulation of any of the five senses (Sprinzeles, 1992). Although they occur without environmental stimuli, they may well occur because of the total environmental impact. Hallucinations arising out of psychologic conflicts tend to be less predominant in old age, whereas those generated as security measures to avoid anxiety tend to increase. These hallucinations are thought to germinate in situations in which one is feeling alone, abandoned, isolated, or alienated. To compensate for insecurity, a hallucinatory experience, often in the form of a companion, is imagined. Imagined companions may fill the intense void and provide some security, but they sometimes become accusing and disturbing.

The character and stages of hallucinatory experiences have not been adequately defined in terms of the aged. Many are in response to neurophysiologic disorders such as dementias, Parkinson disease, and medications. Most often, hallucinations of the aged seem mixed with disorientation, illusions, intense grief, and immersion in retrospection, the origins being difficult to separate. Almeida et al (1995) found that psychotic states arising in late life were predominately associated with cognitive decline.

It is important for nurses to determine whether the hallucinations are a result of dementia, psychoses, deprivation, or overload, because the treatment will vary. An isolated old person who is admitted to the hospital in a hallucinatory state must be carefully and thor-oughly assessed physically and then gradually brought into socializing experiences. He or she should be allowed peripheral participation and retreat when necessary. Persons in the community who develop hallucinations must be assessed in terms of threats to security, severe physical or psychologic disruptions, withdrawal symptoms, medications, and overload of stimuli. Antipsychotic medications are a significant aspect of management for most hallucinations.

SCHIZOPHRENIA

The onset of schizophrenia usually occurs between adolescence and the mid-30s. The occurrence in persons 60 years of age and older is rare and is most likely to include paranoid delusions and hallucinations. These symptoms may be responsive to low doses of antipsychotic medications. Sensory deficits, particularly hearing loss, occur more frequently in persons with schizophrenia than in the general adult population. Those who developed schizophrenia early may have developed a chronic adaptation that is difficult to distinguish from a mood disorder. Unfortunately, those elders with frank psychiatric disorders who had been residing in state hospitals are now among the homeless on the streets of any inner city, frequently victimized by the younger homeless, or they have been placed in nursing homes without appropriate mental health services available to them. These individuals have largely been left to shift for themselves. The plight of elderly schizophrenic persons demonstrates the realities of human needs neglected: they are not protected, have little sense of belonging, and have no self-esteem.

DEPRESSION

Depression is the mental health problem of greatest frequency and magnitude in the aged population. Estimates of prevalence vary radically, depending on the qualitative variables being considered and the definition being used. Although it is estimated that between 1% and 2% of the population over age 65 meet the DSM-IV criteria for a major depressive disorder (Alexopoulos, 1995), numerous others have dysthymic conditions of varying degrees. Some 31 million elders suffer from some degree of depression (Lebowitz, 1996). Katona (1994) reports that although relatively few meet the DSM-IV criteria for depression, many of those considered dysthymic are equally severely distressed. It is useful to think of depression as being on a continuum from mild, brief sadness, to intense reaction to loss, to severe psychotic depression, to the profound regression of pseudodementia (Alexopoulos, 1995).

Bipolar disorders often level out in late life, and individuals tend to have longer periods of depression. An individual with a bipolar disorder is afflicted with a chemical imbalance and must be treated as such. Lithium, the most commonly used substance for individuals with bipolar disorders, disturbs the fluid balance, which may already be a problem for an elder. Balancing the appropriate medication dosage and monitoring side effects is particularly precarious in elders and requires very careful and consistent attention.

Many of the drugs and medical conditions common to the elderly are associated with depression (Boxes 25-9 and 25-10); in addition, the life situations of elders may result in depression. In spite of its prevalence, depression is underrecognized and undertreated. Fortunately, depression is one of the most manageable problems once it is recognized. However, there is a high incidence of relapse after treatment, especially in the very old who have concurrent physical disorders and unrewarding life situations.

Etiology

Factors of health, gender, developmental needs, socioeconomics, environment, personality, losses, and awareness of time running out are all significant to the development of depression in later life. Depressive symptoms in an older adult are complex and may arise from several intersecting situations and conditions: biologic changes of age, sleep cycle changes, neurotransmitter reduction, and alterations in neuroendocrine substances. These all contribute to a predisposition toward depression. The old are thought to be more vulnerable to depression because of the reduced production of mood-controlling neurotransmitters (Kaplan, Sadock, 1994). The helplessness of observing one's slowly deteriorating physical capacities is also depressing. Some factors that have been found to have a high correlation with depression are stroke, physical impairment, vitamin B deficiencies, hearing loss, and pain.

Assessment

Assessment of depression in elders is complicated by the fact that some somatic changes that occur normally in aging, such as tendencies toward constipation, early-morning waking, and slowed motor activity, which would be indications of depression in a young adult,

---

Box 25-9 DRUGS THAT CAN CAUSE SYMPTOMS OF DEPRESSION IN ELDERLY PATIENTS

Antihypertensives
  Reserpine
  Methyldopa
  Propranolol
  Clonidine
  Hydralazine
  Guanethidine
  Diuretics*
Analgesics
  Narcotic
  Morphine
  Codeine
  Meperidine
  Pentazocine
  Propoxyphene
Nonnarcotic
  Indomethacin

Antiparkinsonian agents
  L-Dopa
Antimicrobials
  Sulfonamides
  Isoniazid
Cardiovascular agents
  Digitalis
  Lidocaine†
Hypoglycemic agents‡
Steroids
  Corticosteroids
  Estrogens
Others
  Cimetidine
  Cancer chemotherapeutic
    agents

From Kurlowicz LH, NICHE Faculty: Nursing standard of practice protocol: depression in elderly patients, *Geriatr Nurs* 18(5):192-200, 1997.
*By causing dehydration or electrolyte imbalance.
†Toxicity.
‡By causing hypoglycemia.

---

may be the normal consequences of aging. In addition, certain medications and illnesses predispose the elder to depression. These must be given consideration in reaching an appropriate diagnosis.

Hypochondriasis

Hypochondriasis is a scattering of health concerns that seems to increase when there is a real health problem, but it is often a cardinal symptom of depression. Elderly people tend to express depression through somatic symptoms. Thus the hypochondriacal preoccupation of the elderly may be a signal of the presence of depression, as are frequent visits to general practitioners. Mild, transient bouts of hypochondriasis are frequent and serve as a means of coping with the stress of real illness and loss. These patients are far less likely to view problems as psychologic, interpersonal, or situational; chief complaints are usually of various physical discomforts (e.g., "constipation," "gas pain," or "heartburn"). These sorts of complaints are too readily dismissed as hypochondriacal when a more holistic approach to the patient would re-

---

Box 25-10   PHYSICAL ILLNESSES ASSOCIATED WITH DEPRESSION IN ELDERLY PATIENTS

Metabolic disturbances
  Dehydration
  Azotemia, uremia
  Acid-base disturbances
  Hypoxia
  Hyponatremia and hypernatremia
  Hypoglycemia and hyperglycemia
  Hypocalcemia and hypercalcemia
Endocrine disorders
  Hypothyroidism and hyperthyroidism
  Hyperparathyroidism
  Diabetes mellitus
  Cushing's disease
  Addison's disease
Infections
  Viral
    Pneumonia
    Encephalitis
  Bacterial
    Pneumonia
    Urinary tract
    Meningitis
    Endocarditis
  Other
    Tuberculosis
    Brucellosis
    Fungal meningitis
    Neurosyphilis
Cardiovascular disorders
  Congestive heart failure
  Myocardial infarction, angina

Pulmonary disorders
  Chronic obstructive lung disease
  Malignancy
Gastrointestinal disorders
  Malignancy (especially pancreatic)
  Irritable bowel
  Other organic causes of chronic abdominal pain, ulcer, diverticulosis
  Hepatitis
Genitourinary disorders
  Urinary incontinence
Musculoskeletal disorders
  Degenerative arthritis
  Osteoporosis with vertebral compression or hip fractures
  Polymyalgia rheumatica
  Paget's disease
Neurologic disorders
  Cerebrovascular disease
  Transient ischemic attacks
  Stroke
  Dementia (all types)
  Intracranial mass
    Primary or metastatic tumors
  Parkinson's disease
Other illnesses
  Anemia (of any cause)
  Vitamin deficiencies
  Hematologic or other systemic malignancy

From Kurlowicz LH, NICHE Faculty: Nursing standard of practice protocol: depression in elderly patients, *Geriatr Nurs* 18(5):192-200, 1997.

---

veal the extent and complexity of problems. Fortunately, physicians are beginning to address the psychologic and interpersonal reasons why elders feel symptomatic and seek medical attention (Barsky, 1996).

Illness

Illness is often coexistent with depression, which may intensify illness and delay recovery through the depletion of the immune system. Patients with chronic medical illnesses are frequently subject to secondary depressions related to the disease processes. Studies have shown that the presence of depression impedes healing in hip fractures and myocardial infarctions (Barker, 1990; Fielding, 1991). This is a significant problem and is often related to routine assessment practices that ignore depression as

a possible deterrent to recovery. Older individuals are likely to be judged hypochondriacal when the complications of depression slow their recovery from illness.

Older persons with serious medical problems are at high risk of developing depression. Poststroke depression is so common that it is virtually ignored in treatment because symptoms parallel those of the stroke itself: apathy, amnesia, and pathologic crying (Black, 1995). Borson (1989) found that patients with chronic obstructive pulmonary disease (COPD) are particularly vulnerable to depression. The depression is often accompanied by anxiety and panic. Often physicians do not recognize these as symptoms of depression, and when they do, they may be reluctant to treat the depression because of the adverse reactions to antidepressant drugs of the anticholinergic type. We encourage nurses to routinely assess ill elders for the presence of depression using the simple and reliable tools provided in Chapter 14 and to alert physicians when there is evidence of depression. There are presently excellent drugs to manage depression in the elderly.

Treatment Considerations

Depression is often reversible with prompt and appropriate treatment. Kurlowicz (1997) provides a standard-of-practice protocol for nurses in dealing with depression in the elderly (Box 25-11). This involves a systematic and thorough assessment using a depression screening tool, individualized assessment and interview, determination of iatrogenic or medical causes, and mutual decision making regarding treatment. It is most important that the nurse recognize suicidal potential in the depressed elder, inquire about suicidal thoughts, and provide necessary protection. For those suffering from iatrogenic or medical-induced depression, restoring basic function—sleep, nutrition, hydration, exercise, comfort, and pain control—will often help. Relaxation strategies and scheduled activities with periods of rest may be useful. Maintaining the social and spiritual support systems may be extremely important.

In treating depression in the aged, consider the following:

1. There are several types of depression. It is important that a comprehensive evaluation be made before a conclusion is reached.
2. Biochemical and hormonal changes of aging may intensify depression in the aged (e.g., neurotransmitters change with aging); most hormones, particularly thyroid hormones, are reduced.
3. Drugs that are used for medical problems may intensify depression (e.g., hypotensives, psychotropics, cardiotonics, hypnotics).
4. Antidepressant drugs may have idiosyncratic effects, toxic accumulation, and/or paradoxical effects. They should be used with expert knowledge, discrimination, and adequate observation (see Chapter 15).
5. Knowledge of the presence of depression may be helpful when assisting the older person with understanding and coping with some of the unexplained symptoms that he or she is experiencing. Clients should be involved in assessment and discussion of depression. Having the individual assess the level of depression immediately engages the person actively in examining his or her own feelings. Tools that can be used in this manner are included in Chapter 14.

6. The importance of restoring a sense of control, choice, and mastery needs to be recognized.
7. Often, increased socialization and relief from physical discomfort and ailments will significantly lift depression.
8. One must be alert to early signs of recurrent depression because this is common in major depressions.
9. To decrease depression and raise self-esteem, defensive structures should be supported unless they are clearly detrimental to the client or family.

Self-Care Guidelines for Depressed Persons

Because of the nature of depression and its frequency in late life, it is seldom recognized by the sufferer. When the presence of depression is acknowledged, a nurse can then begin a dialogue to suggest some self-care measures, such as the following:

1. List activities that have been most pleasurable in the past, and contract to engage in one each day.
2. Schedule the day with short periods of activity interspersed with rest periods.
3. Eat several small nutritious meals at regular times each day.
4. Engage in comforting sleep rituals, and establish a regular sleep-wake cycle.
5. Confer with a spiritual advisor or trusted friend regarding fears, concerns, and life review.
6. Begin a dream journal or personal memoir.

Interventions

Interventions are primarily medical (drugs and electroconvulsive therapy), social (family and social support), grief management, and behavioral conditioning.

Medications

Medications are by far the most common approach to the treatment of depression. Miller (1997) lists the commonly used antidepressants (Table 25-3, p. 541), and Buffum and Buffum (1997) provide guidelines regarding the use of antidepressants (Tables 25-4 and 25-5, p. 542). See additional discussion of psychotropic medications in Chapter 15.

The fact that each person's physiology is as unique as his or her voice and facial characteristics must be recognized when using medications. Medications should be used cautiously and titrated carefully: begin with small doses and increase them as needed; if one drug is not effective, allow time for it to be cleared from

Box 25-11   NURSING STANDARD OF PRACTICE PROTOCOL FOR DEPRESSION IN ELDERLY PATIENTS

I. Background
  A. Depression—both major depressive disorder and minor, dysthymic depression—is highly prevalent in community-dwelling, medically ill, and institutionalized elders.
  B. Depression is not a natural part of aging or a normal reaction to acute illness and hospitalization.
  C. Consequences of depression include amplification of pain and disability, delayed recovery from illness and surgery, worsening of drug side effects, excess use of health services, cognitive impairment, subnutrition, and increased suicide- and nonsuicide-related death.
  D. Depression tends to be long-lasting and recurrent. Therefore a wait-and-see approach is undesirable, and immediate clinical attention is necessary.
  E. If recognized, treatment response is good.
  F. Somatic symptoms may be more prominent than depressed mood in late life depression.
  G. Mixed depressive and anxiety features may be evident among many elderly patients.
  H. Recognition of depression is hindered by the coexistence of physical illnesses and social and economic problems common in late life.
  I. Early recognition, intervention, and referral by nurses can reduce the negative effects of depression.

II. Assessment parameters
  A. Identify risk factors/high risk groups.
    1. Specific physical illnesses (stroke, cancer, dementia, arthritis, hip fracture, myocardial infarction, chronic obstructive pulmonary disease, and Parkinson's disease)
    2. Functional disability (especially new functional loss)
    3. Widows/widowers
    4. Caregivers
    5. Social isolation/absence of social support
  B. Assess all at-risk groups using a standardized depression screening tool and document score. The GDS is recommended because it takes approximately 10 minutes to administer, has been validated and extensively used with medically ill older adults, and includes *few* somatic items that may be confounded with physical illness.
  C. Perform an *individualized* depression assessment on all at-risk groups and document results. Note the number of symptoms; onset; frequency/patterns; duration (especially 2 weeks); change from normal mood, behavior, and functioning.
    1. Depressive symptoms
      a. Depressed or irritable mood, frequent crying
      b. Loss of interest, pleasure (in family, friends, hobbies, sex)
      c. Weight loss or gain (especially loss)*
      d. Sleep disturbance (especially insomnia)*
      e. Fatigue/loss of energy*
      f. Psychomotor slowing/agitation*
      g. Diminished concentration
      h. Feelings of worthlessness/guilt
      i. Suicidal thoughts or attempts, hopelessness
    2. Psychosis (i.e., delusional/paranoid thoughts, hallucinations)
    3. History of depression, substance abuse (especially alcohol), previous coping style
    4. Recent losses or crises (e.g., death of relative, friend, pet; retirement; *anniversary dates;* move to another residence, nursing home); changes in physical health status, relationships; roles
  D. Assess for depressogenic medications (e.g., narcotics, sedative/hypnotics, benzodiazepines, steroids, antihypertensives, H_2 antagonists, beta-blockers, antipsychotics, immunosuppressives, cytotoxic agents, alcohol).
  E. Assess for related systemic and metabolic processes (e.g., infection, anemia, hypothyroidism or hyperthyroidism, hyponatremia, hypercalcemia, hypoglycemia, congestive heart failure, kidney failure).

III. Care parameters
  A. For major depression (GDS score 11, 5 to 9 depressive symptoms [must include depressed mood or loss of pleasure] plus other positive responses on individualized assessment [especially suicidal thoughts or psychosis]), refer for psychiatric evaluation. Treatment options may include medication or cognitive-behavioral, interpersonal, or brief psychodynamic psychotherapy/counseling (individual, group, family), hospitalization, or electroconvulsive therapy.
  B. For less severe depression (GDS score 11, less than five depressive symptoms plus other positive responses on individualized assessment), refer to mental health services for psychotherapy/counseling (see above types), especially for specific issues identified in individualized assessment and to de-

From Kurlowicz LH, NICHE Faculty: Nursing standard of practice protocol: depression in elderly patients, *Geriatr Nurs* 18(5):192-200, 1997. *GDS,* Geriatric Depression Scale.
*Somatic symptoms, also seen in many physical illnesses, are frequently associated with No. 1 and No. 2; therefore the full range of depressive symptoms should be assessed.   *Continued*

Box 25-11   **NURSING STANDARD OF PRACTICE PROTOCOL FOR DEPRESSION IN ELDERLY PATIENTS—cont'd**

termine whether medication therapy may be warranted. Consider resources such as psychiatric liaison nurses, geropsychiatric advanced practice nurses, social workers, psychologists, and other community and institution-specific mental health services. If suicidal thoughts or psychosis is present, a referral for a comprehensive psychiatric evaluation should always be made.

C. For *all* levels of depression, develop an *individualized* plan integrating the following nursing interventions:

1. Institute safety precautions for suicide risk as per institutional policy (in outpatient settings, ensure continuous surveillance of the patient while obtaining an emergency psychiatric evaluation and disposition).

2. Remove or control etiologic agents.
   a. Avoid/remove/change depressogenic medications.
   b. Correct/treat metabolic/systemic disturbances.

3. Monitor and promote nutrition, elimination, sleep/rest patterns, physical comfort (especially pain control).

4. Enhance physical function (i.e., structure regular exercise/activity, refer to physical, occupational, recreational therapies); develop a daily activity schedule.

5. Enhance social support (i.e., identify/mobilize a support person[s] [e.g., family, confidant, friends, hospital resources, support groups, patient visitors]); ascertain need for spiritual support and contact appropriate clergy.

6. Maximize autonomy/personal control/self-efficacy (e.g., include patient in active participation in making daily schedules, short-term goals).

7. Identify and reinforce strengths and capabilities.

8. Structure and encourage daily participation in relaxation therapies, pleasant activities (conduct a pleasant activity inventory).

9. Monitor and document response to medication and other therapies; readminister depression screening tool.

10. Provide practical assistance; assist with problem-solving.

11. Provide emotional support (i.e., empathic, supportive listening, encourage expression of feel-

ings, hope instillation), support adaptive coping, encourage pleasant reminiscences but do not "force" happiness.

12. Provide information about the physical illness and treatment(s) and about depression (i.e., that depression is common, treatable, and not the person's fault).

13. Educate about the importance of adherence to prescribed treatment regimen for depression (especially medication) to prevent recurrence; educate about *specific* antidepressant side effects and any dietary restrictions.

14. Ensure mental health community link-up; consider psychiatric nursing home care intervention.

IV. Evaluation of expected outcomes

A. Patient
   1. Patient safety will be maintained.
   2. Patients with severe depression will be evaluated by psychiatric services.
   3. Patients will report a reduction of symptoms that are indicative of depression. A reduction in the GDS score will be evident, and suicidal thoughts or psychosis will resolve.

B. Health care provider
   1. Early recognition of patients at risk, referral, and interventions for depression, and documentation of outcomes will be improved.

C. Institution
   1. The number of patients identified with depression will increase.
   2. The number of in-hospital suicide attempts will not increase.
   3. The number of referrals to mental health services will increase.
   4. The number of referrals to psychiatric nursing home care services will increase.
   5. Staff will receive ongoing education on depression recognition, assessment, and interventions.

V. Follow-up to monitor condition

A. Continue to track prevalence and documentation of depression in at-risk groups.

B. Show evidence of transfer of information to post-discharge mental health service delivery system.

C. Educate caregivers to continue assessment processes.

Table 25-3

Commonly Used Antidepressants

Type	Examples	Trade name
Cyclics	Imipramine	Tofranil
	Desipramine	Norpramin, Pertofrane
	Amitriptyline	Elavil
	Nortriptyline	Aventyl, Pamelor
	Doxepin	Sinequan, Adapin
	Trimipramine	Surmontil
	Amoxapine	Asendin
	Maprotiline	Ludiomil
	Protriptyline	Vivactil
SSRIs	Fluoxetine	Prozac
	Sertraline*	Zoloft
	Paroxetine*	Paxil
	Fluvoxamine*	Luvox
Unique types	Lithium	Eskalith
	Bupropion*	Wellbutrin
	Trazodone	Desyrel
	Venlafaxine*	Effexor
	Nefazodone*	Serzone
	Mirtazapine*	Remeron
MAOIs	Tranylcypromine	Parnate
	Phenelzine	Nardil
Psychostimulants	Methylphenidate	Ritalin

From Miller CA: Keeping up with new developments in antidepressants, *Geriatr Nurs* 18(4):180-181, 1997.
SSRIs, Serotonin-specific reuptake inhibitors; *MAOIs,* monoamine oxidase inhibitors.
*Approved by the Food and Drug Administration since 1990.

the system before introducing a new drug. Involve elders in keeping a log of responses to the drug and recognize that personal biorhythms have a significant influence on drug responses. When is the best time to give the drug to get maximal response?

Some tricyclic antidepressants (TCAs) are notoriously poor selections for the elderly. TCAs fall into the category of class I antiarrhythmic drugs, as well as major anticholinergics. These have been responsible for Sjögren syndrome, increased cardiac disorders, and deaths in persons with ischemic heart disease. Serotonin-specific reuptake inhibitors (SSRIs) are a class that seems at present to be effective for elders, but it is not yet known what the long-range effects will be.

In about 60% of cases, antidepressant medication is helpful in reducing depression. (To produce effects in elderly patients, 6 to 12 weeks of a medication regimen may be necessary.) Active participation in the treatment plan and compliance with medication dosage must be encouraged because clients' motivation may be very low (see further discussion in Chapter 15).

Electroconvulsive Therapy

Electroconvulsive therapy (ECT) has lost favor in recent years, although it has been used very successfully for remission of severe depression. However, it may be necessary to repeat the ECT series (usually six sessions using muscle relaxants, oxygen, and short-acting anesthesia to prevent undesirable effects such as severe seizures) within a few months. The chief advantage is a very rapid response without the anticholinergic side effects of medications. The major disadvantage is an induced mental confusion that persists from a week to 10 days. Historically, ECT was overused with inappropriate controls and had serious effects. When ECT is used with elders, a thorough physical is essential to rule out any complicating factors that may make ECT hazardous, such as osteoporosis, certain cardiac disorders, or Parkinson disease.

Exercise

Physical exercise on a consistent basis has been found to be very helpful in decreasing depression. Short, vigorous workouts (as little as 8 minutes daily) by elders have been shown to significantly reduce depression, tension, and fatigue in 82% of a sample of elders diagnosed with clinical depression (Levine, 1997).

Spirituality

Discovering meanings and developing the spiritual self may be significant to recovery. Many believe that depression involves a spiritual crisis. Stollenwerk and colleagues (1996) suggest that attention must be given to interconnectedness. Where and when has the individual felt most connected with nature, with others, and with a spiritual self? Ask about these aspects of the individual's past, not to judge, but to explore. How can those connections be cultivated again or for the first time? Even a sprouting plant or a singing bird may help one regain a sense of the mysteries of creation.

Humor

Richman (1995) has found humor useful because it increases a sense of sharing and is highly interactive and stress reducing. Obviously, humor must be used with extreme care. Clients must never believe that their misery is taken in a lighthearted manner.

Table 25-4

Classes and Side Effects of Available Antidepressants in the United States

Pharmacologic class	Examples	Side effects
TCA	Amitriptyline, doxepin, imipramine, clomipramine	Dry mouth, constipation, urinary retention, orthostasis, sedation
	Nortriptyline, desipramine	Less of above side effects
SSRI	Fluoxetine, sertraline, paroxetine, fluvoxamine	Nausea, vomiting, dry mouth, headache, sedation, nervousness, anxiety, dizziness, insomnia, sweating, ejaculatory/orgasmic dysfunction
Phenylethylamine type	Bupropion, venlafaxine	Nausea, dry mouth, headache, dizziness, nervousness
Serotonin-2 antagonists/serotonin reuptake inhibitors	Trazodone, nefazodone	Sedation, orthostasis, nausea, dizziness, headache
Alpha$_2$ autoreceptor antagonist/5HT$_2$ antagonist/5HT$_3$ antagonist	Mirtazapine	Sedation, weight gain, dry mouth, dizziness
MAOI	Phenelzine, tranylcypromine	Orthostasis, weight gain, sexual dysfunction (anorgasmia), edema, insomnia

From Buffum MD, Buffum JC: The psychopharmacologic treatment of depression in elders, *Geriatr Nurs* 18(4):144-149, 1997; data from Kaplan HI, Sadock BJ: *Pocket handbook of psychiatric drug treatment*, ed 2, Baltimore, 1996, Williams & Wilkins; Schatzberg AF: Course of depression in adults: treatment options, *Psychiatr Ann* 26:336-341, 1996; and Semia TP, Beizer JL, Higbee MD: *Geriatric dosage handbook*, ed 2, Cleveland, 1995, Lexi-Comp.
TCA, Tricyclic antidepressant; *SSRI*, serotonin-specific reuptake inhibitor; *MAOI*, monoamine oxidase inhibitor.

Table 25-5

Antidepressant Dosages Included in the Geriatric Dosage Guidelines

Antidepressant	Dose	Comments
Amitriptyline	—	All use in elders should be avoided.
Desipramine	10 to 25 mg/day initially, titrate up to 150 mg/day	Titrate dose up by 10 to 25 mg/day every 2 to 4 days (every week for outpatients) to a maximum of 150 mg/day.
Doxepin	Dermatologic use: 10 to 25 mg/day initially; titrate up to 150 mg/day	All psychiatric use should be avoided in elders; care should be used when required for dermatologic use: 10 to 25 mg/day initially; titrate dose up by 10 to 25 mg/day every 3 to 4 days (every week for outpatients) to a maximum of 150 mg/day.
Imipramine	10 to 25 mg/day initially; maximum of 150 mg/day	Titrate dose up by 10 to 25 mg/day every 2 to 4 days (every week for outpatients) to a maximum of 150 mg/day.
Nortriptyline	25 mg/day initially	Titrate dose up by 25 mg/day every 3 days (every week for outpatients) to a maximum of 75 mg/day or serum levels of 50 to 150 ng/ml.
Trazodone	25 to 50 mg/day initially; titrate up to 150 mg/day	Titrate dose up by 25 to 50 mg/day every 3 days (every week for outpatients) to a maximum of 300 mg/day.

From Buffum MD, Buffum JC: The psychopharmacologic treatment of depression in elders, *Geriatr Nurs* 18(4):144-149, 1997.

Dreams and Life Review

A strategy that we developed fully in one of our earlier editions of *Toward Health Aging: Human Needs and Nursing Response* was the use of dreams for self-expression, understanding, and reestablishing control. We have found this useful because many very depressed persons seem to live more fully in their dream time than while awake. We have not corroborated this with studies. Reminiscing serves somewhat the same functions, although a very depressed elder may not reminisce spontaneously. Chapter 5 deals with this topic more fully. Always, in all interventions with depressed elders, the goal is to stimulate them to take control and make the decisions, explain what they want, and what they enjoy or appreciate.

Sharing of Self

Sharing of self has been thought to be inappropriate in nursing and, at best, to take away from the focus on the client; at worst, it uses the client for one's own needs. However, in caring for the aged, and particularly those in long-term care institutions, it is often very helpful to share one's own life experiences and return the elder's consciousness to the experiences outside the institution. The sharing of self may bring about healing through feelings of connectedness with the reality of the other and reduce loneliness. This will also increase the individual's trust in the authenticity and honesty of the nurse.

Self-disclosure must be consciously used for the patient's benefit, and the level of intimacy must not be burdensome for the elder. Nowak and Wandel (1998) report a case of therapeutic sharing with a depressed elder that began with a lighthearted discussion about the nurse's infant and progressed until the elder sought a daily report about the child and began to reconnect with the world beyond her small room.

SUBSTANCE ABUSE

Substance abuse often arises in old age as a coping mechanism to deal with loss, anxiety, depression, or boredom. Although alcohol temporarily alleviates the distress in some situations, it has been found to create significantly more problems in carrying out important social roles (Krause, 1996). Alcohol-related problems in the elderly often go unrecognized, although the residual effects of alcohol abuse complicate the presentation and treatment of many chronic disorders of the aged. In the general population, abuse of alcohol is readily recognized because of social and work problems; however, elders may live alone and not come under scrutiny at work. They may easily hide their drinking.

Late-onset drinking among women over 60 years of age seems to be increasing, although the actual number of cases remains unknown. Those women living alone and abusing alcohol are likely to remain concealed until a fall, gastritis, pancreatitis, or a medication interaction brings them to the attention of an emergency room staff. Even then, the problems with alcohol may not be addressed by the health care providers. Late-life drinking for men and women seems to be associated with a life-changing event, such as retirement or moving into a less desirable living situation. The most predominant episode to trigger excessive use of alcohol among men is loss of their spouse.

Elderly individuals who are drug abusers are most likely dependent on prescribed anxiolytics or over-the-counter (OTC) analgesics. Nicotine and caffeine may be misused by the elderly, but the most common offenders are OTC analgesics (35%) and laxatives (30%) (Kaplan, Sadock, 1994). Unexplained gastrointestinal, psychologic, or metabolic problems may be signs of the abuse of OTC products.

Assessment

It is estimated that 40% of all adverse drug reactions occur in those over 65 years of age, and many are a result of OTC drugs and alcohol (McMahon, 1993). This is thought to contribute to the frequency of suicide among this group, and more older people were hospitalized in 1993 for alcohol-related problems than for heart attacks.

Nurses are often the first to recognize problems of substance abuse and are most likely to see clients in a variety of situations—most important, at home. The more frequent and diverse contact of nurses with clients gives them the advantage of recognizing subtle changes in a client's behavior and appearance.

Morning drinking is seen as particularly indicative of problems in the elderly woman (Schuckit et al, 1995). Symptoms of alcohol abuse include difficulties with gait, balance, and cognition (Clement, 1995). In addition, frequent falls and bruises may alert the nurse to the possibility of alcohol and drug abuse, although bruises may also indicate abuse by others. Often these events are overlapping—an elder may abuse alcohol and also be abused by alcoholic family members. Assessment guidelines are seen in Box 25-12.

Box 25-12	**ASSESSING ALCOHOL PROBLEMS WITH GRAHAM'S SCREENING**

Quantity and Frequency of Alcohol Intake
Typical day description
Evening routine description
Everything eaten and drank in the last 24 hours
Daily taking a drink in the afternoon or evening

Alcohol-Related Social and Legal Problems
Housing problems
Pedestrian or driving accidents
Social isolation
Recent family crises
Spouse illness
Loss of a good friend by moving away or death

Alcohol-Related Health Problems
Coordination changes
Falls
Poor nutrition, eating pattern changes, weight loss
Lack of hygiene or exercise
Feelings of depression
Gastritis
Sleeping pattern changes

Problems With Drunkenness and Dependence
Recent arrest or stop for driving while drinking
Recent driving school attendance
Episodes of forgetfulness or blackouts

Self-Recognition of Alcohol-Related Problems
"My friends said I should cut down on my drinking."
"I spend too much money on alcohol."
"Drinking contributed to my accident."

From Cowart ME, Sutherland M: Late-life drinking among women, *Geriatr Nurs* 19(5):214-219, 1998.

Box 25-13	**PREVENTIVE APPROACHES AND INTERVENTIONS**

Preventive Approaches
Target individuals who are at risk because they are experiencing stressor life events, including:
• Loss of a friend or loved one
• Illness of a spouse
• Change in financial status
• Retirement
• Nursing home admission
Arrange sessions on coping and alcohol use for caregivers who are responsible for spousal care.
When providing nutritional advice, incorporate education about alcohol and its effects.
When supervising over-the-counter and prescription drug use, include specific information about interactive effects of alcohol.
Include screening questions about alcohol use in all routine assessments.
Follow-up on coordination impairment, including falls and driving accidents, with information about alcohol effects and patterns of usage.

Interventions
Teach the effects of alcohol on sleep, nutrition, and co-ordination and how it acts as a depressant.
Integrate nutrition therapy and drug interaction awareness in all alcohol education.
Form a self-directed group composed of compatible peers.
Prescreen established therapy groups for barriers before referring older women.
Explore coping patterns that do not include alcohol in individual counseling sessions.
Identify appropriate social opportunities for alcohol consumption.
Refer clients with such signs as self-neglect to more comprehensive therapy approaches.

From Cowart ME, Sutherland M: Late-life drinking among women, *Geriatr Nurs* 19(4):214-219, 1998.

Changes in drinking patterns should alert nurses to potential coping problems or deterioration of health and/or social outlets. Depression and mental oblivion induced with drugs and alcohol can lead progressively to suicide or apathetic withdrawal. In the arena of drug and alcohol abuse, the tendency of health care providers to judge the behavior as the problem results in a judgmental attitude. Particularly in the case of substance abuse, nurses must search for the pain beneath the behavior. Elderly individuals entering treatment programs report that they do so because they had more problems because of drinking, were feeling more symptoms of depression, experienced more negative life events and stressors, and were distressed as they found alcohol becoming a problem more than a solution (Finney, Moos, 1995).

Treatment

Acute alcoholic withdrawal in an elder is serious and sometimes life threatening. Recommended treatment includes frequent determination of vital signs, maintaining fluid balance without overhydrating, and providing regular dosage with oxazepam (Serax) every 1 to 2 hours (Ketcham, Hayner, 1992).

Elders are likely to feel excessively guilty and regretful about alcohol misuse, and it is important to reach out to them with understanding. It is productive to discuss the issue of substance abuse factually, avoiding judgmental overtones. For example, the nurse might say, "Many elders find that the stresses, loneliness, and losses of aging are very hard to bear. Some retreat into alcohol use as a way of coping. There are treatments and groups that assist individuals in these difficult adjustments. If this is a problem for you or if it becomes a problem, please let us know so that we may provide resources or referrals for you." The notion that alcoholism is a genetic or metabolic disorder that can be cured only by a return to God may be useful to some, but elders are also responsive to activity enrichment and group support.

Those elders who have never had problems with alcohol early in life are particularly able to benefit from treatment. Cowart and Sutherland (1998) provide a screening tool for identifying alcohol-related problems and suggest both preventive approaches and interventions (Box 25-13). An extensive protocol for developing a plan of care for the alcohol abuser is seen in Box 25-14. Long-term self-help treatment programs for elders show high rates of success, especially when social outlets are emphasized and cohort supports are available (Blazer, 1995b).

SUICIDE

Common precipitants of suicide include physical or mental illness, death of one's spouse, substance abuse, and pathologic relationships. Widowers are thought to be most vulnerable because they have often depended on the wife to maintain the comforts of home and the social network of relatives and friends.

White men over 85 years of age commit suicide at an annual rate of 66 per 100,000. In contrast, white women of the same age category commit suicide at an annual rate of 5 per 100,000. Women are most suicidal between ages 45 and 54, with an incidence of 7 per 100,000. Suicide rates for white men and white women over age 75 have slightly but steadily decreased since 1990. Elderly blacks have much lower suicide rates (men, 14 per 100,000; women, less than 1 per 100,000); however, suicide rates of elderly black men have almost doubled since 1980 (US Department of Health and Human Services, 1999). One of the significant differences in suicidal behaviors in the old and young is the lethality of the method. Eight of ten suicides of men over age 65 were with firearms, and most were successful (Kaplan et al, 1994).

Aged white men in America suffer the most status loss because the American white male society is almost wholly devoted to occupational success, often to the neglect of other social roles. As more women identify themselves with the work role and abstain from having children, statistics may shift.

Assessing the Suicidal Risk of an Elder

Aged suicidal clients are encountered in many settings. It is our professional obligation to prevent whenever possible an impulsive destruction of life that may be a response to a crisis or a disintegrative reaction. The lethality potential of an elder must always be assessed when elements of depression, disease, and spousal loss are evident. Delusional and hypochondriacal thinking (discussed earlier in the chapter) are risk factors (Lester, Tallmer, 1994). Many studies have shown that with few exceptions a suicidal individual has seen a physician within a month before the suicide attempt (American Association of Retired Persons, 1994). Unfortunately, few physicians make a suicide assessment.

Nurses are often in a position to assess lethality potential. The clues that are common signals of suicidal intent may be absent, disguised, or misinterpreted in the elderly. However, any direct, indirect, or enigmatic references to the ending of life must be taken seriously and discussed with the elder. Many, having grown up in the era when suicide bore stigma and even criminal implications, may not discuss their feelings in this respect. It is often helpful to depersonalize the subject and discuss it on a more philosophic basis, using questions such as the following:

- Under what conditions do you think a person has a right to take his or her life?
- What are your opinions about the present interest in active euthanasia and assisted suicide?
- Do you think suicide is a sign of weakness or strength?

Box 25-14   NURSING DIAGNOSIS: Ineffective Coping: Alcoholism

The following potential diagnoses must be considered, as well as diagnoses unique to the particular individual:

Denial, ineffective
Knowledge deficit
Noncompliance
Poisoning, risk for
Sensory/perceptual alterations

Sleep pattern disturbance
Social interaction, impaired
Spiritual distress
Thought processes, altered

NURSING PROCESS

Etiologies and Related Factors
Stresses
    Environmental changes
    Losses
    Chronic illness
    Finances
Lack of purpose
Physiologic changes (neurotransmitter depletion)
Physiovulnerability to depression

Defining Characteristics
Denies alcohol use is a problem
Justifies use of alcohol
Argumentative with mate/friends/authority
Unreasonable resentments
Paranoia
Impulsive judgment
Impatience
Daytime fatigue
Unsteady gait
Impaired memory
Apathy
Disorientation
Confusion
Slurred speech
Self-neglect
Social isolation
Blackouts
Falls
Physical pathology: myopathy, diarrhea, malnutrition, gout, decreased lower extremity sensation, tremors
Visual/tactile hallucinations

Knowledge
Alcohol abuse/alcoholism
Effects of alcohol on the older adult
Percentage of alcohol in various alcoholic beverages and over-the-counter medications

2 ounces alcohol
    = 2 shots = 4 ounces 100-proof whiskey
    = 4 glasses = 16 ounces wine
    = 4 mugs = 48 ounces beer
Physical and psychologic assessment skills
Standard alcohol screening tests (e.g., CAGE)
Signs and symptoms of withdrawal
Therapeutic communication skills
Crisis intervention skills
Group therapy
Coping strategies
Treatment of alcoholism
Community resources

Clinical Judgment and Related Skills
Maintain a nonjudgmental approach.
Administer a standard alcohol screening tool.
Perform a physical and mental status examination.
Monitor nutritional status.
Help client to gain an understanding of alcoholism as an illness, its progressiveness, and its effects on the body and interpersonal relationships.
Set realistic short-term goals.
Discuss alternative coping strategies.
Involve family (if there is one).
Conduct group sessions with recovering and recovered persons.
Educate family and community groups on the older adult and alcoholism.
Provide information of resources.
Make referrals as needed.

Evaluation
Admits is alcoholic
Abstains from alcohol use
States recognizes need for continued treatment
Explains the physical and psychologic effects of alcohol
Uses alternative coping mechanisms for stress
Takes pride in appearance
Reintegrates into social activities

The nurse might also say, "Suicide is a taboo subject that many people are uncomfortable discussing, but as a health professional I feel it is very important. Have you ever felt like you would be better off dead?"

Typical behavioral clues such as putting personal affairs in order, giving away possessions, and making wills and funeral plans are indications of maturity and good judgment in late life and cannot be construed as indicative of suicidal intent. Other things such as self-neglect, erratic behavior, suspiciousness, hoarding pills, and personality change are more likely the side effects of illness or progressive dementia than of suicidal intent. Even such statements as "I won't be around long" may be only a realistic appraisal of the situation in old age. Requests to die and statements that life has no meaning may indicate despair and hopelessness but often lack the conviction of planned suicide. In addition, there are great cultural differences in feelings about suicide and how and when it may be a positive action.

In evaluating lethality potential, the informed nurse will recognize the high-risk patient: male, old, widowed or divorced, white, in poor health, retired, alcoholic, and with a family history of unsatisfactory relationships and mental illness. A cluster of these factors should be a red flag of distress to all health professionals. Recent traumatic changes, mild dementia, depression, or cerebrovascular disease also increase the danger. Present relationships that are unsatisfactory, critical, or rejecting greatly enhance the potential for suicide.

The straightforward aspects of a suicide assessment include the following:

- Frequency of suicidal ideations
- A formulated plan for suicide
- Availability of means to complete the plan
- Specificity regarding details (time, place)
- Lethality of the method chosen

The following must also be considered in assessing lethality potential:

- Internal resources (personality factors and coping strategies)
- External resources (money, family, friends, services)
- Communication skills (ability to ask for help and express feelings)

Suicide is a taboo topic for most of us, and there is a lingering fear that the introduction of the topic will be suggestive to the patient and may incite suicidal action. Precisely the opposite is true. By introducing the topic, we demonstrate interest in the individual and open the door to honest human interaction and connection on the deep levels of psychologic need. Superficial interest and mechanical questioning will not, of course, be meaningful. It is the nature of our concern and ability to connect with the alienation and desperation of the individual that will make a difference. No matter how much empathy and concern are conveyed, there will be a number of old people who will quietly and methodically kill themselves with never a clue to their intent.

Interventions With a Suicidal Elder

Community health nurses, visiting nurses, and other professionals have a case-finding role in the community that extends beyond traditional boundaries: first, awareness and use of resources within the high-risk populations and, second, provision of depression screening at nutrition sites, senior centers, industrial health sites, churches, and community clubs.

The approach to the suicidal elder includes establishing lifesaving connections with individuals and groups that can be available on demand and provide ongoing, long-term counseling, emotional support, and reassurance (Arbore, 1995). Arbore established a 24-hour Friendship Line under the umbrella of suicide prevention that was designed especially for elders. Phone call-in counseling is always available by specially trained volunteers, as well as telephone outreach reassurance and a visiting service. The goal is to intervene before suicide becomes a seriously considered option. In other words, we must be concerned about immediate protection for the highly lethal individual while respecting the individual's right to make the most significant remaining decision open to him or her: namely, whether to live or to die. For some, our well-planned interventions may restore a sense of self and purpose so that the suicidal individual will deem preservation worthwhile. For others, their final statement of dignity will be in the control of their death.

Actions to deal with the suicidal elderly include the following:

- Build trust and rapport.
- Overcome fear of responsibility for client suicide.
- Come to terms with own suicidal impulses and feelings.
- Recognize and handle resentment of the client who wants to die.
- Listen intently and with empathy.
- Focus on the individual's perception of the problem.
- Begin to help establish or restore a supportive network.

If suicidal intent has been established, the following interventions, arranged in order of immediacy, are necessary:

1. Reduce immediate danger by removing hazardous articles.
2. Evaluate the need for constant attendance, and arrange for a family member, friend, or professional to be present during the period of imminent danger.
3. Evaluate the need for medication.
4. Focus on the current hazard or crisis that gives the client the most present distress.
5. Extract a promise from the client not to attempt suicide before your next meeting.
6. Mobilize internal and external resources by getting the individual reinvolved with external supports and reconnected with internal capacities. The caregiver may have to find activities, support systems, transportation, and other resources for the individual.
7. Implement a specific plan of action with an ongoing structured program to obviate long periods alone; develop a "lifeline" of individuals who can be called at any hour of distress, and plan regular calls to the individual.

In many cases, interventions with depressed elders can be extrapolated to suicidal elders, since they are often depressed (see discussion earlier in this chapter). Suicide is often a distorted method of regaining control of one's life. Prevention of suicidal behavior is related to alleviation of depression and restoration of a sense of control in one's life. Working with isolated, depressed, and suicidal elders continually challenges the depths of nurses' ingenuity, patience, and self-knowledge.

PROVIDING PSYCHOGERIATRIC CARE

Therapeutic strategies to promote mental health have included psychotherapy that is time limited, with the goal of restoring emotional stability. Lengthy psychotherapy is seldom carried out with the aged, since there are few therapists specializing in that type of psychogeriatric care and even fewer who understand the experience of old age. Psychodrama and group therapies of all types have been used with varying degrees of reported success. Life review (Butler, 1963) is the therapy that is most nearly like psychotherapy. It is the process by which an elder reminisces about painful events and disappointments and works toward acceptance and integration of those events. Much attention has been paid to life review, but in practice it is often confused with simple reminiscing. All of the mental health strategies that have been used are doubtlessly effective in some cases, but there are few well-designed studies that report solid evidence of success with any. Soft, anecdotal evidence is abundant. Life review is discussed in more detail in Chapter 5.

EXERCISING CONTROL IN THE MENTAL HEALTH CARE SYSTEM

The aged, the largest body of health care consumers, could exert considerable pressure to change health care delivery systems. A nursing function is to assist them in doing so. The great majority of mental health care is actually self-generated and self-financed. Little is being done through Medicare or Medicaid to assist the elder with emotionally disabling problems. Elders must learn how to use the health care system to best advantage. Alert the aged client to the following as being important in obtaining satisfactory care and appropriate referral from a physician when psychologic care is needed:

1. Before engaging the services of a private physician provider, find out whether he or she follows Medicare fee schedules and will bill Medicare directly.
2. Get acquainted with the administrative personnel in the health care system; he or she can be a support person and provide assistance in easing through the system with best results.
3. Make notes of questions and symptoms before visiting the physician, since they are often forgotten during a visit.
4. Ask about satisfaction with prior referrals to a mental health provider.
5. Ask about fees before receiving service and about limitations of therapy.
6. Ask the physician to prescribe generic drugs when possible because they are less expensive.
7. Do not accept "old age" as an explanation for any symptom.

To guide others toward mental health through stressful and crisis situations, the nurse must maintain a reliable support system for his or her own needs and develop a range of stress reduction strategies effective for the self (Frisch, Kelley, 1996). Stetson (1997) has worked with faculty and student nurses in stress reduction classes to strengthen their coping skills and ability to relax, as well as to gain personal insight. These sessions consist mainly of participants learning new stress management techniques each week, using the *Creating Wholeness* text (Peper, Holt, 1993). The exercises progress in complexity from muscle relaxation to imagery and cognitive reframing. Daily practice and logs are required to further embed skills and to facilitate skill mastery.

Working with elders who are emotionally distraught is especially challenging. We emphasize, no matter where nurses are working with elders in this day and age, our first charge is, "Nurse, learn to take care of thyself!"

▶ KEY CONCEPTS

- Disturbing emotions experienced over extended periods may result in depletions of the immune system and resulting illnesses.
- Psychoneuroimmunology is attracting considerable attention as the study of the actual relationship of emotions and disease and the particular physiologic responses involved is becoming clearer.
- The crises and stressors experienced by the aged are less frequent than those among younger adults but often have more devastating consequences.
- Crises have the potential for producing individual growth and higher levels of function as a result of successful mastery of the situation.
- If timely support and appropriate interventions are not activated during a crisis situation, the individual is likely to stabilize at a lower level of function than that existing before the crisis.
- Methods of assessing the impact of stressful events are inadequate if they do not consider chronic stressors that may exist over long periods of time, the particular population profile of the individuals being assessed, the individual's personality, and the recency and frequency of events, as well as very early traumatic events that may have eroded the individual's sense of security.
- Stress management strategies must be designed to meet individual needs because some methods may in fact be experienced as an additional stressor; for example, a shy, reticent elder would be unlikely to find body massage soothing and relaxing.
- Reestablishing feelings of adequacy and control is the sine qua non of crisis resolution and stress management.
- Mental health in old age is difficult to determine as the accrual of life experiences makes for great vari-

ations. Mental health must be determined by the gratification or satisfaction that individuals feel within their particular situation.
- Mental health is a fluctuating situation for most individuals, with peaks and valleys of happiness and pain.
- Elders are not well served within the mental health system as it exists today. Neither practitioners nor reimbursement mechanisms are adapted to their needs.
- Psychologic assessment of elders based on the common psychometric instruments will usually show deficits because these instruments, with few exceptions, have been designed to test the mental health of young adults.
- Anxiety disorders are common in late life and are best managed by restoring some sense of control to the situation the individual perceives as out of control.
- Many of the psychologic aberrations observed in the elderly are coping strategies to deal with overwhelming anxiety.
- Posttraumatic stress disorder is finally being recognized in the aged who have been subjected to extremely traumatic events. Programs are now available to provide support and insight for these individuals.
- Substance abuse and addictions may be distorted adaptational methods used by some aged persons to cope with anxiety related to end-of-life concerns. These individuals have been successfully treated by being provided with supportive groups and relationships.
- Depression is the most common emotional disorder of aging and likewise the most treatable. Unfortunately, it is often neglected or assumed to be a condition of aging that one must "learn to live with." Nurses may be instrumental in ensuring that elders are assessed properly and treated for depression.
- Grief is a component of aging for most individuals as they confront various losses. Grief is not a mental illness, but it often requires grief counseling and support for resolution.
- Suicide is a significant problem among old men. Very old white men are highly suicidal and must be assessed for suicidal intent whenever they confront a trauma or catastrophe. Women vastly outnumber men in late life, and they are rarely suicidal.

NANDA and Wellness Diagnoses

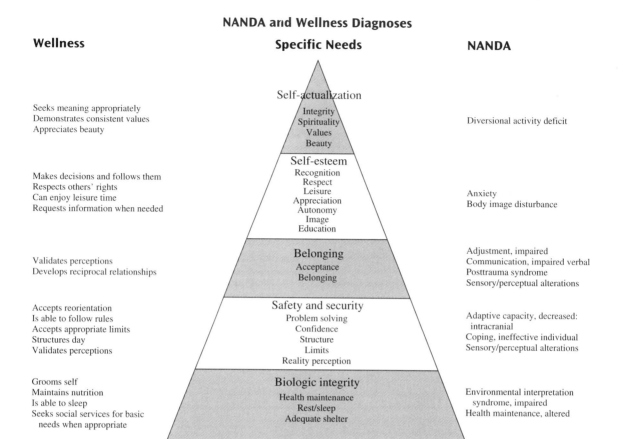

Wellness

Seeks meaning appropriately
Demonstrates consistent values
Appreciates beauty

Makes decisions and follows them
Respects others' rights
Can enjoy leisure time
Requests information when needed

Validates perceptions
Develops reciprocal relationships

Accepts reorientation
Is able to follow rules
Accepts appropriate limits
Structures day
Validates perceptions

Grooms self
Maintains nutrition
Is able to sleep
Seeks social services for basic
  needs when appropriate

Specific Needs

Self-actualization
Integrity
Spirituality
Values
Beauty

Self-esteem
Recognition
Respect
Leisure
Appreciation
Autonomy
Image
Education

Belonging
Acceptance
Belonging

Safety and security
Problem solving
Confidence
Structure
Limits
Reality perception

Biologic integrity
Health maintenance
Rest/sleep
Adequate shelter

NANDA

Diversional activity deficit

Anxiety
Body image disturbance

Adjustment, impaired
Communication, impaired verbal
Posttrauma syndrome
Sensory/perceptual alterations

Adaptive capacity, decreased:
  intracranial
Coping, ineffective individual
Sensory/perceptual alterations

Environmental interpretation
  syndrome, impaired
Health maintenance, altered

These are not all of the possible wellness or NANDA diagnoses that may be identified. The above are frequent examples of nursing diagnoses that should be considered when planning care for the older adult in whatever setting.

▶ Activities and Discussion Questions

1. List the various crises you have encountered with aged persons you have taken care of, and then discuss what was done about them.
2. Discuss several of the unconscious defense mechanisms that serve to help people avoid anxiety states.
3. Discuss the three most common mental disturbances that elders are likely to experience, and describe how these have appeared to you. How did you assess the problem, and what was done about it?
4. What is likely to be different in the appearance of depression in a person who is 70 years old versus the appearance in a person who is 20 years old?

5. What behaviors are indicative of suicidal intent in an elderly person? Discuss the methods of assessment and your reactions to these.
6. Discuss the various situations that may result in elder substance abuse and ways to effectively intervene.
7. Formulate strategies that may be used to provide mental health counseling for vulnerable elders.

RESOURCES

Comprehensive Textbook of Psychiatry, 6th edition, volume 2, by H. Kaplan and B. Sadock (1995, Williams & Wilkins).

Diagnostic and Statistical Manual of Mental Disorders (DSM-IV), 4th edition (1994, American Psychiatric Association).

Public Policy and Aging Report 9(1), winter 1998. Issue focuses on mental health of older adults. *Public Policy and Aging Report* is a publication of the Gerontological Society of America, 1275 K Street NW, Suite 350, Washington, DC 20005-4006.

Mental Health and Aging Network
American Society on Aging
833 Market Street, No. 511
San Francisco, CA 94103-1824

REFERENCES

Alexopoulos GS: Mood disorders. In Kaplan H, Sadock B, editors: *Comprehensive textbook of psychiatry,* ed 6, vol 2, Baltimore, 1995, Williams & Wilkins.

Almeida OP et al: Cognitive features of psychotic states arising in late life, *Psychol Med* 25(4):685, 1995.

American Association of Retired Persons: *Alcohol abuse among older people,* Washington, DC, 1994, American Association of Retired Persons.

American Psychiatric Association: *Diagnostic and statistical manual of mental disorders (DSM IV),* ed 4, Washington, DC, 1994, The Association.

Arbore P: *Suicide in the elderly.* Presentation at the forty-eighth annual scientific meeting of the Gerontological Society of America, Los Angeles, Nov 20, 1995.

Barker S: Does depression impede hip-fracture recovery? *Contemp Senior Health* 2(2):10, 1990.

Barsky AJ: Hypochondriasis: medical management and psychiatric treatment, *Psychosomatics* 37(1):48, 1996.

Battegay R: Psychoanalytic aspects of crisis and crisis intervention, *J Psychosom Med Psychoanal* 41(1):1, 1995.

Benezra EE: Personality factors of individuals who survive traumatic experiences without professional help, *Int J Stress Manage* 3(3):147, 1996.

Black KJ: Diagnosing depression after stroke, *South Med J* 88(7):699, 1995.

Blazer DG: Anxiety disorders. In Abrams WB, Beers MH, Berkow R, editors: *The Merck manual of geriatrics,* ed 2, Whitehouse Station, NJ, 1995a, Merck Research Laboratories.

Blazer DG: Depression. In Abrams WB, Beers MH, Berkow R, editors: *The Merck manual of geriatrics,* ed 2, Whitehouse Station, NJ, 1995b, Merck Research Laboratories.

Boerner RJ: Anxiety disorders in the elderly: diagnostic problems and therapeutic prospects, *Z Gerontol Geriatr* 28(6):435, 1995.

Borson S: Symptomatic depression in the elderly medical outpatient: prevalence, demography and health service utilization, *J Am Geriatr Soc* 34:341, 1989.

Buffum MD, Buffum JC: The psychopharmacologic treatment of depression in elders, *Geriatr Nurs* 18(4):144-149, 1997.

Buffum MD, Wolfe NS: Posttraumatic stress disorder and the WW II veteran, *Geriatr Nurs* 16(6):264-270, 1995.

Butler RL: Life review: an interpretation of reminiscence in the aged, *Psychiatry* 26:65, 1963.

Clement M: Recognizing dependence on alcohol in the elderly, *NurseWeek* 8(20):8, 1995.

Cohen S: Psychological stress and susceptibility to upper respiratory infections, *Am J Respir Crit Care Med* 152(4):S53, 1995.

Cowart ME, Sutherland M: Late-life drinking among women, *Geriatr Nurs* 19(5):214-219, 1998.

Fielding R: Depression and acute myocardial infarction: a review and reinterpretation, *Soc Sci Med* 32:1017, 1991.

Finney JW, Moos RH: Entering treatment for alcohol abuse: a stress and coping model, *Addiction* 90(9):1223, 1995.

Frisch NC, Kelley J: *Healing life's crises: a guide for nurses,* Albany, NY, 1996, Delmar.

Jacobson E: *Progressive relaxation,* Chicago, 1938, University of Chicago Press.

Johnson B: Older adults' suggestions for health care providers regarding discussions of sex, *Geriatr Nurs* 18(2):65-66, 1997.

Kaplan MS, Adamek ME, Johnson S: Trends in firearm suicide among older American males: 1979-1988, *Gerontologist* 34(1):59, 1994.

Kaplan HI, Sadock BJ: *Synopsis of psychiatry,* ed 7, Baltimore, 1994, Williams & Wilkins.

Kaplan HI, Sadock BJ: *Pocket handbook of psychiatric drug treatment,* ed 2, Baltimore, 1996, Williams & Wilkins.

Katona CLE: Approaches to the management of depression in old age, *Gerontology* 40(1):5, 1994.

Ketcham ML, Hayner GN: Safe withdrawal from acute alcohol abuse in the aged, *Geriatr Nurs* 13(5):281, 1992.

Kiecolt-Glaser JK et al: Chronic stress alters the immune response to influenza virus vaccine in older adults, *Proc Natl Acad Sci USA* 93(7):3043, 1996.

Kopin IJ: Definitions of stress and sympathetic neuronal responses, *Ann NY Acad Sci* 771:19, 1995.

Krause N: Stress, gender, cognitive impairment, and outpatient use in later life, *J Gerontol* 51(1):P15, 1996.

Kurlowicz LH, NICHE Faculty: Nursing standard of practice protocol: depression in elderly patients, *Geriatr Nurs* 18(5): 192-200, 1997.

Lebowitz BD: Diagnosis and treatment of depression in late life: an overview of the NIH consensus statement, *J Am Geriatr Soc* 4(suppl 1):S3-S6, 1996.

Lester D, Tallmer M: Now I lay me down to sleep, *Contemp Gerontol* 1(3):91, 1994.

Levine R: *Short, vigorous workouts may reduce depression, increase vigor,* Duke University news release, p 1, April 17, 1997; www.dukenews.duke.edu.

Lindemann E: Symptomatology and management of acute grief, *Am J Psychiatry* 101:141, 1944.

Lusk JT: *30 scripts for relaxation, imagery and inner healing,* Duluth, Minn, 1992, Whole Person Associates.

Martin KS: S.T.R.E.S.S., *Home Health Focus* 2(11):81, 1996 (editorial).

Maslow A: *Motivation and personality,* ed 2, New York, 1970, Harper & Row.

McLean DE, Link BG: Unraveling complexity: strategies to refine concepts, measures, and research designs in the study of life events and mental health. In Avison WR, Gotlib IH, editors: *Stress and mental health: contemporary issues and prospects for the future,* New York, 1994, Plenum.

McMahon AL: Substance abuse among the elderly, *Nurse Pract Forum* 4(4):231, 1993.

Miller C: Keeping up with new developments in antidepressants, *Geriatr Nurs* 18(4):180-181, 1997.

Miller CA: New treatments for erectile dysfunction, *Geriatr Nurs* 18(6):285-286, 1997.

Nowak KB, Wandel JC: The sharing of self in geriatric clinical practice: case report and analysis, *Geriatr Nurs* 19(1):34-37, 1998.

Peper E, Holt CF: *Creating wholeness: a self-healing workbook using dynamic relaxation, images and thoughts,* New York, 1993, Plenum.

Richman J: The lifesaving function of humor with the depressed and suicidal elderly, *Gerontologist* 35(2):271, 1995.

Riley B: Schizophrenia, paranoid disorders, anxiety disorders, and somatoform disorders. In Hogstel MO, editor: *Geropsychiatric nursing,* St Louis, 1990, Mosby.

Schuckit MA et al: The time course of development of alcohol-related problems in men and women, *J Stud Alcohol* 56(2):218, 1995.

Sobel DS: Rethinking medicine: improving health outcomes with cost-effective psychosocial interventions, *Psychosom Med* 57:234, 1995.

Sprinzeles L: Hallucination: the phantom reality, *Parkinson's Disease Foundation Newsletter,* p 5, summer 1992.

Stetson B: Holistic health stress management program: nursing student and client health outcomes, *J Holistic Nurs* 15(2):143, 1997.

Stollenwerk RM et al: Focus on spiritual well-being: harmonious interconnectedness of mind-body-spirit, *Geriatr Nurs* 17(6):262, 1996.

Stratakis CA, Chrousos GP: Neuroendocrinology and pathophysiology of the stress system, *Ann NY Acad Sci* 771:1, 1995.

Ulmer D: Stress management for the cardiovascular patient: a look at current treatment and trends, *Prog Cardiovasc Nurs* 11(1):21, 1996.

US Department of Health and Human Services: *Health, United States, 1999: health and aging chartbook,* DHHS Pub No (PHS) 99-132, Hyattsville, Md, 1999, Centers for Disease Control and Prevention.

Vingerhoets AJ et al: Self-reported stressors, symptom complaints and psychobiological functioning: cardiovascular stress reactivity, *J Psychosom Res* 40(2):177, 1996.

Wolanin MO, Phillips L: *Confusion: prevention and care,* St Louis, 1981, Mosby.

chapter 26

Coping With Loss, Grief, Dying, and Death

Upon completion of this chapter, the reader will be able to:

- Differentiate between loss and grief.
- Explain the different types of grief and the dynamics of the grieving process.
- Explain the characteristics required of the nurse to be able to effectively intervene in grief/bereavement.
- List interventions that are helpful for those whose grief is established.
- Explain the tasks that occur in the dying process.
- Identify and discuss the needs of the dying and appropriate interventions.
- Explain the role and responsibility of the nurse in advance directives.
- Discuss the pros and cons of suicide and physician-assisted death for elders.

▶GLOSSARY

Bereavement overload A number of grief situations in a short period of time (weeks, months, a year).

Euthanasia "Painless death"; "mercy killing."

    Active "The commission of any act that directly leads to the death of a patient. The intent of the act is to mercifully cause the death of the patient" (Minogue, 1996, p. 64).

    Passive Indirectly helping a person to die.

Physician-assisted suicide "When the physician facilitates a patient's death by providing the necessary means and/or information to enable the patient to end his or her life" (Minogue, 1996, p. 80).

▶THE LIVED EXPERIENCE

Losses are the hardest of all experiences. Losing parents is expected; deaths of children hurt. If one lives as long as I have, increasingly others my age, and younger, are dying, and then there is the experience of real loneliness. I sometimes feel like the proverbial last leaf clinging to the tree. Since living at the Meadows I have made and lost many friends; we are constantly reminded of the proximity of death.

Lyn, age 85, in a life-care facility

I know I should have expected this, but I have known so many of these people for several years. Each time one dies, it is as if another very good friend is gone. We really do need some sort of group or ritual or something to help us with our grief. We are always so busy taking care of others.

Isabel, staff member at life-care facility

*L*oss, dying, and death are universal incontestable events of the human experience that one is unable to stop or control. The numerous physical, psychologic, and behavioral responses that are manifested are known as *grief, mourning,* or *bereavement.*

Loss, like death, is an event, whereas dying, grief, and mourning are dynamic processes. Loss for elders generally relates to loss of relationships through death (spouse, friends, at times adult children) and life transitions (retirement, role change, relocation from home to nursing care facility) (Box 26-1). Dying may be the elder's own or that of a significant other. Regardless, grief and grief work, or mourning, facilitate elders in maintaining their lives.

Grief and *mourning (bereavement)* are usually used synonymously. However, grief is an individual's response to a loss. Mourning includes those behaviors that the bereaved uses to incorporate the loss experience into his or her ongoing life. Mourning is an active process rather than one that is reactive to an event. The behaviors associated with mourning are determined by social and cultural norms that prescribe the appropriate ways of coping with loss in a given society. It is important to realize that there is no single way to grieve or respond to loss. Responses will vary widely among individuals and across cultures.

The experience of death (age, place, and manner of death) has been profoundly altered during the twentieth century. Seventy-three percent of deaths each year are of the aged (US Bureau of the Census, 1995), with the leading cause of death attributed to chronic disorders. Increasingly, it is the old who die, making it a pre- dictable and expected function of old age (Hooyman, Kiyak, 1996). The elderly are considered the only group of individuals in which death is culturally acceptable (Godow, 1987). The numbers of elders surviving into very old age have influenced the experience of death and bereavement. Death, unfortunately, is a form of ageist discrimination, a subtle denigration of aging.

CONCEPTUAL BASIS OF THE GRIEF PROCESS

The theories or models are based on the Euro-American perspective of breaking the emotional ties between the bereaved and the dead (DeSpelder, Strickland, 1996). The majority of these grief theories evolved between the early 1900s and early 1980s and have been the foundation of what caregivers and society in general have been taught about the grieving process.

Bowlby (1961) suggests four phases of the grief process: (1) numbness, anger, and distress; (2) yearning and searching for the lost figure; (3) disorganization and despair; and (4) reorganization (Fig. 26-1). Other theorists offer different approaches to the grief process. Regardless of the theorist, it is clear that grief has a beginning with physical and psychologic manifestations; a middle (considered the work of grieving or mourning), during which time the individual is breaking the bonds that tied him or her to the deceased; and an end with the individual emerging refocused, having severed the ties to the dead person.

Current concepts about grief recognize that it is not rigidly structured and is without a predictable pattern of responses. Some responses to grief occur internally and are not visible, whereas other aspects of grief may not occur at all. From the work of Gorer (1965), the following styles of grief were identified by their length of time: (1) little or no grief—including denial and absence of grief, anticipatory grief, and hidden grief; (2) time-limited grief—intense grief followed by a return to the pregrief state; (3) unlimited grief—"I'll never get over this," suggestive of a continuing grief that does not interfere appreciably with daily life; and (4) mummification—the making of a shrine of the deceased's room, indicative of never-ending, deeply painful grief.

Taking Gorer's unlimited grief and expanding on that premise, current thought suggests a newer model that looks at reactions or tasks rather than stages. Worden (1991) modified previous perspectives by offering tasks of grieving. These tasks require (1) accepting the reality of the loss; (2) working through the pain (both

---

Box 26-1   LOSSES OF THE AGED

Loss of Relationships
Significant others
Social contacts through:
  Illness
  Death
  Distance
  Decreased mobility

Life Transitions
Significant roles
Financial security
Independence
Physical health
Mental stability
Life-death

physical and emotional, as well as behavioral pain), the intensity of which will vary with the individual; (3) adjusting to a change in environment; and (4) emotionally relocating the deceased and moving on with life. Doka (1993) added a fifth task, spiritual, to rebuild faith and philosophical systems that challenge loss.

Accepting the reality of the loss can be measured by the use of present or past references to the dead. The individual "is" or "was."

Although working through the pain is an individual process, the individual who is bereaved requires a support network. The danger in this particular task of mourning is the potential for the misuse of pain killers such as alcohol or prescription and nonprescription drugs. The pain needs to be experienced, not deadened.

Adjusting to a changed environment may take a considerable period of time, especially if the relationship with the deceased was a long and close one. Changes in the environment may be physical, emotional, or spiritual, such as rearrangement of furniture, a different seating pattern at the dinner table, or a trip at holiday time rather than observation of a celebration as it always used to be.

The emotional relocation of the deceased and moving on with life produces considerable anxiety. An individual may feel that this is a dishonor to the dead. He

or she may develop a high degree of anxiety about investing emotional energy in other relationships (a letting go of former attachments). It is important to impart to the mourner that letting go does not mean that the individual loved the deceased any less but that there are others still to be loved. This is also true with other losses: there are new avenues to explore.

The newest interpretation of grief and grief work is the pinwheel model of bereavement (Solari-Twadell et al, 1995). Grieving is seen as a dynamic process, the core of which is the griever's personal history. Care themes—(1) being stopped, (2) pain and hurting, (3) missing, (4) holding, (5) seeking, and (6) valuing—surround personal history and are deeply rooted in the inner experience of bereavement. Change, expectations, and inexpressibility revolve around the core of inner experiences. The unique, individual loss experience and its subsequent grief are symbolized by the pinwheel.

Imagine the wind (the loss) spinning the pinwheel. The intensity, or force, of this wind sets in motion a life-changing process of bereavement. Throughout one's life the winds of loss will gently stir recurrent episodes of grief through sights, sounds, smells, anniversary dates, and other triggers. The arms of the pinwheel suggest movement by the bereaved, reaching out of the experience of grief by surrendering (i.e., resting,

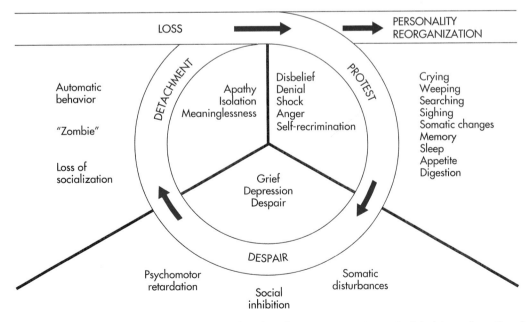

Fig. 26-1 Illustration of John Bowlby's approach to loss. (From Beare PG, Myers JL: *Principles and practice of adult health nursing*, ed 2, St Louis, 1994, Mosby.)

or the lowering of one's defenses toward life and being open to reality or the acceptance of the life event and reaching out to others and rejoining life through change). Each gust of wind may generate a resurgence of the grief experience.

These theories are attempts to specify the dynamics of the grieving process. They are helpful to our understanding of grief, but they should not be imposed on the survivor. Thus there are similarities and differences; the behavior is the same, but the process is explained differently.

TYPES OF GRIEF

Several types of grief need to be addressed briefly—anticipatory grief, acute grief, chronic grief, and disenfranchised grief.

Anticipatory grief is the response to a real or perceived loss before it occurs. One observes this grief in preparation for potential loss of belongings, friends moving away, or knowing that a body part or function is going to change, or in anticipation of the loss of a spouse or oneself through death. In a sense, it is insulation against what will be, a dress rehearsal for the actual event that is destined to occur. Behaviors similar to acute grief are experienced, including preoccupation with the particular loss and anticipation of the mode of adjustment that might be necessary.

Futterman et al (1970) conceptualized anticipatory grief as having five functionally related aspects: (1) acknowledgment—convinced the inevitable will occur; (2) grieving—experiencing and expressing the emotional impact of the anticipated loss and the physical, psychologic, and interpersonal turmoil associated with it; (3) reconciliation of the situation; (4) detachment—withdrawal of the emotional investment from the situation; and (5) memorialization—developing a relatively fixed conscious mental representation of that which will be lost. One frequently sees the struggle of anticipatory grief in families with elders who have been diagnosed with Alzheimer's disease.

Some negative aspects of anticipatory grief should be mentioned. If the loss does not occur when or as expected, those awaiting the actual loss or death may become hostile and impatient. In the event of a relocation, individuals may become angry or hostile toward the agency, institution, or others who are responsible for the delay. Anticipatory grief can result in premature detachment from an individual who is dying. If premature detachment occurs, it prevents the family or others

from reinvesting in the dying individual. This is known as the *Lazarus syndrome.* It may deprive family and friends of a final close relationship and prevent resolution of unfinished business.

Grief after anticipatory grief is no less painful than unanticipated loss, but it does allow for less of an assault on the mourner's adaptive capacity (Parks, Weiss, 1983). It has sometimes been assumed that anticipatory grief work among widows helped them adjust to bereavement when the spouse died. However, the expectancy of death may not be related to adjustment to bereavement (Dessonville, et al, 1983), and in some cases it may actually be associated with a poor adjustment. Anticipatory grief, then, can be helpful or harmful to the griever but is recognized as a legitimate phenomenon.

Acute grief is like a crisis, lasting approximately 4 to 6 weeks. Acute grief has a definite syndrome of somatic symptoms of distress that occur in waves lasting varying periods of time, usually 20 minutes to 1 hour. These symptoms occur every time the loss is acknowledged. Preoccupation with the image (of the deceased, as well as a loss of body function or loss by relocation) is a phenomenon similar to daydreaming and is accompanied by a sense of unreality. Feelings of self-blame or guilt are often present. The feelings of guilt may remain unstated, or a verbalized attempt may be made to seek validation. Hostility or anger toward usual friendships may occur as a result of the griever's inner struggle. The lack of warmth toward others is another internal struggle that also occurs. Outward behavior may be stiff or formal in interactions with persons with whom the griever was previously relaxed socially.

People usually have typical ways of accomplishing activities of daily living, tasks, and responsibilities. The distraction and restlessness created by acute grief cause feelings of being at "loose ends." Motivation and zest disappear; tasks and activities take considerable effort to accomplish. Activities that normally took 30 minutes, such as dressing, now may take hours, and every moment may seem exhausting. The griever becomes overwhelmed with ordinary decisions and activities that have to be performed. These feelings and behaviors are considered loss of patterns of conduct.

Chronic grief has often been called *impaired, pathologic, abnormal,* or *maladaptive grief.* It has been thought that chronic grief begins with normal grief responses, but obstacles occur that interfere with the natural evolution of grieving. Where there should be normal responses, there are exaggerated responses. This type of grief may be fostered by a lack of social involvement with others. Individuals who live alone, socialize little, and have few close friends or have an ineffective support network will be more at risk for chronic grief. Issues of guilt, anger, and ambivalence toward the individual who has died are factors that will impede the grieving process until they are resolved. Behaviors such as irrational anger, social outbursts, and insomnia that linger for an extended time or surface months or years later, or the appearance of mental or physical ailments should be suspected as potential inability to grieve in a healthy, constructive manner. Other behaviors describe maladaptive grief, depending on the interpretation applied to them. This type of grief requires professional intervention of a clinical nurse specialist or hospice nurse trained to deal with it or a psychologist or psychiatrist.

Disenfranchised grief is grief that is not recognized or validated by others. This type of grief occurs when the relationship between the mourner and the dead person is not recognized or the griever is not recognized by others. This has frequently been associated with domestic partnerships in which the family of the deceased does not acknowledge the partner of the dead person. It can also occur in the "black sheep" of the family in situations of family discord, in family members who did not provide support to other family members regarding the care of the individual who has died, or in participants in a secret tryst wherein the involved party cannot tell others of the strong relationship.

The aged can experience this disenfranchisement when persons associated with and close to them do not understand the full meaning of a retiree's retirement or the impact of the death of a pet, or when there are gradual losses caused by chronic conditions that have great impact on the elder but are not seen as important by others. Families coping with a member who has Alzheimer's disease may also experience disenfranchised grief, particularly when others perceive the death of the elder as a blessing but fail to support the griever/caregiver who has struggled for years with anticipatory grief and now must cope with the actual death.

GRIEF WORK

The process or experience of mourning takes time, much longer than anyone anticipates. The pangs of grief continue for years, even though the intensity and the resurgence of the grief may become less frequent. In loss by death it is not unusual for grief to remain with

us. Lund et al (1986) and Arbuckle and deVries (1995) demonstrated that older widows' and widowers' grief is not completed or ended in the prescribed period of time usually considered for grief completion. Horacek (1991) referred to this lingering grief (a form of chronic grief) as *shadow grief*. It may inhibit some normal activity but may be a common response that is not considered to be abnormal. The pain of grief is often exacerbated on anniversary dates (birthdays, holidays, and wedding anniversaries). Grieving or mourning is often viewed as a "weakness," a self-indulgence, or a reprehensible bad habit rather than a psychologic necessity (Parks, 1972).

Grief work takes enormous amounts of physical and emotional energy. It is the hardest work anyone can do. All cultures seem to observe a certain set of behaviors after death, but there do not appear to be a set of behaviors when the loss is of another type. For example, an individual who is seriously ill, who is moved from his or her home (or loses the home), or who retires (willingly or unwillingly) may not realize that feelings being experienced and behaviors displayed in the weeks that follow are natural and normal responses to loss. In most instances the individual is labeled as "depressed" rather than grieving. The essential point is that after any significant loss or change some degree of grief and grief work will occur.

Grief for the older adult may be longer than others might expect. Confusion, depression, or preoccupation with thoughts of the deceased may be mistaken for other conditions such as dementia or deterioration. Initially, positive feelings about the ability to cope may be present, but over time the grief response may be exhibited. An attempt to get the older person into routine activities too soon after a significant loss may complicate the grieving process rather than help it.

Multiple loss experiences through acute and chronic illness may be superimposed on relocation, a shrinking support network, economic changes, and role change. This can lead to a continual state of grieving, known as *bereavement overload*. No sooner has the individual begun to grieve for one loss than another occurs, and so forth. An individual must grieve one loss before he or she can go on to grieve the next.

Grief Assessment

Mortality of the bereaved during the first year of mourning is greater than for those who have not experienced a loss through death. Rees and Lukin (1967) found the mortality rate of the aged surviving spouse to be seven times greater than that of the average population. A higher mortality rate for widowed men after the age of 75 was also noted by Bowling (1989). Another concern is that diseases such as cancer, ulcerative colitis, asthma, congestive heart failure, leukemia, and diabetes may develop or exacerbate during this time (Carr et al, 1970). Mittleman (1996) found that heart attack risk was five times higher than normal 2 days after the death of a significant person and remained elevated for about a month following the death. Pietruszka (1992) notes that bereaved elders may present clinical symptoms that mimic the signs and symptoms of serious medical and psychologic conditions and present a diagnostic challenge to primary care providers. Therefore to anticipate the problems that grief may precipitate, it is important to do a grief assessment.

Assessment is based on knowledge of the grieving process and the subsequent mourning. Data are obtained through observation of behavior of the individual elder, keeping in mind cultural context. Questions should include losses and gains that have occurred within the past year (gains also bring with them some losses), strengths the aged person brings to the situation, what the person values in life, and how grief is unique to the individual. These will help the nurse to develop a plan with the older person that will facilitate physiologic and psychologic manifestations of grieving, regardless of whether they are transient or continuing. Inherent in developing intervention strategies is knowledge about the elder's coping mechanisms (effective and ineffective) and support systems on which he or she can rely. Box 26-2 provides physical, psychologic, and social factors that influence grieving.

Interventions

One of the goals of intervention is to assist the individual (or family) in attaining a healthy adjustment to the loss experience. Actions that can meet this goal are basic and simple; however, the emotional overlay makes the simple often difficult. For the nurse who is confronted with a person's grief for the first time, there is intense discomfort, fear, and insecurity. The tendency is to be sympathetic rather than empathetic. Questions

---

Box 26-2   FACTORS INFLUENCING THE GRIEVING PROCESS

Physical

Illness involves numerous losses
Each loss must be identified
Each loss prompts and requires its own grief response
Importance of the loss varies according to meaning by individual
Sedatives—deprive experience of reality of loss that must be faced
Nutritional state—if inadequate, leads to inability to cope or meet demands of daily living, and numerous symptoms caused by grief
Rest—inadequate leads to mental and physical exhaustion, disease, unresolved grief
Exercise—if inadequate, limits emotional outlet, aggressive feelings, tension, anxiety, and leads to depression

Psychologic

Unique nature and meaning of loss
Individual qualities of the relationship
Role body part/self-image/aspect of self was to the individual and/or family
Individual coping behavior, personality, mental health
Individual level of maturity and intelligence
Past experience with loss or death

Psychologic—cont'd

Social, cultural, ethnic, religious/philosophic background
Sex-role conditioning
Immediate circumstances surrounding loss
Timeliness of the loss
Perception of preventability (sudden vs expected)
Number, type, quality of secondary losses
Presence of concurrent stresses/crises

Specific to Dying/Death (in addition to above)

Role deceased occupied in family or social system
Amount of unfinished business
Perception of deceased's fulfillment in life
Immediate circumstances surrounding death
Length of illness before death
Anticipatory grief and involvement with dying patient

Social

Individual support systems and the acceptance of assistance of its members
Individual sociocultural, ethnic, religious/philosophic background
Educational, economic, occupational status
Ritual

From Hess PA: Loss, grief, and dying. In Beare PG, Myers JL, editors: *Principles and practice of adult health nursing,* ed 2, St Louis, 1994, Mosby.

arise in one's mind: What do I say? Should I be cheerful or serious? Should I talk about or even mention the dead person's name?

The nurse requires four strengths to help someone cope with grief. First, the nurse must have spiritual strength, or strength from within. This does not mean that the nurse must have a specific religious orientation or affiliation but, rather, that the nurse must have a positive belief in self. Second, the nurse must find meaning in life. One needs a philosophy to sustain oneself during difficult times. With age, life experiences grow, and a person's philosophy may change or be amended; but at any particular time, the individual should have a philosophy. Third, the nurse must develop emotional maturity. The individual who has always gotten his or her way will most likely have trouble when confronted with deprivation or loss. Finally, comfort with one's own mortality is essential for working with loss and grief.

The nurse must be ready to listen. Active listening is an important skill for the nurse who serves as a support person for the griever. It is far easier to give advice on how to solve a problem than it is to allow a grieving person time and space to express feelings.

When listening, the nurse soon discovers that it is not the actual loss that is of utmost concern but, rather, the fear associated with the loss. If the nurse listens carefully to both the stated and the implied, what will be heard may be expressions such as the following: "How will I go on?" "What will I do now?" "What will become of me?" "I don't know what to do." "How could he (she) do this to me?" Because the nurse knows there is resolution, such comments may seem exaggerated or melodramatic, but to the one who is grieving there seems to be no resolution. The griever cannot yet look ahead and know that the despair and other feelings will resolve. Therefore in the process of active listening, the nurse will seek to clarify what is said to help the person confront his or her fears about the future.

It is difficult for the nurse and others to listen to the same thing endlessly repeated, but reminiscing is important to the griever. It allows for the working through of the loss. Reminiscence is a means by which denial can fall by the wayside and allow reality of the loss to filter slowly into the conscious mind. Reminiscence helps the griever acknowledge that indeed the loss is real and that life can go on even though it will be difficult.

Kelly (1992) talks about re-forming one's life story. By incorporating the loss and putting the deceased into the life story in a new way (re-forming the story), one can invest energy in all other relationships that exist or may come to be. Drawing out anecdotes and vignettes of the relationship helps the griever to keep control over the story and over his or her own life. Encourage the griever to talk and tell the story of the relationship as it had been. Keeping the continuity of the presence of the deceased alive gives permission for the griever to feel the presence of the dead in life. Spirituality (mystical, beyond humans) is linked with specific beliefs or religions. This is the basis for faith and religious beliefs. Critical to recovery is the ability of the nurse/caregiver to allow the griever to remain in control. Control is crucial to recovery.

A three-point approach that the nurse might use to facilitate the grieving process is "talk out," "feel out," and "act out."

Talking it out requires active listening when the griever is encouraged to talk about his or her grief and express feelings. When feelings are ventilated or shared with others, the momentary panics, hysteria, and other sensations accompanying the grief are less frightening. The belief that those who are grieving want to be left alone is incorrect; in actuality, it is not the usual desire. The person in grief wants to talk about the loss with people who care.

Feeling it out is a cathartic experience. In many instances it is the nurse who guides the griever to cry or otherwise express feelings such as hurt or anger. The nurse may have to say, "It's okay to . . ."—expressing whatever feelings the griever has.

Acting out is a natural extension of feelings. Intense physical activity gives one some control over emotions. Ancients used to rend their clothes or tear their hair. Today, there are numerous ways of acting out feelings—from throwing things, to taking a walk, to busying oneself with tasks, to expressing feelings through creative works. In situations where acting out predominates, it is important to provide a safe means of acting out and a safe environment in which to do so to prevent self-harm.

The nurse's role is as an advocate who displays the behavioral qualities of responsiveness, authenticity, commitment, and competence. Table 26-1 correlates caring behavior with caring actions or interventions.

Outliving those one loves may create an emptiness that can never be fully relieved. Table 26-2 provides a nursing care plan for survivors, whether the survivor is a spouse, sexual partner, friend, companion, or confidant, with suggested interventions. The nurse must be prepared for this most difficult task.

Table 26-1

Caring Behaviors

Behavior	Caring action
Advocacy	Extend oneself to find proper help
	Work to grant reasonable requests
Authenticity	Sharing feelings appropriately
	Honesty
	Use of healing Touch
Responsiveness	Be available
	Interact verbally
	Provide comfort
	Provide privacy
	Be nonjudgmental
Commitment and presence	Provide the little extras
	Grooming
	Quiet for talking
	Time
	Presence
Competence	Perform tasks consistently
	Radiate self-assurance in caregiving
	Teach simply and completely
Give positive meaning to another's life	Listen
	Touch
	Point out reactions to family
	Praise when appropriate
	Help them gain a sense of control

From Krohn B: When death is near: helping families cope, *Geriatr Nurs* 19(5):276-283, 1998.

What is actually helpful to bereaved older persons? Older widows were interviewed to determine the attitudes and actions that they found helpful in coping with grief and that they advised other widows to consider (Rigdon et al, 1987). Their responses included the following:
- Keep busy; accept and extend social invitations.
- Help someone else.
- Learn to enjoy some solitary activities.
- Accept your own grief process as unique and individual.
- Talk to others and express feelings.
- Have faith in recovery and maintain beliefs.

- Take one day at a time, and do not expect to follow a timetable of recovery.

Often help received is crisis oriented and soon stops. Help over time is much needed. Rather than asking, "What can I do?" a person should simply do something. Accompany the bereaved in a new activity or a new situation, and by action invite them to move toward the building of a new life (Rigdon et al, 1987).

As the mourning proceeds toward an integration of the loss and a new beginning or re-forming of the life story occurs, a change in language used by the bereaved often occurs that is suggestive of progress and growth.

The Newly Bereaved

Crisis intervention with the newly bereaved is commonly provided by nurses, since the majority of deaths occur in the institutional setting and most of these deaths are of the aged. Information was sought from newly bereaved persons to determine what nursing actions they found most helpful during the death or immediately thereafter (Richter, 1987). The following comments about what was helpful may assist nurses in gaining a clearer perspective of comfort interventions:
- Kept me informed
- Asked how I was doing and offered support
- Put an arm around me when I cried
- Brought me food
- Knew my name
- Cried with me
- Brought a bed and encouraged me to stay in the room with my dying husband
- Told me to hold my husband's hand while he was dying
- Held my hand
- Got the chaplain for me
- Let me take care of my husband
- Stayed with me after their shift was over

Although we do not know the impact of action as related to overall grief recovery, it is clear that these events stood out as being significant for individuals in their immediate grief.

Grief survivors report great variance in the recovery process and deeply resent a professional's efforts to hurry them through it. Even other widows can be a source of distress when they impose their timetable on a grieving widow. The lesson for nurses is to accept whatever the individual is experiencing and exert extreme caution in urging the person to "get going."

Dysfunctional grief can be assessed only holistically. Is the individual able to maintain self-care? Is the person reaching out to others? Does the individual have

Table 26-2

Nursing Care Plan for Survivors

Nursing diagnosis	Expected outcomes	Interventions
DEPRESSION, LONELINESS, SOCIAL ISOLATION RELATED TO LOSS OF SPOUSE, SEXUAL PARTNER, FRIEND, COMPANION, OR CONFIDANT		
Manifestations: teariness, crying, sleep disturbance, weight gain, compulsive eating, weight loss, anorexia, fatigue, confusion, forgetfulness, withdrawal, disinterest, indecisiveness, inability to concentrate, guilt feelings; displays feelings of detachment, inferiority, rejection, alienation, emptiness, isolation; unable to initiate social contacts; seeks attention	*Short-term/intermediate goals:* The survivor will: Develop or use immediate support systems Express feelings of security Exhibit meaningful social relationships Show decreasing signs of depression *Long-term goal:* The survivor will demonstrate readiness to build a new life as a single person.	Attempt to develop a therapeutic relationship through touch, empathy, and listening. Listen to perceived feelings. Help person realize that grief is a painful but normal transitional process. Encourage use of other women, daughters, widows, men, and friends as support systems. Encourage balance between linking phenomena (mementos, photographs, clothes, furniture) associated with the deceased and the bridging phenomena (new driving skills, evening classes, new job). Establish contact with Widow to Widow Program for counseling if appropriate. Refer to appropriate agencies.
ANXIETY RELATED TO INCREASED LEGAL, FINANCIAL, AND DECISION-MAKING RESPONSIBILITIES		
Manifestations: anger, nervousness, palpitations, increased perspiration, face flushing, dyspnea, urinary frequency, nausea, vomiting, restlessness, apprehension, panic, fear, headache	*Short-term/intermediate goals:* The survivor will demonstrate adequate decision-making skills in financial and legal matters as evidenced by: Seeking legal aid Writing or calling appropriate agencies Formulating a realistic budget *Long-term goals:* The survivor will: Cope with legal, financial, and decision-making responsibilities with only a moderate degree of anxiety Make rational decisions about single life	Assist in obtaining attorney if necessary. Encourage to contact Social Security and/or spouse's employer to assure receipt of all benefits. Encourage to contact insurance agencies if applicable. Discourage immediate decision making regarding assets (e.g., home, stocks, etc.). Encourage to seek advice from individuals who are trusted. Contact proper social agencies if indigent or in need. Assist in seeking employment if health permits and client so desires. Offer alternatives for decision making. Refer to any other proper community agencies that offer needed assistance.

From Alexander J, Kiely J: Working with the bereaved, *Geriatr Nurs* 7(2):85, 1986.

a hope for recovery? Is the person searching for meaning in the event? Widows who use the greatest number of resources were found to be more functional (Gass, 1987), and one's intrapersonal resources had more of an impact in reducing negative effects of spousal bereavement among older adults. In addition, self-help groups seemed to assist those who did not possess the necessary intrapersonal skills by helping them in their efforts to gain self-esteem and an optimistic, meaningful outlook (Caserta, Lund, 1993).

Effects of Grief on Sexuality

The absence of a sexual partner following the death of a spouse temporarily cancels an important expressive role of feelings of femininity or masculinity. The intimacy and closeness of a mate provide strong self-affirmation. The loss of this important role results in asexuality for many of the old. Seldom are they thought to be full sexual beings even when married. When widowed, most older women are effectively neutered. Men may seek and find new sexual partners but are vulnerable to "widower's impotence," a result of guilt, depression, long periods of abstinence from sexual activity, and the strangeness of a new sexual partner. All of these factors may hinder an aged man from consummating a new marriage.

Grief and Gender Differences

Three out of four women will be widowed at one time or other, since women live longer and frequently marry older men. It has been suggested that widowhood is less difficult for women than retirement is for men because there are other widows with whom to share leisure time and activities. In many instances a woman's status increases with widowhood, whereas a man's decreases with retirement (DeSpelder, Strickland, 1996).

The abundance of literature on bereavement, loss, and mourning sheds little light on the bereavement of men, particularly in spousal loss where men are the survivors. The assumption is that men are less emotionally involved in the conjugal relationship than women and therefore less likely to grieve or express their grief. This was found not to be true. Evidence showed that men hurt and knew they hurt but did not reach out to others for help. The magnitude of the loss was felt in hurt, pain, and anger. Men also carried deep lasting attachments to the deceased spouse (Brabant et al, 1992).

Coping With the Death of a Child

It is often thought that the death of an adult child may be the most difficult grief an elder must bear. A small study of 12 Jewish and 17 non-Jewish elders whose child had died seemed to indicate that the Jewish women accepted the death and went on with their lives (Goodman et al, 1991). Although we question this interpretation, the study points out that the manner in which one integrates the death of a child has to do with the centrality of that child to one's existence, the ability to express grief, aspects of generativity in the life-style, and general health and well-being.

Grief and Sibling Death

The death of a sibling is particularly hard to integrate because the close affiliation and identification threaten one's mortality to a greater degree than most relationships. In addition, the death of each sibling removes one more member from one's childhood—those persons who can confirm one's youth and energy (Moyers, 1992). On the other hand, the first sibling who dies may teach the others more about death and coping.

Bereavement as a Growth Opportunity

Survivor coping ability improves when there is awareness that death and bereavement can lead to growth. A change in thinking from limits to potential, from coping to growth, and from problems to challenges are perceptual mind-sets that help move one toward growth. Resolution of loss and working through the grief provide incentives enabling possible important life changes. Transformation from intense focus on self-awareness evolves into a new sense of identity. The loss is placed within the context of growth and life cycles: the lost relationship is changed, not ended. By turning to the inner resources, creativity arises from the experience of grief.

THE PROCESS OF DYING

The Nature of Dying

Dying is the most challenging of life experiences and a very individual and private one. Most of all, dying is coming to terms with being alone. How one reacts to extreme stress, bad news, disappointment, loss, or change governs attitudes and coping with dying. An individual's coping patterns and personality are established early in life; thus most people die as they have lived.

The dying of young and middle-age persons is perceived as tragic, a loss of a not fully lived life. Dying and death of an aged person are frequently regarded as a blessing, a culmination of a full and rich life. That, of course, is presumptive. Many aged persons have not fulfilled their lives, nor are they ready to die. The dying process for one of advanced years can be a period of positive forward movement, a time of fulfillment and growth, a completion of life orchestrated by the individual with the support, understanding, and assistance of those around him or her.

Elders seek to make sense of their lives in the face of impending death. The remaining time may become a time of life review or a time to try to repair former failures, such as resolution of parent-child or sibling-sibling conflict or completion of a task that has been left undone, or a period of transcendence and spirituality.

The Dying Process

Dying may take weeks, months, or years and can be anticipated or, in some instances, predicted. For the aged, dying often arises from degenerative diseases typical of mortality in our society. However, the dynamics of experiencing dying vary greatly based on age, experiences, and culture.

As with the grieving process, the literature on coping with terminal illness and dying has stages and phases associated with dying. These descriptions or expectations are linear in progression and reflect a number of different yet similar variations of the dying process. The frameworks are often used as a cure-all for dealing with the dying. The stage-based approach leads to stereotyping the individual when the person is vulnerable and is coping with dying. Health professionals should not force the terminally ill into preestablished stages; rather, they should take into account the experiences of the individual (Lindley, 1991). What the previously established works provide is a useful vehicle to facilitate sharing of information about dying.

The significant work of Kübler-Ross (1969) focused on untimely dying and death. Those in her study were mainly middle-age and were confronted with an abrupt cessation of their careers, relationships, and tasks that had been planned. The framework continues to suggest a cognitive grid or guideline of possible moods and coping mechanisms, but it does not provide direction for interventions that would be helpful to a caregiver trying to support the dying individual. Keleman (1974) incorporated Kübler-Ross's stages of anger, denial, and bargaining into one of three phases of the dying process. His phases were the resistive phase; the review phase, which dealt with unfinished business and the reclaiming of a part of the self by becoming more in tune with the present rather than the past; and the unconscious phase, in which the individual talked about dying with calmness and which is comparable to acceptance.

Three concepts can be gleaned from previous interpretations of the dying process, especially that of Kübler-Ross: (1) those who are coping with dying are still living and often have unfinished needs that must be addressed; (2) one cannot become an effective provider of care without listening actively to those who are coping with dying and identifying with them and their needs; and finally (3) one needs to learn from those who are dying and coping with dying to come to know oneself better (Corr, 1993). Corr also points out that there are more than five ways in which individuals cope with anything as fundamental as dying. People cope with living and dying in more varied and individualistic ways. One should not assume that the five stages or types of coping are somehow obligatory or prescriptive in how one must or should cope with dying. Insistence on the individual dying in a particular way, considered to be the correct way by others, imposes additional external burdens on the one who is dying.

It is suggested that any approach to coping with dying should consider a basic understanding of all dimensions and all of the individuals involved. The approach should foster empowerment by emphasizing the options available while the individuals are living, emphasize participation in or shared aspects of coping with dying (interpersonal network), and provide guidance for care providers and helpers. To date, there is no such model.

A task-based concept addresses coping with dying from an individual's own perspective and with coping tasks grounded in situational tasks that are fundamental markers of human living (Corr, 1995). The dimensions of coping—physical, psychologic, social, and spiritual—each have a specific function and afford development of interventions.

The physical realm addresses satisfaction of bodily needs and minimization of physical distress in ways that are consistent with other values. These needs include nutrition, hydration, elimination, and shelter. Maslow also considers these as fundamental. Pain, nausea, vomiting, and constipation are among the physical distresses that must be managed. The physical dimension is extremely important because there is still inadequate understanding of the management of pain and other symptoms, misplaced fear of addiction, overemphasis on cure, fear of failure, concern about one's (caregiver's) own mortality, and feelings of frustration and inadequacy in the presence of dying (see Chapter 17).

The psychologic dimension promotes three features: freedom from anxiety, fear and apprehension; autonomy (security); and self-governance or control of one's life (often supported by others) and the texture of one's life that makes it satisfying or bountiful, such as serenity, activity, creativity, and risk or danger (richness).

Relationships with others and with society as a whole are the two aspects of the social dimension. Relationships with others—individuals or groups—sustain and enhance interpersonal attachments. Significant ties continue; others fall by the wayside as death nears. These relationships are ones that the dying person feels are important, not those that others think are important. No matter how much individuals think that they are alone, they are connected to society as a whole through family, culture, congregations, and governmental entities. The dying individual may need to call on these resources at some point.

The spiritual dimension from which one draws spiritual vigor and vitality is dependent on the individual's fundamental values and moral commitments of acceptance, reconciliation, self-worth, meaning, and purpose in living. The latter is reflective of Erickson's integrity or wholeness (1963). The spirituality may be formal or informal religiosity or a life review or both. Spirituality is the manner in which one integrates one's knowledge or belief system, inner life experiences, and exterior life and institutional activities in support of these beliefs (Thibault et al, 1991, p. 29).

Hope is a key element in coping. Hope involves faith and trust, which may or may not have a religious basis. Hope may be related to a cure, a holiday, the birth of a grandchild, or reconciliation. How the dying individual defines *hope* will identify what the meaning of life is to him or her.

Based on task analysis, Corr (1993, 1995), Doka (1993), and Coolican et al (1994) focused on living with life-threatening illness and developed tasks that address the initial diagnosis, the living-dying interval, recovery or death, and the aftermath. These tasks confront general issues and acute, chronic, and terminal phases of the life-death cycle (Table 26-3).

Living While Dying

The time between the diagnosis and the point of death is the living-dying interval or trajectory, composed of acute, chronic, and terminal phases. Science may extend the length of terminal illness for a number of years, thus lengthening the living-dying interval.

The acute phase is associated with recent diagnosis of the terminal illness and is usually the peak time of crisis because there is great uncertainty. Crisis intervention is most effective here because the individual, family, and caregivers are struggling to come to terms with impending death. Impending death, or the chronic living-dying phase (a segment of the trajectory of dying), is a time when work-activity patterns, entertainment, and relationships should be maintained as normally as the individual's condition permits. Martocchio (1982) describes patterns of living-dying as peaks and valleys, descending plateaus, and downward slopes. The patterns may be singular or appear in combination and may or may not be related to the pathologic condition. The terminal phase is ushered in by withdrawal or turning away from the outside world in response to internal body signals that tell the dying person to conserve energy.

The dying process affects all involved. A process of interactional dynamics between those who are terminally ill, family, friends, and health professionals was observed by Glaser and Strauss (1963) that can still be observed today. These interactions are closed awareness, suspicious or suspect awareness, mutual pretense, and open awareness.

Closed awareness is described as "keeping the secret." Medical personnel and the family know that the patient will die prematurely, but the patient does not know it. Generally, caregivers invent a fictitious future for the patient to believe in, in hopes that it will boost the patient's morale.

In *suspicious awareness,* the patient suspects that he or she is going to die. Hints are bandied back and forth, and a contest ensues for control of the information. In truth, the patient wants his suspicions to be wrong.

Mutual pretense is basically a situation of "let's pretend." Everyone knows the patient has a terminal illness and will die, but the patient, family, friends, and medical personnel do not talk about it—real feelings are kept hidden.

Open awareness acknowledges the reality of approaching death. The patient, family, friends, and medical staff openly acknowledge the eventual death of the patient. The patient may ask, "Will I die?" and "How and when will I die?" The patient becomes resigned to dying, and the family grieves with the patient rather than for the patient.

NURSING THE DYING

A major question that arises is, When is an aged person dying? Consensus is that physical deterioration is the prime indicator of dying. The less visible, subtle, and frequently misinterpreted indications of an aged person's terminal process are based on psychologic clues. The aged individual without perceptible physical changes that indicate dying may have a sudden and abrupt change in thought or behavior. Coded communication such as saying "good-bye" instead of the usual "good night," giving away cherished possessions as gifts, urgently contacting friends and relatives with

Table 26-3

Tasks in Life-Threatening Illness

General	Acute phase	Chronic phase	Terminal phase
1. Responding to the physical fact of disease	1. Understanding the disease	1. Managing symptoms and side effects	1. Dealing with symptoms, discomfort, pain, and incapacitation
2. Taking steps to cope with the reality of disease	2. Maximizing health and life-style	2. Carrying out health regimens	2. Managing health procedures and institutional stress
3. Preserving self-concept and relationships with others in the face of disease	3. Maximizing one's coping strengths and limiting weaknesses	3. Preventing and managing health crisis	3. Managing stress and examining coping
4. Dealing with effective and existential/spiritual issues created or reactivated by the disease	4. Developing strategies to deal with the issues created by the disease	4. Managing stress and examining coping	4. Dealing effectively with caregivers
	5. Exploring the effect of the diagnosis on a sense of self and others	5. Maximizing social support and minimizing isolation	5. Preparing for death and saying goodbye
	6. Ventilating feelings and fears	6. Normalizing life in the face of the disease	6. Preserving self-concept
	7. Incorporating the present reality of diagnosis into one's sense of past and future	7. Dealing with financial concerns	7. Preserving appropriate relationships with family and friends
		8. Preserving self-concept	8. Ventilating feelings and fears
		9. Redefining relationships with others throughout the course of the disease	9. Finding meaning in life and death
		10. Ventilating feelings and fears	
		11. Finding meaning in suffering, chronicity, uncertainty, and decline	

From Coolican MB et al: Education about death, dying, and bereavement in nursing programs, *Nurs Educ* 19(6):38, 1994.

whom the person has not communicated for a long time, and direct or symbolic premonitions that death is near are indications that the aged individual is approaching or is experiencing death. Anxiety, depression, restlessness, and agitation are behaviors frequently categorized as manifestations of confusion or dementia but in reality may be responses to the inability to express feelings of foreboding and a sense of life escaping one's grasp.

The elderly do not have a clearly marked trajectory of dying, as do young and middle-age persons. They may harbor multiple illnesses or pathologic conditions; the list may get longer as the person grows older. Elders become accustomed to chronic disorders and repeatedly make adaptations in their life-style to remain active and defy death.

Institutional settings tend to dissect an individual into component parts, dealing with segments rather than with the living whole. Nurses are caught in the biologic and physical aspects of patient care. It is easy and nonthreatening to relieve physical symptoms associated with dying, but to permit oneself to become involved in a meaningful interpersonal relationship to support the dying aged is extremely difficult for most nurses and other caregivers (Box 26-3).

Perhaps because the nurse brings his or her experience with death, perpetuated myths, and values regarding life and death, caring for the dying aged is very difficult. It is also possible that the philosophy of acute care settings, whose goal is to effect cure, governs to some extent care outcomes expected by the nurse. Long-term care facilities, of which there are more than 1 million, are places where the aged are supposed to die and where the decision is made to evaluate or treat a medical problem as the aged face death. However, it is not an uncommon occurrence for an elder not to be allowed to die in the long-term care facility but to be transferred to the acute care facility.

The individual who is dying is a symbol of every person's fears and that which the nurse knows she or he must eventually face: aging and mortality. The nurse follows a social code of living but has none sufficient for dying. The negative cultural norms provide little help in facing death. Many are still not educated in state-of-the-art caring for the dying. The way that caregivers perceive the act of dying—as painful, upsetting, indifferent, or a blessing—influences the treatment the dying patient will receive in the last days whether they are spent in an acute care hospital or a long-term care facility. A study of nursing home personnel demonstrated that nursing personnel who had more negative attitudes toward the aged had a higher level of death anxiety. Therefore they were less able to deal with death of the elderly (Depaola et al, 1992).

Whatever the reason, the nurse may show avoidance behavior when ministering to the dying aged. The nurse must begin to acknowledge the feelings that have been suppressed. When the nurse is able to deal with his or her fears, recognize them honestly, acknowledge the behavior they produce, and begin to act on such behavior, the nurse will be able to approach the dying aged in a more honest and caring way.

The development of the art of being with the dying necessitates inner strength, a strength that may or may not have its basis in religious teachings but that definitely stems from a positive belief in oneself. Formulation of a philosophy and belief about life will help the nurse through difficult times. Emotional maturity and the ability to deal with disappointment and postponement of immediate wants or desires will have a bearing on the nurse's ability to cope with the deprivation that loss brings. Knowledge of the grieving process and the human responses it elicits is also essential for the nurse to effectively and empathetically care for the aged, the family, and himself or herself during the patient's death.

Some nurses are unable to care for the dying because of their own unresolved conflicts and should not be expected to function in these situations. It is important, however, that someone more able to deal with the situation be asked to intervene in the care.

Needs of the Dying

The needs of the dying aged are like threads in a piece of cloth. Each thread is individual but necessary to the integrity and completeness of the fabric. If one thread is

---

Box 26-3	**BILL OF RIGHTS FOR THE DYING**

Nursing Care in Acute Care Hospital

I have the right to be treated as a living human being until I die.

I have the right to maintain a sense of hopefulness, however changing its focus may be.

I have the right to be cared for by those who can maintain a sense of hopefulness, however changing this may be.

I have the right to express my feelings and emotions about my approaching death in my own way.

I have the right to participate in decisions concerning my care.

I have the right to expect continuing medical and nursing attention even though "cure" goals must be changed to "comfort" goals.

I have the right not to die alone.

I have the right to be free from pain.

I have the right to have my questions answered honestly.

I have the right not to be deceived.

I have the right to die in peace and dignity.

I have the right to retain my individuality and not be judged for my decisions, which may be contrary to beliefs of others.

I have the right to expect that the sanctity of the human body will be respected after death.

I have the right to be cared for by caring, sensitive, knowledgeable people who will attempt to understand my needs and will be able to gain some satisfaction in helping me face my death.

From The Terminally Ill Patient and the Helping Person Workshops, Lansing, Mich, Jan 1975.

pulled, it touches the other threads, affecting the material's appearance, the thread placement, and the stability of the piece. It is difficult to separate the physical and psychologic needs of the dying aged to identify specific interventions and approaches, because they are interwoven. Freedom from pain, freedom from loneliness, conservation of energy, and maintenance of self-esteem are four major needs that are most often neglected in the dying older person, and when these needs are unfulfilled, the person's ability to reconcile the remainder of life is impeded. The needs of the terminally ill are listed in Box 26-4.

Freedom From Pain

Pain may be acute or chronic. Acute pain is limited in duration, is diagnostic, and can be relieved by the administration of analgesics given properly (McCaffery, Beebe, 1989), by positioning, and by other physical measures. Chronic pain is a situation, not an event. It is pain that lasts 6 months or longer. The pain becomes the patient's pathologic condition. It frequently expands to occupy the patient's whole attention, isolating him or her from the world. Patients with chronic pain do not respond to the usual methods of relief like those with acute pain. However, most nurses make no distinction between the two types of pain (see Chapter 17).

With any dying person, not just the dying aged, the nurse is placed in conflict. Pain requires the nurse to use a double standard. In the acute pain situation, in which

Box 26-4	**NEEDS OF THE TERMINALLY ILL OLDER ADULT**

To be free of pain
To conserve energy
To obtain relief from physical symptoms
To be secure
To feel that he or she is being told the truth
To trust those who care for him or her
To be given the opportunity to voice hidden fears
To be with a caring person when dying
To be loved and to share love
To be listened to with understanding
To talk
To preserve personal identity
To feel like a normal person, a part of life right to the end
To maintain independence
To maintain respect in the face of increasing weakness
To perceive meaning in death
To share and come to terms with the unavoidable future

pain is expected to dissipate, the nurse is concerned that the patient is weaned from a narcotic analgesic and given a nonnarcotic drug as soon as possible. Chronic pain cannot be treated this way. It requires a regimen of narcotic and adjuvant drug therapy administered on an around-the-clock basis and on time, not just as requested by the patient. Narcotic addiction of a dying patient is not the issue; relief of pain is paramount (see Chapter 17). A study by Cleeland (1994) found that 42% of cancer outpatients still had pain inadequately treated. Patients over the age of 70 were at increased risk of undertreatment of pain because of the health professional's fears of causing addiction, hastening death, and incurring legal liability.

Saint Christopher's Hospice in London demonstrated over the years the effectiveness of a regimen of pain control that is continued by hospices and oncology units in the United States today. When physical pain is controlled proactively, the amount of narcotic medication required by the dying patient does not endlessly increase. The sooner the nurse realizes that imposing his or her values and fears about addiction on the dying patient is negative care, the sooner physical relief for the dying will be effectively met. The key to effective care is knowledge of pain control and management (see Chapter 17). With the methods available today, there are few patients whose pain cannot be relieved.

Only in recent years has a focus on comfort by treating pain and other symptoms associated with dying (palliative care medicine) come into its own. In addition, religious and spiritual concerns are also receiving more attention. However, there are still too few who heed the needs of the dying.

One tends not to think of psychologic pain, but pain induced by depression, anxiety, fear, and other unresolved emotional concerns of the dying is just as strong and just as real. When emotional needs are not met, the total pain experience, physical and psychosocial, may be exacerbated or intensified. Medication alone cannot relieve this pain. Instead, empathetic listening and allowing the dying person to verbalize what is on his or her mind are important interventions that must be based on the energy level of the one who is dying. If tears and sadness are present, silence and touch are worth more than words could ever convey. Gentleness of touch, closeness, and sitting near the person are appropriate. The acknowledgment and sharing of the nurse's own emotions may be meaningful to the dying person.

Sometimes diversional activity can be helpful when there is pain, such as a backrub to ease tension, a foot massage, or access to a radio or television set (see Chapter 17). If hearing is impaired, perhaps an amplifier close to the patient's ear would help. If vision is impaired, talking books can be obtained, or an arrangement for a volunteer reader might be made. Often all that the dying elder needs to feel safe is someone close by to talk with, to listen, and to touch.

Freedom From Loneliness

Loneliness can come from within as well as without. The dying aged have sustained many losses: loss of friends through death, perhaps loss of a spouse, loss of control by institutionalization, loss of meaningful possessions, and loss of physical abilities (sight, hearing, and body functions). Loneliness can also be generated by language barriers and cultural differences.

In the hospital setting the nursing staff can easily intensify loneliness by caring for the aged person with detachment, by surrendering to the mechanical technology of the profession, and by avoiding the death situation. In these ways the nurse truly isolates the old person. Offensive odors coming from the patient's room or body keep people away. Unrelieved pain, physical or psychologic, intensifies loneliness. Behavior meant to attract attention may in fact distance people. The dying person is frequently placed in a single room or curtained off as it becomes more apparent that death is approaching; care is reduced, with decreased tactile and audio stimulation. Lighting in the room is dim, curtains or shades may be drawn, and people speak in hushed tones or not at all. The dying person perceives this as abandonment, the ultimate loneliness. No one wants to die alone; yet knowingly or unknowingly nurses foster this loneliness and aloneness.

Room location and environment are important considerations to reduce or eliminate loneliness. It is critical to assess the rationale for isolating the dying person in a single room. For whose benefit is it . . . the patient's or the staff's? Or is it to protect the uncomfortable visitors to the hospital unit? Some elders confined to bed find it reassuring to see activity. Placing the dying older person in a room with several other persons can provide the opportunity to share conversation and companionship and the security that he or she will not die alone. The patients who remain in the room after a death have the support and solace of each other. When there are only two persons in a room, the remaining occupant is left alone, a situation that can be frightening and a negative experience. These considerations are very individual and must be based on patient preference.

If the energy level of the dying elder allows ambulation, he or she should be free to leave the confines of his or her room and associate with other patients, visitors,

and staff. When physical tolerance is limited to sitting in a chair, a wheelchair can provide mobility and accessibility to the larger environment with the least energy expenditure. Sitting by the nurses' station or desk is sometimes preferable to sitting alone in one's room. If possible, the patient should be encouraged to wear his or her own clothing.

A pleasant room atmosphere with bright colors and diffuse, high-intensity lighting not only protects the aged from visual discomfort but also affords a clearer visual contrast of objects. Gray (1976) noted that in the last hours of the dying process, individuals turned toward light. Perhaps this supports the value of using bright colors and adjusting lights to keep the patient in touch with life until the end of living.

Live plants and flowers are a way of bringing the outside world in. Memorabilia, pictures, cherished objects, or anything that brings solace should be recognized as important in the care of the dying aged. These tangibles are a means of coping with anxiety and furnish a small amount of security and familiarity in an alien environment. A portable radio that is easy to reach or one with headphones conserves energy, staves off loneliness, and provides contact with the outside world. Television, if available, can also be a beneficial outlet.

Visitors should be allowed to be with the dying aged any time of the day or night. Night is the most lonely and painful time for the aged. It is a time of least attention, a time when one reviews the sorrows and joys of life past and thinks about what is to be. It is a time of fear of dying alone and that no one will know. When a friend or relative cannot stay with the dying person, a mature sitter might be the answer. *The sitter's prime responsibility would be psychologic support, not nursing care.* If the dying person is part of a hospice program, a volunteer may be available to stay with him or her. Not all elderly dying patients want this attention, but if they do, it should be available.

Everyone who cares for the dying elderly should be aware of the isolation and loneliness evoked by the dying process. Treating the dying aged person as an intelligent adult, holding a hand, or putting an arm around a shoulder says, "I care" and "You're not alone."

A little time spent listening to the elderly person relieves some of the loneliness of impending death. When caregivers cut the patient off as he or she begins to recall days of long ago, an avenue that helps relieve loneliness has been deliberately blocked. Reminiscence is a means of putting one's life in order. It is a valuable way for the elder to evaluate the pluses and minuses of life. It is a means of achieving closure to life by resolving conflicts, giving up possessions, and making final good-byes. It can provide a new meaning to life.

Some elderly persons have developed a life-style around aloneness. These individuals do indeed prefer solitude. Thrusting any of the nursing care approaches at them would only serve to aggravate the patient. It is important to be sensitive to the patient's clues and to assess and act on them accordingly.

Because of the interactive nature of loneliness and pain (pain may precipitate loneliness, and loneliness can exacerbate pain), the nurse may need to deal with physical and psychologic discomfort separately or together, depending on assessment of the situation.

Conservation of Energy

The dying aged use great amounts of energy in attempting to cope with the physical assault of illness on the body and the emotional unrest that dying initiates.

Nursing interventions should be directed toward conservation of patient energy. How much can the individual do without becoming physically and emotionally taxed? What activities of daily living are most important for the aged person to do independently? Would it be best to bathe the person so that he or she could eat alone or feed the patient so that he or she could wash or receive visitors? How much energy is needed for the patient to be able to talk with visitors or staff without becoming exhausted? The aged person should be involved in answering such questions and making these decisions. When the patient receives care without explanation or is excluded from decision making, the resulting emotional turmoil and anxiety sap the energy that might have been conserved by manipulating the patient's physical requirements.

Anxiety binds energy. Energy can be spared and anxiety reduced by listening, touching, and providing rest and an environment that permits the patient to be dependent when it becomes necessary.

Perhaps conservation of energy is the most tangible patient need the nurse faces when caring for the dying aged. By meeting the needs for freedom from pain, freedom from loneliness, and conservation of energy, the nurse has already begun to intervene in behalf of the maintenance of self-esteem.

Maintenance of Self-Esteem

Pride in oneself is a composite of the physical and psychologic attributes of one's years of living. For the aged person, it is difficult to watch self-image dissolve through loss of independence; loss of the potential for doing (a result of physical disabilities); or loss of body functions such as hearing, seeing, eating, urinating, defecating, or cleaning self. The aged person begins to feel ashamed, humiliated, and like a "burden."

Institutions and caregivers (by their approach and attitude toward the aged) can erode an elder's self-esteem. The aged patient's privacy and dignity are invaded by the number of physicians and others who come to look, prod, and poke in search of diagnoses and learning. Additional insults are imposed by calling the aged person "Mom," "Pop," "Dearie," or "Sweetheart." Bows are put in women's hair, and the old person is treated as if he or she has the mentality of a child. Behavior such as this by caregivers compounds the situation for the dying aged. Withdrawing from the dying aged reinforces the aged person's feeling of worthlessness.

When self-esteem is at an ebb, other factors such as psychologic and physical pain, aloneness, and depletion of energy are intensified. Depression aggravates pain and further isolates the individual. One cannot deny that the way the elderly respond to dying is influenced by their background, past experiences, religious and philosophic orientation, and prior degree of life involvement. If experiences have been negative, the lack of care and attention by caregivers creates a pathetic state of affairs.

Self-esteem and dignity complement each other. Dignity involves the individual's ability to maintain a consistent self-concept. Caregivers frequently take control and dignity away from the dying and impose their expectations on the patient. Essential to the facilitation of self-esteem is the premise that the values of the patient must figure significantly in the decisions that will affect the course of dying. *The important concept for the caregiver to master is that the dying aged individual is a living person with the same needs for good and natural relationships with people as the rest of us.* If this concept can be fully accepted, incorporation of the value of the patient to himself or herself will significantly affect the course of the person's dying process. Including the person in decisions about care encourages the patient to control the most important event in life.

What can be done to help maintain and bolster the self-esteem of the dying aged? Focus on the present and the opportunities that exist in the immediate future. Attention must be paid to the person's hygiene: cleanliness, lack of odors, and personal appearance (without hair ribbons unless asked for). Physical comfort is vitally important because with comfort comes security. Caregivers must become good listeners to allow the dying aged to express their fears of pain and aloneness and their struggles with separation and grief over losses. Caregivers may assume the management of necessary body and ego functions for the aged. This requires emphasis on respect and helpfulness rather than encouraging dependency, guilt, or conflict. Human contact is vital. One quickly falls into the confusional syndrome of human deprivation—loneliness. As early as 1967 it was shown in sensory deprivation experiments (i.e., touch) that a disintegration and loss of ego integrity (dignity) occurred (Pattison, 1967). It is therefore of utmost importance for the caregiver to use auditory, visual, and tactile stimulation appropriately to nurture and foster self-esteem in the dying aged. Verbal and nonverbal communication is necessary to convey positive messages; hand-holding, placing an arm around the shoulder, or sitting on the edge of the bed conveys to the dying person that the nurse or caregiver is prepared to meet the person on his or her own terms and that the aged person is an individual unique unto self and appreciated.

Reconciliation

Many individuals seek reconciliation with God and other persons as death approaches. Pain and other disabilities may interfere with this reconciliation. Symptomatic control in a society that responds to psychologic, social, and religious needs can facilitate this process of adjustment. This requires a multidisciplinary team that includes pastoral care of the dying as a high priority. Serious consideration to the approach deserves attention because an individual must feel involved and in control of treatment and care as long as life persists. Pastoral care seems to facilitate this humanistic approach. Depressed and dying elders often express concerns that have religious overtones. When this is the case, the need for pastoral counseling should be seriously considered and every effort made to assist the elder toward spiritual peace.

• • •

Communication and control are the borders necessary to complete the fabric of needs of the dying aged. Their influence is omnipresent in the other needs. Without them, the cloth can fray, and attempts to meet the needs will be limited.

Talking helps relieve anxiety; it fills time and fosters the sharing of feelings. The dying aged should never be lied to, nor should they be ignored. Lying is betrayal, not listening is interpreted as emotional abandonment, and avoiding the person's room is perceived by the dying as physical abandonment.

Control over one's time of death is a phenomenon that occurs everywhere. If care and institutionalization in life are seen as overwhelming negatives by the dying aged person, death can be hastened through the person's own control. The exact physiologic mechanism is unknown, but it is suggested that hypersensitivity of the sympathetic adrenal system or responses of the parasympathetic nervous system are involved in persons willing their own death (Watson, Maxwell, 1977). Neglect of the needs of the dying aged encourages the aged person to indeed use this last source of control over life, namely, the willing of death.

Conditions have begun to change as death education for health care personnel has become more available; patients insist on being informed about their illnesses; and the public in general exercises the "right to know" and "right to die."

The nurse has great influence on what happens to a dying patient. She or he can influence the social environment by regulating drug use, controlling interactions between the patient and the family, and influencing feelings of patient importance by talking with or ignoring the patient. The nurse can also assume the roles of supporter, facilitator, and advocate of the dying aged.

Spirituality and Hope

Spirituality is the basic human capacity for hope. Without one's own spiritual nourishment, one cannot meet the same needs in others. There is a transcendental relationship between a person and a higher being, which is not necessarily a religious being. In most instances spirituality is two-dimensional: that between the person and God, and that between the person and others. Spirituality may be met through religious acts and/or through human caring relationships. A person's internal beliefs, personal experiences, and religion are expressions of spirituality. This leads to self-discovery, affirmation of self-love, and a connection with all others that is brought about by loving the most unlovable aspects of self and others. Nurses tend to avoid dealing with spirituality needs because they feel they are too personal; however, one can begin to discuss spiritual matters in the following ways:

• Ask the individual his or her source of strength and hope.
• Ask if the individual sees any connection between physical health and spiritual beliefs.
• Discuss sources of spiritual strength throughout life.

Signs of spiritual distress include doubt, despair, guilt, boredom, ennui, and anger at God (Box 26-5). In-

Box 26-5	**ASSESSING AND INTERVENING IN SPIRITUAL DISTRESS**
Assessment	**Interventions**
Brief history:	Create a therapeutic environment.
Losses	Assess support system.
Challenged belief/value system	Assess past methods of decreasing distress (i.e., prayer, im-
Separation from religious and cultural ties	agery, healing, memories/reminiscence therapy, medica-
Death	tion, relaxation).
Personal and family disasters	Determine environmental changes needed to enhance func-
Symptoms (defining characteristics) such as the following:	tioning.
Unmet needs	Assess and assist implementation of coping mechanisms.
Threats to self	Refer to clergy.
Change in environment, health status, self-concept, etc.	Evaluate effects of nursing interventions.
Seeking spiritual assistance	Evaluate medications and their interactions.
Questioning meaning of own existence	Activate and evaluate appropriate community referrals.
Depression	Use techniques to assist client and family in reducing spir-
Feelings of hopelessness, abandonment, fear	itual distress.
Assessment of etiology of spiritual distress:	
Depletion anxiety	
Helplessness/hopelessness	
Perceived powerlessness	
Medication reactions	
Hormonal imbalances	

terventions may involve calling clergy; sharing spiritual readings, poems, and music; obtaining religious articles such as a Bible or rosary; or praying.

Hope is expectancy of fulfillment, anticipation, or relief from something. It is based on belief in the possible, the support of meaningful others, a sense of well-being, overall coping ability, and a purpose in life. Generally speaking, hope is an overall feeling of future good. "Enabling hope" empowers and is an integral thread in one's life.

The multidimensional nature of hope is expressed through thoughts, feelings, and actions. Hope is activated when a crisis occurs and personal resources are exhausted (Herth, 1990). Hope empowers, generates courage, motivates action and achievement, and can strengthen physiologic and psychologic function. Forbes (1994) describes six characteristics of hope that reflect the affective (emotional and sensation), cognitive (imaging, having a future), affiliative (sense of relatedness to others), temporal (time, future, change), and contextual (placing experiences within one's life situation) domains. The characteristics according to Forbes are the following:

• Confidence that change and adaptation are possible
• Relating to others
• A belief in the future

• Spiritual belief
• Active involvement
• Trust

The degree of hope that the dying possess is dependent on caring relationships with others and with caregivers such as health professionals. Love from others is a message of hope. Nurses seldom recognize the small things they may do, routinely and preconsciously, to impart hope. The act of grooming conveys a quiet belief that grooming matters; pain relief and comfort measures reinforce the recognition of an individual's needs and reinforce the value of that individual. Several approaches that may help the nurse to more clearly foster and sustain hope in the physically failing elder are to (1) confirm the value of life, (2) establish a support system, (3) incorporate humor, (4) incorporate religion, and (5) set realistic goals (Hickey, 1986). The nurse is not able to "do" these things for the elder. The nurse becomes the sounding board as the elder sorts through these important elements of survival.

Hope is much more than magical thinking. Hope is delineated as including the following:

• Recognition of a predicament or threat
• Realistic assessment of the severity and implications
• Determination of various methods of resolution or ways out of the dilemma

- Recognition of negative outcomes that may occur and preparation to deal with them
- Realistic optimism about outcomes
- Seeking of supportive relationships and realistic tangible support
- Evaluation of progress toward goals and revisions as necessary
- Determination to endure

The components of hope presented here resemble any problem-solving process, with the added element of the deep belief that problems can be solved and that one can endure and learn from the outcome if it is less perfect than hoped for. Often, leaving a legacy is an extension of elders' hope—if not for themselves, then for those who are left behind.

Legacies

The search for meaning seems to be the basic motivation for leaving a legacy (Birren, Deutchman, 1991) (Box 26-6). A legacy is one's tangible and intangible assets that are transferred to another and that may be treasured as a symbol of the bequeather's immortality. The courage, wisdom, and insight that we perceive in our elders also become part of their legacy (Wyatt-Brown, 1996). Not only the giver but also the receiver is essential to the concept of legacy; reciprocity is essential (Kivnick, 1996).

Legacies are diverse and may range from memories that will live on in the minds of others to bequeathed fortunes. Box 26-7 lists examples of legacies that are as diverse as individual contributions to humanity.

The nurse can assist the older adult in identifying and developing a legacy through the following:
- Find out life-style interests.
- Establish a method of recording.
- Identify recipients (either generally or specifically).
- Record the legacy.
- Distribute as planned.
- Provide a systematic feedback of results to the older person.

It is most gratifying to the older adult if a legacy can be converted into some tangible form, ensuring that it will not readily be dismissed or forgotten. Again, the nurse can facilitate this by assisting the elder in employing any of the following methods:
- Summation of life work
- Photograph albums or scrapbooks
- Written memoirs
- Taped memoirs (video or audio)
- Artistic representations
- Memory gardens
- Mementos
- Genealogies
- Recorded pilgrimages

Box 26-6   SPECIAL CHARACTERISTICS OF OLDER ADULTS

1. Desire to leave a legacy provides a sense of continuity.
2. "Elder" function is a natural propensity of the old to share with the young accumulated knowledge and experience.
3. Attachment to familiar objects gives a sense of continuity; aids the memory; and provides comfort, security, and satisfaction.
4. Change in the sense of time experienced as a sense of immediacy, of here and now, of living in the moment.
5. Personal sense of the entire life cycle.
6. Creativity, curiosity, and surprise may promote active and productive lives in the absence of disease and social problems.
7. Feeling of consummation or fulfillment in life that brings "serenity" and "wisdom."

Box 26-7   EXAMPLE OF LEGACIES

Oral histories
Autobiographies
Shared memories
Taught skills
Works of art and music
Publications
Human organ donations
Endowments
Objects of significance
Written histories
Tangible or intangible assets
Personal characteristics such as courage or integrity
Bestowed talents
Traditions and myths perpetuated
Philanthropic causes
Progeny: children and grandchildren
Methods of coping
Unique thought: Darwin, Einstein, Freud, and others

Transcendence

Transcendence is the desire to go beyond the self, to expand self-boundaries and life perspectives. It embodies aspects of belonging, connecting, giving life, holding commitments, struggling and surrendering ego, turning inward, and becoming free (Forbes, 1994).

Serious illness influences how one perceives the meaning of life. There is often a distinct shift in goals, relationships, and values among those who have survived or who are experiencing life-threatening episodes. There may be a heightened awareness of beauty and of caring relationships, but a long period of emotional "splinting" may be necessary while recovering from the psychic wound of body betrayal. According to Newman (1994), disease can be a manifestation of health as one confronts the crisis and as it reveals special meaning. Certain conditions facilitate the search for meaning in illness (Steeves, Kahn, 1987):

- Suffering must be bearable and not all-consuming if one is to find meaning in the experience.
- A person must have access to and be capable of perceiving objects in the environment. Even a small window on the world may be sufficient to match the energy one has to attend.
- One must have free time from interruption and a place of solitude to experience meaning.
- Clean, comfortable surroundings and freedom from constant responsibility and decision making free the soul to search for meaning.
- An open, accepting atmosphere in which to discuss meanings with others is important.

The following nursing actions may facilitate the search for meaning in suffering:

- Make opportunities for the person to talk.
- Ask how the person has experienced change.
- Accept the process as it unfolds, including anger and bitterness that may accompany the search.
- Listen and facilitate expression of feelings about life and death.
- Recognize and confirm any evidence of a rebirth of a sense of beauty. Often there has been a "peak experience" the patient may share if he or she is made comfortable enough to do so.
- Seek the meaning to self while learning from the elders with whom we are privileged to walk for however brief the time.

Sister Rosemary Donley defines the nursing role in the spiritual search of suffering persons as compassionate accompaniment—entering into another's reality and quietly, attentively sharing the experience. "Nurses need to be with people who suffer, to give meaning to the reality of suffering, and insofar as possible, to remove suffering and its causes. Here lies the spiritual dimension of health care" (Donley, 1991, p. 180).

DYING AND THE FAMILY

Aged persons today may be a member of a multigenerational family. Although they do not necessarily live under the same roof or may be geographically separated, there is some degree of filial tie.

When an elder becomes seriously or terminally ill and cannot uphold his or her role or obligation, the family balance or dynamics can be significantly altered. Even the aged person who is single and relies on friends and neighbors finds a change in the relationships. Depending on the role the individual has in the family constellation, problems often begin at the time of diagnosis or shortly thereafter. Roles and traits of the person who is now considered to be dying may create adjustment difficulties in the to-be survivors whether they are the spouse, the adult children, or the grandchildren. Adult children often begin to see their own mortality through the death of their parent, with the appearance of a new family order.

It can be a constant struggle for a family to remain involved with the dying person as they try to withdraw and try to readjust their lives without the dying member. This requires enormous energy by family members who are already burdened with their own anticipatory grief and daily living and who in many cases are raising their own children. The conflict is in grieving not only for the dying but also for a part of themselves that will be lost with the death of the parent or significant family member. A number of adaptive tasks are required to facilitate healthy resolution of the dying of a family member.

Family members need to remain involved with the patient. This means sharing and responding to the patient's experiences. At times family members have to separate their own identities from that of the patient and learn to tolerate the reality that this family member will die while they live on. The ability of the family members to truly support, love, and provide intimacy may lead to exhaustion, impatience, anger, and a sense of futility as the patient's illness drags on and on. Often family members may be at different points in grief than the patient. This can hinder communication between the patient and family members. As the illness worsens, physical disability increases, and the patient complains more often, intensifying feelings of helplessness and frustration in family members.

Role changes require adaptation and accommodation to new demands within the family as new responsibilities emerge and permanent change occurs. For example, an adult child has to deal with the death of one parent and assumes responsibility for the welfare of the remaining parent.

Bearing the effects of grief requires acknowledgment of the current feelings that surface in anticipatory grief. Coming to terms with the reality of the impending loss means that family members must go through many emotional responses in achieving acceptance of the loved one's approaching death. Because people are supposed to die in old age, the grief responses may not be exceptionally intense, but then, too, many filial relationships that seem superficial can result in very deep and acute grief responses.

Family members may feel extremely pressured during the final days of an aged relative's life. They may be caught between experiencing and remembering the patient as he or she is and was, between pushing for more or letting nature take its course, and at times not wanting to be involved because of a discordant relationship with the patient. These decisions will profoundly affect them for the rest of their lives. Often families feel guilt-ridden because they are thinking more about their own needs instead of those of the dying patient.

Despite the family's grief and pain, the family must give the patient permission to die; they must let the patient know that it is all right to let go and leave. It is the last act of love and dignity the family can offer the dying patient. There are times when there is no family to say, "It's okay to let go." The task then falls to the nurse who has developed a meaningful relationship with the patient throughout care. Rando (1984) summarizes grief work of families with the six R's of grieving: *R*ecognition, *R*eaction to separation, *R*ecollection and reexperience of the deceased and relations, *R*elinquishment of old attachments, *R*eadjustment to moving into a new world without forgetting the old, and *R*einvestment.

DYING AND THE HEALTH PROFESSIONAL

Whenever an individual invests in something or someone and it leaves, is gone, or is lost, there is a need to grieve. Similarly, nurses in their daily work environment are confronted with dying patients. By the very nature of the population that nurses serve, they are forced to confront loss, not only of patients and families, but personal loss as well. Caring for dying patients over time or watching patients go home and repeatedly return involves a degree of emotional investment and a feeling of grief that requires resolution.

A social factor that has long affected the nurse's ability to grieve is the assumption that the role of the caregiver is to be emotionally strong. The nurse has been told that feelings of ambivalence or guilt toward the patient are inappropriate. The nurse attempts to control those feelings by remaining detached, thwarting the acknowledgment or resolution of feelings. The nurse, too, can experience conflict between wanting the dying patient to live and yet wanting the patient to be relieved of suffering if it is a lingering death. A study of nurses in a rehabilitation center found a greater chance of being affected negatively by patient deaths the longer the nurses worked at the facility or if they were recently grieving a loss (O'Hara et al, 1996). The study also suggested that some nurses are at higher risk for negative impact if they have a high personal tendency toward immersing themselves in nursing care. This is an example of an earlier discussion of investing oneself without adequate support systems.

Harper (1977) identified a process of adaptation through which health professionals must pass to cope with the stress of caring for the dying. Intellectualization, which focuses on professional knowledge and facts and at times emphasizes philosophical issues, is the first stage of adapting. At this time conversation with the dying is distant, and a flurry of activity ensues as the caregiver busies himself or herself with physical tasks and reading about the patient's illness in an attempt to allay his or her own anxieties.

The professional in the second stage of adapting is jolted out of this intellectual haven into a confrontation with the realities of the patient's impending death and the professional's own mortality. Grieving is triggered for oneself and at the same time by genuine compassion for the dying patient. Caregivers can feel guilty, frustrated, and hostile. Hostile feelings are not uncommon for caregivers to experience when they attempt to fight their feelings, a situation Harper calls *emotional survival*. Depression, pain, mourning, and grief are crucial in this period for the health professional.

The health professional is said to have arrived at self-mastery when he or she is free from identification with the patient's symptoms and is no longer occupied with personal mortality. Self-mastery allows greater sensitivity to the patient without the incapacitating effects on the caregiver. This phase is called *emotional arrival* and includes moderation, mitigation, and accommodation.

The culmination of previous growth and development enables the caregiver to relate compassionately to the patient and fully accept the impending death. The enhanced dignity and self-respect that the caregiver feels allow him or her to give respect and dignity to the dying patient. Through this growth process, the health professional has learned that living can be more painful than dying. Now concern for the dying can be translated into constructive and appropriate care activities for both the patient and the family. Needless to say, the caregiver must have outside interests and a support network beyond the work setting to maintain a balanced perspective on life. Without this equilibrium, it will be difficult to grow and accept the death of others and oneself. It is realistic that the nurse may experience the stress of grieving and bereavement with the death of a patient for whom he or she gave care. Some of the physical symptoms experienced by others who grieve may occur, such as shortness of breath, palpitations, empty feeling in the stomach, and dry mouth, as well as emotional symptoms such as inability to concentrate, confusion, depression, and sleep disturbance. If there is frequent exposure to death, bereavement overload or caregiver burnout can occur.

Assessment

The Dying Aged

Few, if any, tools are available to assess dying patients. Caregivers for the most part have to depend on their understanding of the grieving and dying processes and draw carefully from behavioral responses outlined in the literature. A danger exists among health professionals of superimposing what they think the patient should feel and do in the dying process. The purpose of knowing about grief and dying theories is to recognize what emotions and behaviors can occur and to plan interventions accordingly as they appear.

As an individual nears the final days and hours of life, physical, psychologic, and emotional events occur that provide clues to the impending death. Too often, nurses, families, and patients are unaware and unprepared for these signs and responses. Tables 26-4 and 26-5 provide guidance for these responses.

The Family of the Dying Aged

The family, whether biologic or chosen by the aged individual, is often neglected when the aged person is dying. Attention paid to family members revolves around their presence as an obstacle or a nuisance to the caregiving staff. As institutions downsize and there are fewer available professional staff to care for patients, patients' families may find themselves beginning to assume more care responsibility. More often than not, animosity toward the family develops, and prejudgments are made about their behavior during this stressful time.

The ability to do a detailed assessment depends on the willingness, availability, and degree of stress of the family, as well as the time constraints of the nurse who may be caring for a group of patients. Using available time, the nurse can make an attempt to acquire information early in the dying patient's illness to help the family cope with the dying process as it progresses.

Values, norms, beliefs, and priorities of the family must be recognized and accepted. Rarely do major changes in behavior and communication patterns occur just because a family member is dying. However, if a health professional plans realistic interventions and outcomes consistent with the existing family system, he or she may be able to foster positive growth.

Interventions

Interventions have many facets and range from the simple act of hand-holding to dealing with a multitude of emotions. The core of interventions focuses on communication, pain and symptom relief, knowledge of available resources, and fostering involvement in and control of decision making by the patient as long as possible. Many interventions have been mentioned throughout the discussion of the needs of the dying patient. Tables 26-4 and 26-5 address interventions that can be done as death nears.

Communication includes the verbal and nonverbal exchange between the nurse, the elder, and possibly the family. Talking with the dying is full of emotional land mines, but it is a vehicle for establishing a trust relationship that can help relieve anxiety. Talking is a way to instruct, explain, divert attention, and amuse. Humor can be very therapeutic. Nonverbal responses are expressed in facial expressions, touch, and behavior. "Touch hunger," or the lack of human contact through tactile stimulation such as holding hands or receiving and giving hugs, is often experienced by the dying. Procedural touch used in bathing and treatments does not fulfill the need for touch.

Table 26-4

Physical Signs and Symptoms Associated With the Final Stages of Dying, Rationale, and Interventions

Physical signs and symptoms	Rationale	Intervention (if any)
Coolness, color, and temperature change in hands, arms, feet, and legs; perspiration may be present	Peripheral circulation diminished to facilitate increased circulation to vital organs	Place socks on feet; cover with light cotton blankets; keep warm blankets on person, but *do not use electric blanket.*
Increased sleeping	Conservation of energy	Spend time with the patient; hold the hand; speak normally to the patient even though there may be a lack of response.
Disorientation, confusion of time, place, person	Metabolic changes	Identify self by name before speaking to patient; speak softly, clearly, and truthfully.
Incontinence of urine and/or bowel	Increased muscle relaxation and decreased consciousness	Maintain vigilance, change bedding as appropriate, utilize bed pads, try not to use an indwelling catheter.
Congestion	Poor circulation of body fluids, immobilization, and the inability to expectorate secretions causes gurgling, rattles, bubbling	Elevate the head with pillows and/or raise the head of the bed; gently turn the head to the side to drain secretions.
Restlessness	Metabolic changes and decrease in oxygen to the brain	Calm the patient by speech and action; reduce light; gently rub back, stroke arms, or read aloud; play soothing music; *do not use restraints.*
Decreased intake of food and fluids	Body conservation of energy for function	Do not force patient to eat or drink; give ice chips, soft drinks, juice, popsicles as possible; apply petroleum jelly to dry lips; if patient is a mouth breather, apply protective jelly more frequently as necessary.
Decreased urine output	Decreased fluid intake and decreased circulation to kidney	None.
Altered breathing pattern	Metabolic and oxygen changes of respiratory system	Elevate the head of bed; hold hand, speak gently to patient.
		ADDITIONAL GENERAL INTERVENTIONS
		Learn to be "with person" without talking; a moist washcloth on the forehead may be soothing; eye drops may help soothe the eyes.

From Hess PA: Loss, grief, and dying. In Beare PG, Myers JL, editors: *Principles and practice of adult health nursing,* ed 2, St Louis, 1994, Mosby.

Knowledge of community resources will help the nurse give direction to the patient and family and help them cope with the physical, emotional, socioeconomic, and religious and spiritual problems that might occur.

Loss of health or deterioration as a result of chronic problems, as well as loss of independence, social contacts, finances, and energy, threatens control over oneself and the environment. The nurse's role is that of supporter, facilitator, advocate, and caregiver. Nurses

Table 26-5

Emotional/Spiritual Symptoms of Approaching Death, Rationale, and Interventions

Emotional/spiritual symptoms	Rationale	Intervention
Withdrawal	Prepares the patient for release and detachment and letting go of relationships and surroundings	Continue communicating in a normal manner using a normal voice tone; identify self by name; hold hand, say what person wants to hear from you.
Vision-like experiences (dead friends or family, religious vision)	Preparation for transition	Do not contradict or argue regarding whether this is or is not a real experience; if the patient is frightened, reassure him or her that it is normal.
Restlessness	Tension, fear, unfinished business	Listen to patient express his or her fears, sadness, and anger associated with dying; give permission to go.
Decreased socialization	As energy diminishes, the patient begins making his or her transition	Express support; give permission to die.
Unusual communication: out of character statements, gestures, requests	Signals readiness to let go	Say what needs to be said to the dying patient; kiss, hug, cry with him or her.

From Hess PA: Loss, grief, and dying. In Beare PG, Myers JL, editors: *Principles and practice of adult health nursing,* ed 2, St Louis, 1994, Mosby.

can facilitate meeting patient needs through patient empowerment and control and by providing choices in care so that the patient remains an active participant. Environmental stimulation through social contacts and diversional activities often relieves the sense of isolation and abandonment. The nurse must realize that some emotions and experiences are inexpressible, but that the nurse's role is his or her presence, being with the person and the family and being able to detect feelings of these individuals.

Hospice: An Alternative

Hospice is a familiar word to health care professionals and the lay public; however, the meaning attached to it is still subject to a variety of interpretations. The model for hospice and its concepts was resurrected more than 35 years ago and implemented at Saint Christopher's Hospice in London under the direction of Dr. Cicely Saunders.

Hospices are now all over the United States; some are affiliated with community hospitals (US Bureau of the Census, 1995). Others are operated by public health agencies, home health agencies, or volunteer groups. The variations in origins and style reflect the particular needs of the community, the style of leadership, fund-

ing sources, political forces, available resources for health and social services, and the spiritual care in each community where hospices are established. Long-term care facilities often have difficulty reconciling the hospice approach to care because of their own rigid interpretation of regulations meant to protect residents from neglect.

Many long-term care facilities provide services that incorporate hospice ideals and are developed using the guidelines of the National Hospice Organization (NHO) (Box 26-8). This organization, formed in 1978, has been in the forefront of promoting standards of hospice care that ensure that the purposes and intents are met. Some facilities offering hospice care may not have appropriately trained staff. Nurses would do well to investigate the quality and staffing of a hospice and compare these with the standards of the NHO.

Efforts to incorporate hospice care into health insurance payments and other third-party reimbursement mechanisms resulted in congressional legislation making hospice a permanent Medicare benefit and granting a modest increase in reimbursement rates. Since then, the number of private insurance companies and health maintenance organizations (HMOs) offering a hospice option has increased. The hope is that in this age of ac-

Box 26-8   PRINCIPLES OF HOSPICE CARE

1. Hospice offers palliative care to all terminally ill people and their families regardless of age, gender, nationality, race, creed, sexual orientation, disability, diagnosis, availability of a primary caregiver, or ability to pay.
2. The unit of care in hospice is the patient/family.
3. A highly qualified, specially trained team of hospice professionals and volunteers work together to meet the physiologic, psychologic, social, spiritual, and economic needs of patients/families facing terminal illness and bereavement.
4. The hospice interdisciplinary team collaborates continuously with the patient's attending physician to develop and maintain a patient-directed, individualized plan of care.
5. Hospice offers a safe, coordinated program of palliative and supportive care, in a variety of appropriate settings, from the time of admission through bereavement, with the focus on keeping terminally ill patients in their homes as long as possible.
6. Hospice care is available 24 hours a day, seven days a week, and services continue without interruption if the patient care setting changes.
7. Hospice is accountable for the appropriate allocation and utilization of its resources in order to provide optimal care consistent with patient/family needs.
8. Hospice maintains a comprehensive and accurate record of services provided in all care settings for each patient/family.
9. Hospice has an organized governing body that has complete and ultimate responsibility for the organization.
10. The hospice governing body entrusts the hospice administrator with overall management responsibility for operating the hospice, including planning, organizing, staffing, and evaluating the organization and its services.
11. Hospice is committed to continuous assessment and improvement of the quality and efficiency of its services.
12. Hospice promotes the development and maintenance of a safe environment for staff, patients, and families.

From The National Hospice and Palliative Care Organization: *Hospice standards of practice,* Alexandria, VA, 2000, The Organization.

celerating costs, hospice care will save money while making more humane care available to terminally ill patients and their families.

Hospice is described as the link between the needs of the terminally ill, their families, and the staff; it employs the medieval concept of hospitality in which a community assists the traveler at dangerous points along his or her journey. It returns nursing to its roots—as humane compassionate care, an ideal that has been the basis of nursing for centuries. The dying are indeed travelers—travelers along the continuum of life—and the community consists of friends, family, and specially prepared people to care—the hospice team.

The philosophy of hospice care is that "the last stages of life should not be seen as defeat, but rather as life's fulfillment. It is not merely a time of negation, rather an opportunity for positive achievement . . ." (Ulrich, 1978, p. 20).

Hospice care is a reorientation in health care for the patient and family. The home usually becomes the primary center of care, and care is provided by family members or friends who are taught basic nursing care, including diet, exercise, and medication needed to care for the dying individual. The patient generally wishes to die at home; the family fears this because they do not know what to do, and they want the patient to die in the hospital. Given the necessary tools and orientation, much anxiety is eliminated, and families, with the emotional support of the hospice team, are able to care for the dying at home.

Hospice is available 24 hours every day of the year for its clients, providing, as needed, the services of physicians, nurses, mental health specialists, therapists, social workers, and chaplains.

Hospice facilitates a redefinition of relationships. The spouse may not always be the caregiver; it could be a friend or child. For those without family, hospice staff and, at times, friends become the patient's family. Someone from hospice is readily available to stay with the patient or family whenever the need occurs. Neither the dying person nor the family is alone during the dying process or during the months of bereavement that follow. There is a great amount of contact, interaction, and sharing between the family and the hospice team. Hospice volunteers provide direct or indirect assistance. They perform chores and provide friendship and companionship to the patient and family.

The unprecedented contribution of hospice continues to be reestablishment of control for the dying person. Through polypharmaceutical means, control of distressful symptoms and pain has been accomplished without denying the patient full alertness and the ability to communicate with others. This gift, so to speak, allows normality for the patient. The crux of accomplishing this end is the anticipation of symptoms and intervention by the caregiver before problems occur (see Tables 26-4 and 26-5).

Pain control, the issue that is discussed most frequently when hospice is mentioned, is not exclusively physical pain but also includes relief of psychologic, social, and spiritual pain. Heightened physical pain may be the only tangible clue to the existence of the other types of pain. Psychologic pain emerges when loss of control over one's life occurs. The equilibrium is disturbed, and the usual coping mechanisms may not be effective. Social pain can be summed up as "man's inhumanity to man," problems stemming from loss of interpersonal relationships, unfinished business, unsaid good-byes, and nonclosure of life.

Spiritual pain may be tied to cultural, racial, and religious aspects from which the dying person feels alienated (e.g., rituals or participation in group prayers). Acceptance of death is thought to be easier for individuals with a strong religious faith regardless of whether they believe in an afterlife (Cartwright, 1991).

Reeducation of the patient and family is another dimension of hospice care. Before teaching is initiated, the hospice team finds out what the patient and family already know, what functional abilities are operant, what unfinished goals remain for the family, and what kind of rehabilitation will facilitate the achievement of the patient's and family's goals.

Pain control and the opportunity to die at home are the key ideas and activities that people associate with hospice. In actuality, hospice represents much more. It supports and guides the family in patient care and ensures that the patient will not die alone and that the family will not be abandoned. Bereavement services for the family extend for a period of time on an emergency and regular basis after the death of the patient. Hospice staff help family members learn care techniques, dietary approaches, medication management, and how to handle an assortment of problems that occur in a family in which a member is dying. Life is made as meaningful as possible.

Nurse's Role in Hospice Care

Nursing practice and hospice incorporate the mind-body continuum. Nursing is considered to be the cornerstone of hospice care. The nurse provides much of the direct care and functions in a variety of roles: as staff nurse giving direct care, as coordinator implementing the plan of the interdisciplinary team or as ex-

ecutive officer responsible for research and educational activities, and as an advocate for the patient and hospice in the clinical and political arena.

The American Nurses Association's Standards and Scope of Hospice Nursing Practice (1987) enumerate the special skills, knowledge, and abilities needed by a hospice nurse:

1. Thorough knowledge of anatomy and physiology and considerable familiarity with pathophysiologic causes of numerous diseases
2. Well-grounded skill in physical assessment and in various nursing procedures such as catheterization, colostomy, and traction care
3. Above-average knowledge of pharmacology, especially of analgesics, narcotics, antiemetics, tranquilizers, antibiotics, hormone therapy, steroids, cardiotonic agents, and cancer chemotherapy
4. Skill in using psychologic principles in individual and group situations
5. Great sensitivity in human relationships
6. Personal characteristics such as stamina, emotional stability, flexibility, cooperativeness, and a life philosophy or faith
7. Knowledge of measures to comfort the dying in the last hours

The Hospice Nurses Association provides guidance in end-of-life care. These guidelines bring geriatric theory, nursing concepts, and knowledge of medical management of acute and chronic conditions of elders together to provide the most sensitive and comprehensive care.

Hope

Hope changes as one is dying. Hope for a cure is never abandoned, but the focus of care is on creating an environment that encourages honesty, compassion, and mutual support. The intimacy of everyone working together establishes an environment where it is safe for the patient, family, and hospice personnel to share sad and wonderful moments with one another.

CURRENT ISSUES IN DEATH AND DYING

Decision making regarding life-prolonging procedures when death is inevitable have become legal, ethical, medical, and professional issues today. The blurring of the lines between living and dying results from technologic advances, the ambivalence of

Table 26-6

Advance Directives*

Type	Characteristics
Durable power of attorney (DPA)	Includes specific legal capacities and incapacities, which must be specified. Similar to a conservatorship without court-oriented procedures to make all decisions. Time limits must be specified (Cohen, 1987; Gilfix, 1987).
Durable power of attorney for health care (DPAHC)	Appointment by the individual of a proxy (of his or her own choice) who is authorized by the individual to express his or her wishes regarding care in acute illness and in dying, and to make medical decisions when the individual is unable to do so by self. The proxy may be kin, friend, or significant other. This is a legal document and must be notarized (Delong, 1995; Berrio, Levesque, 1996, Mezey, 1996; Weenolsen, 1996).
Living will (LW; comparable to directive to physician, instrumental directive, treatment directive)	A personal statement of how one wishes to die. Sets forth choices and instructions for personal end-of-life care. Less specific than DPAHC. There is no provision for proxy (Weenolsen, 1996).
Christian affirmation of life (similar to LW but consistent with Catholic doctrine)	Expresses that the person need not accept extraordinary medical care but must accept ordinary care such as food, water, pain relief, hygiene care (Catholic Hospital Association, 1994, in Weenolsen, 1996).

*Patient Self-Determination Act mandated by Congress in October 1990 preserves an individual's right in decisions related to personal survival.

whether death is to be fought or accepted, and the dilemma brought about by medical technologies. Decision making at the end of life has become increasingly complex because most people die in advanced age from chronic illnesses—dying over a period of years and slowly declining from degenerative conditions, including Alzheimer's disease and Parkinson disease. Seventy-three percent of deaths each year are of elders, making end-of-life decisions a frequent part of this group's needs (US Bureau of the Census, 1995; Mezey, 1996).

Self-determination is at the core of protecting patients from the medical system. Many physicians are unaware of or ignore patients' advance directives. They are inadequately trained to care for the dying and economically deterred from providing humane, compassionate care.

Advance Directives

The Patient Self-Determination Act (PSDA), under which the durable power of attorney (DPA) for health care (DPAHC), the living will (LW), and the directive to the physician (DTP) are subsumed, was created by Congress in October 1990 and implemented in all states in December 1991. The intent of the PSDA is based on belief in the preservation of individual rights in decisions related to personal survival. A DPAHC can relate to any medical situation in which the individual becomes unable to communicate his or her own choices.

All agencies that receive Medicare and Medicaid funds are mandated to disseminate PSDA information to their clients (Mezey et al, 1994; Berrio, Levesque, 1996; Mezey, 1996). Hospitals and long-term care facilities are responsible for providing written information at the time of admission about the individual's rights under law to refuse medical and surgical care and the right to initiate this in a written advance directive. HMOs and home health care agencies are required to do the same at the time of membership enrollment or before the patient comes under the care of the agency. Hospices are obliged to inform patients of their self-determination rights on the initial visit (Berrio, Levesque, 1996; Mezey, 1996; Parkman, 1996). Table 26-6 presents the types of advance directives and their specific characteristics.

Legal planning is essential for the protection of patients with Alzheimer's disease and their families. Unless this planning is done well in advance, there may be serious financial and legal repercussions. Because no one can predict future capacities, everyone should consider establishing certain legal protections. For the elderly this is exceedingly important.

Nurse's Role and Advance Directives

The nurse serves as a resource person ready to answer questions openly and honestly about available options, which requires knowledge and understanding of the PSDA. The nurse is one of the health care professionals who is responsible for ensuring that the individual has the opportunity to learn about and to make an advance directive. The nurse must also ascertain proper disposition of the advance directive if it is completed. For the patient who enters a facility with a directive, the nurse needs to ascertain that it is current and is reflective of the person's choices. The document must be easily available to caregivers (placed on the chart where all can see it).

Nursing home residents with cognitive ability have an opportunity to discuss their thoughts regarding life and death decisions with someone. Residents perceived to have a lack of cognitive capacity do not get the opportunity to do so, nor do those residents with communication disorders. All residents should be given the opportunity to execute an advance directive, including those with a diagnosis of dementia.

In a small study of elderly patients who were diagnosed as demented by standard tests, 30% were found to possess the mental ability to understand the nature of a health care proxy and to designate a relative as their decision maker. Twenty-seven percent of the group were able to express their preference for or against a do-not-resuscitate (DNR) option; 21% could do both a DNR and a health care proxy (Schmitt, 1996). Although this is a limited study, it suggests that decision-making capacity is not always accurately predicted by screening tests such as the Folstein Mini-Mental State Examination (MMSE) or the Global Deterioration Scale (GDS-2). Furthermore, it raises the question of who is making the decision regarding mental capacity. The implication for elders in long-term care facilities is that these elders should not be excluded from consideration in executing an advance directive.

As a provider of information, the nurse needs to be aware of the types of directives that are legally recognized in the state in which the nurse practices and the terminology associated with directives; for example, *surrogate* is not recognized as interchangeable with

Box 26-9	BARRIERS TO COMPLETION OF ADVANCE DIRECTIVES FOR THE ELDERLY

Inability to speak English
Religious/ethnic affiliation
Memory
Inability to concentrate
Eyesight
Hearing
Print size of document/reading material
Family structure and support
Procrastination, or wait to do later
Dependence on family to make decisions
Lack of knowledge about directives
Difficult topic to discuss
Waiting for physician to initiate discussion
Physician waiting for patient to initiate discussion
Believe a lawyer is needed for completion of forms
Fatalism or the acceptance of "will of God"
Fear of signing away life
Fear of being untreated

Modified from Mezey M: Geriatric nursing standard of practice protocol: advance directives—nurses helping to protect patient rights, *Geriatr Nurs* 17(5), 1996; and Berrio MW, Levesque ME: Advance directives: most patients don't have one. Do yours? *Am J Nurs* 96(8):25, 1996.

proxy or *agent* (Weenolsen, 1996). The nurse should also be familiar with the advance directive form(s) used by the organization in which he or she is employed. Forms vary from state to state and from institution to institution, but they may still be recognized as legal documents. It is also important to know that if one is taken ill in a state other than where the directive was executed, reciprocal legislation usually recognizes the original document. The nurse must also be cognizant of the barriers to completion of an advance directive (Box 26-9).

The nurse is expected to be able to answer an elder's questions, such as "Can I just talk about my wishes, or do I have to put it in writing?" or "Does this type of form have to be witnessed?" In addition, the nurse must know how a directive is accomplished. Elders in long-term care facilities usually need two witnesses for their directive, one witness being the ombudsman from the Department of Aging, who serves as a patient advocate.

The nurse may be a patient advocate by bringing family members and the elder together to discuss the difficult issues addressed in making a directive or just to discuss the elder's wishes. It may be the nurse who brings the patient and the physician together to ensure that the patient and the physician agree on the terms of the directive and whether the physician can honor the patient's wishes. It may also be the nurse who obtains the appropriate advance directive form for the elder who is well or ill. Counseling of patients by hospital representatives, nurses, and others has been shown to be an effective and generalizable way of improving recognition and execution of advance directives (Meier et al, 1996).

As a facilitator, the nurse encourages the elder to think about end-of-life decisions before becoming a patient. However, it is not unusual that necessity requires this to be done while one is a patient. Elders in long-term care may be vulnerable to loss of control in their life. Advance directives enable them to have some control over care issues at the end of life.

A values assessment, indicating what the elder holds important in his or her life and how this relates to his or her desires for health care and quality of life, should be encouraged. Does the elder want measures to be taken to prolong life at all costs, or does he or she wish for a natural death if the alternative may mean prolonged maintenance on machines? Are there any persons the elder feels comfortable with who can act as a proxy to ensure that the elder's wishes will be carried out? Answers to these questions are helpful when discussing the elder's wishes. The discussion should include the family and perhaps the clergy and friends, before a directive is completed, to identify if those who are to be involved are comfortable with the decisions and will adhere to the directive. For elders without family, the nurse may become a sounding board.

No one can think of all the possible contingencies that might require decisions with serious illness or a current condition. The nurse can help the elder understand treatments that are available to sustain life and the implications of such interventions as resuscitation efforts (cardiopulmonary resuscitation), intubation, and artificial nutrition, as well as the technical terms associated with them.

Suicide

Suicide by the elderly, per se, is mentioned here only because it is an alternative way of dying that the aged may choose. Suicide no longer holds the societal stigma it once did. In 1994 the suicide rate was 2.6% in the aged population and is thought to be rising (US Bureau of the Census, 1995). The number of successful suicides increases with age, particularly with aged men, who have a suicide rate twice that of the population as a whole. The motive of the aged who attempt suicide is not to attract attention or to gain sympathy but, rather, a genuine desire to end life.

The aged, as mentioned earlier in this chapter, often would rather die than experience the indignities of severe illness, dependency, rejection, and isolation. In their own way, whether in an overt act of suicide or through the insidious culmination of excessive or predetermined drug use (such as alcohol or mixing medications), refusal to eat, or the willing of oneself to die, the suicide presents a final statement, an effort to retain control of life and life decisions. Interestingly enough, if the terminally ill aged have needs met in a hospice or other care environment and are kept in the mainstream of life, suicide, although an option, is rarely considered.

Physician-Assisted Death

Physician-assisted death, physician-assisted suicide, physician-aid in dying, and *active euthanasia* are interchangeable terms. Changes in dying in the latter half of the twentieth century have resulted in the patient's right to refuse life-sustaining medical measures and in the hospice movement. They have also spurred growing debate over physician-assisted suicide and active euthanasia. Reasons for the debate arise from advances in high-tech support systems that maintain cardiac and respiratory function; the increasing aged population; the changing trajectory of illness, with large numbers of patients kept alive for months and years with cancer or other incurable illnesses; limits on health care resources and misconceptions about the rising cost of care of the dying; and greater emphasis on patient autonomy, with policy shifts from societal to individual rights (Foley, 1996).

The Netherlands is the only nation that permits physician-assisted death and active euthanasia. Although it is not legal, it is tolerated (Morrison, Meier, 1994; O'Keefe, 1995; DeSpelder, Strickland, 1996; Hendin, 1996). The contrast between the Netherlands (with its more homogeneous population, with almost all possessing medical insurance) and the United States (with its great heterogeneity of races, cultures, religions, languages, and life-styles) makes it extremely difficult to arrive at a consensus on this issue.

Limited knowledge is available about the circumstances under which physician-assisted death is requested and whether an actual or potential demand really exists. One major question asked is, Why does one request euthanasia? Some answers have indicated that it is because those who are dying fear the loss of dignity, pain, and being dependent on others and are tired of life (Morrison, Meier, 1994).

With passage of Measure 16, the Death With Dignity Act in 1994 and the subsequent referendum in 1997, the Oregon legislature became the first governmental body in the world to pass legislation in favor of physician-assisted dying (Smith, 1999). A report of the Oregon experience with physician-assisted suicide in the *New England Journal of Medicine* looked at the effects of the law 1 year after it was instituted. It compared those who took lethal medication and those who died naturally. The 1998 figures indicated that 23 persons obtained a lethal prescription from their physician; 15 of those died after taking the prescription, 6 died from underlying illnesses, and 2 were still living when the investigation was done. The average age of those who were assisted with the lethal prescription was 69 years. Of the 15 who died after taking the prescription, 8 were white men, and 13 of the 15 had some form of cancer. According to the report findings, the patients were more likely never to have married and were not particularly concerned with inadequate pain control but, rather, with loss of autonomy and loss of control of body functions.

The impact of this law on the public has been an improvement in end-of-life care. Oregon has gone from eleventh place to the second highest per capita in distribution of morphine in the United States; 33% of Oregonians now die in hospice care—this is a 70% increase in Oregonians who die in hospice (national average is 17%) (Lee, 1999).

Nurses have had strong opinions pro and con on this topic. The American Nurses Association position statement on assisted suicide was developed to provide nurses with a point of reference for discussion and understanding of the many difficulties involved in the issue of a patient's request to terminate his or her life. The American Nurses Association advises nurses not to participate in assisted suicide, citing such action a "violation of the *Code for Nurses with Interpretive Statements* and the ethical traditions of the profession" (Canavan, 1996, p. 8; see also American Nurses

Association, 1985). The nurse is involved in many end-of-life care situations because he or she is the primary care provider who implements decisions of others concerning end-of-life care. The position statement of the American Nurses Association does not mean that patients who want their life terminated should be abandoned.

Considerable confusion exists regarding terminology and interpretation of what effects the nurse's role may have. Many nurses believe that turning off the ventilator, turning off tube feedings, stopping intravenous fluids, or giving as much pain medication as is needed, even if the side effect is death, constitutes assisted suicide. It is important for the nurse to understand that withdrawal of such measures as feeding tubes and ventilators is allowing natural death to occur, which is very different from actively doing something to cause death (Murphy, 1996).

The general trend in American law is toward greater freedom for the individual to choose when and how to die. Many believe that physician-assisted suicide could be a reality soon, based on constitutional grounds of the right to privacy (Messinger, 1993) or the due process clause of the Fourteenth Amendment to the U.S. Constitution (Sedler, 1993; Carter, 1996; Wilkes, 1996).

As a means of stimulating thoughtful discussion on this topic, Table 26-7 includes some pros and cons from the work of Morrison and Meier (1994). Murphy (1996) suggests that now is the time for nurses individually among themselves and collectively in professional organizations to consider the implications of physician-assisted suicide and what their role will be while it is still a topic of social debate, rather than be caught unprepared without professional consensus as to their position if it is legalized.

Planning for the Care of Survivors

As discussed earlier in this chapter in relation to grief, outliving those one loves may create an emptiness that never fully goes away. The reader is referred back to Table 26-3, which suggests ways of facilitating the needs of survivors. The nurse must be prepared for this most difficult of all tasks.

• • •

This chapter deals with the peaks and valleys of human experience. The highest levels of nursing function and the deepest feelings are uncovered in the nurse who is privileged to accompany the aged through the processes of fully living the last days before dying.

Table 26-7

Arguments for and Against Physician-Assisted Suicide

For	Against
Physicians have a duty to alleviate uncontrollable pain and suffering, including the obligation to provide an assisted death at a competent patient's request.	Society runs the risk of sliding into a practice of involuntary euthanasia and subtle coercion of vulnerable and disenfranchised patients.
Patients have the right to autonomy, which presently includes the right to forego or have withdrawn life-sustaining therapy.	There is a potential for abuse. Involuntary euthanasia has a higher priority in permissive environments where euthanasia is legal.
It allows the terminally ill to preserve their autonomy and exert final control.	The healing ethos of medical practice may be adversely affected, and public trust in physicians may be eroded.

Data from Morrison RS, Meier DE: Physician-assisted dying: fashioning public policy with an absence of data, *Generations* 18(4):48, 1994.

KEY CONCEPTS

- Grief is an emotional and behavioral response to loss. Grief responses are individual; what is appropriate for one societal group may be considered inappropriate by another.
- One never completely resolves grief. Instead, the individual incorporates the grief as a part of his or her life.
- Dying is a multifaceted active process. It affects all involved: the one who is dying, the family, and the professional caregivers.
- The stages or phases of dying and the type of coping are not obligatory or prescriptive of the way one should die. Such expectations place an added burden on the one who is dying.
- An individual is living until he or she has died.

- The dying older adult is a living person with all the same needs for good and natural relationships with people as the rest of us.
- Hope is empowering. It generates courage and motivates action and achievement. The degree of hope that a dying individual possesses depends on a caring relationship with others.
- The health professional who cares for the dying must have outside interests and support systems before considering care of the dying.
- Living can be more painful than dying.
- Hospice is a process or unique ideology that links the needs of the terminally ill, the family, and staff to fulfill the remainder of the dying individual's life by enabling or returning control to the dying person.
- Advance directives allow an individual control over life and death decisions by written communication and allow (in some instances) an appointed person (a proxy) to be the individual's advocate when he or she is not able to communicate desires personally.

▶ Activities and Discussion Questions

1. Explore your response to being given a terminal diagnosis. What coping mechanisms work for you? With which awareness approach would you be comfortable?
2. Describe how you would deal with a dying person and his or her family when they are especially protective of each other.
3. Describe and strategize how you would bring up the topic of advance directives.
4. What advance directive is legally recognized in your state?
5. Describe how you would introduce the topic of dying with a patient who is critically ill and not expected to live.

NANDA and Wellness Diagnoses

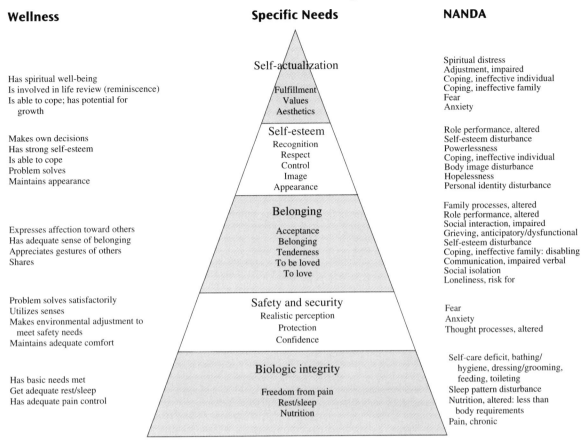

Wellness

Has spiritual well-being
Is involved in life review (reminiscence)
Is able to cope; has potential for
  growth

Makes own decisions
Has strong self-esteem
Is able to cope
Problem solves
Maintains appearance

Expresses affection toward others
Has adequate sense of belonging
Appreciates gestures of others
Shares

Problem solves satisfactorily
Utilizes senses
Makes environmental adjustment to
  meet safety needs
Maintains adequate comfort

Has basic needs met
Get adequate rest/sleep
Has adequate pain control

Specific Needs

Self-actualization

Fulfillment
Values
Aesthetics

Self-esteem
Recognition
Respect
Control
Image
Appearance

Belonging

Acceptance
Belonging
Tenderness
To be loved
To love

Safety and security
Realistic perception
Protection
Confidence

Biologic integrity

Freedom from pain
Rest/sleep
Nutrition

NANDA

Spiritual distress
Adjustment, impaired
Coping, ineffective individual
Coping, ineffective family
Fear
Anxiety

Role performance, altered
Self-esteem disturbance
Powerlessness
Coping, ineffective individual
Body image disturbance
Hopelessness
Personal identity disturbance

Family processes, altered
Role performance, altered
Social interaction, impaired
Grieving, anticipatory/dysfunctional
Self-esteem disturbance
Coping, ineffective family: disabling
Communication, impaired verbal
Social isolation
Loneliness, risk for

Fear
Anxiety
Thought processes, altered

Self-care deficit, bathing/
  hygiene, dressing/grooming,
  feeding, toileting
Sleep pattern disturbance
Nutrition, altered: less than
  body requirements
Pain, chronic

These are not all of the possible wellness or NANDA diagnoses that may be identified. The above are frequent examples of nursing diagnoses that should be considered when planning care for the older adult in whatever setting.

RESOURCES

Legal Assistance

American Bar Association
  1155 E. 69th Street
  Chicago, IL 60637

Hospice

National Hospice Organization
  1901 N. Fort Myer Drive, Suite 402
  Arlington, VA 22209
  (703) 243-5900
  Toll-free hospice referral: (800) 658-8898

Advance Directives

Alzheimer's Disease and Related Disorders Association
  (312) 335-8700
American Association of Retired Persons (AARP)
  Widowed Persons Services (WPS)
  NRTA-AARP
  1901 K Street NW
  Washington, DC 20049
Choice in Dying
  (800) 989-WILL (9455)

REFERENCES

American Nurses Association: *Code for nurses with interpretive statements,* Kansas City, Mo, 1985, The Association.

American Nurses Association: *Standards and scope of hospice nursing practice,* Kansas City, Mo, 1987, The Association.

Arbuckle NW, DeVries B: The long-term effects of late life spousal and parental bereavement on personal function, *Gerontologist* 35(5):637, 1995.

Berrio MW, Levesque ME: Advance directives: most patients don't have one, do yours? *Am J Nurs* 96(8):25, 1996.

Birren JE, Deutchman DE: *Guiding autobiography groups for older adults: exploring the fabric of life,* Baltimore, 1991, Johns Hopkins University Press.

Bowlby J: Process of mourning, *Int J Psychoanal* 42:317, 1961.

Bowling A: Who dies after widow(er)hood? A discriminate analysis, *Omega J Death Dying* 19:135, 1989.

Brabant S, Forsyth CJ, Melanon C: Grieving men: thoughts, feelings and behaviors following death of wives, *Hospice J Phys Psychosoc Pastoral Care Dying* 8(4):33, 1992.

Canavan K: ANA advises nurses not to participate in assisted suicide, *Am Nurs* 96(6):8, 1996.

Carr AC et al: Object-loss and somatic symptom formation. In Schoenberg B et al, editors: *Loss and grief, psychological management in medical practice,* New York, 1970, Columbia University Press.

Carter SL: Rush to a lethal judgment, *New York Times Magazine,* July 2, 1996, p. 28.

Cartwright A: Is religion a help around the time of death? *Public Health* 105(1):79, 1991.

Caserta MS, Lund DA: Intrapersonal resources and the effectiveness of self-help groups for bereaved older adults, *Gerontologist* 33(5):619, 1993.

Cleeland D: Pain and its treatment in outpatients with metastatic cancer, *N Engl J Med* 330:592, 1994.

Cohen E: Durable power of attorney: an overview, *Aging Connection* 8(2):8, 1987.

Coolican MD et al: Education about death, dying, and bereavement in nursing programs, *Nurs Educ* 19(6):38, 1994.

Corr CA: Coping with dying: lessons that we should and should not learn from the work of Elizabeth Kübler-Ross, *Death Stud* 17(1):69, 1993.

Corr CA: A task-based approach to coping with dying. In DeSpelder LA, Strickland AL, editors: *The pathway ahead,* Mountainview, Calif, 1995, Mayfield.

Delong MF: Caring for the elderly, part V, Managing end of life issues, *NurseWeek* 8(9), 1995.

Depaola SJ et al: Death concern and attitudes toward the elderly in nursing home personnel, *Death Studies* 16(6):537, 1992.

DeSpelder LA, Strickland AL: *The last dance: encountering death and dying,* ed 4, Mountainview, Calif, 1996, Mayfield.

Dessonville CL, Thompson LW, Gallagher D: The role of anticipatory bereavement in the adjustment to widowhood in the elderly, *Gerontologist* 23(special issue):309, 1983.

Doka KJ: The spiritual crisis of bereavement. In Doka KJ, Morgan JD, editors: *Death and spirituality,* Amityville, NY, 1993, Baywood.

Donley R: Spiritual dimensions of health care: nursing's mission, *Nurs Health Care* 12(4):178, 1991.

Erickson E: *Childhood and society,* New York, 1963, Norton.

Foley KM: Death in America: a new dynamic for an old reality—the national debate, *Aging Today* 17(1):7, 1996.

Forbes SB: Hope: an essential human need in the elderly, *J Gerontol Nurs* 20(6):5, 1994.

Futterman EH, Hoffman I, Sabshin M: Parental anticipatory mourning. In Schoenberg B et al, editors: *Psychosocial aspects of terminal care,* New York, 1970, Columbia University Press.

Gass K: Coping strategies of widows, *J Gerontol Nurs* 13(8):29, 1987.

Gilfix M: Legal planning is essential for Alzheimer's victims, *Senior Spectrum* 6(12):5, 1987.

Glaser B, Strauss A: *Awareness of dying,* Chicago, 1963, AVC.

Godow S: Death and dying: a natural connection? *Generations* 11:15, 1987.

Goodman M et al: Cultural differences among elderly women in coping with the death of an adult child, *J Gerontol* 46(6):S321, 1991.

Gorer G: *Death, grief, mourning,* London, 1965, Cressett.

Gray VR: Dealing with dying, *Nursing '73* 3:27, 1976.

Harper BC: *Death: the coping mechanisms of the health professional,* Greenville, SC, 1977, Southeastern University Press.

Hendin H: The psychiatrist. In Wilkes P: The next pro-lifers, *New York Times Magazine,* p 25, July 21, 1996.

Herth K: Relationship of hope, coping styles, concurrent losses and setting of grief resolution in the elderly widow(er), *Res Nurs Health* 13:109, 1990.

Hickey SS: Enabling hope, *Cancer Nurs* 9(3):133, 1986.

Hooyman N, Kiyak H: *Social gerontology,* ed 3, Boston, 1996, Allyn & Bacon.

Horacek BJ: Toward a more viable model of grieving and consequences for older persons, *Death Stud* 15(5):459, 1991.

Keleman S: Stages of dying, *Voices* 10:46, 1974.

Kelly JD: Grief: Re-forming life's story, *J Palliat Care* 8(2):33, 1992.

Kivnick HQ: Remembering and being remembered: the reciprocity of psychosocial legacy, *Generations* 20(3):49, 1996.

Krohn B: When death is near: helping families cope, *Geriatr Nurs* 19(5):276-283, 1998.

Kübler-Ross E: *On death and dying,* New York, 1969, Macmillan.

Lee BC: In Oregon's assisted suicide law scrutinized after first year, *Clinician News* 3(7):1, 1999.

Lindley DB: Process of dying: defining characteristics, *Cancer Nurs* 14(6):328, 1991.

Lund DA, Caserta MD, Dimond MF: Gender differences through two years of bereavement among the elderly, *Gerontologist* 26(3):314, 1986.

Martocchio BC: *Living while dying,* Bowie, Md, 1982, Brady.

McCaffery M, Pasero C: *Pain: clinical manual,* ed 2, St Louis, 1999, Mosby.

Meier DE et al: Marked improvement in recognition and completion of health care proxies: a randomized controlled trial of counseling by hospital patient representatives, *Arch Intern Med* 156(11):1227, 1996.

Messinger TJ: A gentle and easy death: from ancient Greece to beyond Cruzan—toward a reasoned legal response to the societal dilemma of euthanasia, *Denver University Law Review* 71(1):229, 1993.

Mezey M: Geriatric nursing standard of practice protocol: advance directives—nurses helping to protect patient rights, *Geriatr Nurs* 17(5), 1996.

Mezey M, Ramsey GC, Mitty E: Making the PSDA work for the elderly, *Generations* 18(4):13, 1994.

Minogue B: *Bioethics: a committee approach,* Boston, 1996, Jones & Bartlett.

Mittleman M: Taking grief to heart, *Harvard Health Lett* 21(8):8, 1996.

Morrison RS, Meier DE: Physician-assisted dying: fashioning public policy with an absence of data, *Generations* 18(4):48, 1994.

Moyers W: *Healing and the mind,* WNET public television, Feb 1992.

Murphy P: In Canavan K: ANA advises nurses not to participate in assisted suicide, *Am Nurs* 96(6):8, 1996.

Newman MA: *Health as expanding consciousness,* ed 2, New York, 1994, National League for Nursing Press.

O'Hara PA et al: Patient death in a long-term care hospital: a study of the effect on nursing staff, *J Gerontol Nurs* 22(8):27, 1996.

O'Keefe M: The Dutch way of dying, *San Francisco Sunday Examiner,* p A8, Feb 19, 1995.

Parkman C: Using advance directives, part II, *NurseWeek* 9(12):10, 1996.

Parks CM: *Bereavement,* New York, 1972, Tavistock.

Parks CM, Weiss RS: *Recovery from bereavement,* New York, 1983, Basic Books.

Pattison EM: The experience of dying, *Am J Psychother* 21:32, 1967.

Pietruszka FM: Management of bereavement in the elderly, *Physician Assist* 16(4):31, 1992.

Rando TA: *Grief, dying, and death,* Champaign, Ill, 1984, Research Press.

Rees WD, Lukin SG: The mortality of bereavement, *BMJ* 4:13, 1967.

Richter J: Support: a resource during crisis of mate loss, *J Gerontol Nurs* 13(11):18, 1987.

Rigdon I, Clayton B, Dimond M: Toward a theory of helplessness for the elderly bereaved: an invitation to a new life, *Adv Nurs Sci* 9(2):32, 1987.

Schmitt L: *The right to choose: capacity study of demented residents in nursing homes,* Executive summary, Chicago, 1996, Franciscan Sisters of the Poor Hospital Systems.

Sedler RA: The constitution and hastening inevitable death, *Hasting Cent Rep* 23(5):20, 1993.

Smith A: Oregon's assisted suicide law scrutinized after first year, *Clinician News* 3(7):1, 1999.

Solari-Twadell PA et al: The pinwheel model of bereavement, *Image J Nurs Sch* 27(4):323, 1995.

Steeves R, Kahn D: Experience of meaning in suffering, *Image J Nurs Sch* 19(3):114, 1987.

Thibault JM, Ellor JW, Netting FE: Conceptual framework for assessing spiritual functioning and fulfillment of older adults in long-term care settings, *J Relig Gerontol* 7(4):29, 1991.

Ulrich LK: The challenge of hospice care, *Bull Am Protestant Hosp Assoc* 21:6, 1978.

US Bureau of the Census: *Statistical abstract of the United States: 1995,* ed 115, Washington, DC, 1995, US Government Printing Office.

Watson W, Maxwell RJ: Elements of the social structure of dying. In Watson W, Maxwell RJ, editors: *Human aging and dying: study in sociocultural gerontology,* New York, 1977, St Martin's Press.

Weenolsen P: *The art of dying,* New York, 1996, St Martin's Press.

Wilkes P: The next pro-lifers, *New York Times Magazine,* July 21, 1996.

Worden JW: *Grief counseling and grief therapy: a handbook for mental health practitioners,* ed 2, New York, 1991, Springer.

Wyatt-Brown AM: The literary legacies: continuity and change, *Generations* 20(3):65, 1996.

chapter 27

Life Space Options for Elders

►LEARNING OBJECTIVES

Upon completion of this chapter, the reader will be able to:

- Explain the significance of personal space to adaptation in late life.
- Identify factors in the environment that contribute to the safety and security of the aged.
- Compare the major features, advantages, and disadvantages of several housing situations available to the aged.
- Name several aspects of relocation stress.
- Describe a desirable long-term care living situation.
- Discuss changes in the environment and the effects on individual function.
- Assist an elder in making an informed choice when planning a move to a protected setting.

►GLOSSARY

Catastrophic reaction An uncoordinated, inappropriate response to a situation. Catastrophic reactions may be triggered by demands beyond one's capability in individuals who have some dementia.
Cognizant Being observant and aware of happenings.

Equitable Just and fair.
Iatrogenic A disorder or condition caused by medical treatments or diagnostic procedures.
Nosocomial Hospital-acquired infections appearing within 72 hours after hospitalization.

►THE LIVED EXPERIENCE

Somehow, I never gave much thought to leaving my home or needing assistance to take care of myself. I should have planned for this move long ago, but I never felt old or weak until I broke my hip. It took me so long to recover, and I'm still not back to myself. I just can't bear moving out of this home that I have lived in for 50 years. My children grew up here, and I still have the marks on the kitchen wall where we measured them each year. It is like leaving a part of myself.

June, age 75

I sort of feel as if I should ask Mother to live with me, but I know neither one of us would really enjoy that. I've always gotten along so well with her, I would hate to ruin that by living together. I just seem to have so much to do right now that I don't know when I'll find time to look for a place for her to live. I wonder where to turn for help.

Janice, June's daughter

A mobile, youth-oriented society may find it difficult to fully comprehend the insecurity that elders feel when moving from one site to another in their later years. In addition to the stress of relocation and the initial anxiety of adapting to a new setting, elders typically move to ever more restrictive environments, often against their wishes. In this chapter the various options along the continuum of care and living environments are considered. The major issues are the degrees of freedom elders have, assistance provided to the elder in making personally appropriate choices, the stress of relocation, and the anxiety surrounding institutionalization. Nursing care is focused on providing orientation, information, resources, advocacy, comfort, and safety in whatever situation the elder is encountering. All of these are considered in this chapter in terms of maintaining per-

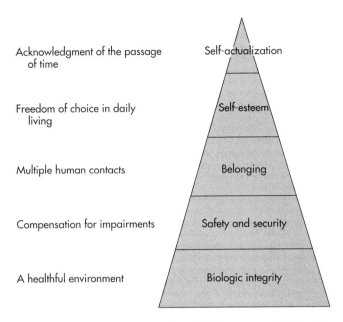

Acknowledgment of the passage of time	Self-actualization
Freedom of choice in daily living	Self-esteem
Multiple human contacts	Belonging
Compensation for impairments	Safety and security
A healthful environment	Biologic integrity

Fig. 27-1 Environmental needs of older Americans. (Modified from Herreth J, Orr P, Jones B: *Environmental needs of older Americans,* Atlanta, 1984, The Exchange.)

sonal space and life space in a safe and satisfactory manner. Fig. 27-1 addresses the basic environmental supports that elders require to function maximally at each level of need.

PERSONAL SPACE

Each person needs an inviolable space for solitude, intimacy, anonymity, and centering oneself. The amount of time needed and the boundaries of this private space are individually and culturally variable. An aged person with no opportunity for privacy may erect psychologic walls for self-protection from personal invasion and will no longer care about seeking enlargement in life space.

Personalized boundaries define one's space and reflect the personality and interests of the inhabitant. Older people characteristically maintain a sense of personal space by saving small items and arranging environmental props (significant personal items) in a particular manner. A thoughtful nurse will respect these territorial boundaries, will not move into private space or thought too rapidly, and will bring together health and illness behavioral needs to establish a secure place for the elder. For example, one elderly woman saved

her paper napkins, cups, and drinking straws. She had grown up in an era of deprivation and needed the security of saving.

Problems such as sensory overload (related to loss of environmental control), medication haze, isolation from significant persons, pain, and biologic disorders all affect one's sense of personal space. These are all discussed in various other chapters throughout this text. Suggestions and nursing interventions throughout this chapter are designed to restore pattern and order and environmental competence, resulting in a sense of safety and security.

LIFE SPACE

Beyond immediate personal space, each person has a defined life space that may diminish as one ages. A person's life space includes the arena in which the individual functions in the neighborhood, community, and world at large. It is dictated by mobility, economics, energy, and status. It is geographically and perceptually defined and subject to enlargement, constriction, and energy exchanges. Although one's personally significant geographic space may be limited to a 5- by 10-foot cubicle, perceptual life space is limited only to the creativity and capacity of the individual. In this chapter we consider older individuals and their personal and geographic life space.

MAINTENANCE IN THE LEAST RESTRICTIVE SETTING

One person may live in abject poverty in an inner-city hotel, although few of these seedy hotels remain after the gentrification of most "downtown" central areas. Another individual will manage nicely in a small "mother-in-law" apartment or cottage on the property of a child or a friend. A few are able to remain in apartments where rent controls have allowed them to beat inflation while landlords wring their hands in despair of ever renting the apartment for its true worth. Many others have found mobile home living in small parks with central recreational and service areas quite fitting for their needs and income. Some have developed a "round robin" tactic in which they live with each child for several months each year and never totally wear out their welcome before they move on to the next. Some remain in their own long-time residence because of property tax advantages; homes they own outright; and/or a grandchild, other relative, or student who is pleased to live on the premises free of charge, providing some minimal assistance, company, and security. There are various arrangements by which an elder may remain in an independent living situation even though he or she is in need of some assistance. The goal of this chapter is to present numerous living situations that may be desirable for individual elders to best meet their needs.

• • •

Personal territories and life space are the fabric of human existence. How people cluster together, where they establish their roots, and how they personally define the limits of their range influence all other aspects of adaptation. When one reaches old age, environmental response is strongly rooted in experiences and the emotional impact of certain houses, areas, and events connecting them. When relocation is essential, the environment should be matched as carefully as possible to previous desirable aspects. The most positive outcomes are seen when the individual has a sense of control and transitional supports. We will be much more effective in dealing with environmental issues if we remember the strong instinctive nature of territorial occupancy.

REMAINING AT HOME

"Home" provides basic shelter, is a place to establish security, and is the place where one "belongs." It should provide the highest possible level of independence, function, and comfort. Most people have basic shelter, but security within that shelter may be minimal. The major task in planning housing for the older adult is to help the older person stay where he or she wants to be with appropriate support. The Program of All-Inclusive Care for the Elderly (PACE) in several sites nationwide provides models for keeping individuals in their own homes with sufficient supports.

The living arrangements of the aged vary tremendously, but more and more, the aged remain in the home. However, the hospital has been brought to the home in the form of equipment needed for high-tech care. Some refer to this as the *hypermedicalization* of the home (Arras, Dubler, 1994). The nurse must adapt to the space of the client and forgo the traditional security of our professional home and institutional care. Even more difficult, the client and family requiring high-tech home care must forgo the security of the hospital and take on responsibilities that they may not feel capable of or willing to manage. In addition to the anxiety provoked by the need to adapt to the client's home and personal space, nurses will also experience some of the patient's anxiety regarding invasion of the home. Arras and Dubler (1994) suggest that patients and their families be informed of the benefits and the burdens of such care and the alternatives. For some people, high-tech home care may not be a reasonable expectation or one that they can accept. Clients in the home need the following:

1. Acknowledgment that the nurse is intruding into the client's domain
2. Assistance in arranging medical equipment comfortably and instruction in safety issues
3. Explanations of rationale and demonstrations of appropriate disposal of potentially contaminated or toxic materials
4. Acknowledgment that home care brings intrusions into the client's surroundings and assistance with life-style modification to produce the most acceptable ambiance
5. Information about alternatives that may be more feasible for the client than those typically recommended
6. Discussion of any modifications needed to ensure safety

7. Ready access to assistance when needed and emergency responses for necessary services

Home Modifications

Minor repairs may present a major problem for older adult homeowners. Those who do not have the strength or skills to make needed repairs often rely on friends and relatives, but many elders have no one to assist them. Some communities have organized a home repair service particularly for the low-income older adult and disabled. Home maintenance service can be managed by retired workers with special skills, and the work can be done by youths who need jobs. The retirees can teach badly needed job skills to youths while providing an inexpensive service to elders in the home. No programs are available across the country; it is therefore suggested that resources might be allotted through Housing and Urban Development (HUD) or by creating a national home modification program modeled after the demonstration funded through HUD (Pynoos, 1992). Until it is recognized that adequate living situations actually promote health and reduce illness costs, it is unlikely that this will be done.

Elders who have planned ahead and have adequate resources often modify their home or buy a more convenient home long before they become frail. Some of the features they seek are absence of stairs in addition to roomy bathrooms with grab bars strategically placed, closets and shelves that are easily accessible without reaching, security systems, lights that may be dimmed at night, and other convenience features. Architectural design and remodeling for individual home owners and institutions have become a thriving business.

Goods and Services

Senior centers, nutrition sites, senior discounts on numerous goods and services, surplus foods, food stamps, Meals on Wheels, homemakers, and family caregiving are only a few of the items that increase the possibility of elders remaining in their own homes regardless of failing health and chronic disorders. Basic services that may keep old people in their homes longer than would otherwise be feasible include the following: (1) home health maintenance; (2) rehabilitation and medical services when necessary; (3) home household help; (4) mobile meals; (5) transportation services; and (6) counseling, crisis intervention, and advocacy (case management).

Function of Senior Centers

The growth and development of senior centers as service centers for the community-residing older adult were developed under Title III of the Older Americans Act of 1975. Effective centers provide assistance, meals, and resources for the aged in the community. The location of the center, availability of transportation, budget, and staff expertise are all critical to the quality and range of services provided.

Keeping the Home

Often a home that has increased immensely in value is the major asset of an elder. However, taxes and maintenance costs have likewise risen. If monthly income is low, a deprived state of existence may be chosen over selling the home. If the elder does choose to sell, some exemptions from the capital gains tax are allowed. This means that a person (over 55 years of age) who wants to sell his or her home and move to a small apartment will be able to use much of the profit from the sale for living expenses rather than losing a large part of the profit through taxes. The IRS information regarding this is available through www.irs.gov. If one does not wish to sell the home and cannot afford the upkeep, a reverse annuity mortgage (RAM) plan may be a reasonable solution. This is designed to allow the use of home equity without forcing the older adult to move. The RAM can be used by a homeowner who owns the home completely to generate monthly payments for a period of 3 to 12 years to a total of 80% of the home's value. The owner retains title to the property, and the monthly payments do not interfere with eligibility for other senior benefits. However, when the term is up, the loan must be repaid with interest. This type of RAM loan is really designed for people with short-term financial needs.

The reverse shared appreciation mortgage (RSAM) is also available in many states. It allows the homeowner to occupy the home for life, and the lender receives a portion of the home's appreciation on the death of the owner and the sale of the home. The monthly check is in direct proportion to the current value of the home and the percentage of appreciation assigned to the loan agency.

In 1989 the Federal Housing Authority (FHA) entered the home conversion market with four different plans. Briefly, the four plans are as follows: (1) a line of credit established based on the borrower's age and the value of the home; (2) a tenure loan that offers lifetime payments not based on shared appreciation; (3) a fixed rate, shared appreciation tenure mortgage based on the life expectancy of the younger spouse and a cap of 25% appreciation contribution to the lender; and (4) a monthly payment similar to the RAM loan but that need not be repaid until the homeowner dies, sells the home, or moves. To qualify for an FHA home equity conversion, one must be at least 62 years old, fully own and live in the home, and receive independent financial counseling from a disinterested party. Additional information can be gained by contacting the FHA or the American Association of Retired Persons (AARP). Banks have various methods and policies regarding reverse mortgages, and interested individuals need to contact several before making a decision.

There are, at this point, numerous arrangements that can be made to activate the equity in a home to fill present needs. Elders should be advised to seek information from several major home loan lenders and counsel from senior legal services before making a decision.

Home Safety

Because community health nurses are in frequent contact with the actual living conditions of the aged, they are responsible for surveying the elder's environment for safety. Home health nurses are responsible for alerting individuals to unsafe situations in the home. One nurse attached red stickers (such as those available in stationery stores) to dangerous areas. Yellow stickers could be used to indicate the need for caution. For example, red tape would indicate when kitchen stove burners or the oven presented hazards; yellow tape would be placed on the risers of steps or jutting corners of objects in the environment. Nurses alert to dangers will find many innovative ways to assist the client in making the environment safe. This is discussed further in Chapter 22.

Fire

There are probably both conscious and subconscious realities in an old person's fear of and respect for fire. Fire symbolizes purification, productivity, punishment, and vigilance, all of which may be subconscious issues of aging. Most of the literature reviewed relates to fire in nursing homes, possibly because the residents of any congregate setting (particularly, frail, immobilized older adults) are vulnerable to fire. However, many independent older adults fear fire. They may reside in dilapidated wooden buildings, walk-up tenements, downtown hotels, or other settings where they are at the

mercy of others' careless behavior. Of course, residents of freestanding dwellings are also victims of fire. Even for those who survive a fire, the loss of treasured belongings can be devastating.

SAFETY IN THE COMMUNITY

In many communities special programs such as escort services, victim counseling, and safety information have been initiated. AARP conducted a national search to identify programs in crime prevention that have proved effective (Leach, 1996). One of the model programs is in Broomfield, Colorado, where a specially assigned police officer presents crime education at senior and community centers within the city, as well as advising individual isolated elders on ways to reduce vulnerability to crime. Another program in Chicago involves low-rent housing occupants who act as representatives of their units to work directly with police to improve building safety. In Dana Point, California, older persons are recruited as volunteers to work with police. They are issued special uniforms and canvas their neighborhoods, performing vacation and neighborhood checks; serve to control crowds and traffic at special neighborhood events; and perform foot patrols in business and shopping areas. Several other creative methods of involving elders and the police in cooperative programs to reduce crime are reported in an AARP Consumer Fact Sheet authored by Leach (1996) (also see Resources at the end of this chapter). Nurses need to learn about programs in crime protection and prevention, how to obtain assistance, and how to obtain legal redress for victims.

RELOCATION

In light of the strong instinctual nature of territorial needs, it is not surprising that much attention has been given to the crisis of relocation. *Relocation* as defined in the *Encyclopedia of Aging* (Maddox, 1995) includes relocation, migration, and residential mobility. Regardless of the type of move and its desirability or undesirability, some degree of stress will be experienced. With each move, if the adaptation is to be satisfying, one must begin to claim personal space by in some way placing one's stamp of individuality on the new surroundings. Because the older adult is particularly likely to move or be moved, the subject of relocation is significant. The first issue to address in any move is whether it is necessary and whether it will provide the least restrictive life-style appropriate for the individual. Questions that must be asked to assess the impact on the individual after a move include the following:

- Are significant persons as accessible in the new location as they were before the move?
- Is the individual developing new and reciprocal relationships in the new setting?
- Is the individual functioning as well, better, or not as well in the new location? This determination cannot be made immediately but must be assessed at least 6 weeks after the move.
- Was the individual given options before the move?
- Was the individual given the opportunity to assess the new environment before making a decision to move?
- Has the individual been able to move important items of furniture and memorabilia to the new setting?
- Has a particular individual who is familiar with the environment been available to assist with orientation?
- Was the decision to move made hastily or with inadequate information?
- Does the new situation provide adequately for basic needs (food, shelter, physical maintenance)?
- Are individual idiosyncratic needs recognized, and is there an opportunity to actualize them?
- Does the new situation decrease the possibility of privacy and autonomy?
- Is the new living situation an improvement over the previous situation, similar, or worse?

Nurses' concerns are with assessing the impact of relocation and determining methods to mitigate any negative reactions. The growing numbers of persons who will spend some of their later years in institutions have made this an urgent issue.

Translocation Confusion

Translocation confusion is a predictable result of abrupt moves to an environment that is vastly different from the one usually occupied. It is often a symptom of anxiety and uncertainty. Many times, drugs and treatments contribute to the confusion. An abrupt and poorly prepared transfer actually increases illness and disorientation. An individual who has functioned quite well before a major move may show previously unrecognized signs of dementia when in an unfamiliar environment. An accurate assessment of mental status before the move must be obtained from family or significant others. If this is not possible, it must be temporarily assumed that the confusion is a transient response. An elder who has been transferred to an institution from a residence in which considerable autonomy was possible may react more intensely than one whose disjunction in life-style has not been so severe. Some, of course, move to a much more comfortable and supportive situation and adapt well.

To avoid some of the translocation confusion, the individual must have some control over the environment, prior preparation regarding new situations, and maintenance of familiar situations to the greatest degree possible. Some familiar and some treasured items must also accompany the transfer. Family members will need considerable support when an elder is moved into an institution. No matter what the circumstances are, the family invariably feels that they have in some way failed the elder. These issues are discussed in more depth in Chapter 23.

Cognitive Maps

One's state of security depends greatly on perceived environmental order or disorder and how it is visualized. People in unfamiliar settings often need assistance developing cognitive maps. Some of the following suggestions may be useful:

1. Maps of buildings and surroundings need to be displayed in centrally accessible areas.
2. Individuals feel more secure with directional orientations (north, south, east, west). These should be given.
3. The locations of important services must be emphasized and color coded.
4. A person familiar with the environment can be asked to orient a newcomer.
5. Discussion of visual points of reference may help (e.g., "Did you notice the large red painting?").
6. Important reference points or services should not be arbitrarily moved without prior information. In a public building a women's restroom was temporarily assigned to men. Several women automatically wandered in and left looking rather bewildered.
7. Preparation should be made before relocation of a familiar item or service.
8. Orientation to new surroundings should be delayed until persons have become settled in their individual space. They need time to establish some security and reduce anxiety. Poorly timed orientation tours are of little help.
9. The nurse should recap and ask for questions at the end of an orientation tour.
10. In a large facility or complex, orientation sessions should be spread out over several days.

Box 27-1   RELOCATION STRESS SYNDROME

Relocation stress syndrome is a physiologic and/or psychosocial disturbance as a result of transfer from one environment to another.

Defining Characteristics
Major
Change in environment or location
Anxiety
Apprehension
Increased confusion (elderly)
Depression
Loneliness

Minor
Verbalization of unwillingness to relocate
Sleep disturbance
Change in eating habits
Dependency
Gastrointestinal disturbances
Increased verbalization of needs
Insecurity
Lack of trust
Restlessness
Sad affect
Unfavorable comparison of posttransfer/pretransfer staff
Verbalization of being concerned/upset about transfer
Vigilance
Weight change
Withdrawal

Related Factors
Past, concurrent, and recent losses
Losses involved with the decision to move
Feeling of powerlessness
Lack of adequate support system
Little or no preparation for the impending move
Moderate to high degree of environmental change
History and types of previous transfers
Impaired psychosocial health status
Decreased physical health status

Sample Diagnostic Statement
Relocation stress syndrome related to admission to long-term care setting as evidenced by anxiety, insecurity, and disorientation

Expected outcomes
1. The resident will socialize with family members, staff, and/or other residents.
2. Preadmission weight, appetite, and sleep patterns will remain stable. If previous patterns were dysfunctional, more appropriate health patterns will develop.
3. The resident will verbalize feelings, expectations, and disappointments openly with members of the staff and/or family.
4. Inappropriate behaviors (i.e., "acting out," refusing to take medicines) will not occur.

Expected short-term goals
1. The resident will become independent in moving to and from areas within the facility during the next 3 months.
2. The resident will react in a positive manner to staff effort to assist in adjusting to nursing home placement in the next 3 months.
3. The resident will express his or her thoughts or concerns about placement when encouraged to do so during individual contacts in the next 3 months.
4. During the next 3 months the resident will not develop physical or psychosocial disturbances indicative of translocation syndrome as a result of the change in living environment.

Expected long-term goals
1. The resident will verbalize acceptance of nursing home placement within the next 6 months.
2. The resident will indicate acceptance of nursing home placement through positive body language within the next 6 months.

Specific nursing interventions
1. Identify previous coping patterns during admission assessment. Clearly document these, and share the information with other staff members.
2. Include the resident in assessing problems and developing the care plan on admission.
3. Adjust for limitations in sensory/perceptual disturbances when planning care for residents. Visual disturbances need special intervention to assist residents in finding their way around.
4. Staff members will introduce themselves when entering the resident's room, indicating the nature of their relationship with the resident. Example: "Hello, Mr. Smith. My name is Nancy. I'll be your nurse attendant today, helping you with your meals and your bath."
5. Each staff member providing care for the resident should make it a point to spend at least 5 minutes each day with new admissions to "just visit."
6. Allow the resident as many opportunities to make independent choices as much as possible.
7. Identify previous routines for activities of daily living (ADLs). Try to maintain as much continuity with the resident's previous schedule as possible. Example: If

Continued

Box 27-1   RELOCATION STRESS SYNDROME—cont'd

Mr. Smith has taken a bath before bed all of his life, adjust his schedule to continue that practice.

8. Familiarize the resident with unit schedules.
9. Encourage family participation through frequent visits, phone calls, and activity sessions. Be sure to let them know schedules.
10. Establish familiar landmarks for the resident when leaving his or her room so that he or she can recognize areas more quickly.
11. Encourage family members to bring familiar belongings from home for the resident's room decorations.

12. Provide reorientation cues frequently. Example: "You are in the dining room. Your room is down the hall three doors just past the window."
13. Encourage the resident to talk about expectations, anger, and/or disappointments and the recent life changes that he or she has experienced.
14. Review the patient's medication list with the physician to verify the need for medications that might promote disorientation.
15. Provide for constructive activities. Initiate activity therapy consultation.

A summary of relocation stress syndrome and nursing actions to prevent relocation stress are noted in Box 27-1.

INNOVATIVE ENVIRONMENTAL DESIGN

Teams of environmental consultants across the nation have begun to take note of the special design needs of congregate living facilities. The owners/investors of such facilities welcome the input of these consultants for several reasons: a well-designed facility will be more effectively operated, services and care will be more easily provided, appearance is important in marketing, and good design may avert accidents and incidents. Residents will also negotiate the environment more easily and have fewer restrictions; restlessness and confusion will be reduced and the residents' quality of life improved.

Architects designing housing for the older adult would be most successful in providing satisfactory arrangements if they consulted the older adult first and then built prototypes to be tested by the aged. There are now several organizations devoted to designing living environments for elders. Two of the most well known are the Society for the Advancement of Gerontological Environment in Huntington Woods, Michigan, and the Center of Design for an Aging Society in Portland, Oregon (Noell, 1996).

The following are some special requirements:
Easily activated emergency and security systems
Phones by beds
Sufficient storage space
Convenient places to obtain meals

Mail drops conveniently placed
Window arrangements that allow for privacy and natural outdoor views
A place to grow things

Whereas in the past architects might dictate design, it is now more common for the design to be a result of interdisciplinary input. The innovative architect listens, reads, tours facilities, and works from the start with functional needs and cost in mind. There is still a great need to look to the future and determine what care should be and how staff should work, and to confer with older persons regarding construction design that will contribute to the quality of life.

CONTINUUM OF HOUSING OPTIONS FOR THE OLDER ADULT

There are currently approximately 32 million people over 65 years of age in the United States, who are living in numerous types of independent, partially dependent, or fully dependent situations. This portion of the chapter examines the continuum of housing options available to the aged, from those who are fully independent to those requiring long-term sheltered care (Fig. 27-2). Questions are being posed as to the effects of managed care on the continuum of housing options for the older adult (American Association of Homes and Services for the Aging, 1995b; AARP, 1996). As Medicare health maintenance organizations (HMOs) continue to expand, managed care providers will find it necessary to establish more networks with housing providers, because the living site of elders will ultimately also be the site where most economical and preventive health services will be dispensed.

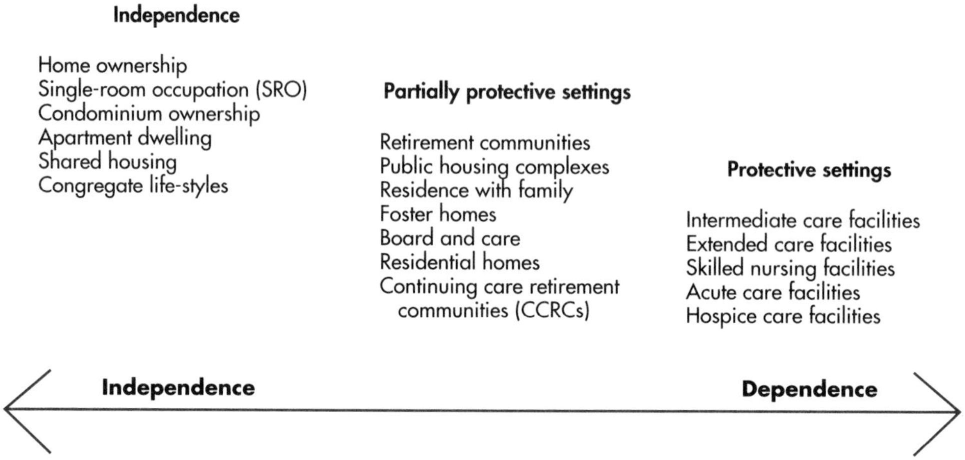

Independence

Home ownership
Single-room occupation (SRO)
Condominium ownership
Apartment dwelling
Shared housing
Congregate life-styles

Partially protective settings

Retirement communities
Public housing complexes
Residence with family
Foster homes
Board and care
Residential homes
Continuing care retirement
    communities (CCRCs)

Protective settings

Intermediate care facilities
Extended care facilities
Skilled nursing facilities
Acute care facilities
Hospice care facilities

Independence ⟵   ⟶ **Dependence**

Fig. 27-2   Continuum of housing security.

Housed With Family Members

The factors most likely to result in shared housing among adult children and dependent elders are widowhood, a small support network, and low economic status. However, strong cultural influences predict the frequency of multigenerational residences. Among Asians and South Americans it is often an expectation, although increasing industrialization in any country changes these traditional patterns. There are many cultural variations, but the important issue is for social policy and supports to provide choices for the individual and the family.

"Granny Flat" Solution

Almost three decades ago the "granny flat" was developed in Australia as a model for providing independent housing for elders with prefabricated small housing units constructed on family property. These units allow families to be close enough to be of assistance if needed but remain separate. They are practical and economical, and their production has continually expanded in Australia. In the United States there has been little indication of this model being used, although existing "mother-in-law" cottages and apartments have served a similar purpose for many families. An additional model that has great popularity in certain areas is the use of mobile homes. These may in fact be mobile and moved onto family property or may in reality be quite immobile and set in es-

tablished mobile home parks that cater to older people and their needs.

Gated Communities

Gated communities are designed for affluent individuals who desire seclusion, protection, maintenance, and high security. These communities tend to be designed for and to cater to older individuals. They often have golf courses, health clinics, entertainment centers, restaurants, gymnasiums, tennis courts, clubhouses, pools, transportation, and convenient services within the compound. One such, characteristic of many, is described thus: ". . . facilities resemble that of a small city. One member of each household must be 55 years of age or older. The resident mix includes currently active and retired professionals. Housing options vary from single family dwellings to single or multi-story condominiums and co-operatives. Health and medical facilities, commercial and retail centers and houses of worship are nearby." (Leisure World, 1996). These communities are flourishing throughout the United States and will undoubtedly increase, because the numerous young-old who can afford them value the advantages they offer. The disadvantages are apparent when one becomes old and frail and must hire from the outside any live-in assistance that may be necessary.

In some ways these are similar to upscale life care communities, but nurses need to be aware of the differences. Health services and nursing care units are not part of the entitlements in these leisure communities as they are in life care communities.

Senior Retirement Communities

Communities designed for elders are proliferating. There are numerous combinations of cottages, apartments, activities, optional services, meals in the home, cafeterias, restaurants, housekeeping, golf, tennis, security, and emergency services and clinics. Some have sections designed especially for assisted living. These are all designed to make independent living feasible with the least effort on the part of the elder. They are usually expensive, and services are purchased outright. The various names for such communities include "retirement community," "independent living centers," and "life care." Considerations important to a client contemplating entering one of these communities include the following:

- Plan far ahead, and anticipate needs. Good facilities have long waiting lists.
- Meals, activities, health care, and housekeeping must be readily available and affordable if desired or needed.
- Examine the compatibility of the residents; look for evidence of interaction and involvement in activities and committees.
- Study the effectiveness of the staff from administrator to maintenance personnel.
- Determine the community's compliance with standards in terms of licenses or certificates, or by other evidence.
- Inquire about the availability of financial statements and marketing projections.
- Contracts should include fixed increases over time or amounts directly related to the inflation index; costs and limits of nursing care should be clearly stated. What amount of the fee is refundable if the client dies or moves?
- Does the resident have a voice in management?
- If a complex is not yet in operation, request a financial incentive before signing up, and put up only a nominal, fully refundable deposit before operation begins.

The Heritage Harbour Retirement Community developed a nonprofit health group founded by the residents of the community for their own use (Ostrowski, 1998). Contracts with various health and service providers allow residents to partake of a full range of services at a reduced cost. Services they are

---

Box 27-2   HERITAGE HARBOUR HEALTH GROUP SERVICES

Cooperating Providers
Pharmacy
Dental plan
Olsten Home Care
Life Line
Meal delivery
Hearing aid services

Health/Medical Services
Professional, licensed, Medicare-certified home care
Annual health fair
Blood pressure clinics
Flu vaccinations
Home aides
Respite training
Personal medical history on file (confidentiality ensured)
RN consultations
Hospital and nursing home calls
Case management

Nonmedical Services
Free tax preparation help
Hospital preregistration
Medicare and insurance form assistance
Physician/attorney/dental referrals
Luncheon socials
Living will/advance directives referrals
Information/library
Support groups (weight, bereavement, caregivers)
Housekeeper referrals

Volunteer Services (Caring Network)
HHHG office
Transportation
Loan closet (medical aids)
Safety Line (phone calls)
Visits
Grocery shopping
Speakers on health-related topics

From Ostrowski MS: The Heritage Harbour Health Group: doing it our way, *Geriatr Nurs* 19(4):225-228, 1998.
HHHG, Heritage Harbour Health Group.

---

able to provide are listed in Box 27-2. It is hoped that health care professionals will find inspiration in this example to encourage resident groups to consider such an approach to meeting health maintenance needs.

Continuing Care Retirement Communities

There are more than 1000 nonprofit continuing care retirement communities (CCRCs) across the country, as well as many corporate for-profit continuing care communities. This mode of service to the aged has chiefly emerged since 1974, although some church-affiliated CCRCs have been in existence for nearly 100 years. These are sometimes called *life care communities* because that is precisely what they guarantee. CCRCs are flourishing. These are designed only for the middle class or wealthy elder. There is a large ($50,000 to $500,000) one-time entrance fee and monthly payments of $800 to $3000 thereafter. There are several basic combinations of service, but the commonality is of lifelong care. The communities usually contract with a nearby hospital for acute care, but aside from that, they are equipped to provide whatever level of assistance and health care is needed by the elder resident. Dining rooms and meals are often exquisite. Residents are predominantly women in their 80s and 90s who entered the community in their late 70s. They are often very involved in the community activities and find this a pleasant life. Resident satisfaction is a major thrust of these communities, and they focus on such things as excellent food and service, comfort, convenience, security, intellectual and artistic pursuits, and socialization.

Increasingly, dynamic and financially secure older women are taking the initiative to move into life care communities while they are active and in good health. They often select them because of the security and the stimulation. The decision to enter a life care facility is often made in response to a growing awareness of the eventual need for more assistance and support. It is also stimulated by observing friends who suddenly lose the capacity for independent living and are abruptly relocated without sufficient time to select a situation to their liking. In making the decision to move to a life care facility, the elder should explore several of them. Selection of the CCRC that best meets the individual's needs and preserves much of the past way of life is important.

Federally Assisted Housing

There are several federally subsidized rental options; most older adults benefiting from this option are assisted through HUD-subsidized rental housing. These are not specific to the aged, but nearly 45% of the units are occupied by elders. Section 202 of the Housing Act,

US Dept. of Housing and Urban Development, approved the construction of low-rent housing units especially for elders. These units also have provisions for health, recreation, and transportation. More than 91% of these apartment units have waiting lists of eight or more applicants for each vacancy that occurs. Under Section 8 of the Housing Act of 1983, tenants locate their own unit. Usually, the tenant pays 30% of his or her adjusted gross income toward the rent, and HUD assists with supplementary vouchers ranging from 30% to 120% of the tenant's contribution to meet the fair market value of the rental.

An ideal public housing complex for low-income aged residents will provide modern facilities, security, accessible services, privacy, and some entertainment and activities. An important consideration in planning low-cost housing units for older adults is the potential for evolution of services. Residents rarely move out, and as they age, their ability and independence are likely to decrease. Retirement communities often solve this dilemma by building semidependent units. For those less affluent people currently in subsidized public housing, the only alternatives may be residential care facilities or nursing homes.

Group Residences

Many housing options are available before one must consider institutionalization (Table 27-1). Facilities for elders who cannot live independently but do not need nursing home care include adult foster care, senior-assisted housing, group-assisted living, domiciliary care, congregate care, supportive housing, continuing care, life care, residential care, board and care, and personal care facilities. These are collectively classed as "assisted living" situations.

Certain fair housing laws have been enacted to protect the rights of frail older persons in group residences (Edelstein, 1995) that are under state and federal jurisdiction. These are primarily focused on antidiscrimination, access accommodations, and health and safety concerns. These are all important in maintaining independence, control, and the quality of life.

The number of individuals in a group residence and the variety and quality of services vary considerably. They may be under local, state, or federal jurisdiction or privately owned and operated. Some accept only private pay, and some are partially or fully subsidized. It would be virtually impossible to define each of these in terms of opportunities, quality, and limitations, but nurses will be asked about them. Elders and their fam-

Table 27-1

Advantages and Disadvantages of Selected Alternative Housing Options

Options	Advantages	Disadvantages
Board-and-care homes	Homelike; economical	Not licensed in some states or concerned with standards; owner/operators often lack training; few planned social activities
Congregate housing	Provides basic support services that can extend independent living; reduces social isolation	Tendency to promote dependency; expensive for most elderly without subsidy
Elder cottages—"granny flats"	Facilitate older persons receiving support from younger family members	Concerns about housing and building code violations
Home equity conversion	Converts lifetime investment into usable income; can be used to finance housing expenses (i.e., make necessary repairs, utilities, taxes)	Reluctance by homeowner to utilize because of lack of information, concern for lien on property, and/or impact on estate for heirs
Life care facilities	Offer prepaid health care; wide range of social activities with health and support systems	Too expensive for many elderly; no guarantees that monthly payment will not rise
Shared housing	More extensive use of existing housing; program inexpensive to operate	Problems with selection of individual to share home; amount of privacy reduced; city zoning ordinances may prohibit

Modified from Mutschler PM: Where elders live, *Generations* 16(2):7, 1992.

ilies should be advised to ask about and carefully consider the following:

- What services are offered?
- What is the out-of-pocket cost?
- What levels of assistance are available?
- What safety factors are in place?
- Are individual preferences respected?
- What range of physical and cognitive impairments can be accommodated?
- What are the security measures?
- What agencies, if any, are responsible for monitoring quality?
- What are the special features designed for the frail or disabled?
- What is the process for reporting abuse, neglect, or exploitation?

Shared Housing

Since so many older adults own their homes, house sharing has been proposed as a feasible way to keep one's home. Older people often live in houses with ample space geared to family life, purchased in their young adult years. It is estimated that half the space is underused. Sharing a house can be easily implemented by locating, screening, and matching older people looking for houses to share with those who have them. The National Shared Housing Resource Center (NSHRC) has established subgroups nationally to assist individuals interested in home sharing. Those who have done so report feeling safer and less lonely. Studies on home sharing need to focus on the effects on well-being, finances, health, social life, and daily satisfaction. Most successful is the intergenerational model, in which an elder with a home locates a younger person to share the home (Bergman, 1994). In each situation the individuals must consider the following:

- Should men and women live together?
- Should the house include aged peers only or people of all ages?
- Should there be equal or reciprocal exchange?
- Should the house provide temporary or permanent residence?
- Should residents sign an agreement form?
- Will residents respect privacy?
- What is the motivation for moving into a shared house: financial need, companionship, or services/assistance?

Shared housing as a method of providing for the needs of several frail older adults in one renovated home has been used with varying degrees of success. Problems arise from long-standing patterns of living, as well as privacy and interpersonal needs. However, small groups of older adults living under the same roof are a growing trend. The following are characteristic of successful group homes:

- They usually have a nonprofit sponsor.
- Services include housekeeping, cooking, maintenance, and social services.
- Spontaneity and interaction are encouraged but not forced.

Foster Care

Adult foster care is meant to provide assistive care in a homelike setting that will enhance function and the quality of life and allow the elder to remain in a community-based setting. This foster care setting is different from other residential care settings in both the size of the homes and the family-oriented care setting (Folkemer et al, 1996). The operational definition of *adult foster care* is as follows: adult foster care offers a community-based living arrangement to adults who are unable to live independently because of physical or mental impairment or disabilities and are in need of supervision or personal care.

Homes providing adult foster care offer 24-hour supervision, protection, and personal care in addition to room and board. They may also provide additional services. Adult foster care serves a designated, small number of individuals (generally from one to six) in a home-like and family-like environment; one of the primary caregivers often resides in the home (Folkemer et al, 1996). A growing number of homes are under corporate ownership, and in these situations the homelike atmosphere tends to be lost. However, with state-regulated outcome-oriented quality assurance strategies focused on achieving maximal function, autonomy, and social integration, adult foster care may fill a real need.

Foster Family Care

The best foster family homes provide personal care, homemaking, transportation, and other services as needed. When families and elders are carefully matched, the elder is nurtured and cared for as if he or she were a member of the family. The foster family is reimbursed by Medicaid in most cases, but there are variations among the states. Costs and outcomes of such care are favorable in comparison with those of institutional settings. Although this model has unlimited potential, it has not been developed to full advantage. Families already caring for an older adult member might find it advantageous both socially and economically to adopt one or two other elders. Problems can be expected if families are not appropriately screened or the care needs of the elder are too demanding.

Board and Care

Board and care is usually provided in small homes serving six to eight residents. These homes serve individuals who are not in need of the professional nursing care provided in nursing homes but need considerable personal care and assistance. This care is often funded by Medicaid, but this varies from state to state. Board and care differs from foster care in that the simulation or reality of a family setting is not the focus of the setting, although the distinction between foster care and board and care in individual circumstances is not at all clear at times. In addition, foster care programs usually provide guidelines, thoughtful matching to family needs, and education for the participants, but this is not the case with board-and-care operations. Most caregivers of the aged in board-and-care settings have not been recruited by agencies but, rather, have taken on this function through their own initiative or at the suggestion of friends or relatives. It is not uncommon that they rent a small house, row house, or flat and maintain it as a business. Although their intentions may be humanitarian, they often need training in the special needs of the older adult.

The National Association of Residential Care Homes is an organization of board-and-care operators that is growing in strength and brings professionalism to its members. Board-and-care regulation and licensing is within the domain of the respective state. It is generally agreed that licensing and provider education should be increased, but few funds are budgeted for the monitoring and improvement of these small facilities. Where these are poorly funded, there is less incentive among operators to meet quality standards. Board-and-care operators cannot provide the quality of care desirable unless there is both financial incentive and continuing supportive resources available to assist them.

Assisted Living

Assisted living is emerging as the option of choice for elders who can no longer remain in their own homes but do not need nursing home care (American Association of Homes and Services for the Aged, 1995a, 1995b). Although some states have developed regulations, there are as yet no federally defined standards. In the absence of such standards the American Association of Homes and Services for the Aged has taken on the challenge of developing prototypes that will provide models for sponsors and developers of such facilities (American Association of Homes and Services for the Aged, 1995a). Assisted living facilities (ALFs) are usually small (average size of 25 residents) congregate living sites that provide help with activities of daily living (ADLs) such as bathing, dressing, and medication monitoring. These facilities may also be designated "personal care." The distinction between these and residential care is often blurred, although residential care most often is limited to independent apartments with meals available, housekeeping, and emergency response systems on site to assist with problems. There are no reimbursement mechanisms for these settings. The costs are borne entirely by the residents.

Subacute Care and Rehabilitation Units

The route taken by many elders has been changed in the current health care system. After spending a few days in an acute care hospital, the elder is often moved to either a rehabilitation hospital for specific therapies expected to increase the elder's function or to a subacute (sometimes called *postacute*) care unit that functions much like the general medical-surgical hospital units of the past, although they are presently most often located in nursing homes. The stay in a subacute care unit is likely to be less than a month and is largely reimbursed by Medicare. The definition of *subacute care* is provided in Box 27-3.

At the present time a 3-day hospitalization is required by Medicare before an elder is moved into a nursing home. The American Health Care Association and other organizations have been trying for some time to have this ruling rescinded. In fact, if the 3 days are used for a thorough workup, it is advantageous because it will facilitate the most appropriate assessment and placement of the elder.

Nursing Homes

Nursing homes provide around-the-clock care for those needing subacute, chronic, and rehabilitative nursing care. They range in size from 10 to over 1000 beds, with most having fewer than 200 beds. Although called

---

Box 27-3	SUBACUTE CARE AS DEFINED BY THE AMERICAN HEALTH CARE ASSOCIATION AND THE JOINT COMMISSION ON ACCREDITATION OF HEALTHCARE ORGANIZATIONS

Subacute care is comprehensive inpatient care designed for someone who has an acute illness, injury, or exacerbation of a disease process. It is goal-oriented treatment rendered immediately after, or instead of, acute hospitalization to treat one or more specific active complex medical conditions or to administer one or more technically complex treatments, in the context of a person's underlying long-term conditions and overall situation.

Generally, the individual's condition is such that the care does not depend heavily on high-technology monitoring or complex diagnostic procedures. Subacute care requires the coordinated services of an interdisciplinary team including physicians, nurses, and other relevant professional disciplines, who are trained and knowledgeable to assess and manage these specific conditions and perform the necessary procedures. Subacute care is given as part of a specifically defined program, regardless of the site.

Subacute care is generally more intensive than traditional nursing facility care and less than acute care. It requires frequent (daily to weekly) recurrent patient assessment and review of the clinical course and treatment plan for a limited (several days to several months) time period, until the condition is stabilized or a predetermined treatment course is completed.

From American Health Care Association, Washington, DC.

---

homes, they resemble hospitals far more than homes, and private rooms are at a premium. Presently there are 14,177 skilled nursing facilities in the United States—nearly triple the number there were in 1980 (US Bureau of the Census, 1998). Costs vary significantly with the location but average $38,000 annually for basic nursing home care. Fees are usually obtained through a combination of Medicare (12.3%), Medicaid (47.6%), out-of-pocket (31%), and insurance (4.9%) payments (US Department of Health and Human Services, 1999). Federal and state regulations have become more onerous and time consuming than the care. The Omnibus Budget Reconciliation Act (OBRA) of 1987 and the frequent revisions and updates are designed to impact the actual quality of resident care, and the system is beginning to show results in this respect and in observation of resident rights and privileges. OBRA laws require that nursing homes do the following:

- Increase their nursing and social work staff.
- Train nurse aides.
- Institute activities programs.
- Set standards for nursing home administrators.
- Expect increased financial sanctions for noncompliance with regulations.
- Guarantee the right to one's own physician.
- Guarantee freedom from drug or physical restraint for convenience or discipline.
- Guarantee resident participation in care and treatment decisions.
- Guarantee resident privacy.
- Investigate the background of individuals applying for work in long-term care facilities.

With the inroads of managed care, block grants, and the shift of responsibility to the states, there is great concern that some of these hard-won gains may be diminished.

Even with the safeguards of OBRA legislation, there is much more to be done to support the quality of life. With institutionalization, individuals are in an environment where the usual noises of life, odors, shifting temperatures and wind patterns, vegetation, and natural diurnal light variations are altered. These changes affect individuals in as yet unknown ways. Elders in restricted living situations and those who are housebound or institutionalized suffer a type of deprivation that is not understood, but we sense that the quality of life is greatly diminished. Disorientation may develop because natural and devised cues are often missing. Most of the devised cues are inexpensive enough to ensure general availability, yet situations still exist where clocks, calendars, locations of important events, facility maps, and individual room identification are missing.

Designing Long-Term Care Facilities

Creating interiors for a changing clientele is an additional challenge for the designers of all long-term care settings and is perhaps the most significant from a nursing perspective. Facilities that are well designed are most likely to operate more efficiently. Benefits are reaped by employees who find their work easier to organize and more satisfying. Most important from a nursing perspective, better layout, facility organization, and technology, as well as convenient furnishings, may reduce the need for restraints while preserving the security of the patient. (Restraints are discussed in Chapter 22.) At present there are numerous "special care units" designed for persons with dementia, but they vary greatly in the efficiency and effectiveness of the design. Throughout the long-term care industry, numerous facilities have established special care units (SCUs). Nurses must be involved in the design of these units and carefully assess the adaptational cues.

Facilitative environmental design is especially important in the care and function of mentally frail elders. When objects and persons in the environment are familiar, less integrative capacity is needed to cope effectively. When mentally frail elders are in unfamiliar places, disorientation and catastrophic reactions may occur. Cues in the environment are fundamental to designing interventions to modify such behaviors.

An environment rich in physical and social cues most helpful to the demented person will have locations and activities labeled with colors and pictures or simple words. Verbal instructions will be congruent and augmented by hand motion or demonstration. Smiling, touching, and direct eye contact provide assurance of interest. Personalization of individual space is also important for orientation, as well as security. For stability and security, cues should remain constant and predictable. Changes in room assignment, staff, furniture arrangement, and interior decoration all elicit confusion. Intercoms, buzzers, continuous music, and excessive light at night are additional distractors.

Evergreen Retirement Community in Oshkosh, Wisconsin, has developed a "home" unit in which the design and activities mimic those of a home and family setting (Green, 1994). Eight resident rooms surround the "farm kitchen," where all activities and meals take place. The results are a close-knit, interactive group of residents and staff. Informality and interaction are stressed. This approach has resulted in greater interest and involvement of the families of those residents as well.

When structural changes are not possible, creative adaptations to individual needs will be a high priority. Individualized care might begin with a psychosocial admission assessment that includes data about the client's preferences, home schedules, strengths, and ability to accomplish ADLs before admission to the facility. Version 2 of the Minimum Data Set (MDS 2.0), now required by OBRA, has made great progress toward individualized care plans. Ideally, the staff who will work up the MDS 2.0 will also obtain a life history of significant roles, events, and activities that have given the individual his or her sense of identity.

Suggestions about ways that family and community members may enhance nursing home life include the following:

1. Donate clothing, supplies, fruit, flowers, art objects, books, televisions, and pianos to nursing homes.
2. Offer positive feedback to the overworked, underpaid personnel.
3. Volunteer your services or special talents.
4. Adopt a grandparent, and include this person in family outings and holidays.
5. Assist children in getting acquainted with individuals in nursing homes. The aged enjoy this immensely, and the children may learn more about the aged than we know.
6. Give input to the director of nursing regarding beneficial services available in the community.
7. Develop forums (schools, city council meetings, religious organizations) for the aged to express their community needs.
8. Educate children to effectively interact with the aged.

9. Provide group meetings for families with aged members to share problems and solutions and to vent their feelings about their situations.
10. Form support groups and a network for counseling older adults in institutional settings to adapt to and work on life issues, such as grieving, stressors, and living situations.

Making a Home

Fifteen factors have been identified in rank order as contributing to satisfaction in a nursing home and improving morale among patients (Fig. 27-3) (Kane et al, 1986). Other studies reinforce the importance of personal possessions in the milieu of the institutionalized older adult. Suggested possessions may include pictures, paintings, photographs, bureaus, bookcases, bedspreads, quilts, lamps, and any items of special significance to the older adult. The following suggestions will help preserve a sense of personal space in a long-term care facility:

1. Patients' rooms need a "Please Do Not Disturb" sign that can be hung on the door when the patient chooses.

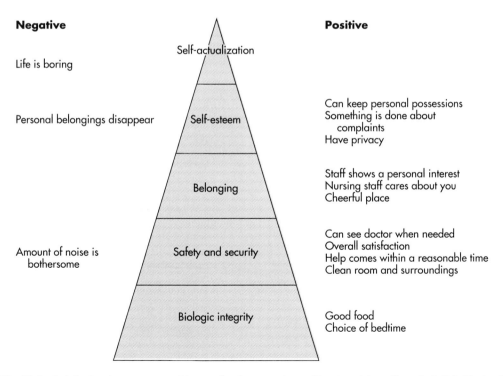

Fig. 27-3 Satisfaction factors reported by nursing home patients. (Developed from Kane R, Bell R, Riegler S: Value preferences for nursing home outcomes, *Gerontologist* 26[3]:303, 1986.)

2. Transfer patients from one room to another infrequently or not at all.
3. Include objects of personal significance in the environment.
4. Respect the arrangement of the patient's space; do not move things without permission.
5. Prepare people for intrusive procedures, even though they are routine to personnel, and verbally assure them that you are aware of intruding into their space. Respect patients' dignity and modesty. Do not leave the patient's body exposed.
6. Ask whether the patient wants the door open or shut and the curtains closed or open.
7. Avoid direct eye contact during care of intimate body areas.
8. Be alert to cues. Touching may increase or decrease anxiety.
9. Communicate territorial preferences of the patient to other health care team members.
10. Confer with patients regarding arrangement of public space.

Pets. Much has been reported about companion therapy with animals, and it has been empirically accepted that they increase morale and provide emotional satisfaction to many older adults. Situations wherein pets may be especially helpful to the older adult include (1) chronic disability or illness, (2) depression, (3) a previous relationship with pets, (4) role reversal, (5) negative dependency, (6) loneliness and isolation, (7) helplessness, (8) low self-esteem, (9) hopelessness, and (10) absence of humor. A pet can often expand the sociability of aged residents, decrease their sense of regimentation, give them some purpose, help them to feel needed and loved, and provide tactile comfort. Rosenkoetter (1992) reported an increase in communication among nursing home residents as they talked about Brutus in anticipation of and after his weekly visits.

The California Veterinary Medical Association Guidelines suggest that it is important to survey staff and resident preferences regarding pets in nursing homes (Bustad, Hines, 1983). Physical space and social space are important in assessments of nursing home characteristics, and certain rules and regulations regarding pets need to be established. If it is not deemed suitable to have a pet continuously in a given facility, there are volunteer programs that provide animals for a short period.

Commonsense considerations concerning including an animal in the facility or as a visitor are that the animal is clean and healthy and has the required immu-

nizations, is kept on a leash or in an appropriate cage, and is kept out of food preparation areas; in addition, people allergic to animals in the nursing home should be warned of their presence, and residents must be protected from injury or tripping because of the antics of a frisky animal.

Creative horticulture in the nursing home. Horticulture, the growing and tending of flowers and plants, can help maintain the physical and mental health of elders in a home for the aged (Bassen, Baltazar, 1997). In the Hebrew Home for the Aged in Riverdale, New York, the residents responded to a horticultural program with increased social and psychologic involvement. The program can be adapted to any resident's level of function. In instituting such a program, goals must be clear and responsive to the needs of the residents and the design of the facility. Various groups may be involved in activities adapted to their abilities. Bassen and Baltazar found many local nurseries and florists willing to donate items or become involved in the program. Box 27-4 provides guidelines for the development of a horticultural program.

Nature hikes for nursing home residents. Morganett (1987), a park naturalist, suggests nature hikes for nursing home residents as a means of heightening awareness and increasing the quality of life. Hikers are encouraged to use all of their senses to experience nature: tasting wild berries; listening to birds,

---

Box 27-4   GUIDELINES FOR DEVELOPMENT OF A HORTICULTURAL THERAPY PROGRAM

- Organize groups according to level of functioning (groups should be homogeneous in nature).
- Adapt activities to meet the needs of a specific group.
- Limit the size of the group by considering the proportion of leaders to participants.
- Determine a schedule and location.
- Have the participants contribute with the planning of activities.
- Include indoor and outdoor projects.
- Document and measure the progress of each participant.
- Apprise your supervisor of the program's progress.
- Evaluate and revise the program.

From Bassen S, Baltazar V: Flowers, flowers everywhere: creative horticulture programming at the Hebrew Home for the Aged at Riverdale, *Geriatr Nurs* 18(2):53-56, 1997.

frogs, and crickets; seeing different colors of soil and sand; touching flower petals and leaves; and smelling flowers and plants. If hiking is too difficult, some of these items can be brought to the nursing home for demonstrations. Morganett gives some directions to follow before beginning such a program: (1) do not contact poisonous plants; (2) do not pick things in state and national parks, since this is illegal; and (3) treat animals gently and set them free immediately after any demonstration.

Morganett suggests careful planning and assembling of materials before departure. An insect box and a magnifying glass are not necessary but will be useful. You may wish to augment the walk with large pictures of birds and recorded bird calls. Berries can be brought back and made into jam. Wild flowers may be placed in pots in the facility. Morganett gives abundant information about special characteristics of plants, animals, and birds. For the neophyte it would be useful to obtain assistance from the park service. Nature hikes can be adapted to many settings in addition to parks.

Responsibility. Many persons believe that the difference between housing and a home is measured by responsibility and caring. In nursing homes residents who have responsibility for the care of a bird, a fish, or a plant remain more active and spontaneous than residents who have nothing to care for. Behaviors reinforcing dependence are frequently noted among nursing home residents. When the interaction patterns between older adult residents and their social partners are looked at, it is often found that the more dependent residents gain more attention from social partners. From these data we might conclude that many residents demonstrate a strong need to care for someone who seems to need them. Studies have previously identified the therapeutic effects of plants in rooms with older adults in nursing homes. A study was done by Roush and Banziger (1982) of the implications and importance of bird feeders outside residents' windows to establish responsibility for the wild birds. It was found that life satisfaction, perceived control, happiness, and activity were significantly improved for those residents. Nurses also rated those individuals as being more active, happy, alert, and sociable.

The current interest in the Eden Alternative (Tavormina, 1999) in nursing homes is based on the responsiveness of elders to plants, children, and pets. These life-enriching elements have always been included in the best facilities.

Consent for Research

Consent for research leads to consideration of other aspects of personal privacy, particularly since Alzheimer's disease is one of researchers' major interests in the geriatric patient. Ideally, a living will or advance directive for health care would designate the willingness of an individual to participate in research, but realistically this is rarely the case. Some researchers (Sansone, Schmitt, 1996) suggest that patients with a diagnosis of senile dementia or psychosis may be competent to consent as research subjects if the information is presented simply and understood by the patient and family. These authors state that consent should not be based on overall competency but on the capacity to understand and consent to a particular study.

Advocacy for Nursing Home Residents

Advocacy organizations for nursing home residents are active throughout the United States. They are engaged in complaint resolution, confrontation and/or negotiation with nursing homes, community education, legal intervention, and legislative reform.

Professional nurses must remain alert to their advocacy role in institutions. Nurses need to be aware of the procedure for filing a complaint against a nursing home. Some may wish to do so and will need the support of the legal system and other nurses in the advocacy of humane care for clients.

A complaint about practices, procedures, physical conditions, or quality of care in a nursing home is initially a request to the state health department to inspect a particular home and determine if a violation exists. Any person may file such a request simply by writing a letter. The letter should specifically detail the incidents of concern. However, even vague complaints such as lack of attention will be investigated. Numbers to call can be found in the telephone book.

Copies of licensing surveys are available to the public through the facilities licensing section of each state. They will show the violations that have been noted. The public has access to these documents simply by requesting them from the administrator of a facility. Copies of regulations are available through the state publications office. These will provide a basis for measuring violations.

Ombudsman. *Ombudsman* as the term is used today most commonly denotes the nursing home advocate prepared to deal squarely but sensitively with the realities of a nursing home resident's life. An ombudsman must view the resident's problem as impartially as possible and act as advocate but not in an adversarial role with the nursing home administration.

In addition to acting as advocate, the ombudsman often locates appropriate resources and links residents to

> **Box 27-5** **WORKING EFFECTIVELY WITH AN OMBUDSMAN**
>
> 1. The administrator should become acquainted with the ombudsman.
> 2. The administrator should introduce the ombudsman to the entire staff.
> 3. The ombudsman should be invited to the facility on a routine basis and on special occasions to become a part of the facility resource rather than an adversary.
> 4. The ombudsman and administrator should share perceptions and facts openly with each other while maintaining confidentiality.
> 5. The administrator should discuss some of his or her concerns and legislative issues that need attention.
> 6. The administrator should inform the residents' council that an ombudsman is available.
> 7. The administrator should likewise inform the family council about the ombudsman.

them, trains friendly visitors, provides a clearinghouse for problems or complaints, gives legislative updates, and provides assistance in conducting family councils and resident councils. The ombudsman must also assist families in transferring or discharging patients from a nursing home to another setting. The ombudsman is concerned about maintaining good relationships with nursing home personnel. Ways that a nursing home can ensure a more collaborative relationship with the ombudsman are summarized in Box 27-5.

The long-term care ombudsman program is mandated by the Older Americans Act (OAA). Each state must have an Office of the State Ombudsman, to which all substate programs report. Models may vary to reflect the needs and conditions within the state. Nursing home and board-and-care residents must have direct and immediate access to an ombudsman when necessary for protection and advocacy. Issues brought to the attention of ombudsmen include abuse, neglect, poor care, poorly trained staff, understaffing, inadequate laundry procedures, roommate conflicts, denial of rights, violation of privacy, and lack of grievance procedures.

CHARACTERISTICS OF ACUTE CARE SETTINGS

Acute care settings largely comprise intensive special care units, extensive surgeries, and day surgeries. Sav-

ing lives is their business, and as soon as an individual is stabilized following surgery and high-tech procedures, he or she will be discharged to the home or a subacute/postacute or rehabilitation unit in a longer-term facility. Hospital equipment and staffing have become prohibitively expensive, and hospitals are dangerous places for elders. Elders frequently become confused, suffer iatrogenic complications, and contract nosocomial infections. Aged patients need protection, continuity of personnel, a consistent advocate, and pain management. All of these are difficult to achieve in the world of medicine today. The John A. Hartford Foundation has funded an Institute for Geriatric Nursing, directed by Mathy Mezey and Terry Fulmer, at New York University. They have developed numerous methods of enhancing the care of the aged in acute care hospitals and have established several model programs to achieve this. In addition, the American Geriatric Society, recognizing some of the effects of the neglect of pain, have established pain management guidelines for physicians.

Various needs should be met in the care of the aged in acute care hospitals, and nurses are at the forefront of these efforts. The major problems for elders remain as follows: too much, too fast, and too expensive. The vast majority of Medicare funds are spent on providing acute hospital care for the last 2 weeks of an aged person's life. However, we must recognize that many elders are alive and functioning well into their 90s because of hip and knee replacements, coronary artery bypass grafts, and pacemaker implants, as well as numerous other procedures. Nurses will always be the major client advocates in the system and can serve elders best by creating a safe and comfortable environment and discharge planning of the most appropriate kind in light of the client's needs and resources.

Meiner (1998) reports a case in which patient transfer from one facility to another was poorly managed, with the ultimate result being the patient's death. In reviewing the case, it was recognized that the death could have been prevented with appropriate nursing assessment, planning, interventions, and evaluation. Specifically, transfer notification to the receiving agency or facility should include the suggestions given in Box 27-6. In addition, the written transfer report must be delivered to the receiving facility by a responsible person (ambulance driver or family member). The receiving facility must make available appropriate medications and meals, make a thorough assessment of the new resident, and provide an orientation to the setting at a time when the individual has been made comfortable.

Box 27-6	**TRANSFER NOTIFICATION**

The hospital agent should give a verbal telephone report to an agent at the receiving facility. This report should include:

- Correct spelling of the patient's full name, age, gender, marital status, medical diagnoses, physician's name, and other demographic information specific to the requests of the receiving facility
- Brief synthesis of hospital course, including surgical procedures and current vital signs
- Activity or mobility orders and special precautions or needs
- Diet orders and special nutritional requirements
- Medications currently prescribed and any special administration needs
- Safety precautions or needs (in bed, sitting, mobility, ADLs, etc.)
- Anticipated time of the transfer

From Meiner SE: Physician's orders and nurses' notes: when time is pressing, details can be lost, *Geriatr Nurs* 19(5):291, 1998.

Consent for Treatment

Consent for medical treatment is traditionally the prerogative of the adult individual of sound mind. The exceptions to this rule are determined by law, regulatory policy, and judicial decision. Usually the patient's wishes prevail if he or she is judged competent. Unfortunately, when individuals are admitted to the hospital for acute illness, they are often functioning poorly and are not in the best position to make thoughtful decisions about their care. The most useful stance is to seek the "most beneficial alternative" as an essential element of the "least restrictive choice."

Rights of Patients

Patients' rights in facilities and institutions of all types are mandated by federal and state laws and the Constitution, as are the rights of the general population. Legal rights vary according to the setting and individual competency. Rights in institutions are to be posted in a place visible to all and are to be reviewed with the individual soon after admission to a facility.

Nursing responsibilities are (1) to ensure that the patient has seen, read, and/or understands the rights; (2) to document explicitly when and why any rights may be temporarily suspended; (3) to observe and record observations attesting to the individual's ability or inability to manage daily affairs; and (4) to be sure that the patient's

Box 27-7	**PRINCIPLES OF ADVOCACY**

1. Gather as much specific data as possible to make your case.
2. Be informed regarding pros and cons of the issue.
3. Know the policies that will influence decisions in the case.
4. Involve others who will support or augment your case.
5. Work with those who have power to make relevant decisions.
6. Make a clear decision regarding risks you are willing to take to win your case.
7. Inform and involve client groups who will benefit from your position in the case.
8. If the client is at risk, be sure he or she is aware of the risk.
9. Take an offensive rather than a defensive position.
10. Be calm and clear when presenting your case.
11. Emphasize positive aspects of the case.
12. Be tolerant of opposing viewpoints.
13. Consider alternatives to your position that would be acceptable.

status is reviewed at appropriate time intervals (these vary from one state to another) and that he or she obtains legal assistance in presenting his or her defense. The rights of patients are enforced largely because of the integrity of nurses and our willingness to act as patient advocates.

ADVOCACY FOR THE AGED

Currently, many senior newsletters and magazines provide a monthly legal advice column. Legal aid to the aged is available in many communities under county health and welfare services. It is often provided by paralegal aides or law students. Most county bar associations also have provisions for brief consultations at a nominal fee. Senior centers provide information and legal assistance, and the local phone book lists legal offices and organizations that can advise seniors about their rights and obligations.

Nurses are advocates of the people they serve and may employ legal representatives to assist in defending their position. No nurse can be entirely exempt from the role of advocate. We have the opportunity and the obligation to plead the cause of our aged clients. Principles of advocacy that are useful in formulating and presenting a case are summarized in Box 27-7.

Geriatric nurses share a responsibility to the young and the old, individually and collectively. Future possibilities will depend on more equitable distribution of resources and protection of rights. We are aware of the remnants of our "child within," but are we as cognizant of the present structuring of our "elder within"? Our children must be adequately supported and treasured as youth if they are to move forward through each developmental stage and reach a satisfying old age. Let us mobilize our strength to enrich the experience of growing and aging for our elders, our own present and future, and that of our children.

▶ **KEY CONCEPTS**

- A familiar and comfortable environment allows an elder to function at his or her highest capacity.
- Relocation has variable effects, depending on the individual's personality, health, cognitive capacities, self-esteem, and preferred life-style.
- Environmental cues such as wall maps, clear directive labels, calendars, and clocks will assist individuals in adjusting to a new setting and remaining oriented.
- Noise pollution and abysmal lighting are seldom given sufficient attention in institutional living.

NANDA and Wellness Diagnoses

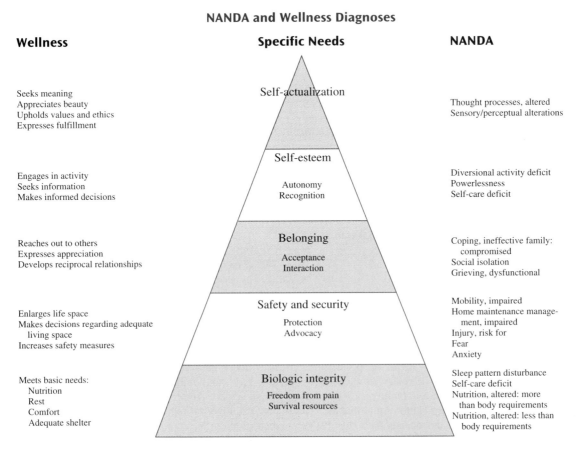

Wellness

Seeks meaning
Appreciates beauty
Upholds values and ethics
Expresses fulfillment

Engages in activity
Seeks information
Makes informed decisions

Reaches out to others
Expresses appreciation
Develops reciprocal relationships

Enlarges life space
Makes decisions regarding adequate
    living space
Increases safety measures

Meets basic needs:
    Nutrition
    Rest
    Comfort
    Adequate shelter

Specific Needs

Self-actualization

Self-esteem

Autonomy
Recognition

Belonging

Acceptance
Interaction

Safety and security

Protection
Advocacy

Biologic integrity

Freedom from pain
Survival resources

NANDA

Thought processes, altered
Sensory/perceptual alterations

Diversional activity deficit
Powerlessness
Self-care deficit

Coping, ineffective family:
    compromised
Social isolation
Grieving, dysfunctional

Mobility, impaired
Home maintenance management, impaired
Injury, risk for
Fear
Anxiety

Sleep pattern disturbance
Self-care deficit
Nutrition, altered: more
    than body requirements
Nutrition, altered: less than
    body requirements

These are not all of the possible wellness or NANDA diagnoses that may be identified. The above are frequent examples of nursing diagnoses that should be considered when planning care for the older adult in whatever setting.

- Individuals residing in long-term care institutions need regularly scheduled opportunities to go outside and participate in natural environments; gardens, lakes, and natural beauty are restorative.
- Quiet, private places for reflection, contemplation, or intimacy should be available to individuals living in congregate settings.

▶ ## Activities and Discussion Questions

1. Identify three objects in your living space that are important to you, and explain why these are significant. Will you take these with you whenever you relocate?
2. Ask an older relative about the items or conditions in his or her home that make him or her feel secure and comfortable.
3. Discuss with this elder various moves he or she has made and how he or she felt about them.
4. Discuss situations with this elder that he or she would find intolerable if it was necessary to move to a protected setting.
5. Select three places listed in your phone book as retirement communities and make inquiries regarding possible placement of an older adult parent. What questions did you ask? What is the cost? What are the provisions for health care? What types of activities and assistance are available? Which would you select for an older person, and why?

RESOURCES

National Center for Assisted Living
    American Health Care Association
    1201 L Street NW
    Washington, DC 20005-4014
    (202) 842-4444
National Center for Home Equity Conversion (NCHEC)
    110 E. Main, Room 1010
    Madison, WI 53703
Public Policy Institute, Research Group
    Consumer Fact Sheets
    American Association of Retired Persons
    601 E Street NW
    Washington, DC 20049
    www.aarp.org

The National Directory of Retirement Residences: Best Places to Live When You Retire by N. Musson. Available from Frederick Fell, Inc, 386 Park Avenue S., New York, NY 10016. (Cost: $9.95.) This book contains brief, concise descriptions of 1000 retirement residences, including villages or single dwellings, groups of apartments, group residences, and multitype facilities built or modernized since 1950. A short description of climatic and geographic conditions for each state is included. The listings include the type of facility, number of units, fees, type of sponsorship, special features and services on the premises, type of locale, and proximity to needed facilities. The directory also includes detailed introductory chapters that provide guidance in choosing a retirement residence; information on financial, legal, and health needs in retirement; and tips on selling a house and surplus belongings when moving to a retirement home.

REFERENCES

American Association of Homes and Services for the Aging: AAHSA creates subsidiary for assisted living, *Provider News* 10(3):1, 1995a.

American Association of Homes and Services for the Aging: Trends and issues, *Currents* 10(9):4, 1995b.

American Association of Retired Persons: *Expanding housing choices for older people,* Conference Papers and Recommendations, AARP WHCoA Mini-Conference, Jan 26, 1996.

Arras JD, Dubler NN: Bringing the hospital home: ethical and social implications of high-tech home care, *Hastings Cent Rep* 24(5, suppl 19), 1994.

Bassen S, Baltazar V: Flowers, flowers everywhere: creative horticulture programming at the Hebrew Home for the Aged at Riverdale, *Geriatr Nurs* 18(2):53-56, 1997.

Bergman G: Shared housing—not only for the rent, *Aging Today* 15(1):1, 1994.

Bustad LK, Hines LM: *Placement of animals with the older adult: benefits and strategies,* Moraga, Calif, 1983, California Veterinary Medical Association.

Edelstein S: *Fair housing laws for group residences for frail older persons,* Washington, DC, 1995, American Association of Retired Persons.

Folkemer D et al: *Adult foster care for the older adult: a review of state regulatory and funding strategies,* Washington, DC, 1996, American Association of Retired Persons.

Green DA: A resident-centered model for nursing home design, *Aging Today* 15(2):15, 1994.

Kane R, Bell R, Riegler S: Value preferences for nursing home outcomes, *Gerontologist* 26(3):303, 1986.

Leach D: *Making your community livable: programs that work,* Washington, DC, 1996, AARP Public Policy Institute.

Leisure World at Laguna Hills: Press release, Laguna Hills, Calif, May 1996.

Maddox G: *Encyclopedia of aging,* New York, 1995, Springer.

Meiner S: A case study of nursing liability: patient transfer from one facility to another, *Geriatr Nurs* 19(5):290-292, 1998.

Morganett B: Nature hikes for nursing home residents, *Geriatr Nurs* 8(4):178, 1987.

Noell E: Design in nursing homes: environment as a silent partner in caregiving, *Generations* 19(4):14, 1996.

Omnibus Budget Reconciliation Act (OBRA) of 1987 (Public Law No 100-203): amendments 1990, 1991, 1992, 1993, and 1994, Rockville, Md, US Department of Health and Human Services, Health Care Financing Administration.

Ostrowski MS: The Heritage Harbour Health Group: doing it our way, *Geriatr Nurs* 19(4):225-228, 1998.

Pynoos J: Strategies for home modification and repair, *Generations* 16(2):21, 1992.

Rosenkoetter MM: Brutus is making rounds, *Geriatr Nurs* 12(6):277, 1992.

Roush S, Banziger G: *Nursing homes for the birds: a control-relevant intervention with bird feeders.* Paper presented at the meeting of the Gerontological Society of America, Boston, Nov 21, 1982.

Sansone P, Schmitt L: *Older adults with dementia can decide own treatment at end of their lives.* Unpublished study conducted at Frances Schervier Home and Hospital in the Bronx, New York, under the auspices of the Bureau of Long Term Care Services of the New York State Department of Health, News release, April 17, 1996.

Tavormina CE: Embracing the Eden alternative in long-term care environments, *Geriatr Nurs* 20(4):158-161, 1999.

US Bureau of the Census: *Statistical abstract of the United States: 1998,* ed 118, Washington, DC, 1998, US Government Printing Office.

US Department of Health and Human Services: *Health, United States, 1999: with health and aging chartbook,* DHHS Pub No (PHS) 99-1232, Hyattsville, Md, 1999, Centers for Disease Control and Prevention.

INDEX

A

AADLs
    definition of, 264
    in functional assessment, 269
AAMI; *see* Age-associated memory impairment (AAMI)
Abandonment, definition of, 505
Aberrant, definition of, 436
Abnormal Involuntary Movement Scale (AIMS), 340-341
Absorption of drugs, 293
Abuse/neglect of aged, 494-498
    assessment of, 497
    dynamics of, 495
    evaluative components of, *497*
    in home care, 496-497
    identification and subsequent action for, *498*
    interventions for, 497-498
    learned dynamic of, 497
    mandatory reporting of, 498
    psychopathologic dynamic of, 497
    stress-related dynamic of, 497-498
Acarbose in diabetes management, 400t
Accidents, 469
Accoutrements, definition of, 1, 342
ACE; *see* Acute care of the elderly (ACE)
Acetaminophen
    for pain relief, 369, 372
    special considerations on, 332
    use of, in elderly, 327t
Acetylsalicylic acid, use of, in elderly, 327t
Acquired immunodeficiency syndrome (AIDS), dementia in, 440
Acting out in grief process, 559
Active euthanasia, definition of, 553
Activities of daily living (ADLs)
    in chronic disorders assessment, 349
    in functional assessment, 269-271, 277
Activity, 217-230
    assessment of, 220-221
    interventions for, 221
    in pain control, 385
    physical, definition of, 217-218
    in physical assessment, 268
    safety considerations for, 229
Activity theory of aging, 114
Acupressure
    for musculoskeletal disorders, 420
    in pain control, 373-374, 375t

Acupuncture
    for musculoskeletal disorders, 420
    in pain control, 373-374, 375t
Acute care of the elderly (ACE), *23*
Acute care settings, characteristics of, 606-608
AD; *see* Alzheimer's disease (AD)
Adapin, toxic characteristics of, 301t
Adaptive/assistive devices
    in chronic illness, 352, 353t
    for hearing impairment, 154-155
    low-vision, 146-147
    for mobility, 468-469
Adjustment reactions, 531-532
Adjuvant, definition of, 360
ADLs; *see* Activities of daily living (ADLs)
Adrenal function in elderly, 97, 111t
Adult protective services, 499
Advance directives, 580-582
    autopsy in, 82-83
    definition of, 69
    documentation of, 77, 81-84
    nurse's role and, 83-84
Adverse reaction(s)
    definition of, 291
    to drugs, 298-299
Advil
    toxic characteristics of, 301t
    use of, in elderly, 327t
Advocacy for aged, 607-608
Aeration in physical assessment, 268
Affectual disturbance in cognitive impairment assessment, 449
Age norms, 122
Age spots, 235
Age-associated memory impairment (AAMI), 120
    word retrieval problems from, 29
Ageism, 2
Agent, 581
    in advance directives, 84
Age-related macular degeneration (ARMD), 145
Agility, mobility and, 471
Aging
    attitudes toward, 2
    biologic theories of, 101, 102t
    cognition and, 117-120
    cohort influences on, 3-4
    cultural influences on, 4
    future of, in United States, 11-12
    gender and, 4, 5t
    health and wellness in, 5-9
    history and, 3
    metaphors of, 12
    physical changes of, 88-103, 106-111t

Aging—cont'd
    postural changes in, 90-91
    sociologic, 120-122
    stereotypes on, 2
    structural changes in, 90-91
    successful, 89
    usual, 89
Agitation
    during bath time, tips for decreasing, *454*
    dealing with, 453
AIDS; *see* Acquired immunodeficiency syndrome (AIDS)
AIMS; *see* Abnormal Involuntary Movement Scale (AIMS)
Akathisia
    from antipsychotics, 315
    definition of, 291
    drug-induced, Barnes rating scale for, 336-337
    global clinical assessment of, 337
Alcoholism, 543-545
    sleep disorders associated with, 209t
Aldactone, special considerations on, 333
Aldomet
    special considerations on, 334
    toxic characteristics of, 301t
    use of, in elderly, 326t
Aloneness, 131
Alpha-glucosidase inhibitors in diabetes management, 400t
Alprazolam, use of, in elderly, 326t
Alternative health care, 9-10
Alternative medicine for degenerative joint disorders, 419-420
Altitude, high, as environmental hazard, 469
Aluminum hydroxide, use of, in elderly, 328t
Alzheimer's disease (AD), 442
    sleep disorders associated with, 209t, 213t
Ambien, use of, in elderly, 326t
American Nurses Association (ANA), geriatric standards of practice of, 16
Amitril, toxic characteristics of, 301t
Amitriptyline
    dose and side effects of, 542t
    side effects of, 330
    special considerations on, 335
    toxic characteristics of, 301t
    use of, in elderly, 326t
Amobarbital, special considerations on, 334

Page numbers followed by t indicate tables.
Page numbers in *italics* indicate illustrations and boxed material.